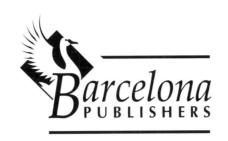

Barcelona
PUBLISHERS

GUIDELINES FOR
MUSIC THERAPY PRACTICE
IN PEDIATRIC CARE

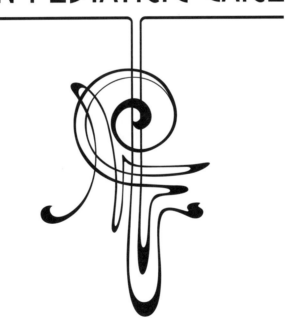

EDITED BY

JOKE BRADT

Guidelines for Music Therapy Practice
in Pediatric Care

Edited by Joke Bradt

Copyright © 2013 by Barcelona Publishers

Print ISBN: 978-1-937440-48-0
E-ISBN: 978-1-937440-49-7

To obtain chapters separately in epub or Mobi formats, please visit:
www.barcelonapublishers.com

Distributed throughout the world by:
Barcelona Publishers
4 White Brook Road
Gilsum NH 03448
Tel: 603-357-0236 Fax: 603-357-2073
Website: www.barcelonapublishers.com
SAN 298-6299

Cover illustration and design: © 2013 Frank McShane
Copy-editor: Jack Burnett

Dedication

To my daughters Gabriella and Elisa Macera
for filling my life with endless love, joy, and creativity.

And

To my husband Felice Macera
for bringing me the moon and the stars

Acknowledgments

I thank Ken Bruscia for his vision for the field of music therapy and the training of music therapy professionals as manifested in this series. His unwavering support and patience throughout the editorial process was greatly appreciated.

I thank each of the authors for the enormous amount of time and work they dedicated to deconstructing their clinical work and that of others so that clear practice guidelines could be articulated in this book. A special 'thank you' to Jennifer Townsend, who even continued to work on her chapter during her initial contractions. Congratulations with your beautiful baby girl!

I thank Claire Ghetti for her feedback and input, even late at night. I highly value your scholarship and wisdom.

I thank Minjung Shim and Noah Potvin, my PhD students, for their help with literature searches.

I thank my colleagues in the Department of Creative Arts Therapies at Drexel University for allowing me the time to work on this project. I am deeply grateful for your support and encouragements for all my scholarly endeavors.

I thank my husband, Felice Macera, and my daughters, Gabriella and Elisa Macera, for their patience with the many hours of editing I put in on evenings, weekends and long car rides.

Permissions

Wong-Baker FACES® Pain Rating Scale reprinted by permission of Connie M. Baker. Originally published in *Whaley & Wong's Nursing Care of Infants and Children.* © Elsevier Inc.

Music Therapy Referral Criteria – Beth Israel Medical Center reprinted by permission of Barcelona Publishers. Taken from J. Loewy (2004). A clinical model of music therapy in the NICU. In M. Nöcker-Ribaupierre (Ed.), *Music therapy for premature and newborn infants* (pp. 166–167). Gilsum, NH: Barcelona Publishers.

Music Therapy NICU Referral Form – Beth Israel Medical Center reprinted by permission of Barcelona Publishers. Taken from J. Loewy (2004). A clinical model of music therapy in the NICU. In M. Nöcker-Ribaupierre (Ed.), *Music therapy for premature and newborn infants* (pp. 171–172). Gilsum, NH: Barcelona Publishers.

NICU Music Therapy Assessment Summary reprinted by permission of the American Music Therapy Association. Taken from D. Hanson-Abromeit, H Shoemark, & J. V. Loewy (2009). Newborn intensive care unit (NICU). In D. Hanson-Abromeit, & C. Colwell (Eds.), *Medical music therapy for pediatrics in hospital settings* (pp. 15–70). Silver Spring, MD: American Music Therapy Association.

Music Therapy Assessment - Beth Israel medical Center reprinted by permission of Barcelona Publishers. Taken from J. Loewy (2004). A clinical model of music therapy in the NICU. In M. Nöcker-Ribaupierre (Ed.), *Music therapy for premature and newborn infants* (pp. 173–175). Gilsum, NH: Barcelona Publishers.

Premature Infant Assessment and Treatment History Form reprinted by permission of the American Music Therapy Association. Taken from J. Standley & D. Walworth, D (2010). *Music therapy with premature infants. Research and developmental interventions* (2nd ed.) (p. 25). Silver Spring, MD.: American Music Therapy Association.

Steven's Standing Song, reprinted by permission of Jessica Kingsley Publishers. Taken from J. Kennelly (2006). Music Therapy in Paediatric Rehabilitation. In F. Baker & J. Tamplin, J. (Eds.), *Music Therapy Methods in Neurorehabilitation* (pp. 232). Jessica Kingsley Publishers, London and Philadelphia.

Steven's Sitting Song, reprinted by permission of Jessica Kingsley Publishers. Taken from J. Kennelly (2006). Music Therapy in Paediatric Rehabilitation. In F. Baker & J. Tamplin, J. (Eds.), *Music Therapy Methods in Neurorehabilitation* (pp. 232). Jessica Kingsley Publishers, London and Philadelphia.

Tracey's Going Home Song, reprinted by permission of Jessica Kingsley Publishers. Taken from J. Kennelly 'Music Therapy in Paediatric Rehabilitation' in Baker, F. and Tamplin, J. (eds.) (2006). *Music Therapy Methods in Neurorehabilitation.* Jessica Kingsley Publishers, London and Philadelphia.

Considerations when Working with Paediatric Patients and their Families reprinted by permission of Jessica Kingsley Publishers. Taken from J. Kennelly (2006). Music Therapy in Paediatric Rehabilitation. In F. Baker & J. Tamplin (Eds.), *Music Therapy Methods in Neurorehabilitation*. London and Philadelphia: Jessica Kingsley Publishers.

Auditory Input from Environment reprinted by permission of Satchnote Press. Taken from K. Stewart (2009). Dimensions of the voice: The use of voice and breath with infants and caregivers in the NICU. In R. Azoulay & J. V. Loewy (Eds.), *Music, the breath & health: Advances in integrative music therapy* (p. 242). New York: Satchnote Press.

13 Areas of Inquiry reprinted by permission of the American Music Therapy Association. Taken from J. Loewy (2000). Music Psychotherapy Assessment. *Music Therapy Perspectives, 18*(1), 47–58.

Table of Contents

Dedication   v

Acknowledgments   vi

Permissions   vii

Table of Contents   ix

Contributors   xi

Preface   xv
    AN EVOLVING PERSPECTIVE
    Kenneth E. Bruscia

Chapter 1   3
    INTRODUCTION
    Joke Bradt

Chapter 2   15
    PAIN MANAGEMENT WITH CHILDREN
    Joke Bradt

Chapter 3   66
    PREMATURE INFANTS
    Monika Nöcker-Ribaupierre

Chapter 4   116
    FULL-TERM HOSPITALIZED NEWBORNS
    Helen Shoemark

Chapter 5   152
    PEDIATRIC INTENSIVE CARE
    Claire M. Ghetti

Chapter 6   205
    SURGICAL AND PROCEDURAL SUPPORT FOR CHILDREN
    John F. Mondanaro

Chapter 7   252
    BURN CARE FOR CHILDREN
    Annette Whitehead-Pleaux

Chapter 8   290
    CHILDREN WITH CANCER
    Beth Dun

Chapter 9   324
    PALLIATIVE AND END-OF-LIFE CARE FOR CHILDREN
    Kathryn Lindenfelser

Chapter 10   356
    BRAIN INJURIES AND REHABILITATION IN CHILDREN
    Jeanette Kennelly

Chapter 11   403
    RESPIRATORY CARE FOR CHILDREN
    Joanne Loewy

Chapter 12   442
    MEDICALLY FRAGILE CHILDREN IN LOW AWARENESS STATES
    Jennifer Townsend

Chapter 13   477
    CHILDREN IN GENERAL INPATIENT CARE
    Christine Neugebauer

Index   513

Contributors

Joke Bradt, PhD, MT-BC is Associate Professor in the Creative Arts Therapies Department at Drexel University. Her work has focused on medical music therapy, particularly in the area of pain management. She has presented extensively at national and international conferences, and has authored and co-authored several music therapy articles and book chapters. She serves as Associate Editor of the *Nordic Journal of Music Therapy*. She is the lead author of six Cochrane Systematic Reviews on the use of music interventions with medical patients. Joke's NIH-funded research focuses on the impact of vocal music therapy on core outcomes in chronic pain management.

Beth Dun, MMus, RMT completed her Bachelor of Music (1988) and her Master's Degree (1999) at the University of Melbourne, Australia. In 1991 Beth Dun was the first music therapist to be employed in a pediatric hospital in Australia where she was the inaugural music therapist at the Royal Children's Hospital (RCH), Melbourne. At RCH she is now Team Leader of Music Therapy, Coordinator of the Music Therapy Clinical Placement Program and Senior Music Therapist for the Children's Cancer Centre and Burns Unit. Beth has lectured in the University of Melbourne's Music Therapy course since 1992.

Claire M. Ghetti, PhD, LCAT, MT-BC, CCLS has extensive clinical experience with children and adolescents in intensive medical settings at the Elizabeth Seton Pediatric Center and the Komansky Center for Children's Health at New York-Presbyterian Hospital. She initiated the PICU music therapy program while at the Komansky Center, and has published and presented on the topic of pediatric intensive care. Claire is Clinical Director for the Creative Arts and Child Life at the Elizabeth Seton Pediatric Center, and adjunct faculty at Molloy College. She has served on the editorial boards of the *Journal of Music Therapy* and *Music Therapy Perspectives*, and has published research regarding music therapy as procedural support, music therapy with emotional-approach coping to improve peri-procedural outcomes, and dual certification of music therapists/child life specialists.

Jeanette Kennelly, BMusEd, PGDipMT is currently completing her PhD in the School of Music, University of Queensland, Australia. She was the Senior Music Therapist at the Royal Children's Hospital & Health Service District, Brisbane between 1995 and 2011. Her main areas of expertise include pediatric rehabilitation (where she has presented nationally and internationally and published several papers and book chapters), tertiary education and professional supervision. The topic of her PhD thesis is professional supervision for Australian music therapists. Jeanette is currently a member of the Education Committee of the Australian Music Therapy Association.

Kathryn Lindenfelser, MMus, MT-BC, FAMI, NCBTMB completed her music therapy education at Augsburg College and her Master's in music therapy at the University of Melbourne. She is also a Fellow of Guided Imagery and Music – Bonny Method completing her training at Appalachian State University. Her master's research investigated bereaved parents' experiences of music therapy with their terminally ill child. Kathryn worked in the pediatric palliative care setting at the University of Minnesota Children's Hospital, Children's Hospitals and Clinics of Minnesota, Monash Children's Hospital, Royal Children's Hospital and Very Special Kids. Kathryn founded and is the executive director of Children's Lighthouse of MN building a children's respite and hospice home in Minnesota.

Joanne Loewy, DA, LCAT, MT-BC, is the Founding Director of the Louis Armstrong Center for Music & Medicine at Beth Israel Medical Center. Her specialties include asthma, sedation, pain, assessment, hermeneutic research, trauma and supervision. The Center serves musicians with chronic fatigue, chemical dependency, performance anxiety and overuse. She is the Co-Editor in Chief of *Music and Medicine* with Ralph Spintge, serves on numerous editorial boards, and is the author, editor, and co-editor of several books, chapters, and articles. She is a Founding Member of the International Association for Music and Medicine, and lectures and teaches at the Albert Einstein College of Medicine, Drexel University, and Molloy College.

John F. Mondanaro, MA, LCAT, MT-BC, CCLS is the Clinical Director of the Louis & Lucille Armstrong Music Therapy Program at Beth Israel Medical Center in New York where he oversees inpatient services and all clinical training. Earning an M.A. in Music Therapy from New York University, and B.A. in Art from St. Ambrose University, John is licensed in New York as a mental health practitioner in Creative Arts Therapy, and maintains board certification in Music Therapy, as well as certification in Child Life. John is a published writer, songwriter, and co-editor of the book, *Music and Medicine: Integrative Models in the Treatment of Pain*, and is a member of the IAMM, AMTA, and ASCAP.

Christine Neugebauer, MS, LPC, MT-BC received her degree in music therapy from Anna Maria College in 1993 after completing her medical music therapy internship at UTMB-Galveston under the directorship of Mary Rudenberg. She worked for 15 years with pediatric burn survivors at Shriners Hospital for Children – Galveston until 2008. In 2009, she established the first pediatric music therapy program at Children's Memorial Hermann Hospital at the Texas Medical Center in Houston. She has published original articles and book chapters, has been an invited speaker at national and international meetings, has served as a music therapy internship director, and is a licensed professional counselor in the state of Texas.

Monika Nöcker-Ribaupierre, Dr.sc.mus., MT-DMtG, PT-HPG did 20 years of pioneering research and practice of her method *Auditory stimulation with the mother's voice after premature birth* in NICU at University Children's Hospital Munich. She is currently a member of the board of the Freies Musikzentrum Munich, Vice-President of the ISMM, member of the Ethics Committee of DMtG, the scientific board of *Musiktherapeutische Umschau,* the Editorial Board of *Music and*

Medicine, and board member of several social foundations. She has published internationally 7 books and more than 50 book chapters and articles.

Helen Shoemark, PhD, RMT is Senior Music Therapist for Neonatology at The Royal Children's Hospital Melbourne and a Career Development Fellow in the Critical Care & Neuroscience Group at the Murdoch Children's Research Institute. She is an Adjunct Professor at the University of Queensland and an honorary senior research fellow at the University of Melbourne. Her own research agenda embraces family-centered practice, and specifically voice and music as a key aspect of healthy development for sick newborn infants. Helen is Associate Editor for the *Australian Journal of Music Therapy*, and is on the review panel for several international journals including the *Journal of Music Therapy*, and *Music and Medicine*. She is published in international texts and journals.

Annette Whitehead-Pleaux, MA, MT-BC works at Shriners Hospitals for Children-Boston, a pediatric burn center. In 2003, she was awarded the Arthur Flagler Fultz Research Grant Award to study the effects of music on pain in the pediatric burn population. In addition, she has written on the use of electronic music technologies in music therapy and multicultural music therapy practice. Prior to SHC-Boston, she worked in psychiatric hospitals for children, adults, and elders, special education classrooms, and a domestic violence program. She has served AMTA since 1997 on the Assembly of Delegates, the Standards of Clinical Practice Committee, Financial Advisory Committee, and the editorial board of *Music Therapy Perspectives*.

Preface

An Evolving Perspective

Kenneth E. Bruscia

Music therapy has grown dramatically in the last 20 years—in theory, practice, and research. New training programs have been founded in many countries, and global networks have been formed through federations, conferences, journals, and online media. The technological revolution has made it possible for professionals and students around the world to communicate their thoughts and discoveries about music therapy in the flash of one simple click. New generations of music therapists have begun to explore the endless horizons of music therapy in different cultures, while the more experienced generations have had the time and resources to reflect upon what has been evolving in the field. Theory, practice, and research can no longer be defined or delimited in terms of a single culture, treatment philosophy, method, training program, or individual.

The traditional modus operandi of music therapists has always been to find or develop the most appropriate methodological approach to meet the unique health needs and resources of each individual client, population, and treatment milieu. This aim has not changed. What has changed, however, is the growing awareness that understanding what these needs and resources are is not as simple as we had previously imagined. Once the strait jackets of a particular theoretical orientation or a single method are removed, and once cultural and individual differences are fully acknowledged, most of the older guideposts disappear, and therapists today are faced with the daunting task of apprehending each client's resources and needs within the full richness and complexity of his or her own unique world.

The primary mission of this series is to provide new, diverse, and more up-to-date guideposts for clinical practice. This mission is based on the belief that music therapy students and professionals have an ethical responsibility to be knowledgeable of *all* approaches to clinical practice that have been found effective for clients within different contexts.

The implications are threefold. First, this series advances the notion that no potentially effective practice should be excluded from the study of music therapy for reasons of personal, organizational, or institutional bias. Gone are the days that music therapists can assert that *only* their own approaches belong within the definitional boundaries of music therapy. Gone are the days when music therapists can assert that music therapy is only improvisational, or that music therapy is only behavioral, or that improvisational or behavioral approaches can be used with every clientele in all contexts. This narrow-mindedness is no longer acceptable. Music therapy is not just what you do, or just what I do—it is what we all do within the boundaries of ethical practice—and within the context of a discipline that also includes theory and research. Moreover, ethical practice can no longer exclude what others do with significant clinical effect.

Second, this series underlines the premise that music therapy is first and foremost a discipline of practice. As such, the practice of music therapy cannot be based solely on theory and research, it must also be informed by what practitioners have learned over the years about what works and what does not work in actual clinical settings. Very often these clinical details and anecdotes cannot be subjected to the rigors of research, yet they have significant practical value. Thus, notwithstanding the contributions of theory and research, clinical practice must be based on the accumulated insights of practitioners who have the experience, expertise, and ethical values needed to serve as our models. In short, music therapy is not merely evidence based or theoretically informed, it is even more essentially clinically based.

Third, this series reinforces the notion that like in other scholarly health care disciplines, music therapists must begin to write about their own clinical work within the context of what others have done in the same area of practice. In the early days, music therapists developed their own ways of working with a particular clientele or method independently of one another, and without the benefit of a world-wide communication network—there were no journals, books, or websites that could provide the wealth of practical information available today. This had a rather bizarre outcome that to some extent still continues today. Not being aware of what had already been done in the field, music therapists often considered and presented themselves as pioneers—touting that their own particular method of working as if it were entirely new—when in fact other music therapists had already been doing the same thing for quite some time. This sometimes made attending a conference a deja-vu experience, where it seemed as if we were proudly re-inventing the wheel and then giving the wheel our own new brand. Mary from Podunk would give a presentation announcing that she had discovered how to use the cello in therapy, when unknown to her, Juliette Alvin had already been doing it for years. Then to further complicate the matter, therapists in Podunk would call it Mary's method, and people in England would call it Alvin's method, even if the methods were practically identical. Of course, this was not the case for the many true pioneers of music therapy who actually invented or created a specific approach or model. But the problem remains: how can one distinguish between ignorant vanity and a truly new contribution to the field? Today there is no excuse for not knowing what others have done, and even less justification for not being interested. All we have to do is a computer search of the rapidly developing literature, and we can find others who are working in the same area of practice. And then our responsibility is quite simple: we have to contextualize what we have discovered about clinical practice in terms of the current state of knowledge in the field. Just like researchers who are expected to review the literature on their research question, modern practitioners are expected to know what they are doing within the context of their discipline.

The specific objectives of the series is to provide practical guidelines for implementing receptive, improvisational, re-creative, and compositional methods of music therapy with major client populations, supported by a comprehensive and critical review of existing literature. These methods are thoroughly defined and discussed in every chapter of the series. The major client populations were identified and categorized by diagnosis and age. As a result, four main areas of practice were identified: developmental health, mental health, pediatric care, and adult medical care. Primary diagnosis was used to distinguish between populations with mental health versus medical needs, and age was used to distinguish between the needs of children, adolescents, and adults.

Authors were carefully selected according to two criteria. First, they had to have extensive clinical experience in the area of practice about which they were writing; and second, they had to acknowledge and recognize significant clinical work done by others in the same area. Their charge then was not to merely write about what they did and believed, but to present a comprehensive picture of a particular area of practice to which they themselves had contributed significantly. Obviously, some areas of practice are more developed than others and in some instances the authors could only rely upon their own experiences. Music therapy is practiced in so many areas that this unevenness in development is to be expected for some time, and also is bound to be evident in the present series.

Given the aims and issues addressed so far in this Preface, it should come as no surprise that unlike many edited books in music therapy that support the "pioneer" syndrome, every chapter in every volume of this series follows the same outline. Authors were not free to determine what would and would not be covered in their respective chapters. A uniform outline was fashioned to ensure not only that the same basic topics would be addressed for each area of practice, but also to ensure that all relevant literature on each area was included. The basic outline is as follows:

1) Diagnostic Information
2) Needs and Resources
3) Assessment and Referral
4) Multi-cultural Issues
5) Overview of Music Therapy Methods
6) Guidelines for Receptive Music Therapy
   a. Method A:
      i. Overview: Definition, indications, goals, contraindications
      ii. Preparation of Session and Environment
      iii. What to Observe
      iv. Procedures for Conducting Session
      v. Possible Adaptations
   b. Method B:
   c. Etc..
7) Guidelines for Improvisational Music Therapy
8) Guidelines for Re-creative Music Therapy
9) Guidelines for Compositional Music Therapy
10) Working with Caregivers
11) Research Evidence
   a. Receptive Music Therapy
   b. Improvisational Music Therapy
   c. Compositional Music Therapy
   d. Re-creative Music Therapy
12) Summary and Conclusions
13) References
14) Resources (Optional)

One of the consequences of following the same outline is that there are bound to be repetitions in the information presented. The editors and authors have done their best to reduce *unnecessary* redundancies, while recognizing that some redundancies are important to keep. For example, many redundancies *between* chapters were left because each chapter will be made available separately in electronic formats, apart from the other chapters. Thus, each chapter had to be a complete presentation in itself, without requiring the reader to consult another chapter that the reader may not have.

Redundancies *within* chapters are another matter. These kinds of repetitions can be quite revealing. Several clinical questions are pertinent. For example, why is it that with a particular population, contraindications or "what to observe" are the same across certain methods but not others, or why are they the same for one population but not others? In some cases, a redundancy can reveal something about the population—that regardless of method, there are certain fundamental considerations that must be made when working with them. In other cases, a redundancy can reveal something about methods and how, though very different, may make the same demands on the client. And lastly, some redundancies can reveal blind-spots in the practitioner, that is when the music therapist can only see certain aspects of the client or clinical situation, regardless of the many complexities or variations present. For this reason, readers are urged to interrogate each redundancy. What does it reveal about the client, method, or therapist?

Another consequence of following the same outline is the opposite problem—disagreements. The authors in these four volumes were sometimes definite about using specific terminology and definitions for music therapy phenomena, even if doing so created disagreements and inconsistencies with other authors or the editors. Sometimes there was good reason, other times there was not. Sometimes it was the "Mary-Podunk" problem of wanting to name and thereby own a particular method or procedure that the author believed that she or he developed; other times it reflected deep theoretical divisions in the field itself; and other times it merely revealed aspects of music therapy that still need further conceptual clarity.

It is important to be aware of these disagreements and inconsistencies, not only to better comprehend what the authors have written, but also to understand the theoretical and practical issues confronting present-day music therapy. Three important differences of opinion became obvious in the planning, writing, and editing of these four volumes—differences that could not always be resolved within the context of the editorial process.

First, there are inconsistencies in how basic terms such as model, approach, method, protocol, procedure, and technique are used and defined. What one calls a model, others call an approach, and what one calls method, others call a technique. In this series, the basic premise was that there are four main "methods" of music therapy: listening (or receptive) experiences, improvisational experiences, re-creative experiences, and compositional experiences, each with their own set of procedural variations. This premise was not shared by all authors.

Second, there are disagreements in how to differentiate these methods. When does improvising become listening, and when does composing a song become improvising? Isn't listening a part of all musical activity, and doesn't listening require activity? So then why and how do we differentiate between receptive and active? An even more important dilemma for music therapy is: Should a method be defined by what the client "experiences" or by what the therapist "does?" If the therapist improvises for the client, is the method improvisational or receptive? Again this dilemma remains unresolved in these volumes.

Finally, there are considerable controversies over what practices a particular "model" (or method, or approach) does and does not include. For example, there is substantive confusion over what practices are legitimately considered part of the "Bonny Method of Guided Imagery and Music (BMGIM)," and which are not, and whether this "method" should be called BMGIM or simply "Guided Imagery and Music" (GIM). Then there is the onslaught of terms for the various "whatevers" that also involve music and imagery. Can anyone explain the procedural differences between the terms "Guided Imagery", "Directed Music Imagery," "Music and Imagery," "Music-imaging," and "Music-assisted imagery?" And do these names actually reflect those procedural differences? This is an example of an area of practice that begs for greater conceptual clarity.

These are not idle or "so what?" questions. How can we communicate about practice if we ignore differences between a model and a method, and if we invent idiosyncratic names for every method and technique? How can we train music therapists in the "discipline" of music therapy if there is no shared vocabulary or common language? How can we develop sensible "protocols" of practice to test through research if we do not understand the basic properties of the music experience that we hope to study, and if we are unclear in specifying what the client experiences and what the therapist does? And, how can we ever imagine an organized body of theory if practitioners and researchers do not use language intentionally and consistently?

It is hoped that this first attempt to present procedural, populational guidelines for practice will highlight the myriad implications of how we talk and write about music therapy. We need to be more aware of our discourses, not only from a philosophical or theoretical perspective (as in feminist and sociocultural streams of thought), but also from a practical point of view. Hopefully, the language problems encountered in this series will lead to a discourse analysis that will spawn more serious efforts to clarify and unify our diverse vocabularies about practice.

One final issue needs to be addressed. This series was envisioned as a teaching tool. Its purpose is to inform students as well as professionals about areas of practice that may not have been studied or experienced previously. The hidden yet obvious assumption is that the way to learn how to practice music therapy is by studying it in reference to each client population rather than by method. This relates directly to the redundancy problem. If the reader scans across "receptive" methods used across different client populations, many redundancies will be found, and the same kinds of repetitions will be found in re-creative, improvisational, and compositional methods. This poses an important pedagogical question: Would it be more economical and effective to first learn how to design music experiences (or use different methods of music therapy), and then learn how to implement or adapt them for different clients? Or is it more economical and effective to first learn about the characteristics and needs of each population, and then learn to design methods within that specific context? Put another way, is it easier and more effective to generalize or extrapolate from method to clients or from clients to method? Should we be training specialists in working with each population, or generalists who master the methods of music therapy? The vote is still out on this because unfortunately these pedagogical issues have not been recognized or discussed widely in the field.

Notwithstanding the decided emphasis given to clinical practice in this series, theory and research are still very much needed in music therapy—and in music therapy education as well. It is hoped that these volumes will stimulate the field to address the myriad research questions and theoretical issues raised by an organized and comprehensive presentation of what we know in practice. Further, it is hoped that this presentation will soon become outdated, and that revised, new, and increasingly more effective methods of practice will be conceived and tested.

GUIDELINES FOR
MUSIC THERAPY PRACTICE
IN PEDIATRIC CARE

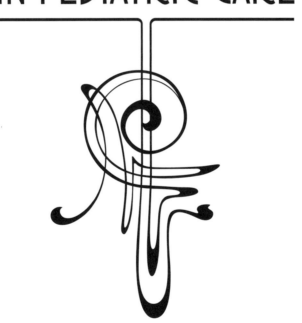

Chapter 1

Introduction

Joke Bradt

AIMS

Music therapy with children in medical settings is a growing area of practice in music therapy. Music therapists working with this population will agree that this work is exciting, stimulating, and enriching. At the same time, it presents several challenges, including the widely diverse needs of hospitalized children and their families; the need for substantive knowledge related to medical diagnoses, treatments, and procedures; the fast pace of the hospital culture; the child's psychosocial well-being (often considered second-tier to their physical well-being); and the therapist's personal well-being in working with significant existential crises likely to be evoked through this work. Music therapists offer an important lifeline to children and their families for effective coping and resilience during a very stressful time.

The aim of this book is to provide student and professional music therapists with a solid foundation for clinical practice with children in pediatric medical settings. The guidelines are based on both the practice wisdom of the contributing authors and a critical review of the existing literature. In addition, each chapter provides an overview of research evidence to date for music therapy practice with the respective populations.

AREAS OF PRACTICE

This book is part of a four-volume series aimed at providing clinical guidelines for receptive, improvisational, re-creative, and compositional methods with major client populations. This volume focuses on the use of music therapy with infants, children, and teens in children's hospitals or pediatric units of general hospitals. The majority of the guidelines focus on the use of music therapy in inpatient care, although outpatient care is addressed in several chapters as well.

The following definition of pediatric medical music therapy is based on Ghetti's definition (2012, p. 6) of music therapy as procedural support:

> Pediatric medical music therapy is the use of music and the therapeutic
> relationship to promote healthy coping and safeguard the child's psychosocial
> well-being during inpatient and outpatient medical treatment.

The following populations and/or areas of care are included in this book: pain management, premature infants, full-term hospitalized newborns, pediatric intensive care, surgery and procedural support, burn care, cancer, palliative and end-of-life care, brain injuries and rehabilitation, respiratory care, medically fragile children in low awareness states, and general inpatient care.

The inclusion of some chapters may surprise the reader, as the populations are not well represented in the literature. The decision to include a separate chapter on full-term hospitalized newborns was based on the fact that music therapy with premature infants has received extensive coverage in the clinical and research literature, with three entire books devoted to this population alone (Loewy, 2000; Nöcker-Ribaupierre, 2004; Standley & Walworth, 2010). Yet, very little has been published on the distinct needs of full-term hospitalized newborns. As pointed out by Helen Shoemark in her chapter, the capacities and needs of full-term infants with medical issues differ substantially from those of premature babies.

Although scant literature exists on the use of music therapy interventions with children in low awareness states, a separate chapter is devoted to this population, as working with these children typically proves to be quite challenging for clinicians new to this area of work. The lack of direct feedback from these children evokes in novice music therapists insecurity about the value of their work. In addition, as pointed out by Jennifer Townsend, the lack of literature in this area only adds to the clinician's insecurity. As a result, these children may become the "forgotten children" in hospital settings where music therapists carry a full caseload. We suspect that, given the limited literature in this area, few training programs prepare students to work with this population. The excellent guidelines provided in this chapter will hopefully lead to increased practice and research in this area.

The chapter on rehabilitation (by Jeanette Kennelly) purposefully focuses on brain injuries only. Rehabilitation is a vast practice area. Many children with physical disabilities (e.g., cerebral palsy, muscular dystrophy, limb malformations) require multiple surgical interventions and rehabilitation throughout their lifetime. However, their daily rehabilitation needs typically take place outside of the hospital environment and are addressed in Volume 3 of this series, *Music Therapy Practice in Developmental Health*. Children with newly acquired brain injuries usually require prolonged hospitalization and present with unique, evolving needs throughout the different rehabilitation phases.

Music therapy for respiratory care is a relatively new area of clinical practice, and here too, there are few reports in the literature. Yet, an extensive clinical practice with this population exists at the Beth Israel Medical Center in New York. Because of their successful interventions with children with respiratory challenges, it was decided to devote a chapter to this population. It is hoped that the guidelines provided by Joanne Loewy will better equip current and future music therapists to offer and advocate for music therapy services for these children.

A chapter on general inpatient care (by Christine Neugebauer) is included. Not all children are hospitalized in specialized care units (e.g., intensive care, burn care, or oncology). Children with a variety of diagnoses who require a lower or less critical level of care may stay on a general unit. Although these children are not in critical condition, they still hold many needs that must be addressed in order to reduce the negative impact of hospitalization on their well-being. In addition, general inpatient units house children with chronic medical conditions who are at risk for developmental delays because of frequent hospitalizations. Most music therapists who work in pediatric hospitals serve general inpatient units, yet very few reports in the literature have addressed work with this population.

Finally, a separate chapter on pediatric pain management (by Joke Bradt) is included, as pain management presents a major area of practice for music therapists working with children in hospitals. To allow for sufficient coverage of pain theories, multidimensional factors influencing pain perception, and pain assessment, it was decided that a separate chapter was warranted. However, the inclusion of such a chapter also presented challenges regarding potential overlap with other chapters, especially those on surgical and procedural support and burn care, as pain management is a dominant need in both of these areas of care. To minimize overlap of content, several of the population-specific pain management interventions (e.g., pain management during debridement with burn patients) are covered in the respective chapters.

THE ROLE AND SIGNIFICANCE OF MUSIC THERAPY

Hospitalization is a chaotic and traumatizing experience for children and teens. They are confronted with an unfamiliar, sterile hospital environment that is unpredictable and beyond their control. The uncertainty about "what will they do next to me?" causes major distress in the child. This frequently leaves children feeling helpless and hopeless, and, in an effort to self-protect, they disengage from the environment. This may inhibit a child's ability to learn and implement effective coping strategies (Robb et al., 2008).

Mondanaro, in his chapter on surgical and procedural support, describes a changing culture in hospitals due to the growing recognition that these stressful experiences negatively impact the child's sense of safety, resilience, and development. This has led to a growing trend toward family-centered care as well as inclusion of nonpharmacological interventions. In order to safeguard the child's psychological well-being, it is indeed important that interventions be provided that help restore the child's sense of security, agency, competency, and connection to others (Robb, 2003).

Music therapy holds great potential for meeting the child's biopsychosocial needs. At the physiological level, music therapy may be used to sedate the child and stabilize physiological responses (e.g., heart rate, respiratory rate) through use of the entrainment principle and/or use of relaxing music. Music interventions can also target arousal or stimulation of the child when needed. Furthermore, through purposeful application of melodic, harmonic, and rhythmic structures, music is able to elongate and deepen the child's breath.

At the psychosocial level, music therapy foremost offers freedom of expression and creative engagement; this stands in stark contrast with coercion, constraints, and the many restrictions that are imposed onto the child in a hospital environment (Robb, 2003). Music furthermore brings structure and familiarity to a chaotic environment, whether through music listening or active music-making. Since music is a temporal experience, it has the potential to sustain a child's attention moment-to-moment. It is this sustained focus that allows for a sufficient refuge from the experience of fear, pain, or chaos. The temporal characteristic of music is a unique aspect of music therapy as a support service for pediatric patients. During hospitalizations, most children undergo many invasive procedures. Some last a few minutes, whereas others may last for hours. Music can accompany the child through this time period, with the music therapist adjusting the musical parameters to match the different phases of the procedures and the developing needs of the child. A well-trained music therapist will be able to seamlessly offer these transitions and create a holistic support experience for the child. Music therapy interventions are also effective in inviting release of tension that builds up in the child as a result of anxiety and fear for painful or invasive procedures, separation from loved ones, and so on.

Another important aspect of music therapy with pediatric patients is that it promotes positive, playful, and supportive interactions not only with the therapist but also with family members and medical personnel. Several music therapists (e.g., Loewy, MacGregor, Richards, & Rodriguez, 1997; Robb et al., 2008; Turry, 1997) have emphasized the importance of a child's connection and interaction with others as a necessary component of adaptive coping. In addition, through the music's beauty, family members can communicate comfort, care, and intimacy during a time when the child may be struggling with understanding why his family cannot protect him against the many procedures.

Music therapy interventions bring many opportunities for enhancing agency and control in the child and fostering independence. Several authors in this book advocate for the child's active role in his treatment, rather than relegating the child to a passive recipient of care. During much of the hospitalization, decisions are made about the child's treatment without direct involvement of the child in the medical decision-making process. In contrast, in music therapy, the child can become an "active agent" by creating music, making decisions, and giving voice to his fears, thoughts, and wishes.

Finally, music can be meaningfully offered to children at various levels of development and consciousness. As an aesthetic and structured auditory stimulus, music possesses unique potential for interaction and communication with children in low awareness states and children under sedation.

Unfortunately, the role of music therapy in medical settings may be perceived by others as one of distraction and entertainment in which the "music lady/man" performs songs for the children. This book demonstrates that music therapy goes far beyond distraction and symptom reduction. Several authors in this book make an excellent case for the music therapist to be an integrated partner in the treatment team, with the ability to clearly articulate a rationale for the use of music therapy, observed effectiveness of the interventions, and implications for the child's overall well-being.

BRIEF HISTORY

Documentation of the use of music with hospitalized children dates from back in the early 1900s. Music was broadcast in pediatric units of hospitals, and nurses used music and dolls to explain procedures (Hanson-Abromeit, 2008). In 1955, the first music therapist was hired to provide services to children in the University of Iowa Hospital. The first journal article on music therapy in pediatric burn care was published by Rudenberg and Royka (1989). Since then, employment for music therapists in pediatric hospitals has steadily increased, as evidenced by a growing number of conference presentations and publications. A review of employment rates by population, as reported in the literature and published annually by the American Music Therapy Association (AMTA) in their sourcebook, reflects this growth. Even though no rates are available specific to pediatrics, a steady growth in medical music therapy is evident. A music therapy survey from 1965 (Michel, 1965) indicated that only 3% of music therapists worked in a general hospital. In 1997, Nolan reported that the National Association for Music Therapy listed less than 3% of its professional members as working with children in medical facilities. In its *Sourcebook of 2000,* the AMTA reported that 9% of its membership works in medical settings. In 2012, this increased to 13%. In contrast, employment rates in mental health dropped from 17% to 11% and in geriatric care from 23% to 16%.

APPROACHES TO MUSIC THERAPY

The music therapy interventions described in this book represent a variety of therapeutic orientations ranging from behavioral therapy in which music is offered as a stimulus to elicit predictable behaviors (e.g., pacifier-activated lullabies) to cognitive therapy in which songwriting is used for cognitive reframing, to existential therapy where meaning-making and empowerment for making choices stand central. Therapists may feel more comfortable with certain orientations. However, it is important that the needs of the child drive the selection of the most beneficial intervention. For example, existential or psychodynamic-oriented therapy may have no place/purpose in addressing the acute stress or acute pain needs of a child. Behavioral interventions may not offer the full potential that music therapy can offer to a child dealing with a chronic illness. An important strength of this series, as emphasized in the preface, is that the four volumes offer guidelines to all interventions that have been reported to be effective, regardless of theoretical orientation.

In the adult and pediatric medical care literature, the term "music therapy" is often used interchangeably to denote interventions delivered by trained music therapists and those delivered by medical personnel. It is important that music therapists continue to advocate for a clear distinction between music interventions administered by medical or health care professionals (music medicine) and those implemented by trained music therapists (medical music therapy). The continuum of care in music in medical settings ranges from performances for patients by musicians to focused individualized psychotherapeutic music therapy interventions. The use of music across this continuum is certainly valued because it enhances patient care and well-being (Bradt & Goodill, 2013). However, when clinical applications and their effectiveness are described, clarity about their distinct features is needed.

In their systematic reviews of controlled clinical trials on the effects of music interventions with medical patients (most of these reviews are inclusive of music therapy and music medicine interventions), Bradt and colleagues (2010) categorized the interventions as follows:

> Interventions are categorized as music medicine when passive listening to prerecorded music is offered by medical personnel. For example, a CD may be offered to a patient for relaxation or distraction; however, no systematic therapeutic process is present, nor is there a systematic assessment of the elements and suitability of the music stimulus. In contrast, music therapy requires the implementation of a music intervention by a trained music therapist, the presence of a therapeutic process, and the use of personally tailored music experiences. These music experiences include (a) listening to live, improvised, or prerecorded music; (b) improvising music spontaneously using voice and/or instruments; (c) composing music; (d) performing music on an instrument; and e) music combined with other modalities (e.g. movement, imagery, art) (2010, p. 6).

Several meta-analyses have indicated that music therapy interventions with medical populations are more effective than music medicine interventions for a wide variety of outcomes (Dileo & Bradt, 2005; Standley & Whipple, 2003). Specifically for pediatric patients, Standley and Whipple (2003) reported that the use of live music resulted in greater health benefits than the use of prerecorded music ($p = .03$). Furthermore, interventions that engaged children in music-making were more active than interventions during which children were asked to passively listen to music ($p = .00$). In Chapter 5 of this book, Ghetti expresses hope that the growing body of music therapists working and publishing in the area of pediatric music therapy will "clarify the beneficial and distinct roles that each discipline can play in meeting the psychosocial needs of children [...]."

Loewy introduced the term "medical music psychotherapy" in her writings and defines it as follows: "Medical music psychotherapy seeks to integrate physical aspects of functioning with behavioral, cognitive, social, and spiritual orientations as presented in a music therapy context. Medical music psychotherapy in a medical setting involves treating the whole person—body, mind, and spirit. The approach warrants clinical interpretation and involves distinct parameters of physiological aspects of functioning that are contextualized within individualized and cultural-centered care" (Chapter 11).

STATUS OF THEORY AND RESEARCH

Theory Development

Several music therapy scholars have emphasized the growing need for theory construction, evaluation, and modification, and theory-based music therapy research (Burns, 2012; Ghetti, 2012; Robb, 2012; Stige & Rolsvjord, 2003). Robb (2012) discussed the movement of behavioral intervention research away from outcome-based research to research that is guided by theoretical frameworks. Most research studies in medical music therapy with adult and pediatric patients have used an outcome-based approach to research (e.g., the use of music therapy to reduce preoperative anxiety). Whereas outcome-based research results in knowledge about the efficacy of the intervention, it does not enhance understanding of why and how an intervention worked or did not work (Robb, 2012). In contrast, theory-based research uses a theoretical framework to identify potential outcomes and the underlying processes that may be mediating the impact of music therapy on the identified outcomes. The use of a theoretical framework in research then allows for (a) identification of variables that may be amenable to change through certain music therapy interventions and (b) meaningful translation of the findings into music therapy clinical practice (Burns, 2012).

Where does pediatric medical music therapy stand in terms of theory development? Music therapists frequently use the Gate Control Theory as an explanation for mechanisms underlying the pain-reducing effects of music therapy, the Iso principle as the underlying process for mood enhancement, and neurophysiological explanations for sedation as well as physical rehabilitation benefits. Recently, music therapists have begun to develop more comprehensive theories of music therapy in pediatric medical care. A few are provided here as an example, but the reader should know that this is not a comprehensive listing.

Sheri Robb (2000, 2003), in her writings on the use of music therapy with children with cancer, has proposed a contextual support model for music therapy pediatric care that is aimed at increasing active coping behaviors. This theoretical model is based on Skinner and Wellborn's (1994) postulation that children's coping behaviors are enhanced by supportive environments. Robb's theoretical model proposes that contextual support influences a child's coping with hospitalization in two ways, namely by buffering the effects of stress and by increasing the child's engagement with the environment. The aim of music therapy interventions, then, is to "reengage children with their environment using music to create three elements of contextual support: (a) Structure: to provide children with opportunities for successful mastery over the environment, (b) Autonomy Support: to afford children opportunities to make choices and direct activities, and (c) Involvement: to express unconditional acceptance of children and reinforce their efforts and actions" (p. 104). The efficacy of Robb's model has been supported by several research studies (Barrera, Rykov, & Doyle, 2002; Robb, 2000, 2008).

Ghetti (2012) has put forth a working model of music therapy for procedural support as a transactional model "reflecting a complex and nonlinear interaction among patient, therapist, music, procedure, and context that unfolds over time. [...] The working model of music therapy as procedural support acknowledges that how one perceives a procedure is not a result of isolated aspects of the procedure itself, but a result of the interrelationships among the person, procedure, context, music, and therapist. Similarly, the music alone does not impact every patient's experience of the procedure in the same way, as the impact of the music is modified by personal variables and the role of the therapist, among other factors" (p. 29). Ghetti uses musical alternate engagement for procedural support as an example (see Chapter 6 for detailed discussion of the intervention): She proposes the need for reflection about whether in this intervention the engagement itself is critical (regardless of the use of music) or whether it is the engagement in music therapy that helps a child reduce anxiety and pain. "With a better understanding of individual mechanisms, we may progress further in the process of discriminating when, for whom, and in which circumstances certain approaches to procedural support will be more effective" (p. 31). For a detailed discussion of both Robb's and Ghetti's theoretical framework, the reader is referred to the respective publications.

Bradt (2001, 2010) discussed the hypothesized mechanisms at work in music entrainment for pain management. Her hypothesized model includes neurophysiological, cognitive, sensory, affective, and social processes underlying the pain-reducing effects of music entrainment.

Loewy, Stewart, Dassler, Telsey, and Homel (2013) explain the underlying mechanisms of the use of live music entrained to premature infants' vital signs to enhance physiological responses and feeding behavior. The hypothesized mechanisms point to the importance of the organized structure of rhythm of the mother's heart and breath pattern, and the overtone vibrations of her voice to the organizational development of the infant.

O'Callaghan (2011, 2012) has contributed to theory-building in pediatric cancer care. Through the use of a constructivist research approach with grounded theory design, she has developed theories about music's role in the lives of children (2011) and adolescents and young adults (2012). Although this research was not solely focused on the role of music within the framework of music therapy sessions, it elucidates potential processes at work in music therapy with pediatric patients with cancer.

Research Evidence

As for the status of research studies in music therapy for pediatric medical care, the contributors to this book were asked to conduct a thorough search of existing music therapy literature on the population of their chapter, including research studies. Studies in quantitative and qualitative traditions are included at the end of each chapter.

Systematic reviews of controlled clinical trials on music interventions with pediatric patients consistently identify and include many more music medicine trials than music therapy trials. Because of the abundance of research studies conducted by medical personnel on the use of music listening on health outcomes in hospitalized children, it is important that music therapists step up their research efforts in this area. More music therapy research is needed that (a) examines the impact of interactive music-making with pediatric patients and (b) builds and/or examines theories that explain the music therapy processes at work. The majority of the music therapy research has focused on the use of receptive music therapy interventions for anxiety reduction. To help others understand (a) the unique contributions of music therapy to the treatment of pediatric patients, (b) the full potential of its applications, and (c) the richness of the experiences that are offered through music therapy, future research needs to focus on interventions that capitalize on the intra- and interpersonal benefits of the child's active engagement in music-making and/or compositions.

Research recommendations resulting from systematic reviews of controlled clinical trials in music therapy have called for improvements of methodological standards, greater transparency in reporting of methodological details, and detailed descriptions of the actual music therapy interventions as per the Consolidated Standards of Reporting Trials (CONSORT) and the Transparent Reporting of Evaluations with Non-randomized Designs (TREND) (Klassen, Liang, Tjosvold, Klassen, & Hartling, 2008; Robb & Carpenter, 2009; Standley & Whipple, 2003; Treurnicht Naylor, Kingsnorth, Lamont, McKeever, & Macarthur, 2011). Accurate reporting is needed for readers to assess the quality of the trial as well as for clinicians to understand how these findings might apply to their clinical work. If music therapy interventions are not adequately described, it is impossible to (a) determine all intervention attributes, (b) compare interventions across studies, and (c) identify which specific intervention component was responsible for efficacy (Robb & Carpenter, 2009).

ORGANIZATION OF THE BOOK

Organization

This volume is divided into 13 chapters. Each author was required to follow the same outline as presented in the Preface. The diagnostic information section provides the reader with definitions and descriptions of illnesses, disorders, and common treatments relevant to the chapter's population. In addition, developmental information is provided where relevant (e.g., the premature infants chapter). Under Needs and Resources, the needs as well as the strengths of the children and their families are addressed. The Referral and Assessment Procedures section presents recommendations for music therapy assessment with each population. This section provides valuable information and many great resources for the novice therapist. Many of the authors included actual assessment forms in the appendix to their chapter. The chapters then provide detailed guidelines for music therapy interventions categorized according to receptive, improvisational, re-creative, and compositional methods.

Receptive music therapy is defined as interventions in which "the therapist engages the client in any kind of listening experience. The experience may focus on physical, emotional, intellectual, aesthetic, or spiritual aspects of the music, and the client may respond through activities such as relaxation or meditation, action sequences, structured or free movement, perceptual tasks, free association, storytelling, drawing or painting, dramatizing, reminiscing, imaging, etc. The music used for such experiences may be live or recorded improvisations, performances or compositions by the client or therapist, or commercial recordings of music literature in various styles (e.g., classical, popular, rock, jazz, country, spiritual, New Age, etc.)" (Bruscia, 2011, pp. 5-6)

Improvisational music therapy is defined as interventions in which "the client "makes up" music while playing or singing, extemporaneously creating a melody, rhythm, song, or instrumental piece. The client may improvise a "solo" or participate in a duet, trio, or ensemble that also includes the therapist, relatives, or other clients. The client may use his/her voice or any musical instrument of choice within his/her capability (e.g., drums, cymbal, xylophone, autoharp, melodica, piano). The therapist helps the client to improvise by creating an ongoing musical accompaniment that stimulates or guides the client's sound productions; presenting the client with a musical theme or structure upon which to base the improvisation (e.g., a rhythm, melody, scale, form); or presenting a nonmusical idea to express through the improvisation (e.g., an image, feeling, story, movement, dramatic situation)" (Bruscia, 2011, p. 6).

In re-creative music therapy, "the therapist engages the client in vocal or instrumental tasks that involve reproducing music in some way. This may include learning how to use the voice or produce sounds on an instrument, imitating melodies or rhythms, learning to sing by rote, learning to use musical notation, participating in a sing-along, rehearsing, taking music lessons, performing a song or instrumental piece from memory, working out the musical interpretation of a composition, performing in a musical show or drama, and more" (Bruscia, 2011, p. 6).

Compositional music therapy involves "the therapist helping the client to write songs, lyrics, or instrumental pieces, or to create any kind of musical product, such as music videos or audiotape programs. Usually, the therapist simplifies the process by engaging the client in the easier aspects of composing (e.g., generating a melody or writing the lyrics of a song) and by taking responsibility for more technical aspects (e.g., harmonization, notation)" (Bruscia, 2011, p. 7).

The chapter ends with a Research Evidence section. This section presents the available research evidence from both quantitative and qualitative research traditions for the given population. The authors were asked to include basic statistical information (e.g., means, standard deviations, p-value or effect size) where available. The inclusion of this type of information is aimed at giving the reader a better understanding of the magnitude of the impact of music therapy. Furthermore, when communicating to other health care professionals about the benefits of music therapy, the music therapist should be skilled in sharing clinical observations of the child's experiences/responses as well as basic scientific details regarding available research evidence.

Finally, the authors were asked to include a section on Working with Caregivers. Some authors included this as a separate section (typically placed after Needs and Resources), whereas other authors incorporated this within the Needs and Resources section.

Challenges

In most cases, the classification of interventions according to the four methods was rather straightforward. However, a few instances evoked interesting debates between the editor and the authors.

For example, Shoemark, in her work with newborn infants with medical needs, views as improvisational some interventions that typically would be classified as receptive. Her argument is that the music therapist and the infant co-construct music together: "[These] methods champion the musicality of the infant's rudimentary communication, the innate musicality of the mother-infant relationship, and the timeless traditions of infant-directed singing. The music therapist can use music-making to acknowledge and promote [the infant's] capacities to interact with an attuned partner" (Chapter 4).

A few authors questioned the validity of organizing the chapter per these methods because sessions with children in medical settings typically evolve organically and include various methods within one session. Therefore, writing about interventions as separate entities felt artificial at times. For example, a music therapist might begin a session by offering a familiar song to a child who appears withdrawn and upset (receptive method). This might move into the child singing along with the therapist and requesting additional songs (re-creative method). Reflective dialogue about the meaning of a given song to the child's current situation might naturally lead to the use of story songs or music-facilitated dramatic play (improvisational method).

The concern of the authors was certainly valid from a clinical perspective. However, from an educational perspective, it is necessary to first teach students interventions as stand-alone interventions. Once they master these interventions, they can begin incorporating multiple interventions within a session. Initially, this happens through creating a session plan that matches specific interventions with specific goals. It is only with sufficient clinical experience that students and novice therapists develop the necessary skills to assess a child's presenting needs (and potential for creative solutions) and organically move from one intervention into the next according to these needs/strengths. As eloquently stated by Ghetti in her chapter: "In practice, therapists will likely transcend these categories by combining various approaches within a session, depending upon client needs and the flow of the ongoing therapeutic process. Furthermore, certain intervention areas, such as the use of music therapy as procedural support for invasive or anxiety-provoking medical procedures, may incorporate several of the approaches described below as the procedure unfolds and the client's needs change from moment to moment. Thus, readers should envision the subsections of clinical approaches [...] as possibilities for clinical intervention and should layer or sequence such approaches in relation to a child and family's ongoing needs and responses."

Another challenge was the lack of supporting literature in certain areas, including respiratory care, full-term newborn infants, medically fragile children in low awareness states, and burn care. The guidelines in these chapters are predominantly based on the clinical experience of the contributing authors.

A major challenge as an editor was coming to terms with some of the repetitiveness across chapters. For example, many chapters include music-guided relaxation, music-guided imagery, songwriting, and so on. However, the authors were asked to write the guidelines for these interventions as specific as possible to their population. A careful comparison of these interventions across chapters indeed highlights important differences, whether in discussions about contraindications, responses to observe, or ways of implementation. Moreover, many authors have included brief clinical examples in the guidelines. These help the reader to contextualize the intervention and better understand the specific needs and resources of the given population. Thus, although the reader may be inclined to quickly glance over guidelines for an intervention that was already covered in a preceding chapter, it is recommended that the reader carefully study the differences in guidelines offered by the authors.

Although the chapters in this volume are available as separate e-chapters, it is recommended that the following chapters be read together:

- Premature Infants & Full-Term Hospitalized Infants

- Pain Management & Burn Care
- Pain Management & Surgery and Procedural Support & Pediatric Intensive Care
- Children with Cancer & Palliative and End-of-Life Care for Children
- Brain Injuries and Rehabilitation in Children & Medically Fragile Children in Low Awareness States

Finally, a few words about grammar. First, to avoid using (s)he and him/her throughout the book, the following gender-specific pronouns rule was employed:

- female authors use she/her when referring to the music therapist and he/him for the child
- male authors use he/his for the music therapist and she/her for the child

Second, it is understood that pediatric hospitals or units serve infants, children, adolescents, and, in some cases, young adults. For the sake of brevity, "children" is used throughout the book except for in the premature infants and full-term hospitalized newborns chapter. In instances where authors provided guidelines specifically for adolescents, the word "adolescents" or "teens" is used.

Concluding Remarks

This book provides practical guidelines for work with children in medical settings. The authors have done an outstanding job in detailing the clinical decision-making process and providing step-by-step instructions for how to implement each music therapy intervention. All contributing authors are experienced clinicians who use and intertwine these interventions in their work naturally. To deconstruct the interventions into detailed, practical guidelines was at times a challenge, but we hope that they will enrich the music therapy practice of many future music therapists in pediatric medical care.

References

Barrera, M., Rykov, M., & Doyle, S. (2002). The effects of interactive music therapy on hospitalized children with cancer: A pilot study. *Psycho-Oncology, 11*, 379–388.

Bradt, J. (2001). The effects of music entrainment on postoperative pain perception in pediatric patients Unpublished doctoral dissertation. Temple University, Philadelphia.

Bradt, J. (2010). The effects of music entrainment on postoperative pain perception in pediatric patients. *Music and Medicine, 2*(2), 150–157.

Bradt, J., Dileo, C., & Grocke, D. (2010). Music for anxiety reduction in mechanically ventilated patients. *Cochrane Database of Systematic Reviews* 2010, Issue 12. Art. no. CD006902. DOI: 10.1002/14651858.CD006902.pub2.10.1002/14651858.CD006911.pub2.

Bradt, J., & Goodill, S. (2013). Creative arts therapies defined: Comment on "effects of creative arts therapies on psychological symptoms and quality of life in patients with cancer. *JAMA Internal Medicine, Online First*. DOI: 10.1001/ jamainternmed.2013.6145.

Bruscia, K. E. (October, 2011). *Conceptualization of the new series: Guidelines for music therapy practice*. Unpublished Manuscript.

Burns, D. S. (2012). Theoretical rationale for music selection in oncology intervention research: An integrative review. *Journal of Music Therapy, 49*(1), 7–22.

Dileo, C., & Bradt, J. (2005). *Medical music therapy: A meta-analysis*. Cherry Hill, NJ: Jeffrey Publications.

Ghetti, C. M. (2012). Music therapy as procedural support for invasive medical procedures: Toward the development of music therapy theory. *Nordic Journal of Music Therapy, 21*(1), 3–35. DOI: 10.1080/08098131.2011.571278.

Hanson-Abromeit, D. (2008). Introduction to pediatric medical music therapy. In D. Hanson-Abromeit & C. Colwell (2008). *Medical music therapy for pediatrics in hospital settings: Using music to support medical interventions.* Silver Spring, MD: American Music Therapy Association.

Klassen, J., Liang, Y., Tjosvold, L., Klassen, T., & Hartling, L. (2008). Music for pain and anxiety in children undergoing medical procedures: A systematic review of randomized controlled trials. *Ambulatory Pediatrics: The Official Journal of the Ambulatory Pediatric Association, 8*(2), 117–128.

Loewy, J., Stewart, K., Dassler, A. M., Telsey, A., & Homel, P. (2013). The effects of music therapy on vital signs, feeding, and sleep in premature infants. *Pediatrics.* Advanced online publication. DOI: 10.1542/peds.2012-1367.

Loewy, J. V. (Ed.). (2000). *Music therapy in the neonatal intensive care unit.* Cherry Hill, NJ: Jeffrey Books.

Loewy, J. V., MacGregor, B., Richards, K., & Rodriguez, J. (1997). Music therapy pediatric pain management: Assessing and attending to the sounds of hurt, fear and anxiety. In J. V. Loewy (Ed.), *Music therapy and pediatric pain* (pp. 45–56). Cherry Hill, NJ: Jeffrey Books.

Michel, D. (1965). Professional profile of the NAMT member and his clinical practices in music therapy. *Journal of Music Therapy, 2,* 124–129.

Nöcker-Ribaupierre, M. (2004). *Music therapy for premature and newborn infants.* Gilsum, NH: Barcelona Publishers.

Nolan, P. (1997). Music therapy in the pediatric pain experience: Theory, practice and research at Allegheny University of the Health Sciences. In J. V. Loewy (Ed.), *Music therapy and pediatric pain* (pp. 57–68). Cherry Hill, NJ: Jeffrey Books.

O'Callaghan, C., Baron, A., Barry, P., & Dun, B. (2011). Music's relevance for pediatric cancer patients: A constructivist and mosaic research approach. *Supportive Care in Cancer, 19(6),* 779–788.

O'Callaghan, C., Barry, P., & Thompson, K. (2012). Music's relevance for adolescents and young adults with cancer: A constructivist research approach. *Supportive Care in Cancer, 20*(4), 687–697.

Robb, S. L. (2000). The effect of therapeutic music interventions on the behavior of hospitalized children in isolation: Developing a contextual support model of music therapy. *Journal of Music Therapy, 37,* 118–146.

Robb, S. L. (2003). Coping and chronic illness: Music therapy for children and adults with cancer. In S. L. Robb (Ed.), *Music therapy in pediatric healthcare: Research and evidence-based practice* (pp. 101–136). Silver Spring, MD: American Music Therapy Association.

Robb, S. L. (2012). Gratitude for a complex profession: The importance of theory-based research in music therapy. [Editorial]. *Journal of Music Therapy, 49*(1), 2–6.

Robb, S. L., & Carpenter, J. S. (2009). A review of music-based intervention reporting in pediatrics. *Journal of Health Psychology, 14*(4), 490–501.

Robb, S. L., Clair, A. A., Watanabe, M., Monahan, P. O., Azzous, F., Stouffer, J. W., Ebberts, A., Darsie, E., Whitmer, C., Walker, J., Nelson, K., Hanson-Abromeit, D., Lane, D., & Hannan, A. (2008). A non-randomized controlled trial of the active music engagement (AME) intervention on children with cancer. *Psycho-Oncology, 17*(7), 699–708.

Rudenberg, M. T., & Royka, A. M. (1989). Promoting psychosocial adjustment in pediatric burn patients through music therapy and child life therapy. *Music Therapy Perspectives, 7,* 40–43.

Skinner, E. A., & Wellborn, J. G. (1994). Coping during childhood and adolescence: A motivational perspective. In D. Featherman, R. Lerner, & M. Perlmutter (Eds.), *Life-span development and behavior.* Vol. 12 (pp. 91-133). Hillsdale, NJ: Erlbaum.

Standley, J. M., & Walworth, D. (2010). *Music therapy with premature infants: Research and developmental interventions* (2nd ed.). Silver Spring, MD: American Music Therapy Association.

Standley, J. M., & Whipple, J. (2003). *Music therapy with pediatric patients: A meta-analysis.* In S. L. Robb (Ed.), *Music therapy in pediatric healthcare: Research and evidence-based practice.* Silver Spring, MD: American Music Therapy Association.

Stige, B., & Rolvsjord, R. (2003). Introduction to "Theory building in music therapy—An international archive." *Nordic Journal of Music Therapy, 12*(1), 67–68.

Thompson, S. W. (1991). Communication techniques for allaying anxiety and providing support for hospitalized children. *Journal of Child and Adolescent Psychiatric Nursing, 4,* 119–122.

Treurnicht Naylor, K., Kingsnorth, S., Lamont, A., McKeever, P., & Macarthur, C. (2011). The effectiveness of music in pediatric healthcare: A systematic review of randomized controlled trials. *Evidence-Based Complementary and Alternative Medicine.* Article ID 464759. DOI: 10.1155/2011.

Wolfe, D. E., & Waldon, E. G. (2009). *Music therapy and pediatric medicine: A guide to skills development and clinical intervention.* Silver Spring, MD: American Music Therapy Association.

Chapter 2

Pain Management with Children

Joke Bradt

INTRODUCTION

Contributing effectively to a child's pain management is a major responsibility for music therapists working in pediatric hospitals. Children expect clinicians to be able to help them with their pain. Parents have similar expectations. Effective management of pain in children is important, especially considering the growing evidence that untreated or inadequately treated pain may have a long-term negative impact on pain sensitivity, immune function, neurophysiology, and health-related behaviors (for a review, see Young, 2005).

In a survey on pain management (Michel & Chesky, 1995), music therapists were asked about the music interventions they used for addressing pain in their clinical work. Ninety-five percent of the respondents reported using music for relaxation, 91% for distraction, 75% as mood enhancer, 52% to stimulate imagery, 14% for "cognitive tasks," 12% for music vibration, and 9% with psychotherapy. Noteworthy is that only a few respondents reported to use "live music activity as part of their protocols" (p. 50). Because children prefer doing over passively receiving, the guidelines in this chapter go beyond music for relaxation or sedation. Instead, most of the interventions presented here seek active participation from the child, if possible.

In the introduction to her book *Music Therapy and Pediatric Pain*, Loewy (1997) emphasizes that "music therapy need not be seen as a replacement for, or an alternative to, a pharmacological approach, but may be used effectively in conjunction with, or as a complement to, a particular treatment plan" (p. 1). In order to work collaboratively with team members toward optimum pain management, it is important that music therapists understand mechanisms underlying the pain-reducing effects of music interventions and are able to adequately articulate these. This will help team members understand the unique role music therapy can play in addressing multiple dimensions of a child's pain experience.

This chapter will enhance the reader's understanding of pain as a multidimensional phenomenon, provide a brief overview of common pain theories, give recommendations for pain assessment, and present guidelines for a wide variety of music therapy interventions for pain management. Several chapters in this book address pain-related needs of specific populations (e.g., burn patients, surgical and procedural support). It is recommended that the reader consult those chapters to learn about music therapy guidelines that meet the specific needs of these populations (e.g., use of music therapy during debridement in burn patients; use of music to reduce agitation and distress in premature infants).

DIAGNOSTIC INFORMATION

Pain as a Multidimensional Phenomenon

For many years, pain was defined solely in terms of tissue damage, namely as a simple transmission of impulses from the nerve receptors at the site of injury to the part of the brain responsible for pain perception, with the intensity of the pain proportional to the extent of tissue damage. However, the fact that people with similar bodily injuries frequently report very different levels of pain led researchers to believe that pain perception was not simply a function of the amount of physical damage alone. Instead, pain became defined as a subjective experience that integrates sensory, emotional, and cognitive information (Brown, Chen, & Dworkin, 1989; Chapman, 1995; Melzack & Dennis, 1978). Besides intrapersonal communication, involving sensation, emotion, and cognition, there is an interpersonal exchange of messages that influences the pain experience. Pain behavior and the emotional expression of pain have as their main function the communication of distress to the immediate environment, in an appeal for increased social support. The reaction of the immediate environment undoubtedly influences subsequent pain behavior and emotions. It is the continuous exchange of information among these four components that results in the experience of pain; it needs to be emphasized that they should be viewed as four concurrent processes, and not as sequential (Chapman, 1995).

The International Association for the Study of Pain (IASP) defines pain as "an unpleasant sensory and emotional experience associated with actual or potential tissue damage, or described in terms of such damage" (IASP, 2011). This definition recognizes the importance of emotions in pain perception. In addition, it emphasizes that pain can be present in the absence of actual injury or tissue damage. With her definition of pain, McCaffery (1968) brought the subjective nature of the pain experience to the forefront: "Pain is what the person says it is and exists whenever he or she says it does" (p. 95). Important in McCaffery's definition is that it gives power to the person who is experiencing pain by giving him or her control over the assessment of the presence, the description, and the intensity of the pain.

Given the understanding that pain is subjective, it is important to distinguish pain from nociception. Nociception refers solely to the processes that regulate the transmission and modulation of noxious stimuli in the nervous system (Craig, 1999). Pain is a broader term, referring to the perceptual state as described above. In order for a noxious stimulus to be considered as pain by the organism, it needs to be processed at a conscious level (Anand, 1998).

Acute, Chronic, and Procedural Pain

Pain can be categorized as acute, chronic, or procedural. This distinction is important since these are very different perceptual states. Acute pain has a sudden onset and usually subsides in less than one month, its main function being to warn the sufferer of noxious internal or external events that may require immediate attention (Selm, 1991). Procedural pain is caused by a medical procedure. This type of pain may subside when the procedure is completed (e.g., venipuncture) or may linger following the procedure.

Pain is considered chronic if it persists beyond the expected period of healing and if the etiology is or is not known. Chronic pain loses its warning function because somatic and psychological adaptation develops. It brings numerous challenges to a child's life, requiring many adaptations and often bringing about existential crises, especially in teens. Despite advances in knowledge of pain mechanisms and treatment, adequate management of chronic pain continues to present a challenge.

Children with a chronic illness often require repeated hospitalization and numerous painful procedures. For example, children with cancer may need several lumbar punctures and bone marrow aspirations. Likewise, children with physical disabilities may require repeated surgeries throughout their childhood.

Chronic cancer-related pain poses its own set of challenges. One of which is the fact that pain exacerbations are often interpreted as signs of a worsening condition by the child as well as his family members. This may evoke heightened anxiety which, in turn, negatively affects the child's pain. Furthermore, pain brings an acute awareness of impending loss of comfort, loss of control, and loss of life (Magill, Coyle, Handzo, & Loscalzo, 1997).

Pain Theories

The literature on the use of music therapy interventions for pain management cites various theories and possible pathways through which music therapy may improve pain perception. These theoretical models recognize the multidimensional nature of pain, including the importance of affective qualities. It is important for music therapists to be knowledgeable about these so that they can serve as a theoretical framework for explicating potential treatment mechanisms.

The Gate Control Theory. The Gate Control Theory was the first comprehensive model of pain perception that incorporated sensory and affective as well as cognitive components. It was developed by Melzack and Wall in 1965. The theory postulates that the information pathway for noxious stimuli, extending from the periphery of our body to the brain, can be significantly altered at the level of the dorsal horns in the spine, modifying the amount of pain stimuli passing through. Regardless of the intensity of the noxious stimuli, little or no pain may be perceived due to the potential inhibitory ability of certain cells along the neural transmission route. It is hypothesized that neural activity in the dorsal horns of the spinal cord acts as a "gate."

It is mainly the activity of the large- and small-diameter sensory nerve fibers that determines to what degree this gate increases or decreases the flow of sensory information. Pain impulses are conducted to the brain by the smaller-diameter, hence slower, fibers. If nothing blocks them, the pain impulses travel up the spinal cord to the thalamus and cerebral cortex. However, increased activity of the large-diameter fibers—because of the activation of peripheral, nonpainful mechanoreceptors—can block the passage of the noxious impulses partially, or even totally (Melzack & Wall, 1965). Thus, by increasing sensory, nonpainful input, especially in the auditory, visual, and tactile domains, the pain perception can be greatly modified (Whipple & Glynn, 1992). This gating mechanism frequently is offered as a rationale for music for pain reduction.

This gate is furthermore influenced by descending pathways stemming from the brainstem and cortex going down the spinal cord. These brain fibers form the "central control mechanism." This mechanism continuously influences the stimulus input at the spinal cord level, facilitating some patterns of input but inhibiting others. Information about the noxious input is interpreted in the higher centers of the brain, and then the reinterpretation is transmitted back down the spinal cord to influence the pain perception (Allen, 1998). Additionally, information on expectation, level of anxiety, locus of control, meaning of the situation in which injury occurs, attention-distraction levels, and emotional state may open or close the gate, partly determining the intensity and quality of pain experiences. Thus, the signal that finally leads to pain perception can be amplified or reduced by higher cognitive processes. Nociception and the experience of pain may, therefore, be totally unrelated: Pain can be reported in the absence of nociception (e.g., phantom pain), or there can be noxious stimulation without pain perception. This notion of bidirectional influence that redefined pain from a purely sensory phenomenon to a multidimensional perceptual experience (Turk & Rudy, 1986) is of great importance to music therapy practice.

Three dimensions of pain are distinguished in the Gate Control Theory and have been widely used in the pain literature and music therapy literature: (a) the sensory-discriminative dimension, which refers to intensity, location, and duration of the pain; (b) the motivational-affective component, including behavioral responses, emotional responses, and a "need state" to limit the pain's duration and intensity; and (c) the cognitive-interpretational dimension, relating the pain experience to contextual biopsychosocial significance and comparing it to previous experiences (Anand, 1998; Ghetti, 2012).

This theory has been instrumental in the acceptance of the interaction between physiological and psychological factors in pain perception and pain behavior. While pain was treated almost solely with pharmacological and surgical interventions for a very long time, it is not surprising that the acceptance of the Gate Control Theory has led to the development of various nonpharmacological approaches to treating pain, using the manipulation of one or more of these contributing variables.

The Neuromatrix Theory of Pain. The Neuromatrix theory was developed by Melzack (1999, 2001) as a further development of the Gate Control Theory. It is important to understand that it does not negate the Gate Control Theory. Growing scientific evidence about the widespread involvement of the brain in pain perception forced Melzack to expand his theory to include extensive neural networks and the concept of neural imprinting. According to the expanded theory, "pain is a multidimensional experience ... produced by characteristic 'neurosignatures' or patterns of nerve impulses generated by a widely distributed neural network: the 'body-self neuromatrix'" (Melzack, 1999, p. 121). The term "body-self" refers to a neural network that consists of loops between the thalamus and cortex as well between the cortex and limbic system. The *neuromatrix* is "the entire network, whose spatial distribution and synaptic links are initially determined genetically and are later sculpted by sensory inputs" (Melzack, 2001, p. 1379). Any inputs (especially repeated sensory inputs) from the body undergo cyclical processing and synthesis and create characteristic patterns in the neuromatrix termed the "neurosignature." Melzack proposes that the neurosignature pattern is modulated not only by genetic factors but also by sensory inputs and cognitive events, such as psychosocial or emotional stress (Melzack, 2001).

The Fear-Tension-Pain Cycle. A theory that is often used to provide a rationale for the use of nonpharmacological pain management interventions is the fear-tension-pain cycle. This cycle is described as a vicious circle: It is a process through which pain produces or increases fear. This, in turn, creates tension in the muscles. Increased muscle tension puts additional pressure on the nerve endings, exacerbating the pain, and increased pain intensity leads, consequently, to greater fear (Cowan, 1991; Fowler-Kerry & Lander, 1987).

The goal of pain treatment is to break this cycle. This can be done in several ways. Refocusing the patient's attention on a pleasant sensory stimulus or an engaging activity may result in decreased fear. A wide variety of relaxation techniques can decrease the muscle pressure on the nerve endings, resulting in pain reduction. Furthermore, enhanced understanding of the cause and meaning of the pain can reduce a person's fear.

Decreased Activation of the Amygdala. Growing evidence suggests that the amygdala, part of the brain's limbic system, plays a mediating role between pain and emotions. The amygdala influences the emotional-affective aspects of behavior as well as the emotional evaluation of sensory stimuli. A section of the amygdala has now been labeled the "nociceptive amygdala" because it contains a large number of neurons that respond to pain (Neugebauer & Li, 2003). Important to music therapists is the fact that pleasure derived from listening to or making music is correlated to decreased activity in the amygdala (Blood & Zatorre, 2001). Neugebauer and Neugebauer (2003) propose that pain-reducing effects of music may be mediated by the amygdala. The decreased activity in the amygdala due to music may, in turn, inhibit the descending neural processes involved in pain perception (Blood & Zatorre, 2001; Neugebauer & Neugebauer, 2003).

Pain in Hospitalized Children

Hospitalized children may experience pain for a wide variety of reasons. In this section, commonly encountered pain conditions and causes for pain are presented. This list certainly is not exhaustive. However, it provides a good starting point for novice therapists.

Procedural and postsurgical pain. The most common cause of pain in hospitalized children is postsurgical and procedural pain. Many surgeries cause moderate to severe pain during the initial postoperative days. Common procedures that cause pain in children include lumbar punctures (a procedure that is performed to collect a sample of cerebrospinal fluid), intravenous line placement, catheter placement, blood draws, and laceration repair. Chapter 6 in this book, by Mondanaro, addresses music therapy interventions for surgical and procedural support. As pointed out by Mondanaro, adequate procedural support and pain management are paramount to the child's well-being and greatly influence the child's coping in subsequent encounters with procedures or surgeries.

Sickle Cell Disease (SCD). SCD is serious disorder in which the body makes sickle-shape instead of disc-shape red blood cells. Sickle cells do not move easily through the blood vessels of the limbs and organs. Blocked blood flow can cause pain, organ damage, swollen limbs, infections, acute chest syndrome, and stroke. Furthermore, the sickle-shape blood cells are not effective in transporting oxygen throughout the body.

SCD is a hereditary disorder. It is more common in certain ethnic groups, including people of African descent, including African-Americans, Hispanic–Americans, and people of Caribbean, and South and Central American Indian descent (National Heart, Lung, and Blood Institute, 2012). Sickle cell anemia is the most common form of SCD, with no widely available cure. However, treatments to improve the anemia and lower complications can help with the symptoms and complications of the disease (National Heart, Lung, and Blood Institute, 2012).

When patients with sickle cell anemia are admitted to the hospital, it is almost always due to "pain crisis" or vaso-occlusive crisis (VOC). These crises cause extreme pain. Narcotics are often administered to help combat the pain, but these have many undesirable side effects. Treatment also includes blood transfusions to dilute the sickle cells.

Hemophilia. Hemophilia is a severe chronic bleeding disorder that impairs the body's ability to control blood clotting or coagulation. It is for the most part managed by coagulation factor replacement. The severe forms of the disease consist of recurrent bleeding episodes which occur most commonly in the joints (hemarthroses). These may start early in life (before the age of two) and can be very painful, to the point of being excruciating when they are not treated properly (Choiniere & Melzack, 1987; Sherry, 2008). Children with hemophilia experience pain from two main causes—bleeding episodes and factor infusions. The frequent joint bleeds may unfortunately lead to structural deficiencies and deformities, orthopedic joint corrections, and chronic pain (Sherry, 2008). Pain management in hemophilia raises serious difficulties, since many analgesic and anti-inflammatory drugs are contraindicated because they may prolong the bleeding time (Choiniere & Melzack, 1987). Therefore, nonpharmacological treatment interventions to help the child manage his pain are important for this population.

Cystic Fibrosis (CF). CF is a genetic disease that causes mucus to build up in the lungs. The disease gets worse over time. As the mucus builds up, it can block airways in the lungs, making it increasingly harder to breathe. In addition, mucus buildup makes it easier for bacteria to grow, causing frequent infections in the lungs. Children with CF frequently suffer from chest pain. Mucus buildup also causes many intestinal problems, leading to recurrent abdominal pain.

Cancer-related pain. Pain is one of the most common symptoms in children with cancer. It can be caused by the cancer itself, diagnostic procedures, or treatments. The most common childhood malignancies, such as leukemia, lymphoma, and neuroblastoma, often produce diffuse bone and joint pain. Treatment-related pain may include postoperative pain, radiation-induced dermatitis or skin inflammation, gastritis from repeated vomiting, prolonged post–lumbar puncture headache, neuropathy (damage to the peripheral nervous system), and infection. Regardless of the source, children often do not receive adequate treatment for their pain. It is best to evaluate every child with cancer for potential pain, because children may experience pain, even though they may not be able to express it. In their Global Year Against Cancer Pain fact sheet, the IASP specifically lists music therapy as one of the nonpharmacological interventions that can be used alone or in tandem with pharmacological pain treatments for cancer-related pain management in children.

Trauma-related pain. Many children sustain injuries that require hospitalization. Injuries may vary from mild to moderate musculoskeletal injuries to severe head traumas and burns. Kennelly (Chapter 10 in this book) writes that acquired brain injuries may impact a child's perception, experience, and communication of pain. An increase in muscle tone with accompanying pain is common with this population. Because of impairments in communication, these children are often unable to clearly articulate the locality and severity of this pain. This presents major challenges for adequate assessment and treatment of pain.

Burn pain is one of the most difficult forms of acute pain to treat. Burn injuries typically result in unusually high levels of pain. In addition, the wound care and rehabilitation interventions typically worsen the existing pain. This high level of pain has been reported to often interfere with wound care and therapies as well as lengthen hospitalization. Moreover, the extreme pain experienced by children with burns appears associated with long-term post-traumatic stress and general emotional distress. Therefore, management of burn pain is of great importance to the well-being of the child during hospitalization as well as for the child's mental health following discharge. Burn pain is usually aggressively treated with potent opioids and anxiolytics (anxiety-reducing drugs) in combination with nonpharmacological methods of pain management (Patterson, Hoflund, Espey, & Sharar, n.d.).

Finally, pain due to abuse and violence (e.g., gunshot wounds) is unfortunately common in children's hospitals. Pain in young victims of violence is quite prevalent in urban pediatric hospitals. Music therapists need to be adequately trained and have significant experience in trauma work and music psychotherapy before working with these children.

Types of Pain Medication

It is beyond the scope of this chapter to present a detailed discussion about the different types of pain medications, their benefits, and their side effects. However, it is important that music therapists know what types of pain medications are available, what their uses are, and what side effects a music therapist may expect to see in a child.

- *Nonsteroidal anti-inflammatory drugs (NSAID):* These pain-relieving and anti-inflammatory medications can be broken into three categories: naproxen, ibuprofen, and aspirin. Naproxen is preferred for chronic pain, whereas ibuprofen and aspirin are better for spontaneous pain. The main side effect of NSAID is irritation of the stomach.
- *Acetaminophen:* Acetaminophen (mostly known as Tylenol) is frequently paired with codeine, hydrocodone, and oxycodone (narcotics) to address more severe pain.
- *Opioids:* This type of medication is reserved for the most severe pain. Opioids are a type of narcotic that can have significant impacts on the body upon initial exposure, including increased sedation and dizziness. They may also cause constipation, which can bring a significant amount of discomfort. Opioid drugs include codeine, fentanyl, hydrocodone, hydromorphone, meperidine, methadone, morphine, and oxycodone.

- *Postsurgical pain management:* For pain following major surgery, it is common practice to give opioids by intravenous injection for the first 24–48 hours. This may be followed by oral narcotics and then non-narcotic analgesics or a combination of both. The child may also receive a patient-controlled analgesia pump (PCA) that delivers pain medication through an IV continuously or through an intermittent dosage. With intermittent dosages, the child decides when he feels bad and pushes a button that administers a dose of pain medication. This system lets the patient have more control over the amount of medication needed to relieve pain and eliminates the anxiety that comes from expecting the return of pain when the dose wears off. The dosage is determined by the child's physician, and the child cannot give himself too much. Children as young as four years old have been shown to use PCA pumps effectively.

NEEDS AND RESOURCES

Many factors may alter pain perception in a child. Some of these factors are relatively constant for a particular child (e.g., sex, age, development), while others may vary greatly, depending on the situation or context in which the child experiences the pain. These variable factors include (a) cognitive-developmental factors such as the meaning ascribed to the pain, locus of control, and an understanding of the pain source; (b) emotional factors such as fear, anxiety, anger, depression, and frustration; (c) sociocultural factors such as parental response, parental expectation, and environment and context in which the child experiences the pain; and (d) spiritual factors (McGrath, 1993).

Cognitive Development

A child's understanding of pain depends on age, cognitive level, and previous pain experience. The dominant theoretical perspective in cognitive-developmental studies of pediatric health and illness has been Piaget's theory of development. Meaningful explanations of children's pain depend on the understanding of what might be a painful event for a child of a certain age, and what that child is likely to perceive as the cause of the pain (Zajdeman & Biedermann, 1991).

Piaget believed that a child's reasoning develops through four broad stages: sensorimotor, preoperational, concrete operations, and formal operations. Each of these is characterized by different types of logic. Studies by Gaffney and Dunne (1986) and Gaffney (1987, 1993), investigating ideas about pain in children, ages 5 to 14, support the hypothesis that children's ideas about pain change with age in a developmental pattern consonant with the Piagetian theory. It is important for music therapists providing pain management services to be knowledgeable about these stages, as they have important treatment implications.

During the preoperational stage (two to seven years of age), children seem to understand pain as a physical entity that has unpleasant qualities and is aversive. Children's descriptions of pain appear to be limited to their simple sensory aspects. Their attitude toward pain is rather passive, and they only know concrete, passive methods of pain relief, including medicine. Furthermore, they tend to rely on their parents for reduction of their pain. There is evidence that children at this stage may attribute pain to the transgression of rules. Therefore, pediatric health professionals should be careful to avoid reinforcing these ideas with suggestions that recovery is dependent on good behavior.

During the concrete operational stage (seven to 12 years of age), children's understanding of pain changes from a purely physical experience to an awareness of negative emotions associated with pain. Pain is further understood to occur within the body; external agents are not the sole causes. A more active attitude toward pain becomes evident, which translates into a more active approach toward pain relief. In addition to the use of medicine, there is the use of simple physical strategies (e.g., rubbing the painful spot) and psychological strategies (e.g., talking to friends or watching TV). Pain is still often linked to transgression of rules, but other, more objective explanations are also given as the child becomes aware of multiple rather than single causes of pain.

Children in the formal operational stage (above 12 years of age) possess the capacity to reflect on pain in a more abstract way; they are even able to recognize the positive, biologically useful aspects of pain as a warning signal. There is a growing emphasis on the psychological aspects of pain and a decreasing emphasis on the physical aspects. Psychological factors are now understood as contributors to the pain experience. Therefore, the child is better able to understand cognitive strategies of pain management. Children at this stage also understand that pain is a subjective experience and that, subsequently, nobody can feel what their own pain is like.

Although there is little research on the understanding of pain of children in the sensorimotor period, studies have shown that very young children have a more sophisticated understanding of pain than previously thought. For instance, children who are 18 months of age can express pain and tell where the pain is. In addition, they can recognize pain in others and try to alleviate that pain (McGrath & McAlpine, 1993).

Gender

The results of studies evaluating gender-related differences in children's pain perception are not conclusive. According to McGrath (1993), boys and girls probably are equally sensitive to pain but differ in their responses to pain. In many cultures, norms for pain behavior are set differently for boys and girls. Boys are often encouraged to suppress their pain complaints, whereas girls may receive subtle reinforcement for verbal expression of their pain. Boys are encouraged to use active pain coping strategies (e.g., physical activity), whereas girls may be encouraged to rely on more passive methods, such as rest and taking medicine. This may explain why boys appear more stoic when they are in pain, whereas girls may express their pain more openly. However, it is important to point out that a few studies have not found significant differences between pain behaviors of boys and girls. For example, a large-scale study involving 994 children (5–12 years) in schools, hospitals, and clinical settings used open-ended questions to determine the extent of their knowledge and understanding of pain, their ability to describe pain, and their use of coping strategies (Ross & Ross, 1984). No clearly defined differences could be found between boys and girls.

Perceived Level of Control

Even more than adults, children perceive much of their medical treatment as unpredictable and beyond their control: they may be uncertain about what to expect, they may not understand the need for a painful treatment, and they may not know any effective strategies to cope with the pain (McGrath, 1993). It is generally accepted that the perception of the controllability of the pain modulates the pain experience in a child. Repeated pain experiences or the development of even low-level persistent pain can lead to a preoccupation with the pain and beliefs concerning its uncontrollability, each of which serves to amplify it (Zeltzer et al., 1997).

Three categories of control-enhancing techniques have proven to be effective in the pediatric setting: behavioral, decisional, and cognitive control. Behavioral control refers to self-pacing procedures in which, for example, the child is given control over when he wants a break during a painful procedure. Decisional control involves giving the child a choice in the pain situation; the child can be asked, for example, which arm should be used for the needle. Finally, cognitive control refers to the children's belief that they are in control of themselves. This belief may be based on past experiences or on a vicarious learning experience (Ross & Ross, 1984).

Coping Strategies

Many coping strategies utilized by children in pain have been discussed in the literature, including distraction, refocusing, thought-stopping, relaxation, fantasy, clenching one's fist, and the defense mechanisms of regression and denial. Children's ability to use coping strategies appears to be greatly influenced by their developmental level. From ages 8 to 10, a shift seems to occur in the kind of coping strategies used by children, namely from behavioral to more cognitive, sophisticated strategies. Children of this age can alleviate some of their pain when they feel they have an increased level of control over the pain and illness (Ross & Ross, 1984). Before the age of five years, cognitive and behavioral coping strategies that require a child to use control strategies such as relaxation or cognitive reframing are generally beyond their capabilities (McGrath & McAlpine, 1993).

McGrath (1990) states that children seem more adept than adults at using nonpharmacological interventions, presumably because they are usually less biased than adults about the potential effects of nondrug treatments. Robb (2003) provides an excellent discussion on children's preferred coping strategies per age group and associated implications for music therapy strategies.

Previous Pain Experience

Children judge the strength and unpleasantness of pain in relation to the types of pain that they have already experienced. The diversity of children's past pain experiences forms "their frame of reference for perceiving all new pain" (McGrath, 1993, p. 41). As children mature, they experience a wider variety of pain that differs in intensity, duration, location, and quality. Children also learn new coping strategies and thus gradually develop a repertoire of methods to alleviate different types of pain (McGrath, 1993).

Emotional Factors

Anxiety and fear. For most children, anxiety and fear are the immediate emotional responses associated with painful stimuli. In fact, it is almost impossible to behaviorally distinguish between children's perceived pain and anxiety. Clinical experience has shown that acute anxiety usually heightens the pain experience. According to Zeltzer et al. (1997), anxiety evoked by pain leads to self-focused attention in the child. When the pain is inescapable, high pain-related anxiety may lead to a fixation of attention on the pain, increasing its perceived intensity and aversiveness. This may lead to a negative cycle of arousal and self-focused attention, which may interfere with attempts to cope with the pain and subsequently intensify pain and distress, thereby reinforcing the child's initial fear. Children with a chronic illness often experience increases in pain because of fears about the possibility of dying, and anxiety about necessary treatments. Also, the anxiety that these children may perceive in their parents' reaction to their illness can cause them to feel guilty, upset, or frustrated, such that the pain experiences become more unpleasant for them (McGrath, 1990).

Depression. Depression is one of the most commonly observed risk factors for poor outcome among children with chronic illness and pain. However, literature about the interaction between depression and pain is almost devoid of empirical studies with children. The child's awareness of his physical limitations may elicit feelings of hopelessness with subsequent reduced coping efforts, thereby exacerbating the pain (Hagglund et al., 1995).

Sociocultural Factors

Parents and siblings are very influential in what children learn about pain, how they express pain, and how they cope with pain. Children learn to evaluate the significance of a noxious event from their parents' reactions. Parents' reactions to their child's pain vary widely. At one end of the spectrum are parents who show little interest in minor pain events, but who are still sensitive to them. At the other end are parents who tend to overreact to minor pain events. At a very early age, children of the latter learn that loud, overt pain responses elicit immediate parental attention (McGrath, 1993; Ross & Ross, 1984).

Parents and other adults can either enhance or impair children's efforts to cope with pain; they can serve as a safety signal and convey reassurance to the child, or they can convey anxiety to the child. It has been found that parents who are highly anxious are less psychologically available to support their child in a medical setting (Zeltzer et al., 1997). Parental support, however, is very important to the child. In the previously cited large-scale study by Ross and Ross (1984), 99.2% of the children indicated that having their parent present is the thing that helps most in dealing with severe pain, regardless of the kind of pain.

Parents may, indeed, have difficulties adjusting to the illness of their child or to invasive medical procedures; this can lead to placing high demands on their children to be compliant and "act like adults" during painful procedures. These demands may lead to restriction of the child's natural pain responses, resulting in a decrease of overt pain behaviors (McGrath, 1987).

Culture undoubtedly plays an important role in shaping patterns of behaviors in response to pain. Although research on the development of pain behavior is limited, there is evidence that pain behavior is learned through mechanisms such as modeling and direct explanation. The culture or ethnic group to which a child belongs teaches the child how to respond to pain, to whom pain should be reported, and what pain relief measures are helpful. The family's religious and spiritual beliefs are also very influential for the child's interpretation of pain; children often believe their pain to be a punishment for misbehavior (Banoub-Baddour & Laryea, 1991). It is important for music therapists to realize that in cultures where complaining or reporting pain is strongly discouraged, a child in pain may not even admit its presence (Banoub-Baddour & Laryea, 1991). At the same time, a child's family's cultural practices may hold great resources for dealing with illness, pain, and hospitalization. For example, families may have daily rituals involving prayer or meditation. A discussion of these practices with the child and family is important because they can provide a healthy construct for coping.

Besides the parental and cultural influences on the child's pain responses, there is the hospitalization itself that may increase pain perception. Hospitalization is never an enjoyable event; it ranks as one of the most stressful events that a child can experience. To children, the hospital is a threatening environment. The strange equipment, unfamiliar sounds and smells, strangers, and technical language encompass the environmental elements that may lead to increased anxiety (Robb, Nichols, Rutan, Bishop, & Parker, 1995). Moreover, it separates them from home, family and friends; it interferes with their routine of daily living; and it is strongly associated with the experience of pain and other aversive events. All these factors may result in feelings of vulnerability, loss of control, anxiety, depression, withdrawal, and regression (Froehlich, 1996).

Undertreatment of Pain in Children

Many myths have led to serious undertreatment of pain in children. For instance, large discrepancies have been reported between the amount of postoperative analgesia administered to adults and that administered to children who have the same diagnoses and who have undergone the same medical procedures (Walco, Cassity, & Schechter, 1997). Even though these myths have been discredited in the literature (Ross & Ross, 1984; Walco et al., 1997), they continue to persist in the clinical assessment and treatment of pain (Stevens et al., 2011).

Young children do not feel pain. Until recently, health care professionals were convinced that young children could not feel much pain. Underpinning this belief was the assumption that the nervous system of young children is immature and, therefore, less sensitive to noxious input. Children's screams were said to stem from fear more than from pain. It has been found, however, that at 30 weeks of gestation, pain pathways and the parts of the brain involved in pain perception are well developed, allowing for a normal conduction speed in the nerves (Kuttner, 1996; Walco et al., 1997).

Children have no memory of pain. It is often assumed that if children do feel pain, they will not remember it and, therefore, it will have no lasting effect. Research evidence, however, has indicated that pain does endure in the memory of infants and children (Walco et al., 1997; Zajdeman & Biedermann, 1991). By the age of six months, infants consistently avoid potentially painful stimuli; this demonstrates infants' memory for pain by that age (McGrath, 1993).

Children get addicted to opioid analgesics. Many studies have found that medical and nursing staff, because of an ill-founded fear of the effects of opioids and addiction, have been giving children and infants significantly less opioid medication than adults for similar pain conditions (Kuttner, 1996). Parents have been found to decline medication for their child's pain possibly because they fear that their child will become accustomed to using drugs to solve other problems (McGrath & McAlpine, 1993). It is important, however, to make the distinction between physical dependence and addiction. When analgesics are administered appropriately, the risk of addiction is minimal. Unlike adults who take drugs for pleasure, children will not become addicted when they take medication to combat pain. A physical dependence may indeed develop, but a gradual reduction in the medication, after the pain has subsided, is used to control withdrawal symptoms (Kuttner, 1996).

A playing child is not in pain. An important misconception that is prevalent is that if a child can be distracted, he is not in pain. Distracting a child from the pain indicates that the child is able to use cognitive strategies to move away from the pain, however, distraction does not exclude the existence of pain (Kuttner, 1996).

REFERRAL AND ASSESSMENT PROCEDURES

Referrals for pain management may happen formally or informally. For pain management during procedures or postsurgically, a referral procedure for supporting services should be in place in each hospital. Ideally, the music therapist wants to meet and assess the child and begin building a therapeutic alliance beforehand. Referrals for other type of pain management often depend on the type of pain (sudden onset vs. chronic) and the anticipated length of hospitalization. For sudden onset pain, a music therapist may get called by the child's nurse with a request to see the child that day. For children with chronic pain or lengthy recoveries from trauma-related injuries, a formal referral is typically completed.

Accurate assessment of pain in children is crucial in guiding pain management interventions. Because of the complex and highly subjective nature of pain perception, an accurate assessment of a child's pain is challenging. An adequate pain assessment calls for subjective assessment tools, requiring input from the child in the form of estimates of pain. The difficulty of assessing pain in children may be magnified in young children or children with developmental delays who may not have the language or cognitive understanding to describe their pain.

A diversity of self-report techniques, including direct questions, self-rating scales, and pain drawings, have been developed to assess pediatric pain. Some have questioned the validity of self-report measures of pain in children, since adult observers' estimates of a child's pain do not always correlate well with the child's self-report. However, to question the child's self-report because of lack of significant correlation is an erroneous concept. Because pain is a subjective phenomenon, it cannot be expected that an individual can assess without measurement error another person's experience of pain. The correlation between the adult patient's self-report and nurses' reports has also been found in several studies to be poor. However, this poor correlation does not lead researchers to question the capacity of these adult patients to assess their pain. Like adults, children should also be considered as the best judges of their pain experience (Varni et al., 1989).

The assessment methods listed below are commonly used to assess children's pain and are categorized as self-report or behavioral observation measures. All measures are well-established standardized measures (Cohen et al., 2008). Where available, an appropriate age range is indicated. Some of the scales have been reprinted with permission in the Appendix. The reader must review copyright permissions for each instrument before commencing use of the instrument for clinical or research purposes.

Self-Report Measures

The Visual Analogue Scale (VAS). The VAS is the most widely used pain rating scale. The VAS is a 100-mm line, the length of which represents a continuum of an experience such as pain. The child is asked to place a vertical mark on the line to indicate how much pain he feels. Verbal descriptors, called anchors, may mark the end of the continuum ("no pain," "severe pain"). The VAS is simple, robust, and sensitive to change in pain perception and is most appropriate for children over eight years of age (Luffy & Grove, 2003; Varni et al., 1989) (Appendix A).

Graphic Rating Scales. Graphic rating scales include numeric rating scales, word-graphic rating scales, pain thermometers, and facial scales:

- *The Numeric Rating Scale (NRS)*: The NRS is one of the most widely used scales for assessing pediatric pain intensity. Children are asked to score their pain intensity from 0 to 10, where 0 represents "no pain" and 10 "very much pain." Age range: 8+ years (Von Baeyer, 2009).
- *Pain Thermometer:* This self-report measure presents the child with a thermometer in a vertical position with the lowest level of the thermometer representing no pain and the highest level the most pain. Sometimes the thermometer is presented in color (with increasingly intense shades of red) or with numbers.
- *Color-Matching*: Pain color-matching requires the child to choose those from an array of colors that best represent the pain. Almost all children choose red for intense pain, orange for milder pain, and yellow for little to no pain (Ross & Ross, 1988a). Varni et al. (1989) recommend, however, that individual children be given the opportunity to make their own developmentally appropriate color/intensity match.
- *Pain Map:* A pain map is an anterior and posterior outline of the human body which is used to assess the location and intensity of a child's pain. The child is asked to mark his specific pain site with colors of his choice which reflect best the intensity of the pain (Ross & Ross, 1988). Similarly, Loewy, MacGregor, Richards, and Rodriguez (1997) developed the *Color Analysis Scale* (CAS) to measure chronic and acute as well as procedural pain. The children are asked to use crayons (red, yellow, blue, green) to color where they feel pain on a human

figure line drawing. In CAS, the children are invited to speak as they color with the therapist recording words verbatim.

- *The Poker Chip Tool* (Hester, 1979; Hester, Foster, & Kristensen, 1990) (Appendix B): This tool uses four red chips that represent "pieces of hurt." One chip represents a little hurt, whereas all chips represent the most hurt one could have. This measure has been used with preschoolers from a wide variety of cultures and is recommended for ages three to four (Cohen et al., 2008).

- *Faces Scales:* Several face scales have been developed to measure pain in children. These scales use drawings or photographs of faces to depict different intensities of pain. Although these scales have generally strong psychometric properties (i.e., validity and reliability scores), some have been criticized for using a smiling face at the lower end of the pain scale. Even if children experience no pain, they typically are not happy in medical situations and therefore may not select the happy face. Similarly, children may not select the crying face (often used as the anchor on the high end of the pain scale) unless they are crying themselves (McCaffery, 2002). The most commonly used face scales are:

    1) *The Oucher*™ (Beyer, 1984; Beyer & Knott, 1998): This face scale provides different photographs for Caucasian, Hispanic, and African-American children and is oriented vertically. Research has suggested that younger children better understand the idea of matching a higher level of pain intensity with a higher point on a scale (Polkki, Pietila, & Vehvilainen-Julkunen, 2003). Age range: 3–12.
    Available at http://www.oucher.org/order.html.

    2) *The Wong-Baker FACES® Pain Rating Scale* (Wong & Baker, 1988) (Appendix C): This scale uses face drawings with word descriptors (e.g., no hurt, hurts a little, etc.). The faces are presented in a horizontal manner. Baker emphasizes that this is a self-assessment tool; it is not to be used with unresponsive patients (personal communication, May 2013). The scale is available in many different languages. Age range: 4–18. Available at http://www.wongbakerfaces.org/.

    3) *Faces Pain Scale–Revised©* (Hicks, von Baeyer, Spafford, van Korlaar, & Goodenough, 2001): The Faces Pain Scale–Revised (FPS-R) uses six drawings of faces. It is recommended for use with younger children. The scale has been translated into 30 languages. Available at www.iasp-pain.org/FPSR.

Multidimensional Pain Scales. The following scales are aimed at measuring multiple dimensions of the pain experience and, because they take longer to administer, are typically used for chronic pain. The Varni/Thompson Pediatric Pain Questionnaire is the most widely used.

- *The Varni/Thompson Pediatric Pain Questionnaire (PPQ)* (Varni, Thompson, & Hanson, 1987): The Varni/Thompson PPQ is considered to be one of the best pediatric pain assessment instruments (Ross & Ross, 1988a). It is a comprehensive, multidimensional questionnaire designed to assess acute and chronic pain in children. The tool has been validated for use with a variety of chronic pain conditions, including sickle cell and chronic musculoskeletal pain.

The PPQ uses the Visual Analogue Scale (VAS), color-coded rating scales, verbal descriptors, and body outlines. Age range: 5–18.
Available at http://www.pedsql.org/index.html.

- *The Abu-Saad Pediatric Pain Assessment Tool (PPAT)* (Abu-Saad, Kroonen, & Halfens, 1990): This tool assesses multiple aspects of pain, including triggers of pain and use of pain medication. It measures sensory, affective, and evaluative components of pain through the use of 30 descriptors. It also measures present pain and worst pain. The tool has been validated in children from different ethnic backgrounds.

Behavioral Observation Measures

Behavioral observation tools assess the patients' display of pain and distress behaviors. These tools have an underlying assumption that anxiety, fear, and other forms of distress coexist with the experience and expression of pain. Behavioral observation methods are the primary approach to accessing pain information from preverbal and nonverbal children, children with cognitive impairments, or at times when the child is too distressed to self-report his pain (Cohen et al., 2008). It is always recommended, however, that, when possible, behavioral observations be combined with self-reports.

- *Children's Hospital of Eastern Ontario Pain Scale (CHEOPS)* (McGrath, Johnson, Goodman, Dunn, & Chapman, 1985) (Appendix D): The CHEOPS is an observational measure of postoperative pain. Age range: 1–12 years.
- *COMFORT Scale* (Ambuel, Hamlett, Marx, & Blumer, 1992): An observational measure that is aimed at measuring pain and distress in intensive care environments. Age range: 0–18 years.
Available at http://painconsortium.nih.gov/pain_scales/COMFORT_Scale.pdf.
- *Observational Scale of Behavioral Distress-Revised (OSBD-R)* (Elliot, Jay, & Woody, 1987): The OSBD-R is one of the most widely used observational tools for pain. It is aimed at measuring pain during medical procedures. Age range: 2–20 years.
- *Premature Infant Pain Profile (PIPPS)* (Stevens, Johnston, Petryshen, & Taddio, 1996): This observational measure was specifically developed to measure acute pain in premature infants.
- *Procedure Behavior Checklist (PBCL)* (LeBaron & Zeltzer, 1984): An observational measure of pain and anxiety to be used during invasive medical procedures. Age range: 3–18 years.

Pain Assessment in Children with Cognitive Impairments

Children with a cognitive impairment (CI) are at greater risk than other children for the undertreatment of pain. They may not have the verbal skills and cognitive capacity to accurately communicate their pain. In addition, they may have behavioral idiosyncrasies such as moaning and facial expressions that may mask their pain expressions (Ely, Chen-Lim, Zarnowsky, Green, Shaffer, & Holtzer, 2012). The interpretation of their pain behaviors is furthermore complicated by motor or sensory disorders (Solodiuk & Curley, 2003). These challenges make accurate interpretation and treatment of their pain difficult (Breau & Burkitt, 2009). Studies have also indicated that children with CI are less often assessed for pain following surgery and receive less opioid pain medication than children without CI (e.g., Malviva, Voepel-

Lewis, Burke, Merkel, & Tait, 2006). The following two assessment tools have been found to be effective for pain assessment in children with CI:

- *Pediatric Pain Profile (PPP)* (Hunt et al., 2004, 2007): The PPP is a 20-item checklist of pain behaviors specific to the child with CI. The behaviors included in this scale were selected through research conducted with parents to identify behaviors indicative of pain in children with CI. The range of scores obtained with this tool is individualized with the caregiver since each child's pain behaviors are unique.
- *Revised Faces, Legs, Activity, Cry, and Consolability (rFLACC)* (Malviya et al., 2006): The scale is specific for use in nonverbal patients with CI. The revised version of this scale allows for health care providers to ask caregivers to identify pain behaviors specific to their child. Thus the scale is individualized for each child.

Both pain assessment tools involve the parents or caregivers in the assessment process. Parents are "the advocates for children with CI and the best historian for their child's behaviors, [and therefore] health care providers need to partner with them to provide for timely and effective pain management" (Ely et al., 2012).

Music Therapy Assessments: More than Pain

It is important to note that while the fast pace typical of a hospital environment often requires a quick method of assessing a child's pain, pain perception is more than pain intensity. If time permits, music therapists must also assess a child's emotional state, developmental level, cognitive understanding of the causes of the pain and/or upcoming painful medical procedures, meaning ascribed to the pain, pain experience history, preferred coping strategies, cultural/familial ideas regarding pain behaviors, and interactions between the child and caregiver. Obtaining this type of information is not always possible—for example, when a therapist is called to offer pain management during a procedure that has already started.

A music therapy assessment should also include information about the musical qualities of the pain. Many attributes that describe pain can be easily translated into musical parameters. For example, if a child says his pain is stabbing and sharp, this can be translated into pulse (how fast is the pain stabbing?) and timbre (sharp-sounding instruments). This type of assessment is an integral part of music entrainment for pain management, as described in the guidelines section. The music therapist should also assess the child's responses to music as discussed in Chapter 7 by Whitehead-Pleaux.

The music therapist can use music therapy experiences and subsequent reflective discussions to uncover information related to the child's understanding of his pain and/or the need for painful procedures, his relationship to his pain, and the meaning assigned to the pain. Through such experiences, feelings and thoughts may be uncovered that had not yet surfaced. These may provide important information about inner resources the child has available as well as unspoken needs the child may have (Loewy, 1997).

Finally, music therapy assessment must include information about the child's music preference and music background and family's music culture, as well as the child's preferred manner of music engagement (e.g., listening to music, singing, playing instruments).

Introduction to Music Therapy Methods

Music therapy interventions can address the multiple dimensions of the pain experience, namely the sensory-discriminative, motivational-affective, and cognitive-interpretational dimensions. The music therapy interventions described in this chapter will vary in their focus in addressing each of these domains. Regardless of whether one or more domains are targeted by the intervention, a shift in one of these dimensions automatically evokes a shift in the others.

The music therapist must carefully consider which pain aspects are addressed in the intervention and verbalize this effectively to the treatment team. To a non–music therapist, the use of live guitar music may seem like good distraction for the child, whereas the music therapist may be using entrainment principles in her playing to calm and sedate the child. Composing a song using software may be interpreted as a great pastime, whereas the intervention is addressing empowerment, meaning-making, and active coping.

An accurate assessment of the child's pain and accompanying psychosocial needs will help guide the music therapist in the selection of suitable music therapy interventions. If the child presents with high anxiety, panic behaviors, and high-pitched crying, asking the child to listen to relaxing music will most likely not be suitable as an initial intervention. A child who prefers to attend to the medical procedure as a way of coping should not be asked to engage in active music-making. For children with recurrent hospitalizations, the music therapist must carefully review the child's chart for a history of the child's coping with past medical procedures, painful injuries, or conditions; the child's preferred coping style; effective (and ineffective) music therapy interventions; and past music or songs used/composed by the child and the therapist.

This section provides guidelines for a wide variety of music therapy methods that are used for pain management in children. Because of the potential overlap between this chapter and subsequent chapters, several interventions specific to a population are addressed in the respective chapters (e.g., music analgesia with burn patients; drumming for release during procedural support). Readers seeking to enhance their understanding of music therapy for procedural support are referred to Chapter 6 by Mondanaro. For guidelines specific to premature infants and full-term infants, the reader is referred to Chapters 3 and 4. For guidelines specific to pain management interventions with burn patients, the reader should consult chapter 7.

Overview of Music Therapy Methods and Procedures

Music therapy methods and procedures included in this chapter are listed below. They are not listed in any specific order.

Receptive Music Therapy

- Music Listening for Sustained Focus: the use of music listening to help the child maintain a prolonged focus away from the pain.
- Music-Assisted Relaxation: teaches the child to use music purposefully to promote relaxation, facilitate sedation, and decrease pain.
- Music-Guided Imagery: the use of imagery supported by music to help a child relax, find refuge from the pain, escape the hospital environment, and be empowered in his healing process.
- Tonal Vocal Holding: the use of purposeful breathing and toning to provide comfort to the child and validation of his vocal expressions.

- Vibroacoustic Therapy: the use of sound in the audible range to produce mechanical vibrations that are applied directly to the body, resulting in relaxation and analgesic effects.

Improvisational Music Therapy

- Tonal Intervallic Synthesis: the purposeful use of tones and timbres that resolve dissonance into consonance to influence circulation, release, integration, pain, and physical perception.
- Vocal Music Therapy for Chronic Pain Management: the use of humming, toning, deep breathing, vocal improvisation, harmonizing, and inspirational songs to enhance coping with chronic pain.
- Improvised Music for Integration: the use of drumming, toning, and chanting in an improvisatory style to help the child integrate the hurt.
- Musical Journey: the use of singing, instrumental improvisation, and verbalization to venture on a journey aimed at having the child experience his pain on a metaphorical level, giving his pain a voice and empowering him to take an active role in his pain management.
- Music Improvisation for Active Engagement and Exploration: using music-making to actively engage the child with his surroundings in a playful manner to restore a sense of control, mastery, and even normalcy.
- Music Entrainment for Pain Management: the creation of live music that progresses from music that matches the child's pain into music predetermined by the child as healing.
- *The Heidelberg Music Therapy Manual for Pediatric Migraine*: the use of interactive music improvisations, creative activation through music, symbols and metaphors, music-guided imagery, relaxation and movement to enhance musical "flexibilization" and expressivity.

Re-creative Music Therapy

- Singing Songs: singing favorite songs to shift the child's focus away from the pain, improve perceived level of control, normalize the sterile hospital environment, and encourage interaction with others.

Compositional Music Therapy

- Songwriting: the use of songwriting to give the child the opportunity to articulate his feelings and direct them into a creative form, to provide cognitive reframing, and to enhance the child's understanding of the pain and/or procedure.
- Instrumental Compositions for Relaxation and Support: composition of instrumental tracks by the child to use for relaxation purposes, procedural support, or motivational and pain management purposes during rehabilitation.

GUIDELINES FOR RECEPTIVE MUSIC THERAPY

The use of receptive music therapy interventions for pain management is based on various rationales. Music has been described as a distractor, a relaxing agent, a mood enhancer, a provider of overriding sensory stimuli, and a mental escape. Although children are "people of action" (Froehlich, 1996, p. 17), for whom active music therapy interventions are thus preferred, there are many instances during a child's hospitalization when active music-making may not be possible (e.g., during certain procedures; when a child is sedated or exhausted). During these times, listening to music may bring pain-reducing benefits. However, when the child is experiencing intense acute pain (e.g., during a procedure) and is beyond himself, music listening may not be an effective intervention.

The type of receptive techniques used will depend on the child's age and the child's presenting need. For young children (ages 3–8), singing familiar songs to enable a focus away from the pain as well as using imagery to activate fantasy stories are appropriate. For older children, longer music-guided relaxation and imagery experiences are possible (Grocke & Wigram, 2007).

Music Listening for Sustained Focus

Overview. Music listening can enable a child to focus on a stimulus different than pain. People in pain, especially intense pain, tend to be preoccupied by the pain experience. Many of this author's clients with chronic pain report that "taking one's mind of the pain" is what helps them get through the day. As a result of the Gate Control Theory and the fear-tension-pain model, the value of distraction in the management of pain is often cited in music therapy clinical and research publications. As described earlier, the Gate Control Theory postulates that efferent nerve fibers exert descending control over the pain perception by transmitting information about attention, emotion, and motivation. A shift in the patient's attention may lead to a decrease in pain perception. Music is an excellent stimulus for holding one's attention and directing it away from the pain. "Cognitively engaging oneself in the music may allow for distraction away from the reality of the moment, away from self-preoccupation" (Brown et al., 1989, p. 56). In her much cited article about music as a nursing intervention, Locsin (1981) argues that to break the fear-tension-pain cycle, the patient's attention to pain should be distracted by refocusing it on a pleasant sensory stimulus, particularly music.

However, unlike with the administration of music by medical personnel, music therapists do more than distract a child when using music for pain management. Several authors have argued against the use of the word distraction (Leeuwenburgh et al., 2007; Loewy, 1997) and have suggested the term "refocusing" instead. Distraction implies a quick diversion, one that can be easily interrupted by another distraction. When using music listening for pain management, it is important that the child's attention to the music can be sustained. Since music is a temporal experience (i.e., it only exists through time), it has the potential to sustain a child's attention moment-to-moment. It is this sustained focus that will allow for a sufficient refuge from the pain experience.

Music listening for sustained focus is indicated for children who are unable to actively engage in music-making because of restraints of the procedures, because their threshold for coping has passed and active engagement is no longer possible (see Chapter 6 for an excellent discussion on the threshold for coping during procedures), because of extreme pain, or because of fatigue. This intervention is not indicated for children who are sedated or drowsy, as it requires an active focus on the music. The music therapist should be aware that the ability to sustain attention on a given stimulus is a developmental skill. Hence, it will be more difficult for younger children to shift their attention away from a threatening stimulus like pain (Robb, 2003).

Preparation. The music therapist reviews the child's music preference information obtained during the music therapy assessment. If live music is used, the music therapist prepares songs or compositions selected by the child. It is important that the music therapist can play the music effortlessly so that her attention can be with the child during the intervention. Too often, students or novice music therapists are overly dependent on sheet music and unable to report on their observations of the child during the music experience.

What to observe. The music therapist must observe the child's nonverbal communication, including facial expression, body language, and physiological responses (e.g., breathing). Sustained focus might be reflected in visible signs of relaxation (e.g., slower breathing, relaxed facial expression, softening of the hands), as well as signs of engagement that suggest that the child is attending to the lyrical or musical content of the music (e.g., smiling, movement of eyebrows, tapping of the fingers or feet, etc.). If the child begins to move around or shows increasing discomfort in his facial expressions or other body language, the music therapist should bring the experience to a close and process the child's experience.

Procedures. Music listening for sustained attention may greatly vary in its delivery depending on the child's emotional and physical state. It therefore requires flexibility and sensitivity from the music therapist. The use of live music is preferred since it allows for in-the-moment adaptations to the child's needs. Moreover, live music allows the music therapist to alter the music frequently so that attentional focus is maintained. Children can easily habituate to a music stimulus. Therefore, the therapist must be ready to change musical parameters and/or the music experience to continuously engage the child's attention (Robb, 2003). At the same time, the therapist should monitor the child's responses for signs of overstimulation and alter the musical characteristics (e.g., drop the accompaniment) to reduce the complexity of the music. Robb (2003) recommends finding a balance between introducing novel elements in the music experience to maintain the child's focus and maintaining predictable and familiar music structures to avoid excessive arousal.

It is important to understand that different types of music can be used for this intervention, not just relaxing music. If this intervention is used during debridement with an adolescent with burns, for example, the adolescent may need music that "is strong enough" to override the onslaught of extremely painful sensations. In this instance, the music needs to be sufficiently engaging to be able to hold the patient's attention. For other children, however, calm and serene music might be preferred. These children may be at risk for overstimulation and may be looking for a reduction in sensory stimulation in order to better cope with the pain (this is not unlike a person with an intense headache having decreased tolerance for environmental noise). These children may be best served by music that communicates care and love (e.g., lullaby-type music) or music that can help structure the sound environment. It is important that the therapist consult with the older child or carefully observe the younger child to find out which music might be most helpful to refocus his attention and help him cope with the pain.

Finally, the music therapist needs to carefully consider which pieces of music are appropriate for live performance. Some songs are better offered as prerecorded music because a live rendition that honors the style of the song may not be possible. Since the goal of the intervention is to engage the child in sustained focus on the music, bringing an unsatisfactory rendition of the song may annoy the child and exacerbate feelings of helplessness and lack of control.

If appropriate, family members present during the session may be involved in the singing and/or selection of the songs and can support the child.

Music-Assisted Relaxation

Overview. Music-assisted relaxation can take on many forms. Some therapists take the child through a brief relaxation induction (e.g., ask the child to focus on his breath) and have this followed by listening to a piece of calming, prerecorded music. Other therapists prefer using live music and use the entrainment principle in their rendition of the music. In entrainment, the music therapist first matches the breathing rate or heart rate of the child and then gradually slows down the tempo of the music to encourage deeper breathing or a slowing down of the heart rate. In the approach described by Bishop,

Christenberry, Robb, and Rudenberg (1996) and Robb, Nichols, Rutan, Bishop, and Parker (1995), the music therapist uses the music to "structure and teach deep diaphragmatic breathing and progressive muscle relaxation, and to facilitate imagery" (p. 92).

Regardless of the approach, the goal is to teach the child to use music purposefully to promote relaxation, facilitate sedation, and decrease pain. With the older child, teaching him how to use music independently to relax his body even when in pain and educating him about the benefits of relaxation for pain management empowers the child to take an active role in his pain management.

Preparation. The music therapist, in collaboration with the child, will select music with sedative qualities. Sometimes the child's preferred genre may not be suitable for relaxation purposes (e.g., hard rock, rap). In these instances, it is important to educate the child about the qualities of music that best promote relaxation and then search for music that meets these qualities and is agreeable to the child.

Sedative music is characterized by a steady pulse, quiet mood, predictable melodic and harmonic structure, and little dynamic change (Grocke & Wigram, 2007). Robb, Nichols, Rutan, Bishop, and Parker (1995) reviewed the literature for recommendations regarding characteristics of music most beneficial for relaxation purposes. The results suggest using music with (a) slow to moderate tempi (i.e., a tempo at or below the resting heart rate, typically around 60 bpm); (b) smooth rhythms without sudden changes; (c) slow, sustained, low-pitched melodies that gradually progress; (d) soft to moderate dynamics (music therapists should consider the ambient sound level in the child's room and make sure that the music can be clearly heard over the environmental sound); (e) consonant harmonies; and (f) softer-quality instruments such as strings and voice.

Patient familiarity with the selected music is desirable, because it provides a sense of security and safety in the chaos and threat caused by the pain. However, this does not mean that the music therapist should limit the music selection to songs that the child knows. Familiarity in music is also achieved by using music in a preferred style of the child or music that is common to the child's culture and offers predictable musical elements. The music therapist also needs to consider existing associations the child may have with the music (e.g., with films, advertisements, significant life events, loved ones, etc.) (Grocke & Wigram, 2007).

The music can be recorded or live. This will depend on the type of relaxation method used and the child's preference, as well as the child's need for interpersonal support.

What to observe. Before starting the intervention, the music therapist should observe the child's behavioral state, observable signs of physical tension and pain, and heart rate and respiratory rate (if the child is connected to monitors). The assessment of the child's developmental level, pain level, anxiety, and procedural requirements, if any, will guide the music therapist in selecting the appropriate relaxation intervention (Neugebauer, 2008). During the intervention, the therapist must continuously assess the child's tolerance for auditory stimuli and reduce the complexity of the music (e.g., drop out the accompanying instrument) or halt the music if signs of agitation are observed.

Procedures. As most chapters in this book contain guidelines for music-guided relaxation, this author decided to present here guidelines based on the MAR protocol as described by Bishop et al. (1996) and Robb et al. (1995), and as derived from the author's experience. As described earlier, it is important to consider the child's developmental level as well as pain and anxiety management needs when selecting an intervention for sedative purposes. For example, for a child who presents as very anxious or fearful, live interactive music based on the Iso principle may be needed before the child is ready to enter into a music-assisted relaxation experience. Alternatively, for a child who is experiencing intense pain and who tends to withdraw from interactions and sensory stimulation, a brief focus on the breath followed by soft a capella singing by the therapist might be indicated.

During the initial visit, the music therapist explains MAR to the child and family, selects preferred music with the child, teaches the child deep diaphragmatic breathing, and introduces the child to progressive muscle relaxation (PMR). PMR is a widely used relaxation technique that asks the patient to tense and release specific muscle groups (e.g., hands, arms, shoulders, face, etc.), slowly progressing through the body. Because the child first experiences tensing certain muscles, the subsequent act of relaxing those muscles brings greater awareness about the sensation of relaxation. If time permits, an imagery journey to a relaxing place is selected and described by the child. If the child easily fatigues, the PMR instructions and imagery may need to be addressed in a subsequent session. The reader is referred to Smith (2005) for detailed instructions and scripts for various relaxation interventions and inductions, including PMR, autogenic training, breathing exercises, and mindfulness.

To teach the child diaphragmatic breathing, the following guidelines may be useful. Children are often told to take a deep breath when they are exhibiting anxiety or reporting that their pain is getting too intense. This often results in a big chest breath, rather than a deep "belly breath." To promote diaphragmatic breathing, the following suggestions may be helpful: (a) imagine having a balloon of your favorite color in your belly that expands as you breathe in and deflates as you exhale; (b) imagine blowing air down the whole length of your body (this helps to prolong exhalation which, in turn, promotes deeper breathing); (c) imagine blowing a feather and keeping the feather afloat in the air; or (d) rest your hands on your belly, take a deep breath in through your nose, slowly and gently, and then release it through your mouth while making a "shhhh" or "ahhhhh " sound.

Children who are too anxious to attend to these instructions—all of these instructions require a rather "quiet" body—can be invited to play some breath games aimed at teaching diaphragmatic breathing. One such game is "ping pong ball." A ping pong ball is placed on the child's tray table. The child and therapist (or a family member) play the ball back and forth using only their breath. After a game of ping pong ball, the child's awareness is brought to his use of breath. The child is then asked to *imagine* blowing the ping pong ball slowly across the table (to promote elongation of the breath).

Once the child is able to engage in diaphragmatic breathing and has received an introduction to PMR, the MAR intervention session can be implemented. The music therapist lowers the lighting in the room, turns off any sources of sensory stimulation (e.g., TV, radio), and asks the child to get into a comfortable position. If parents are present, they are invited to participate in the relaxation experience if they so desire. It is important that the parents understand that this experience will be led by the child's preferences regarding music and imagery, not theirs.

The music therapist invites the child to focus on his breathing (using one of the instructions that was helpful to the child in the preparatory session). The child is then led through PRM instructions. Depending on the child's age, level of fatigue, and attention span, the PMR progresses slowly through the body. As this may take quite some time, the music therapist should feel free to group certain muscle groups to speed up this relaxation exercise if needed (e.g., ask the child to tense his hands and arms at once rather than first focus on the hands and then the arms). In the descriptions by Bishop et al. (1996) and Robb et al. (1995), prerecorded music is used. This author prefers the use of live music during PMR, as it allows for the music to follow the pace of the child. Moreover, the music can support the tension-release sequence through purposeful use of harmonies that suggest a release (e.g., dominant 7th chord is repeated with the instructions "tense, tense, tense" and resolves into a tonic with the word "release"). The novice clinician is forewarned that playing live music and providing verbal relaxation instructions simultaneously is not an easy task. This certainly requires practice outside of the sessions. A willing friend, partner, or colleague makes a good practice subject.

After the PMR, the child is invited to imagine his imagery journey (see the music and imagery section below for guidelines). The music therapist must make a clinical judgment about whether the child is able to handle the addition of the imagery or not. When the child begins to exhibits signs of restlessness, the experience can be closed after the PMR experience.

When using music to help the child relax, it is important that proper closure of the experience is provided. The intervention hopefully brought about a deep state of relaxation, and hence the child is likely to be in an altered state of consciousness. The child needs to be gently guided back into the here-and-now. This "journey back" can be aided by (a) a change in the therapist voice from relaxed to more rhythmic and slightly higher-pitched; (b) ending the music; (c) asking the child to become aware of his body resting on his bed, pillows, etc.; and (d) asking the child to gently wiggle his fingers and toes. If the child has fallen asleep, the therapist should inform the parents or staff and ask them to frequently check in with the child. A note can be left for the child with some words of praise for his ability to relax and to inform him when the music therapist will return.

Music-Guided Imagery

Overview. In this method, the music therapist uses imagery scripts to stimulate imagination and fantasy in the child. The use of imagery is a powerful means to help a child relax, find refuge from the pain, escape the hospital environment, and become empowered in his healing process. This intervention can be used with young children as well as adolescents. Music-guided imagery should not be used with a child who is sedated, as his cognitive functioning may be impaired.

Preparation. The type of music used for imagery is different from that used for relaxation. To best stimulate imagery, the music should have changeable instrumentation, fluctuating dynamics (but no sudden changes), and possibly fluctuations in meter. The music is less predictable in melodic, rhythmic, and harmonic structure than music for relaxation (Grocke & Wigram, 1997). Live improvised as well as prerecorded music is used. The benefit of using prerecorded music is that the child can continue to use this on his own outside of the music therapy session and after discharge. The advantage of live music is that it can be highly individualized to match the imagery selected by the child.

What to observe. The music therapist should observe the child's body language during the imagery experience. Is his body suggesting relaxation? Agitation? Depending on the type of imagery intervention, the child may be asked to dialogue with the therapist about his imagery. The therapist should pay close attention to the metaphors used in these descriptions.

Procedures. It is important to start the imagery experience with an invitation to focus on one's breath. This allows for the child's focus to shift from external to internal. The child can be asked to imagine that he is breathing in his favorite color, imagine blowing on a feather, etc. This will allow for the body and mind to slow down and open itself up for imagery (Snyder Cowan, 1997).

With children, it is helpful to provide them with some suggestions or instructions for the imagery. The therapist can use existing imagery scripts or develop an individualized script together with the child. Scripts can involve imagining a favorite place, a fairy garden, a place in nature, or being held by a loved one. Snyder Cowan (1997) further suggests that physiology-specific imagery can be used with children with specific disorders or illnesses. For example, a child with sickle cell disease may be asked "to visualize the red blood cells easily carrying oxygen-enriched nutrients to all parts of the body" (p. 118). Grocke and Wigram (2007) provide a wide variety of imagery suggestions with accompanying verbal scripts for different age groups. These are a great resource for the music therapist.

Imagery experiences can also include a guided body scan to help the child identify areas of tension and/or pain. The child can then be invited to imagine different types of sensations to alleviate the pain. For example, the child may be instructed to imagine breathing in a beautiful white light and using the light to softly smooth out the painful area; to visualize a colorful ribbon gently swirling over the painful area, scooping up the pain and taking it away high up in the air; or giving the pain a color and then imagining using a different (i.e., comforting) color to color away the pain.

When suggesting imagery, the music therapist must use age-appropriate wording and consider the child's need for concrete vs. more abstract imagery. For a young child, the words "Let's pretend ..." may be easier to understand than asking the child to imagine something (Snyder Cowan, 1997). The very young child (under age six) may not be willing to close his eyes. Novice clinicians may interpret this as the child not yet being able to engage in imagery experiences. This is a false assumption. Even with eyes open, the child can be asked to create an imaginary story stimulated by the music.

Kallay (1997) emphasizes that a child should always be reminded that he is in charge of the imagery and can bring it to an end whenever he desires. It is important to empower the child to use these imagery experiences on his own for pain management. A tape with the child's preferred music for imagery along with recorded verbal instructions or written verbal instructions (depending on the child's preference and age) can be provided to the child for at-home practice after hospital discharge.

Tonal Vocal Holding

Overview. Tonal vocal holding is an intervention that uses purposeful breathing and toning (Loewy, 1995) to provide comfort to the child and validation of his vocal expressions. The therapist purposefully uses the voice to match the tone and timbre of the child's or infant's cry or vocal expressions. The guidelines provided here will focus on the use of this intervention for pain management and for support during painful procedures. Loewy has also published on the use of this intervention with infants and young children (Loewy, 1995, 1997). However, she emphasizes (Loewy, 1997) that vocal holding techniques can also be appropriate for adolescents as regression commonly occurs during hospitalization. Moreover, regardless of age, individuals benefit from being comforted during stressful and painful times.

Procedures. The therapist begins by listening to the child's cry, moaning, or other vocal expressions of pain, discomfort, or fear. The therapist then matches the child's cry with "a long, steady blanket of vocal holding tones" (1995, p. 53), the timbre of which may reflect that of the child's voice. Usually, vocal holding is not accompanied by pitched instruments, as the goal is to establish an intimate connection with the child through the voice. This "close presence" of the therapist's voice can comfort the child. Loewy recommends keeping a tone with a steady airflow and plenty of deep breaths. The use of glissandi may be effective in reflecting the child's cries. It is important that the voice is presented as purely as possible. Therefore, excessive vibrato should be avoided. Finally, the melodic themes should remain simple. Through this tonal vocal holding, the therapist "frames and elongates the child's tonal release" (1995, p. 53).

Turry (1997) emphasizes that the child who is in extreme pain withdraws from interaction with others. An important part of helping the child reintegrate is re-establishing a connection with others. She suggests that the musical framing of the child's vocalizations opens the potential for interaction. Turry eloquently explains:

> The crying is no longer experienced in isolation, as sounds with little form or boundary, a potentially overwhelming expression of the intensity of the impulse. Through the use of musical elements, the crying is framed in an organized form with parameters. A container is created, and the impulse, once ambiguous and infinite in its scope, becomes more manageable, contained, and finite. (p. 93)

Loewy (1997) describes a case in which a five-year-old girl with suspicious scars on her body panicked greatly whenever a staff member approached her for daily care or medical procedures. When the girl needed an IV placement, two music therapists created a safe holding environment through supportive, consonant, vocal toning harmonies. This was followed by singing "Kasey [Dinah], Won't You Blow?," to which Kasey was invited to blow the recorder to "expel her anxiety" (p. 53). Through this intervention, Kasey was able to move from a state of panic to a healthy release. Whereas it typically took Kasey at least 30 minutes to emotionally recover from relatively minor medical procedures, she was now able to immediately resume her normal activities. The staff further reported that the procedure time had been greatly shortened (compared to past procedures).

This clinical case provides a great example of how providing a sense of safety through a low-cost, easily administered music therapy intervention can bring large benefits in terms of a child's emotional well-being, as well as cost benefits for the hospital.

Vibroacoustic Therapy

Overview. Most descriptions of the use of music for pain management in the literature have focused on the auditory aspect of music. However, music is also a source of tactile stimulation. The positive effects of stimulating the skin to alleviate pain are well documented in the literature and include various procedures such as acupuncture, massage, transcutaneous electrical stimulation, and vibration. Vibroacoustic (VA) therapy uses sound in the audible range to produce mechanical vibrations that are applied directly to the body. The analgesic effects of vibrotactile stimulation can be explained by the Gate Control Theory's postulations regarding the pain-reducing effects of large-diameter afferent fiber stimulation. Stimulation of the skin activates particular sensory receptors, the Pacinian corpuscles. When activated, these receptors may suppress the discharge of free nerve endings that are responsible for detection of noxious stimuli. However, the Pacinian corpuscles appear to adapt rather quickly to rigid vibrational frequencies and fatigue, allowing free nerve endings to discharge. Music, composed of ever changing frequencies, allows for a fluctuation in vibration which may postpone the onset of adaptation, fatigue, and habituation in the Pacinian corpuscles (Chesky & Michel, 1991).

Olav Skille from Norway and Petri Lehikoinen from Finland developed vibroacoustic technology over 30 years ago and have been prolific researchers in this field. In the United States, Byron Eakin, as well as Kris Chesky and Don Michel, developed vibroacoustic equipment and have also researched its effects.

The literature includes anecdotal reports on the use of VA therapy for the following pain conditions: colic pains, bowel problems, fibromyalgia, migraine and headache, musculoskeletal pain, and menstrual pain. This intervention is not indicated for patients with acute inflammatory conditions, psychosis, hemorrhaging or active bleeding, thrombosis, hypotension, or cardiac issues (Grocke & Wigram, 2007). VA therapy has been extensively used with children with physical disabilities who suffer from high muscle tone and severe spasticity. It has also been used with children with autism and pervasive developmental disorders (Skille, 1992; Skille & Wigram, 1995). Furthermore, VA therapy has been used to enhance an infants' coping with medical procedures (Burke, Walsh, Oehler, & Gingras, 1995), and some pediatric hospitals have been using VA therapy to help children cope with biopsies, aspirations, and catheter maintenance.

What to observe. As with other receptive interventions, the therapist observes the child's bodily as well as verbal responses to the intervention. The therapist must frequently check in with the child to assess whether the strength of the VA stimulus continues to be well tolerated by the child. At the end of the intervention, it is important that the therapist ask for the child's feedback. Whereas people typically report relaxing effects of VA therapy, this author has experienced that VA therapy may also lead to nausea and headache. Therefore, careful monitoring of the impact of VA therapy is needed.

Procedures. Vibroacoustic therapy is based on universal principles of the effects of music, namely that (a) high frequencies induce tension, whereas low frequencies promote relaxation; (b) music with strong rhythmic beats energizes, whereas rhythmically neutral music calms; and (c) loud music arouses, whereas soft music pacifies (Grocke & Wigram, 1997). VA therapy uses audible frequencies but amplifies the frequency waves that can be most effectively felt in the body as vibrations.

A considerable amount of vibroacoustic equipment has been developed and used for pain relief. Many different types of vibroacoustic equipment are available, including reclining chairs, mattresses, soft furniture, bean bags, and more. Many of these items are manufactured and sold by Somatron®. Grocke and Wigram (2007) even provide detailed instructions to clinicians on how to build their own VA equipment.

When using VA therapy, it is important to follow the protocol as outlined by Grocke and Wigram (2007). This protocol involves the following steps: (a) preparation of the VA equipment for the patient; (b) introducing the patient to the equipment and informing the patient that he can ask for the VA intervention to stop at any time; (c) starting the treatment with a gradual introduction of the VA stimulus and frequent check-ins regarding the strength of the stimulus; (d) monitoring the treatment; (e) ending the treatment, allowing for sufficient time for the client to return from possible altered states of consciousness into an active state; and (f) post-treatment work, which may involve physical therapy, verbal psychotherapy, etc. Treatment length varies at between 20 and 40 minutes. For detailed instructions, the reader should consult Chapter 9 in Grocke and Wigram (2007).

Tension Release

This intervention focuses on the use of musical structures that promote moving from tension to release. This supports the release of tension that may have been building up in the child in response to pain, worrying, or fear of a procedure. The release of tension and the experience of reduced stress are of great importance for effective pain management. The reader is referred to Chapter 6 in this book for detailed guidelines on this intervention.

GUIDELINES FOR IMPROVISATIONAL MUSIC THERAPY

When hospitalized, children feel scared, threatened, and helpless. They often are uncertain about what to expect; they may not understand the need for a painful treatment; and they may not know any effective strategies to cope with the pain. When a child feels threatened and overwhelmed by the fear of pain or actual pain, he may withdraw from the experience and become passive and helpless, adopting an external locus of control. Such strategies have been shown to exacerbate pain perception (McGrath, 1993).

Active music-making can re-engage the child. As the child becomes more present in the moment, his sense of self can be restored. Active music-making enables the child to "regain a sense of himself in a specific time and space" (Turry, 1997, p. 93). During active music-making, many opportunities for choice, control, and mastery can be provided. The child can be asked which instrument to play, how fast to play, how loudly to play, what song to sing, and so on (Bishop et al., 1996; Turry, 1997). Furthermore, children in acute pain often benefit from release through active music-making such as drumming and toning. This allows the children to "move the painful energy out of their bodies" (Loewy, 1997, p. 48).

Music-making brings about change in the child's social role as well. Whereas the child may feel helpless in the hospital environment, resulting in passive/dependent behaviors, active music-making transforms the child into a "doer," enabling the child to experience the benefits of active engagement. The music therapist can help the child transfer this to contexts outside of the music therapy session (Nolan, 1997).

Active music-making also affects the child's perception of time, which typically becomes distorted (i.e., slower) when in pain (Nolan, 1997). Nolan writes that "the time experience in music [...] becomes part of the child's perception and overrides the time component of the pain experience. [...] Once the child is engaged in playing music with the therapist, pain-related distortion of time becomes disrupted as the child attains an orientation to the pulse, rhythmic subdivisions, and tempo of the music" (p. 60).

Playing instruments and responding to music with movement replace the careful and often restricted movements of a child in pain. This author has witnessed many times a patient carefully entering the music therapy room, grimacing in pain with every step. As soon as the patient actively engages in instrumental or vocal music-making, a transformation of the body movements from stiff and restricted to fluid and flowing takes place.

When engaging the child in active music-making, the therapist must be mindful of limitations posed on instrument selection by space availability and sound intensity, as well as by infection control issues. Protocols for disinfecting instruments in adherence to the hospital's infection control policies are typically developed by the hospital's music therapy department. The reader is referred to Chapters 6 and 11 of this book for detailed discussions about and sample protocols for instrument cleaning.

Tonal Intervallic Synthesis

Overview. Tonal intervallic synthesis (Loewy, 2011) is "the purposeful use of tones and timbres combined within and outside of the body and which influence physical functions of the body, including circulation, release, integration, pain, and physical perception" (p. 257). In this intervention, the voice is seen as the primary instrument of release and change. Through the voice, tones and shifting vowel sounds are used within specific intervals to resolve dissonance into consonance.

The intervention is indicated for children, teens, and adults. It may be particularly useful for children who present with extreme pain and have exhausted other modalities of treatment. Maturity and creativity are useful in setting up the toned sounds. The goals are to increase palliation of pain through the tendering of entrained tension-and-release vowel sounds.

What to observe. The therapist carefully observes the child's behavioral, emotional, and physiological responses to the intervention. Although the intervention may initially evoke responses that are indicative of increased perception of pain (e.g., during the initial dissonant intervals), as the toned intervals resolve into consonant harmonies, relaxation and decreased pain should be evident.

Procedures. The guidelines provided here are based on Loewy (2011). The intervention begins with inviting the child to take some cleansing breaths. The Remo ocean drum can be used to lengthen and deepen the child's breathing. The child is encouraged to breathe in through the nose and release the breath with "sh-sh" sounds for as long as possible. The elongated exhale is aimed at promoting relaxation. The music therapist then plays a Paiste gong along the body of the child, carefully listening for overtones and resonant chambers. Loewy describes that "as the gong is vibrated over a part of the body that is in pain, the overtones that are audible are dissonant and the aural movement is fast and arrhythmic" (p. 260). The gong is then purposefully used to influence the vibrational friction of the child's body. Next, the music therapist adds toning to the sounds of the gong, with intervals moving from harmonic tension to harmonic resolution. This brings about a powerful tension-release experience for the patient. The older child might be invited to tone with the therapist, depending on the child's emotional status and his readiness. (See Appendix F in Chapter 11 for the placement of chakra vowels along the body.)

Vocal Music Therapy for Chronic Pain Management

Overview. This author developed a vocal music therapy treatment (VMT) approach for chronic pain management that uses humming, toning, deep breathing, vocal improvisation, harmonizing, and inspirational songs to help patients manage chronic pain. Humming and toning are used to enhance body awareness as an important mechanism in chronic pain management. Patients with chronic pain often use body dissociation and emotional disconnection as a way to cope with physical pain. Singing prolonged vowels produces vibrations that are felt in our bodies, with different vowels and tones resonating with different areas (Loewy, 1997). The deep breathing generated by toning, as well as singing songs that may have a special meaning to the patients, facilitates access to repressed emotions and opportunities for expression. Emotional expressivity plays an important role in stress reduction and mood enhancement. Finally, an important goal of VMT sessions is to energize the patients and provide support through toning exercises, singing, and subsequent reflective discussions.

This intervention is indicated for children with chronic or prolonged pain. As this intervention requires active participation of the child, the child needs to be able and willing to participate in active music-making with his voice. Additionally, sufficient time needs to be available, as this intervention involves multiple steps.

What to observe. The therapist should observe the child's body language and movements. Often, VMT results in the patient's body becoming more relaxed and his movements growing more fluid. During the vocal improvisations, the therapist listens for how the child relates to others, if he dares to venture out and take risks or whether he chooses to stay with the safety of an ostinato pattern, and so on. These behaviors and their underlying meaning can be explored with the child following the improvisations.

Procedures. VMT can be offered to the child alone, or family members can be invited to participate. This author has been successful in engaging family members when a gradual approach to using the voice was used. Teens and adults may feel uncomfortable using their voice in front of others. In contrast, children typically demonstrate less hesitation in using their voice musically.

This intervention begins with a brief deep breathing exercise as a way to bring the child's focus to his body and begin the process of enhanced body awareness. The deep breathing may be accompanied by the therapist playing the Remo ocean drum or a low-pitched native flute. Both instruments have an airy quality, making them perfect for stimulating deeper breathing. The deep breathing is followed by humming a two-note descending interval (second or minor third), accompanied by chordal accompaniment on the piano or guitar to provide a supportive holding environment. The child and family members, if available, are encouraged to feel the vibrations of their humming filling their body. Patients often report a calming and peaceful effect of the humming. This is reinforced by the therapist, and the child is empowered to use soft humming at any time during the day to help manage his pain. The intervention then transitions into toning or singing elongated vowels. Different vowels and different pitches resonate with different parts of the body (see Appendix F, Chapter 11), and some experimenting with these can help the child identify which could provide the best "inner massage" for a painful area in his body. With the older child or when family members are involved, the music therapist may encourage the use of harmonies in the toning experience. This brings a close intimacy and richness to the experience.

The toning stimulates deep breathing, and this, in turn, may facilitate access to repressed emotions. The release of these emotions may be quite intense. It is important that the music therapist be adequately trained to offer psychotherapeutic support.

At this point in the session, the music therapist needs to carefully assess the needs of the child. If emotional release took place and was followed by psychotherapeutic processing, either through music or verbally, the child may be fatigued. In this case, it may be good to end the session by singing a song with a message of comfort, motivation, or inspiration. If the child seems to be able to tolerate more music-making, the session can progress to the use of chants or vocal improvisations. The therapist may teach the child (and family members) a simple vocal melody that can serve as an ostinato. Small percussion instruments may be offered at this time to add a rhythmic layer. It is this author's experience that adding some percussion helps patients to become freer in their use of voice. The child and family can then be encouraged to add a repetitive melodic phrase to the ostinato (e.g., countermelody, harmony, or rhythmic drive). It is best that the music therapist demonstrate a couple of possibilities as the participants continue the ostinato pattern before asking them to take a risk in doing this. It may take some practice before the child dares/is able to deviate from the ostinato pattern. At other times, the child or family members readily engage in creating additional melodic lines. If several family members participate, this has the potential to gradually build up to a beautiful vocal improvisation that is structured and held by the ostinato. Children often appear energized after the vocal improvisation, and lots of laughter may ensue as the child and family members share their experience.

The VMT session should always close with an opportunity to reflect on the improvisation. Often, the child and family members gain insight into the needs of the child, family dynamics, etc. It is important to leave sufficient time to process this.

Improvised Music for Integration

Overview. Integration uses drumming, toning, and chanting in an improvisatory style to help the child integrate the hurt. This technique, developed by Loewy, McGregor, Richards, and Rodriguez (1997), is aimed at "empowering the child in acute or chronic pain to take action in understanding and controlling the hurt and discomfort" (Loewy et al., 1997, p. 48). In contrast to distracting the child's attention away from the pain, integration requires the child to come into the body by focusing on the breath, heart rate, emotions, and feeling of pain itself. Thus, in integration the child has an active role in his own pain management rather than being a passive recipient of distraction stimuli.

Preparation. When this intervention is implemented for procedural support, it is important that the music therapist educate the staff about the purpose and the process of this intervention. If this preparation is ignored, the staff will most likely perceive the "music" as excessive noise that is interfering with the child's ability to cope and that adds stress to the staff. In contrast, if the staff understands the goal of the intervention, they will be able to follow the child's musical process and witness the release experienced by the child.

What to observe. The technique of integration invites the creation of music that reflects the child's pain and stimulates release. This type of music may not always sound musical (Loewy et al., 1997). The music therapist must observe the child's response to this release and ensure that the child is moving toward release rather than being stuck in playing the hurt. The latter may lead to overstimulation and exhaustion without a sense of release.

Procedures. This intervention uses music to integrate breath, heart rate, affect, and pain through "harmonic, rhythmic, and tonal synthesis" (Loewy et al., 1997, p. 48). African drumming is used to provide the child with much needed release. The child is invited to let go of the pain through drumming. This release is musically supported by the therapist. The integration technique also uses toning in which the voice resonates with and vibrates selected areas of the body. Toning is defined as "the conscious use of sustained vocal sounds for the purpose of restoring the body's balance. Sound vibrations free blocked energy and resonate with specific areas of the body to relieve emotional and physical stress and tension" (Austin, 2008). Loewy writes that through toning, air is brought into the body and "opens the area of pain, enabling oxygen to enter, while the drum connects the heart to the intention and spirit of release" (1997, p. 48). The chimes, gong, and cymbal may also be used to stimulate the sound to flow through the body. During integration, "the child's job is to express his physical and psychological needs immediately and authentically and to participate in an active way, if possible" (Loewy et al., 1997, p. 53). Loewy and colleagues emphasize that integration happens at two levels, namely physiologically through enhanced connection because of the vibrations and affectively by connecting the mind to the body through the creation of pain music. The benefits of integration can endure beyond the treatment time period.

Musical Journey

Overview. Loewy and colleagues (1997) have successfully used "musical journey" to alleviate depression and chronic pain in children suffering from chronic illnesses such as sickle cell anemia and HIV/AIDS. In this intervention, the child and therapist use singing, instrumental improvisation, and verbalization to venture on a journey to a destination outlined by the child. The intervention is aimed at having the child experience his pain on a metaphorical level, giving his pain a voice, and empowering him to take an active role in his pain management.

What to observe. The therapist carefully listens to the images and metaphors as presented by the child during his journey, as these often "reveal a rich inner life beneath a presenting flat affect" (Loewy et al., 1997, p. 49). The therapist should also observe the child's movement during his journey. At times, the child may need extra support or musical suggestions by the therapist in order to move forward toward the destination.

Procedures. This intervention begins by inviting the child to choose a destination where he and the therapist should travel. The therapist then uses piano or guitar to reflect the child's presenting affect and energy. During this time, the child is asked to select an instrument to accompany his journey. At the beginning of the journey, rich harmonies and steady rhythms are used to provide a sense of safety and grounding. This communicates to the child that the therapist has confidence in the child's ability to move forward. It is important that the child experience the therapist as a companion who is not afraid of the pain. A therapist who musically suggests moving quickly to the destination may unintentionally communicate to the child that she is unable to tolerate the child's pain and suffering. As the child and therapist improvise together, Loewy and colleagues describe the process as one of emergence from isolation and vulnerability toward the discovery of inner creative powers to assist in the battle for health.

Throughout the journey, the child is asked to describe in word and song what is happening. The therapist interjects reflections as well as guiding questions to encourage the child to be as specific as possible in his descriptions. Central to this intervention is the symbolic transformation of pain. The musical and symbolic expression of pain and emotional hurt facilitates understanding and meaning-making and helps the child move toward acceptance. Emotional expressivity, meaning-making, and acceptance are regarded in the chronic pain literature as important components of effective pain management.

Music Improvisation for Active Engagement and Exploration

Overview. Hospitalized children often experience extreme fear. This fear is evoked by the sterile hospital environment, unknown equipment, unpredictable occurrences of invasive and painful medical procedures, and lack of control. Using music-making to actively engage the child with his surroundings in a playful manner can restore a sense of control, mastery, and even normalcy. As discussed early on in this chapter, negative emotional states such as fear, anxiety, and helplessness can greatly increase a child's pain perception. Music plays an important role in the child's daily life outside the hospital; therefore, participation in music activities is an excellent means to invite active engagement by the child and even normalize the hospital environment for the child (Kallay, 1997). This is true not only for young children, but also for adolescents in whose life music plays a major role in socialization, coping, and emotional expression (Kallay, 1997).

Preparation. The music therapist may need to gather a variety of medical equipment (see below) to use as instruments in the improvisation. If the intervention involves the recording and layering of rhythmic grooves, the therapist needs to bring the necessary recording equipment and software to the session.

Procedures. Music improvisations can enable the child to actively engage with his environment in a meaningful and structured manner. One such way is to incorporate medical equipment and hospital furniture in instrumental improvisations. Although this does not directly address the child's pain, active engagement in music is a powerful intervention to restore a sense of control and safety in the child. Reducing the perceived level of threat calms down neural activation that exacerbates pain perception.

Kallay (1997) describes the use of medical equipment for improvisation with toddlers. This can help the child become familiar with equipment that may be used for medical procedures, potentially reducing reactions of fear when seeing these pieces of equipment in proximity to his body during procedures. She explains that syringes can be used to make "pop" sounds when pulled by the child (with or without help from an adult), elastic bands can used to make plucking sounds, and tongue depressors can be transformed into mallets. In addition, large bins and emesis bowls can be used as percussion instruments.

This author has also incorporated hospital furniture such as the child's bed and tray table in improvisations. With preteens and teens, showing them a YouTube video of youth making cool rhythm grooves with materials in their everyday environment can be quite motivating. With the use of recording equipment, grooves can be created and recorded and then layered on top of each other to provide a rhythmic background track for solo improvisation as well as rapping, beat boxing, or other types of vocal improvisation. This rhythmic track can then be left with the child in a format compatible for one of his electronic devices (e.g., MP3) so that the teen can use this to re-create the experience or create new experiences during times of pain.

This author has also involved staff and family in the creation of these rhythmic improvisations. The teen can ask these people to improvise a brief rhythmic pattern over a four quarter-beat pattern at a preset tempo. These rhythms are recorded by the teen using software such as GarageBand or available apps. They can then be looped and layered. Teens experience great excitement when doing this type of work. They are often so engaged in the creative process that they completely "forget" about their pain. When this happens, it is important to make the child/teen aware of this so that he begins to understand that active engagement in an activity and refocusing one's attention are powerful pain management techniques that are easy to apply.

Music Entrainment for Pain Management

Overview. Music entrainment for pain management involves the creation of live music to match the child's pain. Once resonance is achieved between the pain and the music, the music progresses into music predetermined by the child as healing. Music entrainment is based on a process in physics whereby two previously out-of-step oscillators lock into phase with one another, replacing the vibrational rate of one system with the vibrational frequency of another system (Saperston, 1995). Music entrainment is frequently used by music therapists to manipulate patients' physiological responses, typically the heart rate or respiratory rate. The music therapist first matches the music pulse to the patient's heart rate to establish resonance between the two vibrational systems and gradually changes the music tempo in the therapeutically desired direction (most often, reducing the heart rate). This gradual pull from the music on the physiological response is a crucial aspect of entrainment. Thus, entrainment is not synonymous with synchronizing. Synchronizing music to a patient's behavioral or physiological response means that the music is matched to the external stimulus (e.g., the child's movement or heart rate) and then follows this external pulse (i.e., if the child's movements become faster-paced, the music's tempo grows faster). In entrainment, a reverse process takes place: After the music is matched to the external stimulus, the music is gradually manipulated so that a pull is exerted on the external stimulus and the external stimulus follows the music. These two terms are often confused in the music therapy literature, but it is important for the music therapist to understand the differential goal and outcome of these distinct interventions.

For pain management purposes, entrainment is sought between the music stimuli and the noxious neural stimuli. Because all the chemical and electrical responses in the body have rhythms, many, including noxious nerve transmission, can be entrained by first musically matching their physiological rhythm and then gradually changing the music in the desired direction, modifying the oscillatory patterns of the physiological responses (Rider, 1997). However, since pain perception is a complex phenomenon, music entrainment for pain reduction is more complex than simply matching musical stimuli with neural stimuli. As pointed out at the beginning of this chapter, the pain experience is determined not only by tissue damage, but also by cognitive, affective, and social factors. The healing components of music entrainment for pain, indeed, extend beyond physiological entrainment; many factors at the cognitive, affective, and social level are involved in this pain reduction technique. It should be noted that changes at these four levels continuously interact with each other and cannot be separated.

Music entrainment is indicated for children with acute or chronic pain who are at least eight years of age. This intervention is not appropriate for procedural support. Instead, it can be used to help a child manage postsurgical, postprocedural, or chronic pain.

Preparation. The music therapist needs to bring a wide variety of melodic and nonmelodic instruments to the session representing different timbres and pitches so that the child is able to create music that represents his pain. It is recommended that a keyboard with a large database of timbres be available.

What to observe. As outlined below, the entrainment process begins with musically matching the child's in-the-moment pain experience. Once resonance is achieved between the pain and the music, the pain typically intensifies. One 15-year-old patient who had undergone a spinal fusion surgery two days before the music entrainment session described the moment of resonance as the music pressing onto the wound like a finger. However, once the music transitioned into the healing music, the teen reported that the music "released its finger." The music therapist should observe the child's body language closely throughout the entrainment process but particularly during the matching of the pain. Often, the child's facial expression, tensed shoulders, and tight fists will indicate increased pain perception.

Procedures. The music entrainment process for pain reduction was first described for use with adults by Rider (1997) and Dileo (1997). This author has described the entrainment process specifically for use with children (2001, 2010). The entrainment intervention typically takes place over two sessions. In the first session, an in-depth assessment of the pain is conducted and the pain music is created. To familiarize the child with the instruments, he is given the opportunity to play each instrument or, where severe pain restricts the child's movement, to listen to the therapist play each instrument. After exploration of the instruments, the child is asked to describe his pain in as detailed a manner as possible. This description gives the therapist a first impression of how the pain music may possibly sound. The child is then told: "I am wondering if we could make some music that sounds exactly like the pain you are feeling right now." The following questions, each related to a specific musical parameter, may be useful to help develop an accurate auditory image of the child's pain:

Instrumentation and timbre
- Which instruments sound most like the pain you're having right now?
- What does your pain feel like? (pinching, stinging, pounding, throbbing, shooting, stabbing, tingling, piercing, ...)
- Does your pain have a deep, dark sound or a high, sharp sound to it?
- You just told me your pain feels very sharp (dull/...). Is it as sharp (dull/...) as the sound of this instrument?

Rhythm and tempo
- How fast does that [stabbing pain] go?
- Does your pain have a beat?
- Can you play me that beat?

Dynamics
- How strong/intense is your pain?

Whenever the therapist learns new information about the auditory aspect of the child's pain, she improvises accordingly and asks the child for feedback. It is important to remind the child that he can modify the music at any time. Once the child is satisfied with the auditory image of his pain, an auditory pain-healing image is created in a similar way.

After the creation of accurate auditory images—a pain image and a pain-healing image—the child is asked to recline, close his eyes, and find a comfortable position. The therapist should make sure that the child is warm, preferably covered with a light blanket. The therapist then starts the improvisation with the child's auditory pain image, gradually moving into the pain-healing sounds. The improvisation itself takes approximately 5–10 minutes. When all music has faded, the child is asked to bring his awareness back to the room and slowly open his eyes. The child is then given the opportunity to give feedback regarding this experience and its effects on the child's pain.

The first music entrainment session typically takes 60–75 minutes; subsequent sessions may take about 30 minutes. In subsequent sessions, it is important to reassess the child's pain to see if it still matches the pain music created in the previous session. Most of the time, minor adjustments are needed before the entrainment improvisation can begin. This is especially true in postoperative pain, as this pain reduces over time. For chronic pain patients, the pain experience is more stable and therefore the auditory pain image typically remains quite similar.

As a pain management technique, music entrainment affects several aspects of human functioning simultaneously. Physiologically, the music entrainment of nerve impulses, combined with an increased sensory input, is of importance for pain reduction. At the cognitive level, music entrainment has the potential to increase the child's perceived level of control by helping the child to musically "manipulate" the pain. Also, the gradual change in the music, namely from pain music to soothing music, may possibly create a shift in the cognitive perception of the presence of pain. By its focus on the sensory aspects of the pain, this technique also helps the child to directly confront the pain instead of trying to escape from it. Research has indicated that processing a noxious stimulus as a primarily sensory experience (rather than an affective one) reduces pain and distress (Leventhal & Everhart, 1980). During the creation of the pain sounds, the child's focus is guided toward the sensory aspects of his pain as per the questions provided above. At the affective level, the creation of auditory pain and healing images provides the child with a means for emotional expression, possibly influencing the experience of the pain. The shift from pain sounds to healing sounds may also induce relaxation, reducing the pain. Finally, at the social level, there is the therapist's resonance with the patient's pain. By helping the patient create an auditory reflection of the pain and by taking part in the music improvisation of the pain, the therapist enters directly into the child's pain and resonates with this pain in a very unique way. This provides enormous support and validation for the patient (Dileo, 1997).

The Heidelberg Music Therapy Manual for Pediatric Migraine

Overview. The German Center for Music Therapy Research in Heidelberg, Germany, has developed several treatment interventions for chronic pain. Although most of their work has focused on adult populations, a treatment manual for the reduction of pain due to migraine in children was developed about 10 years ago (Nickel, Hillecke, Oelkers, Resch, & Volker Bolay, 2003). This treatment is indicated for outpatients. Many hospitals have pain management centers in which outpatient care is provided for people with chronic pain. Moreover, children with conditions associated with chronic or recurrent pain (e.g., sickle cell disease) undergo frequent hospitalizations. Although this 12-week treatment manual cannot be applied in inpatient pediatric settings, several of the interventions used in this treatment manual are valuable for music therapy work with these patients during hospitalization.

The concepts of "emotional inflexibility" and "inhibited expressiveness" in pain patients (Traue, 1998) are central to the Heidelberg treatment approach. "Musical flexibilization" can be achieved through interactive music improvisations, emotional and creative activation through music, the use of symbols and metaphors in music, music-guided imagery and relaxation, and music-guided movement.

The treatment manual is divided into three phases, namely (1) the remoralization phase, which focuses on improving the subjective well-being of the child; (2) the remediation phase, which is aimed at symptom reduction; and (3) rehabilitation, which focuses on the child's general functioning. The guidelines below include a brief description of two interventions included in this treatment manual, namely symptom improvisation and reality improvisation. For a complete description of the manual, the reader should consult Nickel et al. (2003).

Procedures. Symptom improvisation is used to symbolically externalize the child's migraine headache. The child is asked to choose an instrument as an acoustic representation of his symptom. Next, the child is asked to select an instrument that can fight the pain. The music therapist and the child then engage in an improvisation, with the music therapist playing the pain instrument and the child, the pain-battling instrument. Nickel provides the following clinical example:

> In a symptom improvisation experience, nine-year-old Daniel chooses the bass drum as the acoustic representation of his symptom. The headache is played by the therapist, while Daniel plays the piano, fighting the headache. Daniel "wins" and seems to profit from the possibility of converting the painful physical symptom into sound, thus relating to it and making it tangible. He learns that he does not have to passively endure the pain, but can actively influence it. (Nickel et al., 2003, p. 12)

Patients who are experiencing intense pain often report feeling overwhelmed or taken over by the pain. They feel as if they have no control over the pain. Giving a child the opportunity to externalize that pain and musically role-play a battle with the pain, resulting in a victory over it, can be an empowering experience. The role of the music therapist is of course to help the child "win the battle" by musically "succumbing" under the child's play. The child may need encouragement to play his instrument in a strong, persistent manner and to not allow the pain sound to be in charge.

A second intervention taken from the Heidelberg treatment manual is called "reality improvisation." This improvisation is also based on the idea of role-playing and focuses on musically creating solutions for a conflict with which the child may be dealing. Research evidence suggests that emotional stress and stressful situations are triggers for migraine attacks in children. Chronic pain literature has also indicated that stress, worrying, and anxiety increase pain perception. Therefore, an assessment of common stress situations in the child's daily life is essential in music therapy work with children with chronic pain. Such assessment can then inform the content or theme of the reality improvisation. In the clinical example presented above, Daniel was reported to have had frequent fights with his three-years-older brother. Nickel writes:

> In a reality improvisation, Daniel practices saying "no" and handling arguments. His musical expression is loud and definite. In musical contact, Daniel always wants to have the last word. In musical role-plays, Daniel learns to deal more adequately with fights, conflict situations, and aggression. Daniel reports finding it easier to stand up to his older brother now. In reality improvisations, self-confidence–boosting experiences are induced. Daniel is encouraged to explore and name things he likes about himself. (Nickel et al. 2003, p. 12)

Needless to say, both interventions may need to be offered to the child on multiple occasions in order for the child to reap benefits. Playing a symptom improvisation may bring immediate short-term pain relief to the child, but it seems unlikely, in this author's opinion, that this would result in long-term effects. Children with chronic pain often internalize fixed ideas and emotions about their pain and may be "stuck" in certain pain behaviors. It is unlikely that a one-time improvisation will bring about change in these fixed patterns. Rather, repeated musical role-plays are needed to begin introducing a shift in the child's perception.

Tension Release Through Drumming

This intervention uses active drumming to help a child release built-up tension. In contrast to the tension release discussed under Receptive Methods, this intervention requires active and energetic participation of the child. The reader is referred to Chapter 6 for guidelines on this intervention.

GUIDELINES FOR RE-CREATIVE MUSIC THERAPY

Singing Songs

Overview. Singing favorite songs can be an effective way to help the child shift his focus away from the pain. Allowing the child to select the songs gives a sense of control over the environment. Singing songs furthermore normalizes the sterile hospital environment and gives parents an opportunity to playfully interact with the child. This intervention is indicated for children of all ages and abilities.

Preparation. Depending on the age of the child, the music therapist should bring song sheets, props (e.g., finger puppets), and an accompaniment instrument to the session. The therapist should have a large and varied repertoire of songs committed to memory. She can also bring an iPad (or other small storage device) with a database of sheet music.

Procedures. When singing songs with the child for pain management purposes, it is important to keep specific goals in mind that will help with pain management. One such goal is to increase the child's perceived level of control. To this end, this author would often make a "pact" with the child, saying that whenever a medical staff member entered the room, I would require them to sing, hum, or play along with whatever song we were singing at the time before the staff member would be allowed to touch the child. To the children's great delight, most staff members and doctors would sing along when requested, as they understood that this would lead to a more cooperative child. Whenever possible, the music therapist must inform the nursing staff and doctors about this beforehand so that they understand the purpose of this request. In the fast-paced hospital environment, medical personnel may otherwise react with some opposition because it may appear to be a waste of valuable time.

Having fun is also an important mediating factor in pain reduction. Singing songs can be a lot of fun and can truly transform a child.

Dayla, a five-year-old girl with sickle cell, was hospitalized for a vaso-occlusive crisis and presented with extreme pain. Her mother came to find me and said that her daughter had been asking for the music lady since her hospitalization earlier that afternoon. I followed the mother to Dayla's room, to find her in bed crying. I walked up to Dayla and strummed my guitar. This caused her to halt her crying momentarily and offer me a faint smile, after which she continued to sob quietly. I quickly consulted my little notebook to see what songs Dayla had liked during previous hospitalizations and noticed that "Old MacDonald" "with jungle animals" was her favorite. I began to hum the beginning of the song, pausing after the first line. Dayla motioned with her leg as if to say, "Continue." I continued the song and waited for Dayla to suggest the first animal. Dayla said "elephant," looking at my face for a reaction. She giggled as I reacted surprised. Within a few minutes, Dayla, her mom, and I were rocking out on "Old MacDonald," naming all the jungle animals we could think of, with Dayla jumping up and down her bed as we sang about monkeys on the farm. To an outsider, this may have appeared as the "music lady" just singing some songs, but we witnessed the transformation that singing songs can bring to a child in extreme pain.

Music Alternate Engagement (MAE)

MAE (Bishop et al., 1996) is used to help a child cope with the anxiety and pain of medical procedures. The intervention focuses on active engagement of the child in specific, achievable tasks associated with a procedure. The use of music or musical components with the therapist provides opportunities for a child to participate in an activity that offers alternate points of focus. Guidelines for this intervention are provided in Chapter 6.

Music-making to Assist with Rehabilitation

Re-creative and improvisational methods are also used to help children manage pain and enhance their endurance during physical therapy. Chapter 10 in this book provides detailed guidelines for several such interventions.

GUIDELINES FOR COMPOSITIONAL MUSIC THERAPY

Songwriting

Overview. As discussed in the first part of this chapter, the meaning that a child ascribes to pain may reduce or increase his pain perception. Songwriting gives the child the opportunity to articulate his feelings and direct them into a creative form (Turry, 1997). It offers the child an avenue for telling his story. This can be powerful for children who have experienced a long journey of painful medical procedures. As the therapist accepts the child's feelings and thoughts, she is able to reframe the situation, enhance the child's understanding of the pain and/or procedure, or merely listen to the child's story and validate his feelings.

Micci (1984) used song composition as a means for pediatric patients hospitalized for cardiac catheterization to gain an understanding of the procedure and to be allowed to take an active role in creating, understanding, and experiencing hospitalization. During the actual procedure, listening to familiar songs was used to promote relaxation. Several children requested hearing their self-composed songs. It was concluded that music was an effective aid in preparing children for cardiac catheterization as well as an effective means for relaxation.

Procedures. Many chapters in this book give guidelines for songwriting specific to the different populations. Therefore, the reader is referred to the individual chapters for instructions. Here, a brief discussion is provided of how songwriting and the performance of self-composed songs may bring relief to children in pain.

In her work with adolescents with sickle cell disease, Charlton (2013) describes how songwriting helped a teenager transform her experiences of pain. First, the song she wrote served as a testimony of her experience and helped people around her better understand her pain. Second, through singing and rehearsing the song, she found her voice and was able to reclaim her identity. Third, the songwriting process helped her move from a position of desperation and frustration to one of empowerment and transformation.

Songwriting with children and teens typically involves a lot of verbal reflection about the themes and metaphors that emerge in the lyrics. Themes that frequently return in songs composed by children and teens in pain (especially those with chronic pain conditions) include control vs. powerlessness, independence vs. dependence, loneliness vs. support, hope vs. fear, and feeling "broken" vs. strength and resiliency. Furthermore, themes related to existential crisis often emerge (Charlton, 2013).

This author has witnessed many times the value of the actual recording of the song and of sharing the recording with others. The recording of the song may involve creating multiple tracks for instrumentation and adding special effects. This very process continues and deepens the process of reflection. Teenagers are quite tuned in to the symbolic meaning of different parts of the sound track. For example, a teen may use voice distortion effects during the first verse of his song to represent the existential crisis caused by his chronic illness and pain. As the song progresses, the distortion is removed and replaced by a clear singing voice supported by backup voices singing in harmony with the teen. A teen may add a driving 8th note base pattern in the bridge of his song to represent his determination to not give up and to take charge of his life in spite of debilitating pain.

Instrumental Compositions for Relaxation and Support

Overview. Children and teens can be encouraged to make their own instrumental track to use for relaxation purposes, procedural support, or motivational and pain management purposes during rehabilitation. The patients are active participants in the composition process that uses electronic music technologies (EMTs) such as GarageBand and GrooveMaker. As per the Neuromatrix Theory outlined at the beginning of this chapter, this active focus can help mediate (i.e., reduce) the brain's processing of noxious stimulation (Whitehead-Pleaux, Clark, & Spall, 2011).

This intervention is not indicated for children who are sedated, unable to communicate, or very fatigued. Furthermore, when a child is experiencing moderate to severe pain, the use of EMTs is contraindicated, as the child may not be able to sustain the necessary focus to engage with these EMTs. As a result, the experience may become unsuccessful and frustrating for the child. This may exacerbate his pain (Whitehead-Pleaux, Clark, & Spall, 2011). Whitehead-Pleaux and colleagues further emphasize that a child who is experiencing moderate to severe pain may not be able to actively participate in music-making and may be limited to music listening instead.

Preparation. The music therapist must be well versed in the use of recording software such as GarageBand, knowledgeable about editing tracks, applying special effects, looping, etc. The therapist should also be familiar with the different types of instrumentation and rhythmic and melodic loops available in the software so that she can guide the child in selecting what he wants.

Procedures. Teens and children are typically easily excitable about the idea of creating a CD with their own music. When introducing this idea to the child, it is best to have a computer with the software available so that a brief demonstration can be given to the child. Teens as well as younger children are amazingly well versed in the use of software. An intuitive program like GarageBand literally takes a few minutes of demonstration before the child is ready to jump in and begin working on a sound track.

Before starting the actual composition, it is important to have the child identify the purpose of the composition. Will the music be used to help him relax? Help him go to sleep? Motivate him during physical therapy? Help him focus his attention away from the pain? Once a purpose is identified, the therapist and the child discuss what characteristics the music should have to meet this purpose.

It is this author's experience that most children need guidance by the therapist at the onset of the project because of the multitude of options in instrumentation, style, and rhythms in these software programs. However, once a melody and/or bass track is developed with the help of the therapist, the child grows increasingly independent in the composition process. The therapist remains available as a sounding board for the decision-making, to help resolve problems, and to demonstrate specific editing tools. In addition, as many children connect imagery to their sound tracks (especially sound tracks for relaxation purposes), the music therapist processes the meaning of the imagery with the child.

The composition process typically takes place over the span of multiple sessions. When the child is satisfied with the track, it is burned onto a CD or downloaded on the child's MP3 device, smart phone, or other device the child has available for playback. When the child intends to use the music during physical therapy, the music therapist should arrange for speakers so that the music can be played free-field and be heard by the treating therapists. This is important so that the therapist can adjust instructions for movement to the tempo of the music, for example.

Children feel greatly empowered by using music that they have created themselves for their pain management and rehabilitation. In addition, they enjoy the praise they receive from family, medical staff, and peers about their compositions.

RESEARCH EVIDENCE

With only a few exceptions, the receptive use of music has been the primary type of music experience used in research studies examining the impact of music interventions on pain management. Several reasons account for the reliance on receptive interventions in pain management research. The first one points to the issue of music therapy vs. music medicine interventions as described in the Introduction of this book. Most studies on music and pain relief have been conducted by medical personnel and not by music therapists.

Second, the use of prerecorded music is often preferred as a stimulus in controlled clinical trials because it allows for standardization. However, it is possible to develop music therapy protocols that will allow for individualization according to patient needs while still adhering to RCT research standards (Bradt, 2012). This author recently received an NIH grant to study the impact of vocal music therapy (VMT) on core outcomes in chronic pain management. The treatment protocol targets specific pain management mechanisms (see the VMT description in the guidelines section) but is not standardized. Music therapists are urged to conduct research studies on music therapy interventions that truly represent the clinical work we do in pain management. "Listening to prerecorded music without therapeutic interactions and reflective discussions is not what music therapists practice in their clinical work. What sets us apart from a CD or MP3 player is the therapeutic relationship and process that develop through music interactions, the use of live music to adapt to the in-the-moment needs of and responses by the patient, and the clinical decision-making based on the individual needs of the patient (Bradt, 2012, p. 137).

Additionally, an erroneous belief may be held that patients in pain cannot engage in active music-making and may not be willing to sign up for a research study that involves active engagement.

Unfortunately, it seems that this has resulted in a strong association of music for pain management with "passive" music experiences.

In 1997, Nolan reported that very few reports existed on the effects of music therapy interventions on pediatric pain. Unfortunately, little progress has been made in this area since then. Although several music therapy studies targeting pediatric pain have been published since then, there is an urgent need to grow the research in this area.

A Cochrane Systematic Review by Cepeda is much cited in the literature and should be mentioned here even though the review mostly included music medicine studies. This review sought to evaluate the effect of music on acute, chronic, or cancer pain intensity, pain relief, and analgesic requirements. Fifty-one controlled clinical trial studies with a combined sample size of 3,663 participants met the inclusion criteria for this review. Eight of these studies evaluated children and neonates. However, only four of these studies provided quantitative data. The others reported improvement (or lack thereof) due to music listening but did not report statistical results. Unfortunately, the results of the studies that included statistical results could not be pooled because of the diverse methods used to assess pain intensity. The study by Arts et al. (1994) that examined the effect of music listening vs. lidocaine-prilocaine (EMLA) emulsion on children's pain responses to intravenous cannulation showed a difference of 0.1 units on a 0 to 10 scale in favor of the EMLA group. This suggests that music listening was nearly as effective as applying EMLA cream in managing a child's pain. Fowler-Kerry (1987), in a study on injection pain using a four-point pain scale from 0 to 3, found a pain difference of 0.44 units in favor of the music group. Joyce (2001) examined the effects of music listening on neonates' pain during circumcision and reported a difference of 0.75 units using the same scale as Fowler-Kerry. A study by Gawronska (2002) found that patients who received music interventions were 1.6 times more likely to report at least 50% pain relief than patients who did not receive music during oral surgery. For a detailed report on the entire review, including adult pain studies, the reader is referred to Cepeda (2006).

The results of single research studies for the management of anxiety and pain—these outcomes are typically both included in research studies with pediatric patients—are described in detail in the chapters that deal with the population at hand in these studies. They are briefly mentioned here to give the reader an overview of the types of studies that are available on music therapy for pediatric pain. The reader is referred to subsequent chapters in this book for further detail on these studies and their findings.

For children with cancer (Chapter 8), two music therapy research studies have included pain as an outcome variable. Sahler, Hunter, and Liesveld (2003) explored the effects of a combined music therapy and relaxation imagery intervention on frequency and intensity of pain and nausea in patients in a bone marrow transplant (BMT) unit. Pfaff, Smith, and Gowan (1989) evaluated the effect of music-assisted relaxation on the fear and pain of six pediatric patients undergoing bone marrow aspirations (BMA).

For pain reduction in children in the Pediatric Intensive Care Unit, one study by Hatem, Lira, and Mattos (2006) is included in Chapter 5. This study examined the effect of music listening on the postsurgical pain in 84 children.

Several music therapy research studies have been conducted with burn patients (Chapter 7). Fratianne et al. (2001) explored the effects of music-based imagery and musical alternate engagement on pain experiences and anxiety with children in an inpatient burns unit during dressing changes and wound debridement. Whitehead-Pleaux, Baryza, and Sheridan (2006), using a two-arm randomized controlled trial, studied the effects of live receptive music experiences using patient-selected music on children with burns receiving reconstructive surgery. An exploratory study by Whitehead-Pleaux, Zebrowski, Baryza, and Sheridan (2007) explored the effects of receptive experiences composed of improvised songs on pain in nine pediatric burn patients during medical procedures.

The chapter on music therapy with premature infants includes several studies on the influence of music on pain responses and excessive agitation in infants.

Finally, music therapy studies that are not included in the other chapters are discussed here. Oelkers-Ax et al. (2007) used a randomized three-arm parallel-group study to explore the effects of music therapy (N = 20), butterbur root extract (N = 19), or placebo (N = 19) on childhood migraine. Music therapy interventions principally comprised music-aided relaxation training, body awareness techniques, and conflict training in musical role-play, and were provided in weekly sessions over 12 weeks. Outcomes measured included medication doses and efficacy, adverse events, reduction of migraine attack frequency, intensity of headache, and psychiatric comorbidity. Music therapy was found to be the most effective intervention during both post-treatment (p = .005) and follow-up (p = .018) in reducing symptoms. For the primary outcome, attack frequency, the music therapy intervention resulted in an average reduction of 65.7% (±31.0) compared to 36.1% (±57.3) in the butterbur group and 28.8% (±39.5) in the placebo group.

Noguchi (2006) explored the effects of music on distress and perceptions of pain in pediatric injection patients ages 4–6.5 (N = 64) using a three-arm parallel-group design. The children were randomized to a musical story, a spoken story, or a standard care control group. The mean Observational Scale of Behavioral Distress score for the music group was 4.64 (SD = 4.82) compared to 5.10 (SD = 3.78) in the spoken story group and 6.12 (SD = 4.64) in the control group, with higher scores representing greater distress. The differences between the groups, however, were not statistically significant. As for pain scores, participants in the musical story group reported less pain (M = 2.67, SD = 2.79) than participants in the spoken story group (M = 4.00, SD = 2.55) and the control group (M = 3.53, SD = 2.76) as scored on the six-point Faces Scale, but again, these differences were not statistically significant. This lack of statistical significance may have been due to the small sample size.

Steinke (1991) examined the effects of music listening (M), relaxation/imagery (RI), and combined music and relaxation/imagery (MRI) on postsurgical pain and anxiety in patients who had undergone surgical correction of scoliosis. The music condition consisted of musical compositions in the "New Age" style. Results indicated that none of the treatments significantly reduced observed pain and anxiety levels from pre- to posttest. However, differences between groups were found in the mean levels of self-reported pain and anxiety. The RI group exhibited lower mean scores on measures of subjective pain and anxiety than did the M group; the MRI group reported the highest scores. The author stated that it is possible that patients experiencing intense pain may not be able to attend to the extra stimuli of both verbal instructions and music and, consequently, end up attending to neither one effectively.

SUMMARY AND CONCLUSIONS

Most children who are hospitalized experience pain. The continuous fear of painful procedures and the actual experience of pain make hospitalization a stressful and even traumatizing event. Inadequate treatment of children's pain during hospitalization may have long-term negative effects on their future pain responses and their emotional well-being. Despite the vast growth in knowledge of pediatric pain, its assessment, and its treatment, the literature continues to point to inadequate treatment of pediatric pain due to enduring misconceptions about children's pain perception. In addition, fear of side effects and addiction to opioid pain medication continues to fuel the undertreatment of severe pain in children.

Music therapists play an important role in ensuring that children's pain management needs are adequately addressed. To best serve hospitalized children, music therapy for pain management must go beyond listening to music for relaxation and sedation. In contrast to the commonly held belief that children in extreme pain are not able to actively engage in music-making, reports in the literature and the experience of seasoned music therapists in the field of pediatric pain management indicate that children in pain may greatly benefit from active engagement. By taking charge of some of the factors contributing to a painful experience, children may learn to reconceptualize the pain experience as one they can partly control. This chapter provides many guidelines for active engagement of the child in music-making to help him manage his pain.

ENDNOTES

1. Wong-Baker FACES® Pain Rating Scale reprinted by permission of Connie M. Baker. Originally published in *Whaley & Wong's Nursing Care of Infants and Children.* © Elsevier Inc.

REFERENCES

Abu-Saad, H. H., Kroonen, E., & Halfens, R. (1990). On the development of a multidimensional Dutch pain assessment tool for children. *Pain, 43,* 249–256.

Allen, F. (1998). *Health psychology: Theory and practice.* Australia: Allen & Unwin.

Ambuel, B., Hamlett, K. W., Marx, C. M., & Blumer, J. L. (1992). Assessing distress in pediatric intensive care environments: The COMFORT scale. *Journal of Pediatric Psychology, 17,* 95–109.

Anand, K. J. S. (1998). Neurophysiological and neurobiological correlates of supraspinal pain processing: Measurement techniques. In G. A. Finley & P. J. McGrath (Eds.), *Progress in pain research and management: Vol. 10. Measurement of pain in infants and children* (pp. 21–46). Seattle: IASP Press.

Arts, S. E., Abu-Saad, H. H., Champion, G. D., Crawford, M. R., Fisher, R. J., & Juniper, K. H. *(1994).* Age-related response to lidocaine-prilocaine (EMLA) emulsion and effect of music distraction on the pain of intravenous cannulation. *Pediatrics, 93(5),* 797–801.

Austin, D. (2008). *The theory and practice of vocal psychotherapy: Songs of self.* Philadelphia, PA: Jessica Kingsley.

Banoub-Baddour, S., & Laryea, M. (1991). Children in pain: A culturally sensitive perspective for child care professionals. *Journal of Child and Youth Care, 6(1),* 19–24.

Beyer, J. E. (1984). *The Oucher: A user's manual and technical report.* Evanston, IL: The Hospital Play Equipment Company.

Beyer, J. E., & Knott, C. B. (1998). Construct validity estimation for the African-American and Hispanic versions of the Oucher Scale. *Journal of Pediatric Nursing, 13,* 20–31.

Bishop, B., Christenberry, A., Robb, S., & Tooms Rudenberg, M. (1996). Music therapy and child life interventions with pediatric burn patients. In M. A. Froehlich (Ed.), *Music therapy with hospitalized children* (pp. 17–24). Cherry Hill, NJ: Jeffrey Books.

Blood, *A. J.,* & Zatorre, *R. J. (2001).* Intensely pleasurable responses to music correlate with activity in brain regions implicated with reward and emotion. *Proceedings of the National Academy of Sciences, 98,* 11818–11823.

Bradt, J. (2001). *The effects of music entrainment on postoperative pain perception in pediatric patients.* Unpublished dissertation. Temple University, Philadelphia.

Bradt, J. (2010). The effects of music entrainment on postoperative pain perception in pediatric patients. *Music and Medicine, 2(2),* 150–157.

Bradt, J. (2012). Randomized controlled trials in music therapy: Guidelines for design and implementation. *Journal of Music Therapy, 49(2),* 120–149.

Breau, L. M., & Burkitt, C. (2009). Assessing pain in children with intellectual disabilities. *Pain, Research and Management, 14,* 116–120.

Brown, C. J., Chen, A., & Dworkin, S. F. (1989). Music in the control of human pain. *Music Therapy, 8(1),* 47–60.

Burke, M., Walsh, J., Oehler, J., & Gingras, J. A. (1995). Music therapy following suction: Four case studies. *Neonatal Network, 14,* 41–49.

Cepeda, M. S., Carr, D. B., Lau, J., & Alvarez, H. (2006). Music for pain relief. *Cochrane Database of Systematic Reviews. 2006 Apr 19*(2), CD004843.

Chapman, C. R. (1995). The affective dimension of pain: A model. In B. Bromm & J. E. Desmedt (Eds.), *Advances in pain research and therapy: Vol. 22. Pain and the brain: From nociception to cognition* (pp. 283–301). New York: Raven Press.

Charlton, M. (2013). "Hear My Song": Giving Voice to Adolescents with Sickle Cell Disease. In J. F. Mondanaro & G. A. Sara (Eds.), *Music and Medicine: Integrative Models in the Treatment of Pain* (pp. 335–346). New York: Satchnote Press.

Chesky, K. S., & Michel, D. E. (1991). The music vibration table (MVT): Developing a technology and conceptual model for pain relief. *Music Therapy Perspectives, 9,* 32–38.

Choiniere, M., & Melzack, R. (1987). Acute and chronic pain in hemophilia. *Pain, 31,* 317–331.

Cohen, L. L., Lemanek, K., Blount, R. L., Dahlquist, L. M., Lim, C. S., Palermo, T. M., McKenna, K. D., & Weiss, K. E. (2008). Evidence-based assessment of pediatric pain. *Journal of Pediatric Psychology, 33*(9), 939–955.

Cowan, D. S. (1991). Music therapy in the surgical arena. *Music Therapy Perspectives, 9,* 42–45.

Craig, K. (1999). Emotions and psychobiology. In P. D. Wall & R. Melzack (Eds.), *Textbook of pain.* London: Churchill Livingstone.

Dileo, C. (1997). Reflections on medical music therapy: Biopsychosocial perspective of the treatment process. In J. V. Loewy (Ed.), *Music therapy and pediatric pain* (pp. 125–144). Cherry Hill, NJ: Jeffrey Books.

Elliott, C. H., Jay, S. M., & Woody, P. (1987). An observation scale for measuring children's distress during medical procedures. *Journal of Pediatric Psychology, 12,* 543–551.

Ely, E., Chen-Lim, M. L., Zarnowsky, C., Green, R., Shaffer, S., & Holtzer, B. (2012). Finding the evidence to change practice for assessing pain in children who are cognitively impaired. *Journal of Pediatric Nursing, 27,* 402–410.

Fowler-Kerry, S., & Lander, J. R. *(1987)*. Management of injection pain in children. *Pain, 30(2),* 169–175.

Fratianne, R. B., Prensner, J. D., Hutson, M. J., Super, D. M., Yowler, C. J., & Standley, J. M. (2001). The effect of music-based imagery and music alternative engagement on the burn debridement process. *Journal of Burn Care and Rehabilitation, 22*(1), 47–53.

Froehlich, M. A. (1996). Music therapy with hospitalized children: A crisis intervention model. In M. A. Froehlich (Ed.), *Music therapy with hospitalized children* (pp. 17–24). Cherry Hill, NJ: Jeffrey Books.

Gaffney, A. (1987). *Pain: Perspectives in childhood.* Unpublished dissertation. University College, Cork, Ireland.

Gaffney, A. (1993). Cognitive developmental aspects of pain in school-age children. In N. L. Schechter, C. B. Berde, & M. Yaster (Eds.), *Pain in infants, children and adolescents* (pp. 75–85). Baltimore: Williams & Wilkins.

Gaffney, A., & Dunne, E. A. (1986). Developmental aspects of children's definitions of pain. *Pain, 26,* 105–117.

Gawronska, S. J., Zienkiewicz, J., Majkowicz, M., Szwed, E., Kiewlicz, W., & Soroka Letkiewicz, B. (2002). Music therapy before and during oral surgeries as a positive relaxing influence on the young patients. *Annales Academiae Medicae Gedanensis, 32,* 161–172.

Ghetti, C. M. (2012). Music therapy as procedural support for invasive medical procedures: Toward the development of music therapy theory. *Nordic Journal of Music Therapy, 21*(1), 3–35. DOI: 10.1080/08098131.2011.571278.

Grocke, D., & Wigram, T. (2007). *Receptive methods in music therapy: Techniques and clinical applications for music therapy clinicians, educators and students*. Philadelphia, PA: Jessica Kingsley.

Hagglund, K. J., Schopp, L. M., Alberts, K. R., Cassidy, J. T., & Frank, R. G. (1995). Predicting pain among children with juvenile rheumatoid arthritis. *Arthritis Care Research, 8*(1), 36–42.

Hatem, T. P., Lira, P. I., & Mattos, S. S. (2006). The therapeutic effects of music in children following cardiac surgery. *Jornal de pediatria, 82*(3), 186–192. DOI: 10.2223/JPED.1473.

Hester, N. K. (1979). The preoperational child's reaction to immunization. *Nursing Research, 28*(4), 250–255.

Hester, N. O., Foster, R., & Kristensen, K. (1990). Measurement of pain in children: Generalizability and validity of the pain ladder and the poker chip tool. In D. C. Tyler & E. J. Crane, *Advances in pain research and therapy* (pp. 79–84). New York: Raven.

Hicks, C. L., von Baeyer, C. L., Spafford, P., van Korlaar, I., & Goodenough, B. (2001). The Faces Pain Scale–Revised: Toward a common metric in pediatric pain measurement. *Pain, 93*, 173–183.

International Association for the Study of Pain. (2009). *Global Year against Cancer Pain: Cancer Pain in Children*. Retrieved from http://www.iasp-pain.org/AM/Template.cfm?Section=Fact_Sheets1&Template=/CM/ContentDisplay.cfm&ContentID=9138

International Association for the Study of Pain. (2011). *IASP Taxonomy*. Retrieved from http://www.iasp-pain.org/Content/NavigationMenu/GeneralResourceLinks/PainDefinitions/default.htm

Joyce, B. A., Keck, J. F., & Gerkensmeyer, J. *(2001)*. Evaluation of pain management interventions for neonatal circumcision pain. *Journal of Pediatric Health Care, 15(3),* 105–114.

Kallay, V. (1997). Music therapy applications in the pediatric medical setting: Child development, pain management and choices. In J. V. Loewy (Ed.), *Music therapy and pediatric pain* (pp. 33–44). Cherry Hill, NJ: Jeffrey Books.

Kuttner, L. (1996). *A child in pain: How to help, what to do*. USA: Hartley & Marks.

LeBaron, S., & Zeltzer, L. (1984). Assessment of acute pain and anxiety in children and adolescents by self-reports, observer reports, and a behavior checklist. *Journal of Consulting and Clinical Psychology, 52*(5), 729–738.

Leeuwenburgh, E., Goldring, E., Fogel, A., Kanazawa, M., Lynch, T., & Mondanaro, J. (2007). Creative arts therapies. In S. Chisolm (Ed.), *The health professions: Trends and opportunities in U. S. health care* (pp. 397–424). Sudbury, MA: Jones and Bartlett.

Leventhal, H., & Everhart, D. (1980). Emotion, pain and physical illness. In C.E. Izard (Ed.), *Emotions and Psychopathology*. New York: Plenum Press

Locsin, R. (1981). The effect of music on the pain of selected postoperative patients. *Journal of Advanced Nursing, 6*, 19–25.

Loewy, J. V. (1995). The musical stages of speech: A developmental model of pre-verbal sound making. *Music Therapy, 13(1)*, 47–73.

Loewy, J. V. (1997). Introduction. In J. V. Loewy (Ed.), *Music therapy and pediatric pain*. Cherry Hill, NJ: Jeffrey Books.

Loewy, J. V. (1999). Music psychotherapy assessment in pediatric pain. In C. Dileo (Ed.), *Applications of music in medicine, vol. II: Theoretical and clinical perspectives*. Silver Spring, MD: AMTA.

Loewy, J. V., MacGregor, B., Richards, K., & Rodriguez, J. (1997). Music therapy pediatric pain management: Assessing and attending to the sounds of hurt, fear and anxiety. In J. V. Loewy (Ed.), *Music therapy and pediatric pain* (pp. 45–56). Cherry Hill, NJ: Jeffrey Books.

Luffy, R., & Grove, S. K. (2003). Examining the validity, reliability, and preference of three pediatric pain measurement tools in African American children. *Pediatric Nursing, 29,* 54–59.

Magill, L., Coyle, N., Handzo, G., & Loscalzo, M. (1997). Cancer and pain: A creative multidisciplinary approach in working with patients and families. In J. V. Loewy (Ed.), *Music therapy and pediatric pain* (pp. 45–56). Cherry Hill, NJ: Jeffrey Books.

Malviya, S., Voepel-Lewis, T., Burke, C., Merkel, S., & Tait, A. R. (2006). The revised FLACC observational pain tool: Improved reliability and validity for pain assessment in children with cognitive impairment. *Pediatric Anesthesia, 16,* 258–265.

McCaffery, M. (2002). Choosing a faces pain scale. *Nursing, 32,* 68.

McGrath, P. A. (1987). An assessment of children's pain: A review of behavioral, physiological and direct scaling techniques. *Pain, 31*(2), 147–176.

McGrath, P. A. (1990). *Pain in children: Nature, assessment and treatment.* New York: The Guilford Press.

McGrath, P. A. (1993). Psychological aspects of pain perception. In N. L. Schechter, C. B. Berde, & M. Yaster (Eds.), *Pain in infants, children and adolescents* (pp. 39–63). Baltimore: Williams & Wilkins.

McGrath, P. J., & McAlpine, L. (1993). Psychologic perspective on pediatric pain. *The Journal of Pediatrics, 122*(5, part 2), S2–S8.

McGrath, P. J., Johnson, G., Goodman, J. T., Dunn, J., & Chapman, J. (1985). CHEOPS: A behavioral scale for rating postoperative pain in children. In H. L. Fields, R. Dubner, & F. Cervero (Eds.), *Advances in pain research and therapy* (pp. 395–402). New York: Raven Press.

Melzack, R. (1999). From the gate to the neuromatrix. *Pain, 6*(S), 121–126.

Melzack, R. (2001). Pain and the neuromatrix in the brain. *Journal of Dental Education, 65*(12), 1378–1382.

Melzack, R., & Dennis, S. G. (1978). Neurophysiological foundations of pain. In R. A. Sternbach (Ed.), *The psychology of pain.* New York: Raven Press.

Melzack, R., & Wall, P. (1965). Pain mechanisms: A new theory. *Science, 150,* 971–979.

Micci, O. N. (1984). The use of music therapy with pediatric patients undergoing cardiac catheterization. *The Arts in Psychotherapy, 11,* 261–266.

Michel, D. E., & Chesky, K. S. (1995). A survey of music therapists using music for pain relief. *The Arts in Psychotherapy, 22*(1), 49–51.

National Institute of Heart, Lung, and Blood Institute. (September, 2012). *What is Sickle Cell Anemia?* Retrieved from http://www.nhlbi.nih.gov/health/health-topics/topics/sca/

Neugebauer, C. T. (2008). Pediatric Burn Recovery: Acute care, rehabilitation, and reconstruction. In D. Hanson-Abromeit & C. Colwell (Eds.), *Medical music therapy for pediatric in hospital settings* (pp. 195–232). Silver Spring, MD: American Music Therapy Association.

Neugebauer, C. T., & Neugebauer, V. (2003). Music therapy in pediatric burn care. In S. L. Robb (Ed.), *Music therapy in pediatric healthcare: Research and evidence-based practice* (pp. 31–48). Silver Spring, MD: AMTA.

Nickel, A., Hillecke, T., Oelkers, R., Resch, F., & Volker Bolay, H. (2003). Music therapy in the treatment of children with migraine. *Music Therapy Today* (online), *4*(4). Available at http://musictherapyworld.net

Noguchi, L. K. (2006). The effect of music versus nonmusic on behavioral signs of distress and self-report of pain in pediatric injection patients. *Journal of Music Therapy, 43*(1), 16–38.

Nolan, P. (1997). Music therapy in the pediatric pain experience: Theory, practice and research at Allegheny University of the Health Sciences. In J. V. Loewy (Ed.), *Music therapy and pediatric pain* (pp. 57–68). Cherry Hill, NJ: Jeffrey Books.

Oelkers-Ax, R., Leins, A., Parzer, P., Hillecke, T., Bolay, H. V., Fischer, J., Bender, S., Hermanns, U., & Resch, F. (2007). Butterbur root extract and music therapy in the prevention of childhood migraine: An explorative study. *European Journal of Pain, 12*, 301–313.

Patterson, D. R., Hoflund, H., Espey, K., & Sharar, S. (n.d.). *Pain management*. International Society for Burn Injuries. Retrieved from http://www.worldburn.org/documents/painmanage.pdf

Pfaff, V. K., Smith, K. E., & Gowan, D. (1989). The effects of music-assisted relaxation on the distress of pediatric cancer patients undergoing a bone marrow aspiration. *Children's Health Care, 18*(4), 232–236.

Rider, M. S. (1997). Entrainment music, healing imagery, and the rhythmic language of health and disease. In J. V. Loewy (Ed.), *Music therapy and pediatric pain* (pp. 81–88). Cherry Hill, NJ: Jeffrey Books.

Robb, S. L. (2003). Coping and chronic illness: Music therapy for children and adults with cancer. In S. L. Robb (Ed.), *Music therapy in pediatric healthcare: Research and evidence-based practice*. Silver Spring, MD: AMTA.

Robb, S. L., Nichols, R. J., Rutan, R. L., Bishop, B. L., & Parker, J. C. (1995). The effects of music assisted relaxation on preoperative anxiety. *Journal of Music Therapy, 32*(1), 2–21.

Ross, D. M., & Ross, S. A. (1984). Childhood pain: The school-aged child's viewpoint. *Pain, 20*, 179-191.

Ross, D. M., & Ross, S. A. (1988). Assessment of pediatric pain: An overview. *Issues in Comprehensive Pediatric Nursing, 11*, 73–91.

Sahler, O. J., Hunter, B. C., & Liesveld, J. L. (2003). The effect of using music therapy with relaxation imagery in the management of patients undergoing bone marrow transplantation: A pilot feasibility study. *Alternative Therapies in Health and Medicine, 9*(6), 70–74.

Saperston, B. (1995). The effects of consistent tempi and physiologically interactive tempi on heart rate and EMG responses. In T. Wigram, B. Saperston, & R. West, *The art & science of music therapy: A handbook* (pp. 55–82). Switzerland: Hardwood Academic.

Selm, M. E. (1991). Chronic Pain: Three issues in treatment and implications for music therapy. *Music Therapy Perspectives, 9*, 91–97.

Sherry, D. D. (2008). Avoiding the impact of musculoskeletal pain on quality of life in children with hemophilia. *Orthopedic Nursing, 27*(2), 103–108. DOI: 10.1097/01.NOR.0000315623.59385.2b.

Smith, J. (2005). *Relaxation, Meditation and Mindfulness: Training Manual*. Available at: http://www.lulu.com/items/volume_11/126000/126612/13/preview/Relaxation_Meditation_Mindfulness_Self-Study_Program.VERSION_2..FINAL_LULU_VERSIONwpd.pdf

Snyder Cowan, D. (1997). Managing sickle cell pain with music therapy. In J. V. Loewy (Ed.), *Music therapy and pediatric pain*. Cherry Hill, NJ: Jeffrey Books.

Solodiuk, J., & Curley, M. A. Q. (2003). Pain assessment in nonverbal children with severe cognitive impairments: The Individualized Numeric Rating Scale (INRS). *Journal of Pediatric Nursing, 18*, 295–299.

Steinke, W. R. (1991). The use of music, relaxation, and imagery in the management of postsurgical pain for scolioses. In C. Dileo-Maranto (Ed.), *Applications of music in medicine* (pp. 141–162). Silver Spring, MD: NAMT.

Stevens, B., Johnston, C., Petryshen, P., & Taddio, A. (1996). Premature infant pain profile: Development and initial validation. *Clinical Journal of Pain, 12*, 13–22.

Stevens, B. J., Abbott, L. K., Yamada, J., Harrison, D., Sinson, J., Tadio, A., Barwick, M., Latimer, M., Scott, S. D., Rashotte, J., Campbell, F., & Finley, A. (2011). Epidemiology and management of painful procedures in children in Canadian hospitals. *Canadian Medical Association Journal, 183*(7), E403–E410.

Turk, D. C., & Rudy, T. E. (1986). Assessment of cognitive factors in chronic pain: A worthwhile enterprise? *Journal of Consulting and Clinical Psychology, 54,* 760–768.

Turry, A. E. (1997). The use of clinical improvisation to alleviate procedural distress in young children. In J. V. Loewy (Ed.), *Music therapy and pediatric pain* (pp. 89–96). Cherry Hill, NJ: Jeffrey Books.

Varni, J. W., Thompson, K. L., & Hanson, V. (1987). The Varni/Thompson Pediatric Pain Questionnaire: I. Chronic musculoskeletal pain in juvenile rheumatoid arthritis. *Pain, 28,* 27–38.

Varni, J. W., Walco, G. A., & Katz, E. R. (1989). Assessment and management of chronic and recurrent pain in children with chronic diseases. *Pediatrician, 16,* 56–63.

von Baeyer, C. L. (2009). Numerical rating scale for self-report of pain intensity in children and adolescents: Recent progress and further questions. *European Journal of Pain, 13,* 1005–1007.

Walco, G., Cassidy, R., & Schechter, N. (1997). Pain, hurt and harm: The ethics of pain control in infants and children. In J. V. Loewy (Ed.), *Music therapy and pediatric pain* (pp. 23–32). Cherry Hill, NJ: Jeffrey Books.

Whipple, B., & Glynn, N. J. (1992). Quantification of the effects of listening to music as a noninvasive method of pain control. *Scholarly Inquiry for Nursing Practices, 6*(1), 42–59.

Whitehead-Pleaux, A., Baryza, M. J., & Sheridan, R. (2006). The effects of music therapy on pediatric pain and anxiety during a donor site dressing change. *Journal of Music Therapy, 43*(2), 136–153.

Whitehead-Pleaux, A. M., Clark, S. L., & Spall, L. E. (2011). Indications and counterindications for electronic music technologies in a pediatric medical setting. *Music and Medicine, 3,* 154–162.

Whitehead-Pleaux, A. M., Zebrowski, N., Baryza, M. J., & Sheridan, R. (2007). Exploring the effects of music therapy on pediatric pain: Phase 1. *Journal of Music Therapy, 44*(3), 217–241.

Wong, D. L., & Baker, C. (1988). Pain in children: Comparison of assessment scales. *Pediatric Nursing, 14,* 9–17.

Young, K. D. (2005). Pediatric procedural pain. *Annals of Emergency Medicine, 45,* 160–171.

Zajdeman, H. S., & Biederman, H. J. (1991). North American pediatric pain concepts, assessment procedures and treatment strategies: Overview and critique. *Archivio di Psicologia, Neurologia e Psichiatria, 52*(4), 505–513.

Zeltzer, L., Bursch, B., & Walco, G. (1997). Pain responsiveness and chronic pain: A psychobiological perspective. *Developmental and Behavioral Pediatrics, 18*(6), 413–422.

APPENDIX A

VISUAL ANALOGUE SCALE

VAS without anchors*

_____

VAS with verbal anchors

_____
No Pain   Severe Pain

*Important: all VAS lines must be exactly 100mm in length, not as shown here.

APPENDIX B

Poker Chip Tool Instruction Sheet[†]

English Instructions:

1. Say to the child: *"I want to talk with you about the hurt you may be having right now."*
2. Align the chips horizontally in front of the child on the bedside table, a clipboard, or other firm surface.
3. Tell the child, *"These are pieces of hurt."* Beginning at the chip nearest the child's left side and ending at the one nearest the right side, point to the chips and say, *"This* (first chip) *is a little bit of hurt and this* (fourth chip) *is the most hurt you could ever have."*

   For a young child or for any child who may not fully comprehend the instructions, clarify by saying, *"That means this* (one) *is just a little hurt, this* (two) *is a little more hurt, this* (three) *is more yet, and this* (four) *is the most hurt you could ever have."*

   - o Do not give children an option for zero hurt. Research with the Poker Chip Tool has verified that children without pain will so indicate by responses such as, "I don't have any."
4. Ask the child, *"How many pieces of hurt do you have right now?"*
   - o After initial use of the Poker Chip Tool, some children internalize the concept "pieces of hurt." If a child gives a response such as "I have one right now," *before* you ask or before you lay out the poker chips, proceed with instruction #5.
5. Record the number of chips on the Pain Flow Sheet.
6. Clarify the child's answer by words such as, *"Oh, you have a little hurt? Tell me about the hurt."*

Spanish Instructions[††]:

1. Tell the parent: *"Estas fichas de poker son unamanera de medir dolor. Usamos cuatro fichas rojas."*
2. Say to the child: *"Las fichas son como pedazos de dolor: una ficha (pedazo) es un poquito de dolor, mientras cuatro fichas (pedazos) significa el dolor máximo que tu puedes sentir. ¿Cuántos pedazos de dolor tienes?"*

[†]Developed in 1975 by Nancy O. Hester, University of Colorado Health Sciences Center, Denver, CO.

[††]Spanish instructions by Jordan-Marsh, M., Hall, D., Yoder, L., Watson, R., McFarlane-Sosa, G., & Garcia, M. (1990). The Harbor-UCLA Medical Center Humor Project for Children. Los Angeles: Harbor-UCLA Medical Center.

APPENDIX C[1]

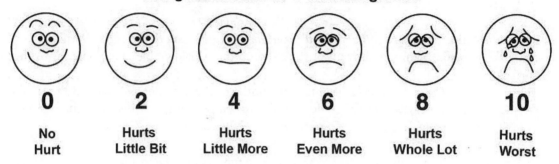

APPENDIX D

Children's Hospital of Eastern Ontario Pain Scale (CHEOPS) in Young Children

Overview: The CHEOPS (Children's Hospital of Eastern Ontario Pain Scale) is a behavioral scale for evaluating postoperative pain in young children. It can be used to monitor the effectiveness of interventions for reducing pain and discomfort.

Patients: The initial study was done on children 1 to 5 years of age. It has been used in studies with adolescents, but this may not be an appropriate instrument for that age group. According to Mitchell (1999), it is intended for ages 0–4

Parameter	Finding	Points
cry	no cry	1
	moaning	2
	crying	2
	screaming	3
facial	smiling	0
	composed	1
	grimace	2
child verbal	positive	0
	none	1
	complaints other than pain	1
	pain complaints	2
	both pain and nonpain complaints	2
torso	neutral	1
	shifting	2
	tense	2
	shivering	2
	upright	2
	restrained	2
touch	not touching	1
	reach	2
	Touch	2
	Grab	2
	Restrained	2
legs	Neutral	1
	squirming, kicking	2
	drawn up tense	2
	Standing	2
	Restrained	2

Definitions of Finding Terms:

- no cry: child is not crying
- moaning: child is moaning or quietly vocalizing silent cry
- crying: child is crying but the cry is gentle or whimpering
- screaming: child is in a full-lunged cry; sobbing may be scored with complaint or without complaint
- smiling: score only if definite positive facial expression
- composed: neutral facial expression
- grimace: score only if definite negative facial expression
- positive (verbal): child makes any positive statement or talks about other things without complaint
- none (verbal): child not talking
- complaints other than pain: child complains but not about pain ("I want to see Mommy" or "I am thirsty")
- pain complaints: child complains about pain
- both pain and nonpain complaints: child complains about pain and about other
- things (e.g., "It hurts"; "I want Mommy.")
- neutral (torso): body (not limbs) is at rest; torso is inactive
- shifting: body is in motion in a shifting or serpentine fashion
- tense: body is arched or rigid
- shivering: body is shuddering or shaking involuntarily
- upright: child is in a vertical or upright position
- restrained: body is restrained
- not touching: child is not touching or grabbing at wound
- reach: child is reaching for but not touching wound
- touch: child is gently touching wound or wound area
- grab: child is grabbing vigorously at wound
- restrained: child's arms are restrained
- neutral (legs): legs may be in any position but are relaxed; includes gently swimming
- squirming, kicking: definitive uneasy or restless movements in the legs and/or striking out with foot or feet
- drawn up tensed: legs tensed and/or pulled up tightly to body and kept there
- standing: standing, crouching, or kneeling
- restrained: child's legs are being held down

CHEOPS pain score = SUM (points for all 6 parameters)

Interpretation:
     Minimum score: 4
     Maximum score: 13

REFERENCES FOR APPENDIX D

Beyer, J. E., McGrath, P. J., & Berde, C. B. (1990). Discordance between self-report and behavioral pain measures in children aged 3–7 years after surgery. *Journal of Pain Symptom Management, 5,* 350–356.

Jacobson, S. J., Kopecky, E. A., et al. (1997). Randomised trial of oral morphine for painful episodes of sickle-cell disease in children. *Lancet, 350,* 1358–1361.

McGrath, P. J., Johnson, G., et al. (1985). CHEOPS: A behavioral scale for rating postoperative pain in children. *Advance in Pain Research and Therapy, 9,* 395–402.

McGrath, P. J., & McAlpine, L. (1993). Physiologic perspectives on pediatric pain. *Journal of Pediatrics, 122,* S2–S8.

Mitchell, P. Understanding a young child's pain. (1999). *Lancet, 354,* 1708.

Chapter 3

Premature Infants

Monika Nöcker-Ribaupierre

INTRODUCTION

Premature infants are special patients. They are so vulnerable physically and emotionally that they cannot survive on their own. After being delivered prematurely, these babies begin their lives in the highly mechanical environment of a Neonatal Intensive Care Unit (NICU), where they are confronted with intense and medically invasive care. The outcome of their hospital stay is highly dependent on their gestational age (GA) at birth: the more immature the infant is at birth, the more challenging and invasive the intensive medical care he receives. Preterm infants have to cope with deprivation, stress, and overstimulation, and the loss of their predictable and safe prenatal environment. A premature baby is also traumatizing for the parents because of uncertainty about both their child's survival and the impact the premature birth will have on their child's development. In addition, witnessing the invasive care their child needs can be very upsetting to parents.

Music therapy for those in neonatal care is a complex area of clinical practice requiring a range of professional competencies. Music therapists who provide services in NICU for preterm infants must possess basic knowledge in developmental psychology, be aware of the latest in neonatal research, and have an understanding of music medicine, music psychology, and music therapy practices for neonatal care. Effective music therapy services should be geared not only toward the infants but also toward the parents. In addition, the music therapist may work with the nursing staff as well, since working in a NICU environment is stressful and emotionally demanding.

This chapter will first provide basic knowledge regarding diagnostic information about premature infants. This will be followed by an overview of brain development, auditory development, and emotional development of a premature infant. It will then provide clinical guidelines for music therapy assessment and treatment in the neonatal intensive care environment. Finally, a summary of the available music therapy research involving preterm infants is presented.

DIAGNOSTIC INFORMATION

The NICU Environment

Intensive Care Units (ICUs), in general, are not open to the public. It should come as no surprise that those specifically established for premature and newborn infant care are also restricted. Nevertheless, NICUs can be noisy, busy, high-stress environments. During the last decade, there have been increasing efforts to reduce noise levels in the NICU (e.g., by using light alarms instead of acoustic ones) and to make the environment more private for families. Unfortunately, there are still many NICUs where noise and lack of privacy present significant challenges to the infants, caregivers, and staff. Although a few large NICU units have private rooms for nurses and parents, this is not common in most hospitals and some units may have the added discomfort of many incubators in close proximity of each other. It is often difficult for parents to have quiet time with their infant. In addition, the NICU environment remains rather dystopian because of all the mechanical equipment and commotion needed to ensure the survival of the infants staying there.

Today, family-centered care is a major focus of NICU care. There has been an increasing effort to facilitate interactions and attachments between parents and their infant by providing supportive transition services from the delivery room to the NICU and from the NICU to the home environment. Long gone are strictly enforced visiting hours. Now, parents are encouraged to visit their baby at any time, around the clock, and to stay as long as they wish. Many NICUs also encourage parents to hold their baby and enjoy skin-to-skin contact.

Clients after Preterm Birth: Infants, Parents, and Nursing Staff

A music therapist who works in the NICU serves multiple clients: the infant, the mother, the father, the family as a unit, and the nursing staff.

Infants. Preterm infants referred to a neonatal intensive care unit are born prior to 37 weeks' gestation. They frequently have a birth weight of less than 2,500 g (approximately 5.5 pounds). Continuous advancement in neonatal medicine during the last 30 years has ensured the survival of more extremely low birth weight infants. Today, the official limit of viability is around 23 weeks of gestation, although babies of slightly less than 22 weeks' gestation have survived.

Clinically we can differentiate subcategories of premature infants according to their birth weights (Rais-Bahrami & Short, 2013):

- Extremely low birth weight infant (ELBW) (typically infants 23–24 weeks)
- Very low birth weight infant (VLBW) (typically infants 25–28 weeks)
- Low birth weight infant (LBW) (typically infants 29–33 weeks)
- Late preterm infant(infants 34–37 weeks)

For the infant, premature birth can cause physical and mental trauma (Fischer & Als, 2004, 2012; Linderkamp & Skuroppa, 2008). Preterm infants are prematurely withdrawn from the rhythms created biologically (the cadenced sounds produced by their mother's heartbeat, breathing, blood flow through the placenta, etc.), the pace of their mother's movements, the closeness of her voice, and her constant physical and emotional presence. This trauma can lead to biophysical and social stress reactions.

Because of their developing autonomous nervous system, these infants have decreased self-protective and self-regulatory abilities. This means that they cannot filter or process harmful stimuli. As a result, they are extremely vulnerable to sensory stimuli such as noise, touch, and light, including the invasive and painful treatments they need to survive (Als, 1985; Fischer & Als, 2004, 2012; Wachman & Lahav, 2012; Zahr & Balian, 1995). This is problematic since many of these infants must stay in the NICU for several weeks or months. This unfamiliar, nonphysiological, highly mechanized environment is often chaotic and filled with bright lights and unpredictable noises. This overstimulation causes stress, anxiety, and agitation in the infant (Schwartz, Ritchie, Sacks, & Phillips, 1999). In order to deal with these stresses, the infant uses an enormous amount of energy, which he would normally invest in his growth and development (Schwartz, 2004). Often, the infant is sedated to help him reduce the stress-induced physiological effects and conserve energy. Moreover, in the NICU incubator environment, the baby has to live and grow while being deprived of the normal sensory experiences that surrounded him in his mother's womb.

The parents as a unit. During pregnancy, parents develop a strong attachment and desire to meet their baby after viewing him through ultrasounds, listening to heartbeats, checkups, and fetal movement. With the constant presence of the child in their lives, they were able to nurture their fantasies and their love toward him. The actual baby, who will be fragile, too small, covered with IVs and tubes, and housed in a plastic incubator, is completely different from what any parent will expect. In the first days after the delivery and the hospitalization of their baby, mother and father may be incapable of adapting to the situation. Like other families dealing with trauma, they may repeatedly ask the nurses the same questions, unable to register the answers. They are confronted with the typical ICU uncertainties: The baby's physical condition may change from one hour to the other. In addition, the clinical outcome and the length of hospitalization are unpredictable, especially in early stages, causing high anxiety. Several times, the parents may witness alarms and emergency, lifesaving efforts performed on their child.

Research suggests that parents feel overwhelmed and helpless in the high-tech NICU environment and often suffer from disappointment, depression, anger, and anxiety. Without adequate psychological support, this may lead to subsequent social and emotional problems within the family (Jotzo & Poets, 2005; Treyvaud, Doyle, Lee, Roberts, Cheong, Inder, & Anderson, 2011; Vonderlin, 1999; Wereszcak, Shandor Miles, & Holditch-Davis, 1997). In addition to combined fears and stresses, each parent has their own unique reactions to a preterm infant.

The mother. Mothers of premature infants are vulnerable to developing post-traumatic stress disorder (Jotzo & Poets, 2005). For a woman, premature birth is a situation of unexpected bodily and emotional separation from her child. Research suggests that the profound stressors caused by this separation are akin to experiencing trauma firsthand. Moreover, these mothers experience feelings of guilt and depression, mourning, lack of self-worth, and fear for the survival and development of their baby. These feelings create a barrier that makes it difficult for a woman to develop a positive emotional relationship with her child (Caplan, Manson, & Kaplan, 1965; Jotzo & Poets, 2005; Klaus & Kennell, 1976; Nöcker-Ribaupierre, 1998; Vonderlin, 1999). Mothers of multiple births have been prepared for the possibility of premature birth and as a result seem to accept the NICU situation better. Although they may be physically weakened, it has been this author's observation that they tend to be mentally more stable and active.

Because NICU care primarily focuses on the survival and development of the infant to term outside of the womb, the mother's emotional needs are often overlooked by staff. The impact of the premature delivery may be compounded by the mother's own personal vulnerability and even genetic propensity to developing depression. Her emotional symptoms can be as diverse as fear, insecurity, withdrawal, emotional paralysis, restlessness, and overprotectiveness. Fortunately, recent research has helped to build a more complete picture of mothers' experiences and has underlined the necessity to establish psychological support for them (Aagaard & Hall, 2008; Coppola & Cassibba, 2010; Nöcker-Ribaupierre, 2004; Ravn, Smith, Aarhus Smeby, Kynoe, Snadvic, Haugen Bunch, & Lindemann, 2011; Zimmer, 2004).

Consider the following scenario, which gives a brief glimpse of a mother's experiences with her premature NICU baby: Tracy feels her pregnancy was not yet finished; she had not grown into her maternal identity. Her baby is not real; it does not resemble those she saw in the baby books. Her womb is empty, and so are her arms because Tracy's baby is too medically compromised for her to hold him. She cannot protect her baby from the threatening, chaotic environment or the many invasive procedures of the NICU. She feels completely helpless. She cannot help her baby stay alive; the safety of her womb has been replaced by doctors, nurses, and equipment. She can neither communicate with her baby nor convey her love through the hard incubator that separates them. She cannot see her baby's smile beneath the medical tape and tubes helping him to breathe or feel her baby wrap his delicate fingers around hers. Without any outward responses to her, she deeply questions if he loves her or even realizes she is there waiting to hold him for the first time.

The father. After a premature delivery, the father becomes preoccupied and concerned with the survival of both mother and child. Initially, he may feel compelled to act like an emergency manager, attempting to organize this unpredictable situation. When the mother is not physically stable enough to visit her baby, he develops into an important link between the maternity ward and the NICU. At the same time, he must also continue to support the whole family emotionally and financially while maintaining the home and potentially taking care of older siblings. He has to find a balance between his job, his home, and the hospital during the transition to a new and stressful fatherhood. Because of his different social role and because he has not experienced the pregnancy or delivery physically, a father has different strategies for dealing with this situation. His job may be the only thing that offers him a sense of normality and refuge from the chaotic and uncertain situation.

In the NICU environment, the father tends to focus on understanding the technical equipment, without necessarily interacting with the infant or striving for emotional attachment to his child. Observations of a father's behaviors in the NICU are encouraging nurses to strive for a better understanding of the father' s needs, to develop ways to support him, and to help him better cope with this life event (Nagorski-Johnson, 2008). The literature and current clinical practice clearly demonstrate important benefits of supporting both mother and father to develop positive interactions with their child, to encourage emotional bonding, to actively participate in caring for their baby, and to experience unconditional love. Both parents need to be included in NICU family-centered care whenever possible to strengthen their identity as partners.

The nursing staff. Members of the nursing staff report that they are often negatively affected by the constant NICU noise and stress. This can lead to desensitization to the environment and to their work with the infants (Aagaard & Hall, 2008). Music therapists need to be aware of these needs. Since NICU nurses play a crucial role in the development of mother–child bonding, it is important that their emotional well-being is safeguarded. An increasing number of studies have suggested that the mother's ability to learn how to mother a preterm infant is dependent on her professional relationship with the nurses. The nurses are primary caregivers for the baby, they attend to the infant around the clock, and they provide security when the mother is handling the baby. Although this professional care is necessary, it may highlight the mother's feelings of inadequacy and of not truly being the baby's mother. To help counteract these feelings, it is important for the nurses to establish a relationship with the mother and include her in the baby's care at least verbally, by continuously answering the mother's questions, sharing knowledge, or just friendly chatting.

The nurses' readiness to promote the relationship between parents and infant supports the music therapist's family-centered work. But the music therapist also has to be sensitive to the nurses' problems concerning the acoustic stressors. This involves close contact and exchange of information about the music therapy approach, procedures, expectations, and limits (Hanson-Abromeit, 2004, 2012).

The Infant's Development

When looking at intrauterine development, it is obvious that a fetus is capable of taking in sensory impulses long before regular-term birth. That means that the sensory organs are able to influence the structural, functional, and emotional development of the fetus (Fischer & Als, 2004, 2012).

Brain development. Knowledge of brain development has been rapidly increasing during the last 10 years. The thesis of experience-dependent brain development has been substantiated by a large number of international studies (De Graaf-Peters & Hadders-Algra, 2006; Elliot, 2000; Fox,

Levitt, & Nelson III, 2010; Linderkamp, Janus, Linder, & Skoruppa, 2009; Turkewitz, 2007). This data is of prime interest for neonatal care.

Several studies on fetal brain development have revealed that environmental factors are influential in brain development even from the beginning of gestation. As postgestational age increases, the role these factors play becomes increasingly important. In the course of brain development, there are four distinct milestones related to defined developmental periods:

1) From 7 to 22 weeks, 20 billion neurons form and then move to their final positions in the brain.

2) From 20 to 35 weeks, the foundation of the cortex develops. In fetal brain cells, this is a critical period classified by high plasticity prior to the neurons becoming mature brain cells. This transitional time period is most important for brain development.

3) Beginning at 24 weeks and continuing throughout life, the neural network begins its organization by forming nerve fibres and synapses, and half the neurons are destroyed in an effort to shape the brain and reduce overlap that can make communication more organized and accurate.

4) During the last weeks of gestation, axonal myelination (or sheathing) begins in order to speed signal transmission; this continues for the first few decades of life. (Linderkamp et al., 2009)

Neuroscientific evidence suggests that early brain development, namely the neurogenesis (6–23 weeks of gestation) and neuronal migration (22–34 weeks of gestation), is largely determined by genes. However, early adverse environmental conditions, such as stress or sensory deprivation, can change, hinder, or affect this development (Bergmann, Sarkar, O'Connor, Modi, & Glover, 2007; Linderkamp, Janus, Linder, & Skuroppa, in press). This means that both fetal experiences and fetal environmental factors influence preliminary neural connections (Fox, Lewitt, & Nelson III, 2010). As a result, the developing neural network adapts to environmental and individual needs. This phenomenon is referred to as brain plasticity.

There are three types of brain plasticity:

1) *Experience-independent plasticity* refers to the fact that the basic structural brain development (e.g., neurogenesis, neuronal migration, and early neurite and synapse formation) is determined primarily by genetic factors.

2) *Experience-expectant plasticity* refers to the assimilation of environmental data received through channels such as the basic sensory perceptions. Because this input of information will only trigger the change during the critical period of sensitivity (in this case, from 24 weeks until birth), without appropriate environmental feedback during this time, certain neural functions, like vision, will not develop normally.

3) *Experience-dependent plasticity* describes how the brain is modified after exposure to sensory input. Unlike experience-expectant plasticity, which requires sensory input in order for the brain to develop normally, experience-dependent plasticity is centered on learning unique attributes. It influences the development of special skills (e.g., memory, association, social competence) from birth until the end of life. (Linderkamp et al., in press)

Neuroscientific evidence confirms that these different types of brain plasticity are the basis for human development and acquiring specific human abilities (Linderkamp et al., in press; Neves, Cooke, & Bliss, 2008). Experience-dependent plasticity works as a double-edged sword and can make the developing brain vulnerable to adverse experiences. For example, deprivation from sensory experiences can hinder development. Therefore, any treatment or therapy created for premature infants should focus on experience-expectant plasticity and the challenge of providing appropriate environmental conditions and stimulation.

The complex interactions between genes and environment guarantee the individuality of each person. A prematurely born infant, deprived of appropriate experiences and exposed to severe stress, may suffer from long-term sensory, behavioral, and cognitive impairments (Fischer & Als, 2004, 2012; Hüppi, Schuknecht, Boesch, Bossi, Fusch, & Herschkowitz, 1996).

Earlier follow-up studies and special care like NIDCAP have verified that the antenatal stress of mothers is easily transferred to the fetus as premature stress (Achenbach, Howell, Aoki, & Rauh, 1993; Als, Duffy, McAnoulty, Rivkin, Vajapeyam, & Mulkern, 2004; Als & Gilkerson, 1999). Recent neuroscientific studies conclude that maternal stress has many adverse effects on fetal brain development. There are critical development periods, which are sensitive to the neurobiological effects of specific stressors, especially maternal stress. Maternal stress releases corticosteroids to the fetus that influence hippocampus development (the part of the brain where memories are stored) (Fenogli, Brunson, & Baram, 2006). Maternal stress beginning at 22 weeks and continuing to birth has been linked to developmental delays, lowered IQ, and behavioral problems (Bergmann, Sarkar, O'Connor, Modi, & Glover, 2007).

Developmental follow-up studies show that in comparison to full-term infants, preterm infants have a significant risk for neurodevelopmental problems. These include serious educational problems, such as attention deficit disorders, language comprehension and speech problems, emotional vulnerability, specific learning disabilities, consistently lower IQ, visual–motor impairments, and difficulties in self-regulation. There is increasing evidence that these impairments result from permanent high stress levels (Fischer & Als, 2004; Hüppi et al., 1996; Linderkamp & Skoruppa, unpublished; Volpe, 2008).

Since NICU preterm infants usually suffer from both deprivation and stress, they are at high risk to develop cognitive and behavioral problems due to functional impairment of the prefrontal cortex, the hippocampus and amygdala (of the limbic system), and of the fiber tracts connecting these centers (Anderson & Doyle, 2008).

Hearing development. Human beings develop hearing ability very early in their development. In the developing embryo, the initial structure of the ear is laid out within the third week. At the same time, the cochlear nucleus also appears where the auditory nerve has its origin. Then, beginning in the fourth week, one can observe the development of the cochlear duct, where the sensory cells of the organ of Corti are situated. The cochlea begins functioning at the age of 18 weeks (Rubel, 1984).

This means that the fetus has a working auditory system for the entire last trimester of pregnancy. This was verified through early physiological measurements: Fetal responsiveness to outside stimuli has been measured either by observation of eye blink responses to vibro-acoustic stimulation (Birnholtz & Benacerraf, 1983) or by the monitoring of fetal pulse rate after 24 weeks of gestation (Hepper & Shahidullah, 1994). In fact, at only 19 weeks' GA, a fetus has been observed changing body activity or inactivity in response to a 500 Hz tone (Hepper & Shahidullah, 1994). After 28 weeks of gestation, consistently present responses indicate the maturation of the auditory pathways in the central nervous system.

Research concludes that, after this week of development, those fetuses in whom no observable responses to auditory stimuli occur typically are diagnosed later with severe sensorial hearing loss or with nonauditory anomalies (Birnholtz & Benacerraf, 1983). Recent research shows that although auditory functioning begins after about 20 weeks, adultlike auditory threshold levels are not mature until by about 35 weeks' gestation. At term, the newborn infant's sensitivity and frequency resolution has reached adult levels (Gooding, 2010; Graven & Browne, 2008; Lasky & Williams, 2009).

The background sounds (or sound floor) of the uterus are predominantly produced by maternal blood flow, respiration, digestion, and movement. These sounds are the backdrop above which maternal vocalisations and externally generated sounds emerge. What actually is discernible for the fetus is determined by attenuation of sound levels in the different frequency ranges. The high-pass filter function of the tissues and fluids of pregnancy shapes any external stimuli before they reach the fetal auditory system and thus protects the fetus from being overwhelmed by noise. The maternal womb reduces frequency ranges above 500 Hz by 40 to 50 dB and below 500 Hz by 10 to 20 dB before they reach the inner ear of the fetus. Within the frequency range below 500 Hz, he cannot hear speech and music when the intrauterine noise floor sound level exceeds the external sound level by about 10 dB. In other words, the fetus can hear outside sounds only when the airborne sound levels exceed 60 dB (Gerhardt & Abrams, 2004).

Researchers conclude that this prominence of lower frequencies helps focus the fetus on the frequency range of speech (Standley, 2003a). The mother's voice has an immediate effect on the fetus; this may provide an idea of fetal ability to process sensory information (Fifer & Moon, 1988). Researchers postulate that prenatal experience with auditory stimulation, especially with the mother's voice, is the precursor to postnatal linguistic development (Nöcker-Ribaupierre, 1999; Maiello, 2004; McMahon, Wintermark, & Lahav, 2012; Wachman & Lahav, 2010). Specifically, studies have shown that newborn infants:

- distinguish the words they heard repeatedly during their prenatal life from unfamiliar words (DeCasper & Fifer, 1980);
- prefer female voices to male voices, the mother's voice to other female voices, and voices from the same ethnic group to those of other groups (Casper & Spence, 1986; Moon, Cooper, & Fifer, 1993);
- discriminate between ascending and descending intonation if both scales are sung by the same voice on the same vowel (Fernald, 1989).

Emotional development. Decades ago, researchers verified that the mother's biological and psychological conditions influence the physical and emotional well-being and development of the unborn child. This makes sense knowing that the mother and child are connected biologically and emotionally while the infant is developing. They also found that the mother's emotional or psychological disturbances during pregnancy increase heart rate activity in the fetus and affect the reactions of newborns after birth. In addition, metabolic instability (e.g., through maternal drug abuse) causes endocrinological changes in the infant (Ferreira, 1965; Rottman, 1974). The stressful environment of the NICU has been compared to in vivo maternal stress and has similar effects on fetal development.

Psychologists agree that the capacity for self-regulation is set in motion with the exchange of social behavior, or the communication and interaction between the infant and his mother, which begins prenatally. Right after birth, the full-term infant demonstrates the ability to recognize an object with the help of one sense (e.g., seeing) with which he became familiar through another sense (e.g., hearing) (Eagle, 1984). The infant researcher, Daniel Stern, labelled this ability "cross-modal awareness" (1985, 2010). He recommends that voices and faces (e.g., of mother and father) should come together in order to support the infant's development and social communication. This recommendation extends to the last weeks of preterm infant development; it can be observed in premature infants from about 36 weeks onward (in other words, four weeks ahead of normal birth date). At this point, the baby is no longer happy being exposed to his mother's recorded voice alone; he becomes increasingly agitated to see her face at the same time (Nöcker-Ribaupierre, 1995, 2004).

Infant researchers, prenatal psychologists, and psychotherapists theorize that the development of an infant must be regarded from a holistic viewpoint, requiring both the mother, with her bodily and emotional presence, and the rest of the family.

NEEDS AND RESOURCES

The music therapist must have a clear understanding of normal infant neurological and functional development, as well as preterm infant behavior, stressors, and behavioral responses to those stressors. With this knowledge in mind, she can address the preterm infant's needs and resources.

Stressors after Premature Birth

Inside the mother's womb the fetus is highly protected from outside noise and light. In addition, the womb offers a controlled space of ideal warmth and humidity. This environment allows all sensorial and cortical systems to develop at an appropriate pace before being required to manage uncensored life outside the intrauterine world.

A premature birth forces the infant's immature sensorial and cortical systems to develop with interference. Unprotected, the infant is extremely vulnerable to all kinds of environmental stressors, which may have a harmful impact on his development.

Premature infants react to stress-inducing noises with observable and measurable physiological stress responses. These include reduced oxygen saturation, increased rates of apnea and bradycardia, wide fluctuations in blood pressure, increased excitement and agitation, crying, and sleep disturbances. Consequently, premature babies are often treated with sedatives in order to handle and to reduce these effects.

Acoustic stressors. In NICUs, the preterm infant is exposed to a spectrum of unexpected noises, from the constant low frequencies of the incubator motor to the unfiltered high-frequency sounds from monitor alarms and ventilation devices. This aversive ambient noise is accompanied by the telephone ringing, staff conversation, housekeeping, equipment movement, other infants crying, and sometimes radio music, which combines into an unpredictably chaotic sound field. In addition, when the preterm infant cries, the noise is amplified within the incubator (Wachman & Lahav, 2012).

The noise level in an intensive care unit may range from a very low 38 dB to 75–90 dB; this is equivalent to the sound level of a vacuum cleaner or heavy traffic. Inside the incubator, sound levels vary from the base 45 dB to impulse noise peaks of 120 dB (e.g., Philbin, 2000). Although recent technology has developed closed incubators, which diminish the ambient NICU noise by 10% (compared to the 45% noise reduction of the mother's womb), the closed incubator cannot protect from outside noise (Wubben, Brueggeman, Helseth, & Blaschle, 2011).

The noise spectrum inside the incubator can be summarized as follows:

- NICU noise is mostly produced by technical equipment such as ventilation and alarms, as well as by human inattentiveness (Beyers, Waugh, & Lowman, 2006; Philbin, 2000).
- In general, the incubator itself increases noise levels (Fischer & Als, 2004; Philbin, 2000).
- Impulse noises, such as tapping a finger on the outside of the incubator, can produce noises of 80 dB inside the unit, which is comparable to heavy traffic; placing an object on the Isolette or closing the solid plastic portholes becomes a 100 dB noise; a ringing telephone can create a 114 dB noise, which is categorized as a painful sound

level (American Academy of Pediatrics, Committee on Environmental Health, AAP, 1997).

- Constant noise in NICU above 45 dB can lead to cochlear damage (Lasky & Williams, 2005; Nzama, Nolte, & Dorfling, 1995; Zahr & Balian, 1995)

The effects of these high sound levels are comparable to the effects of ototoxic drugs. They result in constant sleep disturbance and even sleep deprivation for the baby (Fischer & Als, 2004, 2012). It should come as no surprise that congenital hearing loss in preterm infants increases as the GA of a birth decreases. This trend could be caused by the fact that the younger premature infants have more immature auditory systems being exposed to unfiltered noise or that they have longer periods of exposure to the ambient noise of the NICU due to prolonged mechanical ventilation, lengthened hospital stays, and additional physical problems requiring noisy interventions (Gooding, 2010). Noise-induced hearing loss and severe hearing problems are linked to ambient noise exposure (Lasky & Williams, 2005; Wachman & Lahav, 2010; Zahr & Traversy, 1995).

Recent research has focused on the influence of NICU noise upon the well-being and long-term development of premature infants. For example, it has been suggested that the high number of speech and language problems found in children born prematurely may be related in part to auditory processing dysfunction associated with NICU ambient noise (Gorski, Huntington, & Lewkovicz, 1990; Graven, 2000; Wachman & Lahav, 2010). Others have reported that the loud transient noise also has short-term, aversive effects on the respiratory and cardiovascular systems of premature infants. This, in turn, leads to multiple episodes of bradycardia and apnea, as well as brief changes in heart rate and blood pressure (Doheny, Hurwitz, Insoft, Ringer, & Lahav, 2012; Wachman & Lahav, 2010).

Due to increasing concerns about long-term exposure to aversive auditory stimuli and the possible resulting hearing loss, the AAP Committee on Environmental Health (1997) and the National Consensus Committee (White, 2007) highly recommend that environmental noise levels within NICU should be as far below (and not exceed) an hourly level of 45 dB on an A-weight scale (dBA) as possible. Unfortunately, no NICU (with the exception of some Swedish NICUs) has been able to document meeting these recommended sound levels. In addition, despite the vast technological improvements over the years, incubators may still produce or amplify noise levels above what is recommended.

Environmental stressors. As stated before, the earliest possible time for surviving is at around 19 weeks' gestation. By 23 to 24 weeks, all sensory organs are sufficiently mature enough to receive input. At 24 weeks, most neurons may be poorly connected, but they have, for the most part, developed and migrated to their final location inside the brain. In extremely low birth weight infants (ELBW), each neuron is connected, on average, to one other neuron. In contrast, full-term neonates generally have each neuron connected to 1,000 other neurons. Since ELBW infants may live up to two months in the incubator and four months in the hospital, their fundamental brain development occurs in a highly abnormal, physiologically stressful environment. Furthermore, it occurs while experiencing separation from their mother, psychoemotional deprivation, environmental overstimulation, invasive painful experiences, and multiple caregivers. Thus, these children may "learn" on an implicit level that their environment is stressful during a time when their brain is less conditioned to work on a high-stress level.

Emotional stressors. Infants exposed to permanent stress tend to withdraw or to develop high irritability. Since little can be done by caregivers to help the infant regulate himself, the infant does not learn to seek help or to self-regulate. In addition to the impact of stress on the infant's development and on his behavior, exposing preterm infants to stress can also create transitioning issues, such as having an impaired ability to transition from irritability to calm or from awake to sleep. These situations can be influenced with the help of music therapy (see the section on guidelines).

Infant reactions to stress. Infants communicate their stress and self-regulatory behavior through visible cues from their autonomic nervous system, as well as motor- and self-regulation systems. The infant's vital signs, such as heart rate, respiration rate, and oxygen saturation, are predictors of his behavior and are constantly monitored. On the physical level these signs indicate the primary survival needs of the infant. Any therapy and stimulation program can be applied only with careful monitoring and response to these signs. In addition to measured signs, the infants show clear, observable expressions of stress and self-regulation (Fischer & Als, 2004, 2012; Hanson-Abromeit, Shoemark, & Loewy, 2008; Standley, 2003a).

The following overview defines what type of infant behaviors (autonomic nervous and motor systems, self-regulation) indicates distress (beyond crying) and what type of behaviors suggests appropriate self-regulation:

Autonomic Nervous System
- Indicators for stability: smooth respiration; a pink, healthy-looking skin color; and visceral stability.
- Stress signals: seizures, apnea (respiratory pauses), rapid or slow breathing, holding the breath, color changes (jaundiced, pale, red-purple-blue), spitting up, hiccupping, burping, gasping, yawning, sighing, and sneezing (frequency-dependent).

Motor System
- Indicators for stability: regulated muscle tone, smooth movements, sucking, hand clasping, hand-to-mouth movement, grasping, and holding.
- Stress signals: flaccid hands and legs, extension of trunk (stretch, arch), active and posture-extended arms and legs, finger moving, facial grimacing, hyperflexion, and activity.

Self-regulation/Subsystem
- Indicators for stability: clear sleep states, rhythmical crying, ability to self-quiet, alertness, animated facial expression, smiling, and cooing.
- Stress signals: irritability, crying, hyperalertness, staring, roving, and sleeplessness.

The Needs of the Premature Infant

The development of the infant's senses and inner organs increases rapidly by the time of the third trimester of pregnancy, when extrauterine life in NICU is possible. During this developmental period, the infant's capacity to tolerate different levels of stimulation is rapidly increasing. Stimulation programs during this time need to be adapted to and follow the developing neurological and functional patterns of the baby. If the infant is ill or too distressed, the music therapist has to accept in a nonjudgmental way parental and staff decisions about treatment or nontreatment. At any developmental stage, the therapist must recognize the infant's warning signs of distress and decreasing desire for interaction. The main purpose of the music therapist is to provide a musically calming and soothing environment with voice and soft instruments—and to help the baby develop an awakening interest in social interaction.

One must recognize that the parent's emotional states will stabilize with the infant's increasing development. The music therapist can support the parents' discovery of their resources and strengths by helping them to accept their fears and anxieties and by encouraging them to talk about the real or imagined problems they may have. The music therapist should offer enough time in each session to support the parents' needs for communication. She has to be aware and accept that she is part of a sometimes problematic developing process, and she needs empathy and patience for the parents. The music therapist may sometimes feel that the parents are not really listening to her when they ask repetitive questions, but the true reason for this behavior is that they often understand answers only according to their capability to bear and to cope with their situation. By supporting the parents in overcoming their acute stress and anxiety, the therapist strengthens their resources and helps the infant to better regulate his physiological systems because he is dependent upon his caregiver's emotional feedback (Winberg, 2005). This works in reverse as well: If the music therapist provides musical tools that help the infant to calm down, to relax, to increase positive parental interactions, this will help the parents to accept their new child as he is and to bond with him.

The needs of the infant and his parents are obvious: Their resources are undeveloped, hidden, or buried. This can be addressed through music therapy. Providing music therapy in the NICU should be based on the assumption that each premature infant is an individual, and, together with his respective family, he forms a unique unit. Music therapy provides increasing assistance for developing family attachment while, at the same time, decreasing the multiple stress factors in the environment.

To ensure that clinical quality therapy is provided, detailed referral and assessment procedures have been formulated.

REFERRAL AND ASSESSMENT

Referrals for music therapy may be made by individual staff or family members or may be based on predetermined criteria (Hanson-Abromeit et al., 2008). Several music therapists have created research- and practice-based referral and assessment forms to be used in music therapy practice in NICUs (Hanson-Abromeit, 2004, 2012; Hanson-Abromeit et al., 2008; Loewy, 2004, 2007, 2012; Shoemark, 2004; Standley, 2003a).

This section will present the forms created by these authors for review. These forms require music therapy–specific information, as well as information provided by the medical staff, in order to obtain a complete assessment profile. Since most academic music therapy training programs do not provide advanced instruction on the assessment of premature infant responses to music stimuli and medical knowledge related to NICU care, it is important that music therapists wishing to work in NICUs participate in a specialized NICU training course.

Referral Criteria and Forms

In general, the referral criteria for music therapy are dependent on the philosophy of the treatment team, on available research, and on hospital-specific procedures (e.g., need for physician approval, individually generated vs. criteria-based approval) (Hanson-Abromeit et al., 2008).

The following referral criteria are based on research and extensive clinical practice.

- *Medical music therapy referral:* The first set of referral criteria were developed by Standley and are based on medical parameters: The infant must be a minimum of 28 weeks' GA, must be at least one week old, and must be either medically stable or have been referred by the professional team and the family. The medical indications for music therapy interventions are, for example, agitated or disorganized behavior, a need for prolonged or high oxygen ventilation, and events which may require prolonged hospitalization (Standley, 2003a; Standley & Walworth, 2010).
- *Beth Israel Medical Center Music Therapy Referral Criteria* (Loewy, 2004, 2012): An important criterion for music therapy referrals at the Beth Israel Medical Center is that no music therapy practice can be offered to an infant without the prior informed consent of the family. This standard is based upon the growing emphasis of family-

centered care in the NICU. However, the family does not necessarily need to be involved in the music therapy sessions.

The referral criteria consider different issues related to the infant's state of being: if the infant is irritable or has trouble in making transitions from being awake to sleep, for example. It also draws attention to when the infant has limited opportunity for developmental activities, such as when the infant is unable to react or to respond vocally or physically to stimuli because of intubation. In addition, it gives referral weight to infants who do not have both parents available, to the nursing staff, and to those in need of psychoemotional and/or social support.

Two referral forms are included in the Appendix as they are currently used in the NICU at Beth Israel Medical Center. One form lists the specific referral criteria (Appendix A), and the other form is used to document the referral (Appendix B). These forms are based upon the music therapy experiences that Loewy acquired while working exclusively with live music, voice, and different instruments. The referral criteria include to support bonding; to reduce irritability, pain, crying, and respiratory difficulties; to support feeding procedures; and to promote sedation, sleep, and self-regulation. It also includes music therapy approaches for providing a safe and calm environment by using the music therapist's voice and diverse instruments.

Assessment

Since music therapists provide extra stimulation to the infant, it is important for the therapist to be able to accurately interpret the infant's responses to this stimulation. This requires knowledge of how and to what extent music can elicit and regulate the infant's physical and physiological responses and affect the development of his sensory system. This knowledge will allow the well-trained NICU music therapist to appropriately apply sensory stimulation.

Specific NICU assessment forms have been developed by Deanna Hanson-Abromeit, Joanne Loewy, and Jane Standley and Jennifer Whipple:

- *NICU Music Therapy Assessment Summary* (Hanson-Abromeit, 2003; Hanson-Abromeit, Shoemark, & Loewy, 2008): This assessment form gathers information about the infant's physical and sensory responses, the course of his hospital stay, and his prognosis. It also includes information about the infant's family and strategies for how to support them (Appendix C).
- *Music Therapy Assessment at Beth Israel Medical Center* (Loewy, 2004, 2007, 2012): This assessment tool gathers information about the infant's physiological responses, crying behavior, psychosocial needs, feeding behavior, responses to sensory and proprioceptive stimulation, pain, and need for sedatives. This assessment tool is used in the NICU Music Therapy Treatment Program at Beth Israel Medical Center (New York) (Appendix D).
- *Premature Infant Assessment and Treatment History* (Standley, 2003a; Whipple, 2001): This assessment tool gathers information about the infant's auditory, visual, motor, and social/communicative responses. The form is used at the Music Therapy Program at Tallahassee Memorial Hospital (Appendix E).

Introduction to Music Therapy Methods

Longitudinal studies have shown that premature infants have a significantly higher risk for neurodevelopmental problems than their full-term peers (e.g., Anderson & Doyle, 2008; Fischer & Als, 2004, 2012; Volpe, 2008). As a result, the goal of neonatal care has shifted from merely survival to prevention of major disabilities by safeguarding normal brain development as much as possible. As a result of this shift, the three main goals for NICU music therapy practice are to

1) support the infant's neurobehavioral and sensory system development by providing individualized music therapy interventions;
2) increase social, emotional, cognitive, motor, and communication developmental competencies by providing balanced sound/sensory stimulation and avoiding overstimulation;
3) engage and support the infant's parents by providing opportunities for culturally appropriate infant–parent interaction and bonding. (Hanson-Abromeit et al., 2008)

Music therapy in neonatal intensive care is based on 20 years of music therapy research and clinical practice as well as cumulative knowledge of premature and newborn infant development and human responsiveness to music. In addition, NICU music therapy practices are influenced by different treatment philosophies (e.g., behavioral, psychodynamic).

The literature regarding the use of music with premature infants has predominantly focused on the use of receptive techniques (i.e., listening to prerecorded music). However, during the last decade, music therapy interventions have increasingly included many possibilities for human interactions and communication through live music such as singing or humming by the music therapist a cappella or with soft instrumental accompaniment as well as the inclusion of the parents in providing musical interactions to their infant. It is important to distinguish the use of prerecorded music by the NICU medical staff from the use of music by a trained music therapist: Music therapists provide individualized music to premature infants, and the interventions are based on a detailed assessment of the infant and careful observation of the infant's response to sensory stimulation.

In general, music therapy work with premature infants requires

- a clear understanding of normal fetal and neonatal development, the impact of preterm birth on infant development, and stress responses in preterm infants (Shoemark, 2011);
- specialized music skills (especially vocal) to meet the premature infant's needs in stressful situations and to support, contain, and enhance the infant's development;
- knowledge about appropriate voice and instrument use in the NICU environment so as to avoid overstimulation;
- knowledge about the infant's capacities to respond to musical elements on a physiological, behavioral, and psychological level (Hanson-Abromeit et al., 2008);
- knowledge of established parameters for recorded music presentation: volume, level, duration, and individual applied frequencies (Shoemark, 2011);
- understanding of the physiological and emotional impact of the NICU environment on the infant, the parents, and the staff (Shoemark, 2011);
- insight into the potential emotional distress and trauma that a premature delivery may bring to the parents and skills in music psychotherapeutic interventions to support them (Nöcker-Ribaupierre, 2004, 2011; Stewart, 2009; Zimmer, 2004);

- skills in engaging parents in musical activities that enable them to communicate musically with their infants (Hanson-Abromeit, 2006; Hanson-Abromeit et al., 2008; Loewy, 2011; Shoemark, 2004; Standley, 2000; Whipple, 2005).

As this work is quite demanding for the music therapist in various ways, emotionally and physically, supervision is required to help the music therapist understand her involvement in the therapeutic process and to stabilize her involvement physically, mentally, and emotionally. Supervision should be provided by a NICU music therapist. RBL (Rhythm, Breath, and Lullaby) Training is currently being grandfathered in 13 countries. A monograph defining specific guidelines and training modules accompanies the yearlong supervision leading to certification in the application of these interventions.

Music Therapy Interventions According to Stages of Sensory Development

A premature infant who is between 23 and 40 weeks' GA in the NICU follows the same developmental sequences as a fetus in the womb. Even in infants with extreme prematurity (23–24 weeks' GA), sensory systems are capable of processing and reacting to various stimuli. However, premature babies react more slowly to sensory stimulation than full-term babies; the younger the infant, the slower the reaction. As the infant matures, so does his ability to tolerate sensorial interventions. When providing routine care as well as sensory stimulation programs, one must carefully consider the current developmental state of the infant. Therefore, music therapy programming in the NICU must adhere to the following developmental guidelines:

23–24 weeks: This is the earliest possible age of survival. The infant needs pacification. Musical stimulation must not be offered to infants this young.

25–28 weeks: The infant remains in various sleep states. He may react with minimal startles to sound. The soft toning voice of the therapist may have soothing effects. The mother's voice (recorded or live) is preferred to support bonding. Instrumental stimulation is not appropriate.

28–31 weeks: Prerecorded musical stimulation can cautiously be provided but must be carefully monitored for signs of overstimulation.

32 weeks: Increased tolerance for acoustic and multimodal stimulation. Toning, humming, and lullaby-singing by the mother and the music therapist, preferably in combination with kangaroo care and massage, are recommended. The infant begins to show state regulation.

34 weeks: The infant begins to socially respond to parents and caregivers. The mother's and father's voice and the therapist's interactive singing support social interaction.

36 weeks onward: Responses to auditory stimuli are now predictable and state-dependent (i.e., an infant who is asleep will respond less than when awake). The infant begins to habituate to lower-frequency sound stimuli and develop cross-modal capacities in integrating various stimuli (visual, auditory, tactile): he seeks voice in combination with touching, holding, being carried, for example. The infant reciprocates social interactions and may begin to smile in response to positive stimulation. (Hanson-Abromeit, 2006; Loewy, 2012; Nöcker-Ribaupierre, 2004; Standley, 2010; Whipple, 2000)

Regardless of the infant's age, constant and careful observation of the infant's responses is needed. Before beginning any music interventions, approval must be obtained from the infant's nurse.

When the infant is ill or has gone through medical procedures, the infant's nurse may decide that music is not indicated at this moment. In addition, the timing of the administration of the music is coordinated with the medical staff so that the intervention will not be interrupted.

The following section addresses music therapy guidelines that are predominantly based on the clinical work and research by music therapists in the United States, Australia, and Germany, and represent various theoretical orientations, including behavioral, developmental, and psychodynamic.

Even though most NICUs include the care of full-term hospitalized infants, the discussion in this chapter will continue to focus on music therapy interventions with premature babies. For a discussion about the use of music therapy with full-term hospitalized infants, the reader is referred to Chapter 4.

OVERVIEW OF MUSIC THERAPY METHODS AND PROCEDURES

Since premature infants are not active partners in music therapy interventions, most of the music therapy methods described in this section are categorized under receptive music therapy. However, some interventions are categorized under improvisational music therapy because the music therapist is reacting vocally to the infant's cues and thus developing the infant's interaction capacities.

Receptive Music Therapy

- Individually Provided Sustained Music: the use of prerecorded or live music for brief intervals to provide a soothing environment, help the infant to calm down, and reduce his stress-related behavior.
- Music and Multimodal Stimulation: This intervention combines soft humming or singing of lullabies with tactile, visual, and vestibular stimulation to stimulate neurological development, increase the infant's tolerance for stimulation, and improve the infant's capacity for homeostasis.
- Music-Reinforced Nonnutritive Sucking: the use of lullabies as contingent reinforcement for sucking through the use of a Pacifier-Activated Lullaby (PAL) mechanism.
- Breathing Entrainment: the creation of womblike sounds entrained to the infant's breath through use of the ocean disc, Gato box, and familiar voices and/or melodies.
- Singing as Entrainment: matching of the singing voice to the infant's physiological and behavioral responses to meet the infant vocally and thus provide a feeling of being heard and supported.
- Environmental Music Therapy: the use of live music to address the noise of the NICU and provide for a quieter, more aesthetically pleasing, and safer environment.
- Contingent Singing: the use of infant-directed singing by the music therapist to promote interaction between the infant and his caregiver.

Improvisational Music Therapy

- Creative Music Therapy for Premature Infants and Their Parents: an interactive, resource-oriented intervention that uses improvisational infant-directed singing to increase relaxation, stabilization, and pacification, as well as adequate stimulation, development, and apperception.

- PATTERNS (Preventive Approach to Traumatic Experience by Resourcing the Nervous System): a preventive multilayered treatment model that addresses traumatic experiences connected with premature birth.

Re-creative Music Therapy

- Auditory Stimulation with the Mother's Voice: the use of a recording of the mother's voice in the form of talking to the infant, reading a book, telling a story, or singing to provide the infant with a connection to the lost maternal environment.
- Song of Kin for Caregiver Support: the use of Song of Kin and lullabies to offer support to the caregivers.

GUIDELINES FOR RECEPTIVE MUSIC THERAPY

Receptive music therapy in the NICU includes listening to prerecorded or live instrumental and vocal music. Recommendations for musical characteristics in the NICU have been described by Standley (1998) and Hanson-Abromeit (2003):

- Dynamics: consistent dynamic level (about 60 dB), no crescendo
- Form: structured, constant repetition, long pauses
- Harmony: simple harmonies (major/pentatonic)
- Melody: simple, lilting, flowing, and lyrical melodies (like a lullaby)
- Rhythm: simple, often 3/4 or 6/8 meter, minimal changes, steady flowing meter
- Tempo: about 70 beats per minute (bpm), which corresponds to a relaxed heartbeat of the mother; no abrupt changes
- Timbre: vocal, soft tone and/or with limited accompaniment by soft string instruments

It is recommended to select music according to these musical characteristics rather than emotional or personal intuitive preferences by parents, staff, or music therapist (Calabro, Wolfe, & Shoemark, 2003; Hanson-Abromeit, 2003, 2006; Loewy, 2012; Shoemark, 1998, 2006).

Because of the cultural diversity among premature client families, Loewy works with Songs of Kin. A Song of Kin is a popular tune or song familiar and meaningful to the parents, originating from the parent's cultural or religious tradition. A Song of Kin accompanies the infant and the caregivers through this intensive care time and may serve as a bond between them (Loewy, 2006).

Musical toys are often too loud and not well-tuned and the sound cannot be easily manipulated. Therefore, these toys should be avoided in the NICU. Music played free-field for the ward may not be appropriate for all infants and therefore should be avoided as well. Open space sound transmission close to the infant is preferred because of possible difficulties in appropriately regulating the sound level when using ear cups or earphones (Gray & Philbin, 2004; Philbin, 2000).

When using prerecorded music, appropriate technical audio equipment that ensures high-quality recording and playback is of prime concern. In addition, the sound level should regularly be evaluated by means of a sound meter placed near the infant's ear and should not exceed 65–70 dB, according to recommendations by the AAP (1997). When using a decibel meter, the volume settings should be based on the predetermined dB level in the unit, less than or equal to the average ambient dB level of the unit (e.g., if the average level in the unit is 70 dB, then the dB level measured at the infant's ear should be equal or less than 70 dB when the music is playing). Based on our knowledge of infant hearing development, the bass sounds should be amplified, whereas the higher frequencies should be decreased. When using prerecorded music, the therapist needs to carefully consider the placement of the playback unit or speakers. Ideally, the speakers are placed at 20 cm from the infant's head.

During the music intervention, the music therapist will monitor the physiological responses of the infant as shown on the monitor (respiratory rate, oxygen saturation, and heart rate) and behavioral signs such as restlessness, changing skin color, body movements, or grimacing.

Individually Provided Sustained Music

Overview. Individually provided sustained music (Standley, 1991, 2002) is the use of prerecorded or live music for brief intervals with premature infants. This music intervention is indicated for medically stable premature infants of at least 28 weeks' GA. The primary goals of this method are to provide a soothing environment, help the infant to calm down, and reduce his stress-related behavior. This may enhance respiration and social development, and facilitate growth.

In case of documented or observed inability to hear, and if the infant reacts with hyper-responsiveness to music as opposed to ambient sounds, any music application should be avoided.

Preparation. The music therapist needs to carefully select lullaby music according to the recommendations provided in this chapter.

What to observe. The therapist must watch for signs of overstimulation, including sneezing, hiccupping, struggling movements, yawning, halt hand, heart rate or respiratory rate that exceeds normal limits, reduced oxygen saturation (particularly below 87%), startle/Moro reflex, crying, red face, or grimace. When the infant shows one of these reactions, the intervention must be halted for a few seconds until the infant calms down. The music can then be restarted with careful monitoring of the infant's reactions.

Procedures. This intervention is best delivered when the infant begins to fall asleep, immediately after stressful experiences, or following daily care and feeding procedures. Standley (2003a) recommends the use of lullaby music sung by a female voice (mother or other female voice), heartbeat sounds, or nature sounds. Prerecorded music is often used simply because it enables the administration of the music stimulus by medical staff or caregivers. However, live, unaccompanied humming or singing is recommended when possible because it allows for social reciprocity between the singer and the infant.

The total music administration time per day should not exceed 1.5 hours. This time is divided into 20–30 minutes of music alternated with 15 minutes of silence. It is important that nurse approval is sought before the administration of the music stimulus and that the infant's vital signs and behavioral states (awake, sleeping, drowsy, and restless) are documented during the music provision.

Music and Multimodal Stimulation (MMS)

Overview. Music and multimodal stimulation (Standley, 1998, 2003a; Standley & Walworth, 2010; Whipple, 2005) combines soft humming or singing of lullabies (a cappella or accompanied) with tactile, visual, and vestibular stimulation. This method is indicated for clinically stable premature infants of at least 32 weeks' GA and a weight of 1700g or more.

The goals of this intervention are to stimulate neurological development, increase the infant's tolerance for stimulation, and improve the infant's capacity for homeostasis. The literature does not report any contraindications for this intervention. MMS is particularly useful for infants with hearing deficits because it promotes the opportunity to integrate multiple sensory experiences.

What to observe. The music therapist has to carefully observe the infant's reactions to the cumulative stimulation. A pause is recommended when the infant exhibits hiccupping, sneezing, grimacing, frowned forehead, clinched or averted eyes, finger play, struggling movements, or startle reflex in arms or legs. The intervention should be stopped when the following is observed: change in skin color (from pale to flush), cry face/crying, spitting/vomiting, or hands-in-halt position.

Procedures. After permission has been obtained from the nurse, the music therapist removes the infant from the incubator or open crib. It is possible to provide a modified MMS procedure to infants who cannot be removed from the incubator or crib for medical reasons (e.g., need for uninterrupted phototherapy, placement of a central or PICC line). In those cases, auditory, tactile, and visual stimulation can still be provided, but not vestibular.

When the infant is in a quiet state, the music therapist starts to softly hum a lullaby. The music is meant to pacify the infant and also to obtain his attention. The therapist can add tactile stimulation as soon as the infant has adjusted to the auditory stimulation and demonstrates homeostasis. The tactile stimulation must follow a prescribed pattern, namely the cephalocaudal/proximodistal pattern. This pattern begins at the infant's head, progressing from his back to his neck, arms, legs, and feet. The music therapist may not progress to the next body area until touch to the preceding area is tolerated by the infant. The tactile stimulation consists of moderate pressure (i.e., not too soft and not too hard) to avoid aversive sensations. Next, vestibular stimulation is added in the form of slow and steady rocking. During the rocking, the auditory and tactile stimulation continue. Throughout the procedure, continuous eye-to-eye contact is encouraged.

The multimodal stimulation program is cumulative: New stimulation is added after approximately 30 seconds and is separated by brief intervals, thus allowing the infant to calm down. If the program has to be interrupted because of signs of overstimulation, the program can be resumed after an interval of 15 seconds, with careful observation of any further signs of overstimulation. A session length of 15–30 minutes is optimal. If an infant continues to demonstrate signs of overstimulation, the procedure must be stopped immediately. MMS should be limited to a daily maximum of 60 minutes, but in practice, it is unusual for an infant to receive more than one 15–30 minute session per day (Whipple, personal communication). After each session, the music therapist must document the infant's physiologic reactions and observe parents' interactions with the infant.

If the parents show readiness, they can be trained to apply multimodal stimulation to their baby. The training program consists of two or three 30-minute instructional sessions during which parents learn to hum or sing a lullaby while holding their infant and use a slow, steady rhythm while rocking their baby. In addition, parents are taught to recognize the signs of stress and overstimulation and the need for rest in their infant. The parent-training program is aimed at teaching parents how to use musical and tactile stimulation to soothe their infant, helping the infant to develop his capacity to better respond to the environment and ensuring continued appropriate stimulation after hospital release.

Adaptation. A multisensory stimulation program (Hanson-Abromeit, 2009; Shoemark, 1998, 2006, 2012) with live singing has been developed based on Standley's MMS. It is designed for younger and more fragile infants from 28 weeks' GA onward who are ready for live singing and multimodal stimulation. In contrast to MMS, the infant remains in his bed.

Music-Reinforced Nonnutritive Sucking (NNS)

Overview. A fetus typically develops a coordinated suck-swallow-breathe response around the 34th week of gestation. Premature infants may lack coordinated sucking behavior and, in addition, may develop an aversion to oral feeding because of prolonged gavage feeding (Palmer 1993, as cited in Standley 2003b). Music-reinforced nonnutritive sucking (Standley, 1999, 2000; Whipple, 2008) uses lullabies as contingent reinforcement for sucking through the use of the Pacifier-Activated Lullaby (PAL) mechanism.

This intervention is indicated for medically stable infants (>34 weeks) with ineffective nutritive sucking (so-called poor feeders). It is also indicated for infants for whom nipple feeding results in change of heart rate and respiration or for whom the transition from tube feeding to nipple feeding is too stressful. Finally, it is recommended for infants who are not successfully bottle- or breast-feeding and who are still requiring some tube feeding. The goal is to support the infant in developing his sucking capacities, to increase sucking duration, and to transfer the infant's sucking behavior from nonnutritive to nutritive sucking.

If the infant's medical condition prevents sucking (e.g., if the infant is still ventilated), this intervention is contraindicated. In a situation where the infant withdraws, ceases to suck, or shows signs of overstimulation, the music therapist must end the intervention and possibly wait several days before administering the NNS program again.

Preparation. This intervention uses a selection of prerecorded lullabies sung by a professional female singer that are played free-field. The music therapist prepares the pacifier which is adapted with a pressure transducer to ensure that a suck of a given strength activates the music recording. A strong enough suck activates 10 seconds of the recorded lullaby music.

What to observe. The music therapist has to carefully observe the infant's reactions during the intervention, watch for overstimulation, and record observations of the infant's sucking behavior.

Procedures. Music-reinforced NNS uses the Sondrex® Pacifier-Activated Lullaby (PAL) System®. "The PAL system uses the Wee Soothie®, Soothie®, or Super Soothie® pacifier by Children's Medical Ventures. This pacifier is connected to a wired or wireless transmitter and plays music contingent on infant sucking. The transmitter sends a signal to the Sondrex® Sound CD System and the baby is rewarded with music, provided he or she generates a certain threshold of pressure. The PAL system has also the capability to play continuous music with or without the use of the pacifier and transmitter" (Whipple, 2008, p. 238). The device has received FDA approval as a device to improve poor feeding behaviors (Whipple, 2008).

The PAL intervention requires prior approval from the infant's primary caregiver and the infant's nurse. The recommended duration for the daily intervention is 15 minutes in length, 30–60 minutes prior to any bottle-feeding.

Adaptation. PAL has also been used for pain management (Whipple, 2008). Whipple reports using PAL for three minutes or more prior to a heel stick, throughout a heel stick, and for three minutes following the heel stick. Reports of a research study on the use of PAL for pain management with premature infants is reported in the final section of this chapter.

Breathing Entrainment

Overview. Breathing entrainment is the creation of womblike sounds through use of the ocean disc, Gato box, and familiar voices and/or melodies (Loewy, 2009; Loewy et al., 2013). This intervention is designed for infants older than 32 weeks who are referred because of problems with irritability, respiratory distress, or feeding. The goals are to improve physical behavior via regulation of cardiac or respiratory irregularities. No contraindications are reported in the literature for this intervention.

Preparation. The music therapist has to take care that during the session the environment is as quiet and undisturbed as possible. A sound meter is used to ensure that the decibel level remains below 65 dB. It is strongly recommended that Songs of Kin (Loewy, 2005, 2008) be the primary lullaby intervention, rather than music selected by someone outside of the parent–family life world. This means that the music therapist needs to meet with the parents or caregivers beforehand to prepare for a proper music selection.

What to observe. The music therapist observes if the live music reduces the infant's stress responses (e.g., heart rate, respiratory rate).

Procedures. The guidelines provided here are based on Loewy (2009) and Loewy et al. (2013). This intervention uses the voice, ocean disc, or Gato box to replicate intrauterine womb sounds. The first step is to assess if the use of the voice, ocean disc, or Gato box entrained to the infant's live vital sounds can assist in regulating the infant's vital signs. This occurs with careful observation of the infant as well as continuous attention to the infant's monitors. It is recommended to evaluate the impact of the live presentation of each sound. The instrumental sounds, reflective of the intrauterine sound environment, combined with the soft vocal toning of the parent or the music therapist, provide a steady acoustic basis to comfort the infant and sustain a homeostatic environment.

The music therapist plays the Gato box with the index finger (not a mallet) in a slow and steady rhythm entrained to the infant's heartbeat. This predictable and steady rhythm may provide a feeling of safety and comfort. The Gato box rhythm, in combination with soundscaping (i.e., musically controlling the sounds that make up the auditory environment) in meter to the infant's suck, can activate the sucking response. When used just prior to feeding time, this may help perpetuate the sucking movements throughout the feeding procedure and lead to a more successful feeding.

The music therapist plays the ocean disc at the infant's midline in a gentle swirling pattern. The perpetual motion of the ocean disc replicates the fluid sounds of the womb. By imitating and entraining with the infant's breath rhythmically, the ocean disc can be used to support respiratory irregularities (e.g., Respiratory Distress Syndrome).

Although breathing entrainment is first implemented using the ocean disc and Gato box, these sounds are soon taught to parent/s and caregivers. They are instructed to hold the infant over their heart, use the "ah" and breath sounds of the ocean disc, and pat the rhythm of the heart.

Singing as Entrainment

Overview. Singing as entrainment (Loewy, 2004, 2007, 2012; Stewart, 2009a, 2009b) matches the singing voice to the infant's physiological and behavioral responses. It can be used with infants of 32 weeks' GA or older. It is indicated for infants who demonstrate long periods of distress, high irritability, and inconsolable crying (e.g., infants with Neonatal Abstinence Syndrome). The goal for the music therapist is to meet the infant vocally and thus provide a feeling of being heard and supported. Parental involvement is encouraged, and work with parents separate from their infants, prior to using the music with parent and infant, can support their process and attend to ways in which having an infant in the NICU may affect them. Training in music psychotherapy is recommended for music therapists who will treat parents who may have postpartum depression and/or traumatization related to having premature infants.

Preparation. Loewy (2012) recommends musical preparation individualized to each infant through identification of familiar songs and lullabies and Song of Kin/lullaby. In addition, the music therapist will use simple consonant intervallic, vowel-toned rhythmic responses, without lyrics.

What to observe. The therapist should observe whether the entrainment helps the infant relax and aids in developing interactive communication with the music therapist.

Procedures. The music therapist begins by matching the infant's crying tone, pitch, and intensity vocally with her voice. Here within, she orients herself to the infant's audible breathing by releasing the same vocal tone in synchrony with the infant. The music therapist works by being constantly aware of the infant's emotional expressions and gives the infant time to respond by providing many grand pauses. The therapist may then change her vocal expressions (e.g., into lullabies) and develop interactive music behaviors with the infant (Loewy, 2012).

Environmental Music Therapy (EMT)

Overview. Typically, an NICU environment, inclusive of the infants, caregivers, and staff, can be experienced as acoustically intrusive. If there is a noisy environment and medical activity inclusive of talking, and monitors and other equipment are not attended to, the healing environment is threatened. A quieter and safer environment can be achieved through increased awareness of the sound environment in personnel and parents. Live music can help modulate the experience of environmental noise and chaos. EMT addresses the noise of the unit and provides for a quieter, more aesthetically pleasing, and safer environment (Canga, Hahm, Lucido, Grossbard, & Loewy, 2012; Loewy, 2004; Stewart & Schneider, 2000).

Preparation. The music therapist first uses a sound meter to assess the noise level of the unit. Consultation with the nurse manager is recommended. The therapist observes the noise and its source/s. In addition, the therapist identifies favorite lullabies or Songs of Kin in collaboration with parents and staff. In this way, a medley of familiar music can be included in the EMT program. Typically a guitar or wind or other string instrument is used to avoid loud dynamics or cluttering of the environment. The music therapist adapts each program anew every time a live music program is prepared within the NICU environment.

What to observe. During EMT, parents and staff may be asked to observe changes in individual infants' behavior (e.g., infant becomes quieter, falls asleep).

Procedures. The music therapist works with voice and instruments within the sound environment to lower the ambient noise and the environmental stress. The sound environment includes specific pitches of medical monitors as well as the rhythm of the chaos and the staff's expressed moods. These combinations of environmental factors may vary from moment to moment, from day to day, and the music therapist must have the flexibility, agility, and musical skill to react musically and sensitively to these sounds. The sound environment is reflective of the important needs of many people who must function with and coordinate the give-and-take of medical care and human compassion amidst difficult and stressful circumstances (Stewart, 2009a).

The music therapist may use a hammered dulcimer, string or wind instruments, and voice (with vowels and phonemes, lyrics are not recommended). The music is matched to the keys of the beeping of medical monitoring equipment and is used to modulate the stressful environment of the unit. Singing and/or playing music that is preferred by the parents and staff is most useful for this purpose. Additionally, the music therapist encourages the parents to identify a Song of Kin (Loewy, 2005, 2006, 2012) that reflects their culture. This communicates to the parents that their input is important and that their cultural preferences are respected. A time frame of 30 minutes or less per EMT session is recommended.

During and after the intervention, it is recommended that the music therapist stay in close communication with staff and parents. Supervision of the music therapist is strongly recommended to help her understand what occurs in-the-moment within the unit, with consideration given to all of the people involved. Supervision should be provided by a music therapist who has had NICU training.

Contingent Singing

Overview. Contingent singing (Shoemark, 2006) is a therapist-led intervention that uses infant-directed singing to promote interaction between the infant and his caregiver. This intervention is presented in great detail in Chapter 4 of this volume. The full-term infant develops social maturity that allows him to seek nurturing care and companionship at the same time. This development starts in late preterm infants (>36 weeks' GA). The goal is to expand periods of meaningful interaction between the infant and the caregiver. The development of relationship and interaction between infant and parents are often disturbed because of the infant's poor reactions due to medical problems (e.g., esophageal atresia, mechanical ventilation). With contingent singing, the music therapist provides a safe tool to develop reciprocal interaction.

If the infant is sedated or receives pain medication, mutual interaction is not possible. The music therapist will need to wait until the infant is again available for interplay.

Preparation. The music therapist has to find a quiet time within the daily routine during which the addition of live singing is acceptable. The infant may remain in his bed or open crib, but does need to be awake for this work.

What to observe. The music therapist observes the infant's communicative interest and assesses the infant's availability for increasing interplay and joy.

Procedures. When the infant is ready for interplay, the music therapist entices the infant's attention first by being in the infant's visual field. This is followed by the presentation of her voice and facial expression and by offering highly intonated speech leading to short vocal sequences. The therapist provides space for the infant to respond and maintains this level of interaction until the infant indicates a readiness for more. In this work, the music therapist depends on the infant's ability to show communicative signals through facial expression, movements, and, for more mature infants, even voice. The therapist responds to the infant's communicative expressions in order to develop mutually regulated communicative experiences.

GUIDELINES FOR IMPROVISATIONAL MUSIC THERAPY

Creative Music Therapy for Premature Infants and Their Parents

Overview. Creative music therapy (CMT) (Haslbeck 2004, in press) is an interactive, resource-oriented intervention which includes improvisational infant-directed singing. It is based on the "creative music therapy" approach initially developed by Nordoff and Robbins (1977) and the principles of CMT used with patients in a coma (Aldridge, Gustorff, & Hannich, 1990). It has been adapted by Haslbeck (2004) for the specific needs of premature infants and their parents in the NICU setting. This method is meant for medically stable infants. The goals are to increase relaxation, stabilization, and pacification, as well as adequate stimulation, development, and apperception. The parents are often included through participating in interactive singing or just by listening and observing their baby. The goals for parents are to promote their autonomy and self-confidence, and support the intuitive parent–infant interaction and bonding process. This approach is not indicated if the infant is medically unstable or too heavily sedated.

Preparation. The music therapist must assess the optimal time for interaction with the infant during which a minimal number of interruptions are likely. Before starting the intervention, the music therapist must assess infant's individual needs and in-the-moment behavioral state. If appropriate, the intervention starts with therapeutic touch while observing the infant's breathing, heart rate, gestures, and facial expressions. The music therapist also checks in with the parents to assess their individual needs and their musical preferences and wishes.

What to observe. The music therapist observes the infant's behavioral responses and breathing pattern. In late preterm infants, the music therapist observes whether the intervention increases alertness, orientation, behavioral participation, and engagement (eyes/face open or smiling, smooth finger movements). Often, the infant shows interactional synchrony with the therapist's musical rhythms and expressions.

The therapist also observes the parents' responses to the intervention (e.g., Do they appear to be more relaxed? Do they express a sense of empowerment?). In addition, the parents' level of attention to and sensitization for their infant's needs is observed.

Procedures. The music therapist carefully observes the infant's "music" (i.e., the infant's breathing patterns, facial expression, and gesticulations) and transforms it into improvised infant-directed humming. The improvised humming is continuously adjusted to the infant's rhythms and subtle expressions. Thus, a musical interplay is created between the infant's behavioral and vocal expressions and the music therapist's music. Because the infant truly is a "musical partner" in this intervention, it is included under improvisational methods. The parents are instructed to carefully observe the therapeutic intervention with the infant, to listen to the therapist's humming and/or singing and to observe the infant's reactions/interactions. When they wish to participate in the singing, the therapist supports their singing.

Since CMT with premature infants and their parents is an interactive, resource-oriented music therapy approach, the therapist identifies culturally specific, preferred music or songs of the families for adaptation into the therapeutic process. Support for the parents can vary from conducting the intervention during kangaroo care to encouraging the parents in their own unique ways of singing (e.g., in creating and singing a song for their infant).

PATTERNS (Preventive Approach to Traumatic Experience by Resourcing the Nervous System)

Overview. PATTERNS (Stewart, 2009a, 2009b) is a preventive multilayered treatment model that addresses traumatic experiences connected with premature birth. "PATTERNS in NICU music therapy integrates theory and best practices from NICU music therapy, trauma, high-risk infant development, and transpersonal psychology and is based on the use of trauma renegotiation and music therapy principles to develop, restore, or otherwise engage absent and/or latent human resiliency processes" (Stewart, 2009a, p.31). PATTERNS is based on current NICU music therapy best practices related to sound environment, individualized bedside interventions for the infants, and interventions for the caregivers, as well as standards for safety for the acoustic environment and developmentally based infant care (Stewart, 2009a).

The goals are to enhance stabilization, integration, and relational development. In addition, the intervention seeks to enhance interactions between staff, infants, and parents, and improve the mood and attitudes of staff and caregivers so that their approach with the infant is attuned and regulated. This method is intended for medically stable infants after approval from the medical staff. No recommendations for minimum age have been reported in the literature.

Preparation. Therapist awareness of and attunement to her personal mental, emotional, and physical state, and her acute awareness of the environment, are important conditions for this intervention. The therapist must work to enhance homeostasis in self to develop a stable therapeutic relationship with the infant. This will enable physiologic stability in the infant and will provide a sound "container" through which development of resiliency is possible.

What to observe. The therapist carefully observes the present environment of the NICU (e.g., architectural design, the unit's ecosystem, and its ambient sounds) as well as the individualized infant care, and the caregivers' experience of distress, mood, and tensions within the unit. Observations are to be conducted in every area of treatment, including the infant, parent/primary caregiver, staff, and NICU environment, structurally and culturally. Regarding the human relational areas, the therapist must first identify any acute signs of distress present: disorientation, confusion, frantic behavior, panic, extreme withdrawal, extreme irritability and anger, and excessive worry (Brymer, Jacobs, Layne, Pynoos, Ruzek, &

Steinberg, 2006). Further assessment will help to evaluate whether observations of such distress are epidosic in nature or a part of baseline behavior. It is important to ascertain whether observations indicate hyperarousal in the form of peak/spike in physiologic response or a collapse. Physiologic as well as mental/emotional collapse is indicative of the highest form of arousal, though the outward appearance indicates the contrary. The infant's physical cues for acute distress include but are not limited to rapid and/or erratic heart rate and respiration rate, increased and/or uncoordinated movement, muscle constriction/tension (as per arching in infants), sweating, hypersensitivity to startle, hyperalert eyes, crying, aversion, defensive postures, depressed physiologic and/or mental and emotional states, lack of response, lack of engagement, and difficulty in being roused (Stewart, 2009b).

It is important to note that these cues may reflect a multitude of causes, particularly for the preterm infant. Thorough history gathering and collaboration with the treatment team, in conjunction with observation and assessment, will help the therapist to develop a clear understanding of influencing factors.

Procedures. PATTERNS follows a phase-oriented treatment approach and includes the following sequential phases: (a) stabilization, (b) self-regulation, (c) integration, (d) attachment/social engagement, (e) restorative experiences, and (f) future planning. These phases are applied across the different areas of treatment [i.e., infant, caregiver(s), and staff], and, again, are based on NICU music therapy practices, many of which are included in this chapter. Because of the complexity and comprehensiveness of the model, it is beyond the scope of this chapter to present it here in detail. This author strongly encourages readers to consult Stewart (2009a) and Stewart (2009b), as these publications provide in-depth coverage of this NICU treatment model.

Because this is a psychotherapeutic clinical model, psychotherapeutic knowledge, education, and accompanying supervision by a trained music therapist or a psychotherapist is strongly recommended.

GUIDELINES FOR RE-CREATIVE MUSIC THERAPY

Auditory Stimulation with the Mother's Voice

Overview. Auditory stimulation with the mother's voice (Nöcker-Ribaupierre, 1998, 2004, 2011; Zimmer, 2004) provides the infant with a connection to the lost maternal environment by using his mother's voice as a familiar "bridge." The intervention uses a recording of the mother's voice in the form of talking to the infant, reading a book, telling a story, or singing. For the mother, this method offers the opportunity to convey something personal to her infant in the intensive care environment that is not replaceable by any other caregiver. The method can be applied as soon as the infant has reached clinical stabilization or if requested by the parents or neonatal team. It is also offered on a case-by-case manner for medically fragile infants, as soon as the mother is available after delivery. The intervention can be used with infants from 26 weeks' GA onward. Goals for the infants are to increase homeostasis, optimize long-term development, and promote bonding and interaction. Cevasco (2008) and Shoemark (2004, 2012) have also reported on the use of recordings of the mother's voice with premature infants.

For the mother who has experienced a traumatic delivery, psychotherapeutic support, including trauma intervention, is important to help her overcome the experiences connected with the preterm delivery. The music therapist, with appropriate training in psychotherapy and trauma work, may help the mother to understand her history, address her unwanted feelings of fear, guilt, anger, and shame, and understand the experiences related to premature delivery and the NICU environment. These insights will enable activation of inner resources, development of her feeling of being a mother, and re-establishment of the interrupted bonding process with her baby. Furthermore, it may enhance her communication with the staff and other mothers of premature infants.

Preparation. The music therapist must be trained in music psychotherapy. The first contact with the mother happens preferably at the infant's bedside, as this provides the opportunity for joint observation of the infant. If the mother is not present in the unit, the therapist may initiate contact through a note posted to the incubator so that a meeting can be arranged. At this meeting, the music therapist introduces the method and explains its intention and procedures.

For the voice recording, the music therapist arranges for a quiet environment and sets up the recording equipment. The music therapist provides storybooks and songbooks in the parents' native language, if available. Before presenting the recording to the baby, the music therapist has to carefully install the playback equipment, with the speaker placed at an appropriate distance to the infant's ear. In addition, she must ensure, with help of a sound meter, that the sound of the mother's voice can be heard slightly above the ambient noise.

What to observe. The music therapist and the mother jointly observe the infant's reactions to the mother's recorded voice. It is important to understand that seeing her baby's first responses to her voice may be an overwhelming experience for the mother. Additionally, the infant's physiological responses (heart rate and respiratory rate) are monitored by the music therapist.

Procedures. The first recording typically takes place at a time when the mother is still overwhelmed with adapting to the premature delivery and is dealing with disappointment, grief, and anxiety. Therefore, it is meaningful to suggest that she talk to her baby for the initial recording. For example, she could read a letter that she has prepared in advance, read from a book, tell a story, or talk about her wishes and dreams. The actual singing of a lullaby or song is not recommended for the first recording because she is still too overwhelmed by the situation and may emotionally be very vulnerable. Through the work on the first recording, the mother may develop more stability and may then be ready to sing. The music therapist encourages her to sing her song in her own way even if she is not able to carry a tune. The music therapist supports her throughout the process to help her find her own way of communication and rediscover her own resilient resources. During the recording, the music therapist is not present because mothers are often insecure and may be embarrassed to record their voice in the presence of others. This could prevent the expression of intimacy to her baby.

The mother has to take a central role in the first recording because she is the one who is traumatically involved and physically and emotionally affected by the premature delivery. In her womb, the baby was living with her voice, so her voice can bring about a sense of safety. Besides making the actual voice recordings, the music therapist provides the mother with an opportunity to meet on a regular basis to process her current experiences as well as events in her past that may impact her feelings toward her baby. Periodic review, together with the music therapist, of the recordings made over time can help the mother to reflect on changes in her emotional and physical well-being. In subsequent recordings, the father can be included. It is important to provide support for the father as well in this process.

The voice recordings are played for the infant at quiet and undisturbed times, depending on daily routine, medical care, and mother/parent visits. The timing of the playback is determined in collaboration with the mother and staff and may occur several times a day. The duration should not extend beyond 30 minutes each. The frequency is determined for each infant based on his stability, medical procedures, and the parent visits. The recording should be stopped when any disturbance occurs or when the parents are present. Their presence and their live interactions with their baby are always preferred.

As this work is emotionally demanding for the music therapist, supervision is required to help the therapist to understand her involvement in the process and to strengthen her resources.

Adaptation. After the music therapist has worked with the mother and the father for a prolonged period of time, other family members (e.g., siblings) can be included in the recordings.

Auditory stimulation with the mother's voice is an important method at the beginning of life for the most prematurely born infants. When the infant reaches an age when communicative cues can be observed, it is important that the music therapist begin to use more interactive music therapy methods.

Song of Kin for Caregiver Support

Overview. This intervention uses Song of Kin and lullabies to offer support to the caregivers (Loewy, 2006, 2008, 2009, 2011). It is aimed at helping parents to bond with their infants. The separation of parents from their infant often results in feelings of being out of control and helpless. In addition, the separation results in feelings of shame, guilt, fear, and anger. In this intervention, the therapist develops a relationship with the parents through music, and, in particular, through accessing their favorite song or lullaby. The therapist encourages the parents to identify their fears, which can be allayed through accessing their inner resources, in particular the music that was used in their own heritage. The music therapist provides support and comfort by use of musical memories of the parents' childhood. The music therapist encourages parents to use their voices directed at the baby.

Preparation. Before starting the intervention, the music therapist must assess the parental level of stress by talking and being with them, accompanying them during visits with their infant, and exploring the impact that this unexpected life event has on their relationship.

What to observe. The music therapist observes the subtleties of the parents' relationship and attentively looks for collaborative aspects of their relationship that can be enhanced through music-making and lullaby-singing. The therapist also identifies any blame or anxiety that may exist within the relationship as result of the unexpected and possibly traumatic moments of the current neonatal experience.

Procedures. Music therapy support is carefully provided in a music psychotherapy context. The Song of Kin is harvested in therapy with the parents prior to it being implemented with their infant. The use of Song of Kin can palliate not only the difficulties that parents may experience between one another but also may serve as an impetus of bonding with the infant, lessening fear and anxiety in the developing relationship and shaping a new family context that is both as novel and historic as it is inclusive of their family's heritage. Showing parents how a Song of Kin can be used sedatively, for sleep, or in times of irritability or stress can be useful.

A selected Song of Kin can be shifted to a lullaby (soft, ¾ or 6/8 meter with simplified sequences) to enhance a quiet alert state in the infant, to induce a sleep state, or to assist with transitions.

Adaptation. This work may lead to use of compositional methods in which the music therapist helps the parents to change the lyrics by, for example, expressing their own wishes, dreams, or prayers, or to include the infant's name.

NICU TRAINING

Working in an NICU requires specialized training so that music therapists can practice safely and effectively. At the time of this writing, two specialized training programs are offered.

Jayne Standley from the National Institute for Infant & Child Medical Music Therapy at Florida State University in Tallahassee offers a three-component training course leading to NICU-MT certification. The training course consists of lectures, clinical fieldwork, and reading. The lecture component is typically held in conjunction with the National Conference of the American Music Therapy Association.

Joanne Loewy at the Beth Israel Medical Center in New York offers the Rhythm, Breath, Lullaby (RBL) NICU Music Therapy Training Program. The RBL training is offered to board-certified or equivalent music therapists who wish to train in NICU music therapy with the focus on live music interventions and psychotherapy. The training consists of three parts: NICU Orientation, Music Therapy in the NICU—learning and observation (infant session observations; parent/infant session observations), and Integration and Intervention (music therapy and case studies with supervision).

Additionally, music therapists wishing to develop a NICU music therapy program should consult the guidelines formulated by Hanson-Abromeit (2004, 2012).

RESEARCH EVIDENCE

In the late 1970s, health care professionals in nursing science, medicine, and behavioral science began to observe the physiological reactions of premature infants to the exposure to music (e.g., recording of Brahms' lullaby, female singing voices, the mother's singing voices). This interest in premature infants' responses to music continues today and has had a major influence on the development of music therapy research and clinical work. Therefore, music therapy in the NICU is considered an interdisciplinary area in research and clinical practice.

Until this century, research mainly focused on the immediate and short-term outcomes of receptive music intervention on the infant. The results of this line of research indicated that music interventions have observable and measurable positive effects on premature infants.

This section will present an interdisciplinary overview of empirical research on music in the NICU and demonstrate how medical, nursing, and music therapy research can mutually influence and stimulate each other.

A meta-analysis by Standley (2002) pooled the results of 10 studies that examined the impact of music on physiological, physical, and behavioral outcomes in premature infants. Studies that met the following inclusion criteria were included: (1) experimental studies using group or individual subject designs, (2) participants are premature or low birth weight infants receiving treatment in the NICU, (3) music is the independent-variable, and (4) the study/report is published in English. The 10 studies included are shortly described here:

- Caine (1991): recorded lullabies vs. ambient auditory stimulation led to greater daily weight gain, formula intake, and significant earlier discharge.
- Cassidy and Standley (1995): recorded lullabies vs. ambient noise positively affected physiological measures, including oxygen saturation, heart rate, respiratory rate, and apnea/bradycardia episodes.
- Coleman, Pratt, Stoddard, and Abel (1997): male and female singing vs. male and female speaking resulted in earlier discharge and significant increased caloric intake and weight gain.
- Collins and Kuck (1991): the use of womb sounds combined with female lullaby-singing significantly improved oxygen saturation and behavioral state in agitated infants.
- Flower, McCain, and Hilker (1999): examined the effects of soft rock ballads vs. music with womb sounds. Music with womb sounds resulted in significant better oxygen saturation, respiratory rate, and sleep time.
- Moore, Gladstone, and Standley (1994): compared mother's reading poetry vs. female lullaby singing vs. white noise vs. uterine sounds vs. silence. All auditory types resulted in significantly higher oxygen saturation levels compared to silence.
- Standley and Moore (1995): Female sung lullabies vs. mother's voice reading resulted in inconclusive findings.

- Standley (1998): Live lullaby singing with MMS resulted in a significantly earlier discharge and increased weight gain.
- Standley (1999, 2000): Music-reinforced NNS with a lullaby sung by a female resulted in a significant increase in sucking rates and feeding rates.

The pooled effect sizes on various outcomes ranged from .49 to 1.95, reflecting the difference between the music and nonmusic results in standardized units. The overall effect size for the meta-analysis was d = .83 and was statistically significant (Standley, 2002). A widely accepted guide to interpreting effect sizes is provided by Cohen (1988): An effect size of d = .2 is considered a small effect; .5, a medium effect; and .8, a large effect.

In 2012, Haslbeck conducted an integrative review of clinical trials that examined the impact of music on premature infants. This review included 19 studies by music therapists, 16 by nurses, 6 by medical doctors, and 2 by behavioral scientists. For details, the reader is referred to Standley's meta-analysis (2003) and Haslbeck's integrative review (2012).

We will now review single research studies on music in the NICU categorized according to receptive or active music therapy methods.

Receptive Music Therapy

As stated earlier, neonatal music therapy research has predominantly focused on the effects of listening to prerecorded and live music on the infants' physiological responses and has mainly employed quantitative research designs. In general, the results suggest that music is effective in calming the infant and reducing observable stress behaviors.

The majority of the medical and music therapy studies have focused on effects of music on behavioral states and have reported the following results:

- Statistically significant increase in oxygen saturation and improved respiration rate (Arnon et al., 2006; Bo & Callaghan, 2000; Butt & Kisilevsky, 2000; Cassidy & Standley, 1995; Chou, Wang, Chen, Pai, 2003; Collins & Kuck, 1991; Courtnage, Chawla, Loewy, & Nolan, 2002; Farhat, Amirib, Esmailyd, & Mohammanzadeha, 2010; Keith, Russel, & Weaver, 2009; Nöcker, Güntner, & Riegel, 1987; Nöcker-Ribaupierre, 1995; Standley & Moore, 1995). Positive but not significant effects on increasing oxygen saturation and respiration rate were observed by Burke et al. (1995), Cassidy and Standley (1995), Ingersoll and Thoman (1994), and Lorch, Lorch, and Diefendorf (1994).
- Statistically significant decrease in motor activity and heart rate (Arnon et al., 2006; Bo & Callaghan, 2000; Butt & Kisilevsky, 2000; Nöcker-Ribaupierre, 1995; Loewy et al., 2013). A positive but nonsignificant effect on heart rate was reported by Cassidy (2009), Coleman et al. (1997), and Lorch, Lorch, and Diefendorf (1994).
- Significant effects on growth parameter, including caloric intake (Caine, 1991; Coleman et al., 1997), weight gain (Caine, 1991; Coleman et al., 1997; Malloy, 1979; Standley, 1998; Whipple, 2000), and feeding abilities and sucking rates (Cevasco & Grant, 2005; Standley, 2000, 2003; Loewy et al., 2013).
- Decreased stress level results in increased pacification and stability and leads to earlier discharge from the hospital. This trend was observed by Caine (1991); Coleman et al. (1998); Malloy (1979); Schwartz et al. (1999); Standley (1998); Standley & Walworth (2010); Thoman, Ingersoll, & Acebo (1991); and Whipple

(2005). Earlier discharge means a reduction of the high daily costs for intensive care (Schwartz, 2004). This may increase the economic interest in music therapy intervention.

- Some studies reported a statistically significant effect of music on the premature infant's sleep quality and resting energy expenditure (Lai et al., 2006; Lubetzky, Minouni, Dollberg, Reifen, Ashbel, & Mandel, 2010), whereas others reported a trend but no statistically significant results (Arnon et al., 2006; Thoman et al., 1991)

A two-arm randomized controlled trial evaluated the influence of music (instrumental version of Brahms' lullaby) on EEG activity in 20 neurologically healthy newborns from 32 weeks of gestation onward. The study reported a trend toward more discernible sleep-wake cycles in infants exposed to music (Olischar, Shoemark, Holton, Weninger, & Hunt, 2012).

Studies that involved the mothers or parents reported a trend to better coping and self-reported increased time spent with their infant in the hospital (Cevasco, 2008; Nöcker-Ribaupierre, 2004; Whipple, 2000).

A handful of studies have dealt with long-term effects of rhythmic therapeutic interventions on premature infants. These behavioral and nursing studies suggest that rhythmic interventions with a "breathing bear" result in improved sleeping patterns in infants five weeks of age (Ingerson & Thoman, 1994). Furthermore, results indicate that rhythmic interventions with a rocking bed and heartbeat sounds improve mental development at 24 months (Bernard & Bee, 1983).

The influence of music on pain response and excessive agitation in infants has been the topic of some research since 2000. Results suggest that music is able to attenuate excessive agitation and responses to acute stress exposure (e.g., medical procedures). Infants demonstrated significantly lower levels of stress and higher levels of oxygen saturation during and after medical procedures when listening to music compared to infants who did not (Bo & Callaghan, 2000; Butt & Kisilevsky, 2000; Chou et al., 2003; Johnson, Filion, Campbell-Yeo, Goulet Bell, McNaughton, & Byron, 2009; Keith et al., 2009; Whipple, 2008). Whipple (2008) examined the effectiveness of the use of PAL for pain management in which infants received the PAL for three minutes or more prior to a heel stick, throughout the heel stick, and for three minutes following the procedure. The results suggested the greatest benefit during the postprocedure period, when infants regained homeostasis. Behaviorally, the infants receiving PAL returned to optimal behavior states faster than those infants who did not receive the music intervention; physiologically, the oxygen saturation levels improved and the heart rate and respiratory rates stabilized more quickly in infants receiving PAL than those who did not. The research study used heel stick as the procedure, since it is the most common painful or stressful intervention experienced by hospitalized preterm infants. However, these results may be able to be generalized to other stressful or painful caregiving procedures (eye exams, dressing changes, etc.) common to the NICU environment.

Two studies using the taped mother's voice during NICU time reported positive results in infant development after hospital release. A nursing study (Katz, 1971) and a music therapy study (Nöcker-Ribaupierre, 1999) measured long-term effects in mother's behavior and infant development at the age of five, 20 months, and six years. The results indicated a significant increase in breast-feeding and improved well-being of the mothers as well as significantly advanced motor and verbal development in the infants.

Active Music Therapy

During recent years, there has been a shift from the use of receptive music interventions to active music therapy interventions. Music therapists increasingly involve the parents in the music therapeutic treatment and care for their infant. Research has shown that this shift positively affects parents in terms of dealing with trauma, grief, and anxiety by enhancing parental stability, self-confidence, and well-being (Hanson-Abromeit, 2004; Loewy, 2004; Stewart & Schneider, 2000). The parent's training as part of the MMS program has been shown to lead to positive changes in parent behavior and parent–infant interaction (Whipple, 2008). Additionally, in music therapy there has been a growing interest in supporting the mother individually. After the premature delivery, the mother is the person who is physically and emotionally affected in a traumatic manner, and she is the prime attachment person for the infant. Therefore, she needs to be supported as soon as possible after the delivery.

A two-arm repeated measures study by Teckenberg-Jansson, Houtilainen, and Pölkki (2011) examined the effects of combined kangaroo care with live music interventions (e.g., use of the pentatonic lyre and the music therapist's singing or humming voice) compared to kangaroo care alone on physiological outcomes in 61 premature infants. Participants in the music group received six music therapy sessions. The treatment led to statistically significant improvements in heart rate, respiratory rate, oxygen saturation level, and blood pressure ($p < .05$). No statistically significant results were found for height or weight.

Some studies report positive effects of music psychotherapeutic support for mothers in terms of their well-being, coping, bonding, and ability to sing for their infant in the NICU as well as at home after discharge (Blumenfeld & Eisenfeld, 2006; Cevasco, 2008; Haslbeck, in press; Nöcker-Ribaupierre, 1995, 2004; Whipple, 2000; Zimmer, 2004). One RCT (N = 30) investigated the influence of music during kangaroo care on maternal anxiety and preterm infants' responses. The mother–infant dyads in the treatment group received music during kangaroo care for 60 minutes/day for three consecutive days. The results indicated that mothers in the treatment group had significantly lower anxiety scores than those in the control group ($p < .05$). As for the infants, the music group had significantly more occurrences of quiet sleep ($p < .01$) and fewer occurrences of crying than the control group ($p < .05$) (Lai et al., 2006).

To summarize, the research suggests that music interventions have beneficial effects on the premature infants' physiological and behavioral responses. Research also supports the use of active music therapy interventions to support mother–infant bonding and attachment.

SUMMARY AND CONCLUSIONS

The music therapy guidelines provided in this chapter detail evidence-based music therapy techniques to address the premature infant's needs. The premature infant who was taken away from his protected, safe intrauterine environment and placed into an ambient, highly technical environment needs to be supported and protected to survive and to grow. In contrast to the chaotic and irregular ambient noise characteristic of the NICU, music offers predictability and structure. The predictable characteristics of the music help the premature infant to stabilize his behavioral responses, including organizing his behavior, calming into a quiet alert state or sleep, and learning to regulate himself. In the course of his maturation, the infant is capable to express cues of readiness for interactive music play.

The methods provided here differ in their orientation (e.g., medical, behavioral, psychotherapeutic), in their use of active vs. receptive music interventions, and in their focus on the infant and/or caregivers.

The practice of music therapy in the NICU is based on a wealth of clinical and empirical evidence. Scientific interdisciplinary and quantitative studies show that music has significant effects on the premature infants' physical behavior and stabilization. Ongoing quantitative clinical trials on the impact of receptive music therapy underline and expand this knowledge.

However, our theoretical knowledge about the impact of music and music therapy on the human psyche at the beginning of life and how this supports attachment and development is quite limited. During the last decade, infant and developmental research has increasingly focused on the importance of bonding and attachment. Stern (1985, 2010) and Schumacher, Calvet, and Reimer (2011) state that the infant is born a social being, necessarily depending on communication, interaction, and attachment with a primary care person. It is unknown when this connectedness on the emotional level begins, but it undoubtedly begins via physiological parameters during the embryonic state. More research is needed to further develop this scientific area.

Ongoing research is needed to understand the mechanisms of music to enhance bonding and attachment in the premature infant. We need to understand how and where and under which circumstances bonding processes originate and how music can contribute to this development. This could be best addressed by qualitative research. Future research designs may include the differentiation of processes which enable emotional regulation, bonding, attachment, and synchronization.

REFERENCES

Aagaard, H., & Hall, E. (2008). Mother's experiences of having a premature infant in the neonatal care unit: A meta-synthesis. *Journal of Pediatric Nursing, 23*(3), 26–36.

Abromeit, D. (2003). The newborn individualized developmental care and assessment program (NIDCAP) as a model for clinical music therapy interventions with premature infants. *Music Therapy Perspectives, 21*(2), 60–68.

Achenbach, T.M., Howell, M. S., Aoki, M. F., & Rauh, V. A. (1993). Nine-year outcome of The Vermont Intervention Program for low birth weight infants. *Pediatrics, 91*(1), 45–55.

Aldridge, D., Gustorff, D., & Hannich, H. J. (1990). Where am I? Music therapy applied to coma patients. *Journal of the Royal Society of Medicine, 83*, 345–346.

Als, H. (1982). Toward a synactive theory of development: Promise for the assessment and support of infant individuality. *Infant Mental Health Journal, 3*(4), 229–243.

Als, H., Duffy, F. H., McAnulty, G. B., Rivkin, M. J., Vajapeyam, S., & Mulkern, R. V. (2004). Early experience alters brain function and structure. *Pediatrics, 113*, 846–857.

Als, H., & Gilkerson, L. (1997). The role of relationship-based developmentally supportive newborn intensive care in strengthening outcomes of preterm infants. *Seminars in Perinatology, 21*, 178–189.

Altuncu, E., Akman, I., Kulekzi, S., et al. (2009). Noise level in neonatal intensive care unit and use of sound absorbing panel in the isolette. *International Journal of Pediatric Otorhinolaryngology, 73*, 951–953.

American Academy of Pediatrics. Committee on Environmental Health. (1997). Noise: A hazard for the fetus and newborn. *Pediatrics, 100*, 724–727.

Anderson, P. J., & Doyle, L. W. (2008). Cognitive and educational deficits in children born extremely preterm. *Seminars in Perinatology, 32*, 51–58.

Arnon, S., Shapsa, A., Forman, L., Regev, R., Bauer, S., Litmanovitz, I., & Dolfin, T. (2006). Live music is beneficial to preterm infants in the neonatal intensive care unit environment. *Birth, 33*(2), 131–136.

Barnard, K. E., & Bee, H. L. (1983). The impact of temporally patterned stimulation on the development of preterm infants. *Child Development, 54*, 1156–1167.

Barreto, E., Morris, B., Philbin, M. K., Gray, L., & Lasky, R. (2006). Do former preterm infants remember and respond to neonatal intensive care unit noise? *Early Human Development, 82*(11), 703–707.

Baker, F., & Mackinlay, E. (2006). Sing, soothe and sleep: A lullaby education programme for first time mothers. *British Journal of Music Education, 23*(2), 147–160.

Bergmann, K., Sarkar, P., O'Connor, T. G., Modi, N., & Glover, V. (2007). Maternal stress during pregnancy predicts cognitive ability and fearfulness in infancy. *Journal of the American Academy of Child and Adolescence Psychiatry, 46*, 357–372.

Birnholtz, J. C., & Benaceraff, B. R. (1983). The development of human fetal hearing. *Science, 222,* 516.

Blumenfeld, H., & Eisenfeld, L. (2006). Does a mother singing to her premature baby affect feeding in the neonatal intensive care unit? *Journal of Clinical Pediatrics, 45,* 65–70.

Bo, L. K., & Callaghan, P. (2000). Soothing pain-elicited distress in Chinese neonates. *Pediatrics, 105*(4), 1–5.

Start Bozzette, M. (2008). Healthy preterm infant response to taped maternal voice. *The Journal of Perinatal & Neonatal Nursing, 22,* 307–316.

Brazelton, T. B. (2011). *Neonatal Behavioral Assessment Scale* (4ᵗʰ ed.). *(Clinics in developmental medicine, no. 50).* Philadelphia: J. B. Lippincott Co.

Brymer, M., Jacobs, A., Layne, C., Pynoos, R., Ruzek, J., & Steinberg, A. (2006). *Psychological first aid: Field operations guide* (2nd ed.). Retrieved from The National Child Traumatic Stress Network website: http://www.nctsn.org/content/psychological-first-aid

Burke, M., Walsh, J., Oehler, J., & Gingras, J. (1995). Music therapy following suctioning: Four case studies. *Neonatal Network, 14*(7), 41–49.

Butt, M. L., & Kisilevsky, B. S. (2000). Music modulates behaviour of premature infants following heel lance. *Canadian Journal of Nursing Research, 31*(4), 17–39.

Byers, J. F., Waugh, W. R., & Lowman, L. B. (2006). Sound level exposure of high-risk infants in different environmental conditions. *Neonatal Network, 25,* 25–32.

Caine, J. (1991). The effects of music on the selected stress behaviors, weight, caloric and formula intake, and length of hospital stay of premature and low birth weight neonates in a newborn intensive care unit. *Journal of Music Therapy, 28,* 180–192.

Calabro, J., Wolfe, R., & Shoemark, H. (2003). The effects of recorded sedative music on the physiology and behaviour of premature infants with a respiratory disorder. *Australian Journal of Music Therapy, 14,* 3–19.

Canga, B., Hahm, C. L., Lucido, D., Grossbard, M. L., & Loewy, J. V. (2012). Environmental music therapy: A pilot study on the effects of music therapy in a chemotherapy infusion suite. *Music and Medicine, 4*(4), 221–230.

Cassidy, J. W. (1998). Presentation of aural stimuli to newborns and premature infants: An audiological perspective. *Journal of Music Therapy, 35*(2), 70–87.

Cassidy, J. W. (2009). The effect of decibel level of music stimuli and gender on head circumference and physiological responses of premature infants in the NICU. *Journal of Music Therapy, 46,* 180–190.

Cassidy, J. W., & Standley, J. M. (1995). The effect of music listening on physiological responses of premature infants in the NICU. *Journal of Music Therapy, 32,* 208–227.

Cevasco, A. M. (2008). The effects of mothers' singing on full-term and preterm infants and maternal emotional responses. *Journal of Music Therapy, 45*(3), 273–306.

Cevasco, A. M., & Grant, R. E. (2005). Effects of the pacifier-activated lullaby on weight gain of premature infants. *Journal of Music Therapy, 42,* 123–139.

Chou, L., Wang, R., Chen, S., & Pai, L. (2003). Effects of music therapy on oxygen saturation in premature infants receiving endotracheal suctioning. *Journal of Nursing Research, 11,* 209–215.

Cohen, J. (1988). *Statistical power analysis for the behavioral sciences* (2nd ed.). Hillsdale, NJ: Lawrence Earlbaum Associates.

Coleman, J. M., Pratt, R. R., Stoddard, R. A., Gerstmann, D. R., & Abel, H. H. (1997). The effects of male and female singing and speaking voices on selected physiological and behavioral measures of premature infants in the intensive care unit. *International Journal of Arts Medicine, 5,* 4–11.

Collins, S. K., & Kuck, K. (1991). Music therapy in the neonatal intensive care unit. *Neonatal Network, 9,* 23–26.

Coppola, G., & Cassibba, R. (2010). Mothers' social behaviours in the NICU during newborns hospitalization: An observational approach. *Journal of Reproductive and Infant Psychology, 28*(2), 200–211.

Courtnage, A., Chawla, H., Loewy, J., & Nolan, P. (2002). Effects of live infant-directed singing on oxygen saturation, heart rate, and respiratory rates of infants in the neonatal intensive care unit. (Abstract 23469). *Pediatric Research, 51*(4), 403a.

DeCasper, A. J., & Fifer, W. P. (1980). Of human bonding: Newborns prefer their mother's voices. *Science, 208,* 1174–1176.

DeCasper, A. J., & Spence, M. J. (1986). Prenatal maternal speech influences newborns' perception of speech sound. *Infant Behavior and Development, 9,* 133–150.

De Graaf-Peters, V. B., & Hadders-Algra, M. (2006). Ontogeny of the human central nervous system: What is happening when? *Early Human Development, 82,* 257–266.

Doheny, L., Hurwitz, S., Insoft, R., Ringer, S., & Lahav, A. (2012). Exposure to biological maternal sounds improves cardiorespiratory regulation in extremely preterm infants. *Journal of Maternal-Fetal and Neonatal Medicine, 25*(9), 1591–1594.

Eagle, M. N. (1984). *Recent development in psychoanalysis: A critical evaluation.* New York: McGraw-Hill.

Elliot, L. (2000). *What's going in there? How the brain and mind develop in the first five years of life.* New York: Bantam Books.

Farhat, A., Amirib, R., Karbandic, S., Esmailyd, H., & Mohammadzadeha, A. (2010). The effect of listening to lullaby music on physiologic response and weight gain of premature infants. *Journal of Neonatal-Perinatal Medicine, 3,* 103–107.

Fenoglio, K. A., Brunson, K. L., & Baram, T. Z. (2006). Hippocampal neuroplasticity induced by early-life stress: Functional and molecular aspects. *Frontiers in Neuroendocrinology, 27,* 180–192.

Fernald, A. (1989). Intonation and communicative intent in mothers' speech to infants: Is the melody the message? *Child Development, 60,* 1497–1510.

Ferraiuolo, A., Loewy, J., et al. (in press). *The rhythm, breath and lullaby compendium.* New York: United Music World Press, Independent Hospital.

Field, T., Hernandez-Reif, P., Feijo, L., & Freedman, J. (2006). Prenatal, perinatal and neonatal stimulation: A survey of neonatal services. *Infant Behavior and Development, 29*(1), 24–31.

Fifer, W. P., & Moon, C. M. (1994). The role of the mother's voice in the organization of brain function in the newborn. (Supplemental material). *Acta Paediatrica, 83*(s397), 86–93. DOI: 10.1111/j.1651-2227.1994.tb13270.x.

Fischer, C. B., & Als, H. (2004). Trusting behavioral communication. Individualized relationship-based developmental care in the newborn intensive care unit—a way of meeting the neurodevelopmental expectation of preterm infant. In M. Nöcker-Ribaupierre (Ed.), *Music therapy for premature and newborn infants* (pp. 1–20). Gilsum, NH: Barcelona Publishers.

Fischer, C. B., & Als, H. (2012). Was willst du mir sagen? Individuelle beziehungsgeführte Pflege auf der Neugeborenen Intensiv-Station zur Förderung der Entwicklung des frühgeborenen Kindes [Trusting behavioral communication: individualized relationship-based developmental care in the newborn intensive care unit—a way of meeting the neurodevelopmental expectation of preterm infant]. In M. Nöcker-Ribaupierre (Ed.), *Hören—Brücke ins Leben. Musiktherapiemit früh- und neugeborenen Kindern* (pp. 19–40). 2.akt.Aufl. Wiesbaden: Reichert.

Flowers, F., McCain, A. P., & Hilker, K. A. (1999). *The effects of music listening on premature infants.* Paper presented at the Biennial Meeting, Society for Research in Child Development, Albuquerque, NM.

Fox, S. E., Levitt, P., & Nelson III, C. A. (2010). How the timing and quality of early experiences influences the development of brain architecture. *Child Development, 81*(1), 28–40.

Gerhardt, K. J., & Abrams, R. M. (2004). Fetal hearing: Implications for the neonate. In M. Nöcker-Ribaupierre (Ed.), *Music therapy for premature and newborn infants* (pp. 21–32). Gilsum, NH: Barcelona Publishers.

Gooding, L. F. (2010). Using music therapy protocols in the treatment of premature infants: An introduction to current practices. *The Arts in Psychotherapy, 37*, 211–214.

Gorski, P. A., Huntington, L., & Lewkovicz, D. J. (1990). Handling preterm infants in hospitals: Stimulating controversy about timing of stimulation. *Clinical Perinatology, 17*(1), 103–112.

Graven, S. (2000). The full-term and premature newborn: Sound and the developing infant in the NICU: Conclusions and recommendations for care. *Journal of Perinatology, 20*, 88–93.

Graven, S., & Browne, J. (2008). Auditory development in the fetus and infant. *Newborn and Infant Nursing Review, 8*(4), 187–193.

Gray, L., & Philbin, M. K. (2004). Effects of the neonatal intensive care unit on auditory attention and distraction. *Clinics in Perinatology, 31*, 243–260.

Hanson-Abromeit, D. (2003a). The newborn individualized developmental care and assessment program (NIDCAP) as a model for clinical music therapy interventions with premature infants. *Music Therapy Perspectives, 21*(2), 60–68.

Hanson-Abromeit, D. (2003b). *Naturalistic observation sheet for mt assessment—Adapted from Als, 1995*. Iowa City, IA: Department of Rehabilitation Therapies, University of Iowa Hospitals and Clinics and the Children's Hospital of Iowa.

Hanson-Abromeit, D. (2004): A resource guide for establishing a neonatal music therapy program. In M. Nöcker-Ribaupierre (Ed.), *Music Therapy for premature and newborn infants* (pp. 177–190). Gilsum, NH: Barcelona Publishers.

Hanson-Abromeit, D. (2006). Developmentally based criteria to support recorded music selections by neonatal nurses for use with premature infants in the neonatal intensive care unit. Doctoral dissertation. University of Kansas. *Dissertation Abstracts International Section A: Humanities & Social Sciences, 67*(4), 1143.

Hanson-Abromeit, D. (2012). Aufbau eines Musiktherapie-Programms für neugeborene Kinder [A resource guide for establishing a neonatal music therapy program]. In M. Nöcker-Ribaupierre (Ed.), *Hören—Brücke ins Leben. Musiktherapie mit früh- und neugeborenen Kindern* (pp. 209–218). *2.akt.Aufl*. Wiesbaden: Reichert.

Hanson-Abromeit, D., & Colwell, C. (Eds.). (2008). *Effective clinical practice in music therapy: Medical music therapy for pediatrics in hospital settings*. AMTA Monograph Series. Silver Spring, MD: American Music Therapy Association.

Hanson-Abromeit, D., Shoemark, H., & Loewy, J. V. (2009). Newborn intensive care unit (NICU). In D. Hanson-Abromeit & C. Colwell (Eds.), *Medical music therapy for pediatrics in hospital settings* (pp. 15–70). Silver Spring, MD: American Music Therapy Association.

Haslbeck, F. (2004). Music Therapy with preterm infants—Theoretical approach and first practical experience. *Music Therapy Today, 5*(4).

Haslbeck, F. B. (2012). Music therapy for premature infants and their parents: An integrative review. *Nordic Journal of Music Therapy, 21*(3), 203–226.

Haslbeck, F. B. (in press). The interactive potential of creative music therapy with premature infants and their parents: A qualitative analysis. *Nordic Journal of Music Therapy*.

Hepper, P. G., & Shahidullah, B. S. (1994). Development of fetal hearing. *Archives of Disease in Childhood, 71*, 81–87.

Hüppi, P. S., Schuknecht, B., Boesch, C., Bossi, E., Felblinger, J., Fusch, C., & Herschkowitz, N. (1996). Structural and neurobehavioral delay in postnatal brain development of preterm infants. *Pediatric Research, 39*, 895–901.

Ingersoll, E. W., & Thoman, E. B. (1994). The breathing bear: Effects on respiration in premature infants. *Physiology & Behavior, 56,* 855–859.

Johansson, B., Wedenberg, E., & Westen, B. (1964). Measurement of tone response by the human foetus: A preliminary report. *Acta Otolaryngology, 57,* 188–192.

Johnston, C., Filion, F., Campbell-Yeo, M., Goulet, C., Bell, L., McNaughton, K., & Byron, J. (2009). Enhanced kangaroo mother care for heel lance in preterm neonates: A crossover trial. *Journal of Perinatology: Official Journal of the California Perinatal Association, 29*(1), 51–56.

Jotzo, M., & Poets, C. F. (2005). Helping parents cope with the trauma of premature birth: An evaluation of a trauma-preventive psychological intervention. *Pediatrics, 115,* 915–919.

Katz, V. (1971). Auditory stimulation and developmental behavior of the premature infant. *Nursing Research, 20,* 196–201.

Keith, D. R., Russel, K., & Weaver, B. S. (2009). The effects of music listening on inconsolable crying in premature infants. *Journal of Music Therapy, 46,* 191–203.

Keller, L. (2008). Preterm infants exposed to maternal voice. *Journal of Undergraduate Research, 9,* 1–4.

Kemper, K., Martin, K., Block, S., Shoaf, R., & Woods, C. (2004). Attitudes and expectations about music therapy for premature infants among staff in a neonatal intensive care unit. *Alternative Therapies in Health and Medicine, 10*(2), 50–54.

Klaus, M. H., & Kennell, J. H. (1976). *Maternal-Infant-Bonding.* St. Louis MO: Mosby.

Krueger, C. (2010). Exposure to maternal voice in preterm infants: A review. *Journal of Advances in Neonatal Care, 10,* 13–18.

Lai, H. L., Chen, C. J., Peng, T. C., Chang, F. M., Hsieh, M. L., Huang, H. Y., & Chang, S. C. (2006). Randomized controlled trial of music during kangaroo care on maternal state anxiety and preterm infants' responses. *International Journal of Nursing Studies, 43,* 139–146.

Lasky, R. E., & Williams, A. L. (2009). Noise and light exposures for extremely low birth weight newborns during their stay in the neonatal intensive care. *Pediatrics, 123,* 540–546.

Linderkamp, O., Janus, L., Linder, R., & Skoruppa, D. B. (2009). Time table of normal foetal brain development. *The International Journal of Prenatal and Perinatal Psychology and Medicine, 21*(1/2), 4–16.

Linderkamp, O., Janus, L., Linder, R., & Skoruppa, D. B. (in press). Development of the fetal brain. Genetics and experience driven plasticity. *The International Journal of Prenatal and Perinatal Psychology and Medicine.*

Linderkamp, O., & Skoruppa, D. B (2008). The foetal brain. Effects of maternal stress and sensory deprivation. Unpublished manuscript.

Loewy, J. (2004). A clinical model of music therapy in the NICU. In M. Nöcker-Ribaupierre (Ed.), *Music therapy for premature and newborn infants* (pp. 159–176). Gilsum, NH: Barcelona Publishers.

Loewy, J. (2007). Developing music therapy programs in medical practice and healthcare communities. In J. Edwards (Ed.), *Music: Promoting health and creating community in healthcare contexts* (pp.17–28). Cambridge, UK: Cambridge Scholars Press.

Loewy, J. (2009). Musical sedation: Mechanisms of breathing entrainment. In R. Azoulay & J. Loewy (Eds.), *Music, the breath & health: Advances in integrative music therapy* (pp. 223–232). New York: Satchnote Press.

Loewy, J. (2011). Music therapy for hospitalized infants and their parents. In J. Edwards (Ed.), *Music therapy and parent-infant bonding* (pp. 179–190). London: Oxford University Press.

Loewy, J. (2012). Ein Modell klinischer Musiktherapie in der Neugeborenen Intensiv—Station. [A clinical model of music therapy in the NICU]. In M. Nöcker-Ribaupierre (Ed.), *Hören—Brücke ins Leben. Musiktherapie mit früh- und neugeborenen Kindern* (pp. 193–208). *2.akt.Aufl.* Wiesbaden: Reichert.

Loewy, J., Stewart, K., Dassler, A. M., Telsey, A., & Homel, P. (2013). The effects of music therapy on vital signs, feeding, and sleep in premature infants. *Pediatrics, 131*(5), 1–17.

Loewy, J. V. (Ed.). (2000). *Music therapy in the neonatal intensive care unit.* Boston, MA: The Louis & Lucille Armstrong Music Therapy Program, Beth Israel Medical Center.

Lubetzky, R., Mimouni, F. B., Dollberg, S., Reifen, R., Ashbel, G., & Mandel, D. (2010). Effect of music by Mozart on energy expenditure in growing preterm infants. *Pediatrics, 125,* e24–e28.

Maiello, S. (2004). On the meaning of prenatal auditory perception and memory for the development of the mind: A psychoanalytical perspective. In M. Nöcker-Ribaupierre (Ed.), *Music therapy for premature and newborn infants* (pp. 85–96). Gilsum, NH: Barcelona Publishers.

Malloy, G. B. (1979). The relationship between maternal and musical auditory stimulation and the developmental behavior of premature infants. *Birth Defects: Original Art Series, 15,* 81–98.

McMahon, E., Wintermark, P., & Lahav, A. (2012). Auditory brain development in premature infants: The importance of early experience. *Annals of the New York Academy of Sciences, 1252,* 17–24.

Meves, A. U., Hüppi, P. S., Als, H., Rybicki, F. J., Inder, T. E., McAnulty, G. B., Mulkern, R. V., Robertson, R. L., Rivkin, M. J., & Warfield, S. K. (2008). Regional brain development in serial magnetic resonance imaging of low-risk preterm infants. *Pediatrics, 118,* 23–33.

Moon, C., Cooper, R. P., & Fifer, W. P. (1993). Two-day-olds prefer their native language. *Infant Behavior and Development, 16,* 495–500.

Moore, R., Gladstone, I., & Standley, J. (1994). *Effects of music, maternal voice intrauterine sounds and white noise on the oxygen saturation levels of premature infants.* Paper presented at the National Conference of the National Association for Music Therapy, Orlando, FL.

Nagorski-Johnson, A. (2008). Engaging fathers in the NICU. Taking down the barriers to the baby. *Journal of Perinatal & Neonatal Nursing, 22*(4), 302–306.

Neves, G., Cook, S. F., & Bliss, T. V. (2008). Synaptic plasticity, memory and the hippocampus: A neural network approach to causality. *Nature Reviews. Neuroscience, 9,* 65–75.

Nöcker, M., Güntner, M., & Riegel, K. P. (1987). The effect of the mother's voice on the physical activity and the tcPO^2 of very premature infants. *Pediatric Research, 22,* 21.

Nöcker-Ribaupierre, M. (1995*). Auditive Stimulation nach Frühgeburt* [Auditive stimulation after premature birth]. Stuttgart: G. Fischer Verlag.

Nöcker-Ribaupierre, M. (1998). Short- and long-term effects of the maternal voice on the behaviors of very low birth weight infants and their mothers as a basis for the bonding process. In R. R. Pratt & D. Grocke (Eds.), *MusicMedicine 3: Expanding horizons* (pp. 153–161). Victoria: University of Melbourne.

Nöcker-Ribaupierre, M. (Ed.). (2004). *Music therapy for premature and newborn infants.* Gilsum, NH: Barcelona Publishers.

Nöcker-Ribaupierre, M. (2011). When life begins too early: Music therapy in a newborn intensive care unit. In A. Meadows (Ed.), *Developments in music therapy practice: Case study perspectives* (pp. 30–48). Gilsum, NH: Barcelona Publishers.

Nordoff, P., & Robbins, C. (1977). *Creative music therapy: Individualized treatment for the handicapped child.* New York: John Day Company.

Nzama, M., Nolte, A. G., & Dorfling, C. S. (1995). Noise in the neonatal unit: Guidelines for the reduction or prevention of noise. *Curationis, 18,* 16–21.

O'Gorman, S. (2005). Music therapy for premature and newborn infants. *Australian Journal of Music Therapy, 16,* 120–122.

Olischar, M., Shoemark, H., Holton, T., Weninger, M., & Hunt, R. (2011). The influence of music on EEG activity in neurologically healthy newborns >32 weeks' gestational age. *Acta Paediatrica, 100*(5), 670–667.

Palmer, M. M. (1993). Identification and management of the transitional suck pattern in premature infants. *Journal of Perinatal and Neonatal Nursing, 7*, 66–75.

Philbin, M., & Evans, J. (2006). Standards for the acoustic environment of the newborn ICU. *Journal of Perinatology, 26*, S27–S30.

Philbin, M. K. (2000). The influence of auditory experience on the behavior of preterm newborns. *Journal of Perinatology, 26*, S76–S86.

Philbin, M. K. (2004). Planning the acoustic environment of a neonatal intensive care nursery. *Clinics in Perinatology, 31*(2), 455–460.

Rais-Bahrami, K., & Short, B. L. (2013). Premature and small-for-dates infants. In M. L. Batshaw, N. J. Roizen, & G. R. Lotrecchiano (Eds.), *Children with disabilities* (7th ed.) (pp. 87–104). Baltimore, MD: Paul H. Brookes Publishing Co.

Ravn, I. H., Smith, L., Aarhus Smeby, N., Kynoe, N. M., Snadvic, L., Haugen Bunch E., & Lindemann, R. (2011). Effects of early mother-infant intervention on outcomes in mothers and moderately and late preterm infants at age 1 year: A randomized controlled trial. *Infant Behavior and Development, 35*, 36–47.

Rottmann, G. (1974). Untersuchungen über die Einstellung zur Schwangerschaft und zur fetalen Entwicklung [Studies on attitudes about pregnancy and fetal development]. In H. H. Graber (Ed.), Pränatale Psychologie (pp. 68–88). München: Kindler.

Rubel, E. W. (1984). Ontogeny of auditory system function. *Annual Review Physiology, 46*, 213–229.

Samra, H. A., McGrath, J. M., & Wehbe, M. (2011). An integrated review of developmental outcomes and late-preterm birth. *Journal of Obstetric, Gynecologic, & Neonatal Nursing, 40*(4), 399–411.

Schumacher, K., Calvet, C., & Reimer, S. (2011). Das EBQ-Instrument und seine entwicklungs-psychologischen Grundlagen. [The EBQ-Instrument and its development-psychological basics]. Göttingen: Vandenhoeck & Ruprecht.

Schwartz, F. J. (2000). Music and sound effect on perinatal brain development and the premature baby. In J. V. Loewy (Ed.), *Music therapy in the neonatal intensive care unit* (pp. 9–19). New York: The Louis & Lucille Armstrong Music Therapy Program.

Schwartz, F. J. (2004). Medical music therapy. In M. Nöcker-Ribaupierre (Ed.), *Music therapy for premature and newborn infants* (pp. 85–96). Gilsum, NH: Barcelona Publishers.

Schwartz, F. J., Ritchie, R., Sacks, L. L., & Phillips, C. E. (1999). Music, stress reduction, and medical cost savings in the neonatal intensive care unit. In R. R. Pratt & D. E. Grocke (Eds.), *MusicMedicine, vol. 3: Expanding horizons* (pp. 120–129). Victoria: University of Melbourne.

Shoemark, H. (1998). Singing as the foundation for multi-modal stimulation of the older preterm infant. In R. R. Pratt & D. Grocke (Eds.), *MusicMedicine, vol. 3: Expanding horizons* (pp. 140–152). Victoria: University of Melbourne.

Shoemark, H. (2004). Family-centered music therapy for infants with complex medical and surgical needs. In M. Nöcker-Ribaupierre (Ed.), *Music therapy for premature and newborn infants* (pp. 141–158). Gilsum, NH: Barcelona Publishers.

Shoemark, H. (2006). Infant-directed singing as a vehicle for regulation rehearsal in the medically fragile full-term infant. *Australian Journal of Music Therapy, 17*, 54–63.

Shoemark, H. (2011). Contingent singing: The musicality of companionship with the hospitalized newborn infant. In F. Baker & S. Uhlig (Eds.), *Voicework in music therapy* (pp. 233–254). Philadelphia, PA: Jessica Kingsley.

Shoemark, H. (2012). Familienzentrierte Musiktherapie für Kinder mit komplexen medizinischen und chirurgischen Problemen. [Family-centered music therapy for infants with complex medical and surgical needs]. In M. Nöcker-Ribaupierre (Ed.), *Hören—Brücke ins Leben. Musiktherapiemit früh- und neugeborenen Kindern* (pp. 175–192). *2.akt.Aufl*. Wiesbaden: Reichert.

Shoemark, H., & Dearn, T. (2008). Keeping parents at the centre of family-centered music therapy with hospitalized infants. *Australian Journal of Music Therapy, 19,* 3–24.

Standley, J., & Walworth, D. (2010). *Music therapy with premature infants. Research and developmental interventions* (2nd ed.). Silver Spring, MD: American Music Therapy Association.

Standley, J. M. (1991). Long-term benefits of music intervention in the newborn intensive care unit: A pilot study. *Journal of the International Association of Music for the Handicapped, 6,* 12–22.

Standley, J. M. (1998). The effect of music and multimodal stimulation on responses of premature infants in neonatal intensive care. *Pediatric Nursing, 24*(6), 532–538.

Standley, J. M. (1999). Music therapy in the NICU: Pacifier-activated-lullabies (PAL) for reinforcement of nonnutritive sucking. *International Journal of Arts Medicine, 6,* 17–21.

Standley, J. M. (2000). The effect of contingent music to increase non-nutritive sucking of premature infants. *Journal of Pediatric Nursing, 26*(5), 494–499.

Standley J. M. (2002). A meta-analysis of the efficacy of music therapy for premature infants. *Journal of Pediatric Nursing, 17*(2), 107–113.

Standley, J. M. (2003a). *Music therapy with premature infants. Research and developmental interventions.* Silver Spring, MD: American Music Therapy Association.

Standley, J. M. (2003b). The effect of music-reinforced nonnutritive sucking on feeding rate of premature infants. *Journal of Pediatric Nursing, 18*(3), 169–173.

Standley, J. M., & Madsen, C. (1990). Comparison of infant preferences and responses to auditory stimuli: Music, mother, and other female voice. *Journal of Music Therapy, 27*(2), 54–97.

Standley, J. M., Cassidy, J., Grant, R., Cevasco, A., Szuch, C., & Nguyen, J. (2010). The effect of music reinforcement for non-nutritive sucking on nipple feeding of premature infants. *Pediatric Nursing, 36,* 138–145.

Stern, D. (2010). The issue of vitality. *Nordic Journal of Music Therapy, 19*(2), 88–102.

Stern, D. N. (1985). *The interpersonal world of the infant.* New York: Basic Books.

Stewart, K. (2009a). PATTERNS—A model for evaluating trauma in NICU music therapy: Part 1—Theory and design. *Music and Medicine, 1*(1), 29–40.

Stewart, K. (2009b). PATTERNS—A model for evaluating trauma in NICU music therapy: Part 2—Treatment parameters. *Music and Medicine, 1*(2), 123–128.

Stewart, K., & Schneider, S. (2000). The effects of music therapy on the sound environment in the NICU: A pilot study. In J. V. Loewy (Ed.), *Music therapy in the neonatal intensive care unit* (pp. 85–100). New York: The Louis & Lucille Armstrong Music Therapy Program.

Teckenberg-Jansson, P., Huotilainen, M., & Pölkki, T. (2011). Rapid effects of neonatal music therapy combined with kangaroo care on prematurely-born infants. *Nordic Journal of Music Therapy, 20*(1), 22–42.

Thoman, E. B., Ingersoll, E. W., & Acebo, C. (1991). Premature infants seek rhythmic stimulation, and the experience facilitates neurobehavioral development. *Journal of Developmental & Behavioral Pediatrics, 12,* 11–18.

Treyvaud, K., Doyle, L. W., Lee, K. J., Roberts, G., Cheong, J. L, Inder, T. E., & Anderson, P. J. (2011). Family functioning burden and parenting stress 2 years after very preterm birth. *Early Human Development, 87,* 427–431.

Turkewitz, G. (2007). The relevance of the fetal and neonatal period for the development of novelty preferences, learning, habituation and hemispheric specialization. *Developmental Psychobiology, 49,* 780–787.

Volpe, J. J. (2008). *Neurology of the newborn* (5th ed.). Philadelphia, PA: W. B. Saunders.

Vonderlin, E. (1999). *Frühgeburt: Elterliche Belastung und Bewältigung* [Premature birth: parental burden and coping]. Heidelberg: Schindele.

Wachman, E. M., & Lahav, A. (2010). The effects of noise on preterm infants in NICU. Retrieved from http://fn.bmj.com

Wereszcak, J., Shandor Miles, M., & Holditch-Davis, D. (1997). Maternal recall of the neonatal intensive care unit. *Neonatal Network, 16*(4), 33–40.

Whipple, J. (2000). The effect of parent training in music and multimodal stimulation on parent-neonate interactions in the neonatal intensive care unit. *Journal of Music Therapy, 37,* 250–268.

Whipple, J. (2005). Music and multimodal stimulation as developmental intervention in neonatal intensive care. *Music Therapy Perspectives, 23*(2), 100–105.

Whipple, J. (2008). The effect of music-reinforced nonnutritive sucking on state of preterm, low birthweight infants experiencing heelstick. *Journal of Music Therapy, 45*(3), 227–272.

White, R. D. (2007). Recommended standards for the newborn ICU. *Journal of Perinatology, 27,* 4–19.

Winberg, J. (2005). Mother and newborn baby: Mutual regulation of physiology and behavior—A selective review. *Developmental Psychology, 47*(3), 217–229.

Wubben, S. M., Brueggeman, P. M., Helseth, C. C., & Blaschke, K. (2011). *The sound of operation and the acoustic attenuation of the Ohmedas Medical Giraffe OmniBed.* Poster presented at the 22nd Annual Gravens Conference on the Physical and Developmental Environment of the High Risk Infant. University of South Florida.

Zahr, L. K., & Balian, S. (1995). Responses of premature infants to routine nursing intervention and noise in the NICU. *Nursing Research, 44,* 179–185.

Zimmer, M. (2004). Premature babies have premature mothers: Practical experiences with premature infants and their mothers using auditive stimulation with the mother's voice. In M. Nöcker-Ribaupierre (Ed.), *Music therapy for premature and newborn infants* (pp. 113–128). Gilsum, NH: Barcelona Publishers.

APPENDIX A

MUSIC THERAPY REFERRAL CRITERIA
BETH ISRAEL MEDICAL CENTER[1]

Referrals may be made by the nurse practitioner, patient care manager, and residents but must have the consent of the attending physician and the parent/caretaker.

Age: >32 weeks unless approved by the attending on a case-by-case basis.

I. BONDING:
Parents and infants (identified by the team) who are in need of collaborative experiences may be referred. Incorporating Brazelton's Neonatal Behavioral Assessment Scale, musical focus will emphasize infant–parent attachment. Music and soft singing with skin-to-skin contact will be encouraged. Melodic (3–5 note) vocalizations will be modeled and simple lullabies will be encouraged for use by mother/dad/caretaker. The parent–infant dynamic will be strengthened as the use of soft sounds (repeated sung phrases) will be patterned for use during times of sleep, transitions, and/or separations.

II. IRRITABILITY — CRYING (INTENSE HIGH-PITCHED):
Music (lullabies and toning) will be offered as a means to contain the sound environment for the infant in distress. Toning will be provided as a blanket of steady sound to comfort and sustain a homeostatic environment. Tones enable the infant to trust his/her surroundings and offer an atmosphere of predictability. Human voice sounds made through vocal tones provide an atmosphere of safety which induces sleep and assists in relaxation.

III. RESPIRATORY DIFFICULTIES:
The Gato box (also called a tongue or slit drum) and breath sounds can be useful in helping the infant synchronize and regulate the rhythm of his/her breath. The Gato box provides a predictable rhythm that mimics the sound of a human heart. The infant can entrain to the provided rhythm which can lengthen and ease the meter of the breath. The breath voice is soothing and provides a flowing release of oxygen which can enhance the breathing process. The ocean drum is an interuterine sound environment that provides safety and familiarity, stimulating the infant's breathing process.

IV. FEEDING—SUCKING—WEIGHT GAIN:
Comfort sounds may be a catalyst for inducing gurgles and vegetative sucking. Soft, rhythmic soundscaping (mouth and vegetative clicking) prior to feeding may assist in the infant's coordination with sucking, swallowing, and breathing. Nutritive sucking with rhythmic reinforcement may help infants maintain steady mouth motion which can be further sustained through melodic holding during feedings.

V. SEDATION—SLEEP—PAIN:
Music therapy can provide an environment of safety during painful procedures. Tonic tones that match the pitch of the infant's cry, entrained with the meter of the breath, can ease and alter the experience/perception of pain. Using the Attia (et al., 1987) infant pain scale, the music therapist can assess the level of pain and distract the infant from focusing on the painful stimuli. Music can assist the infant in reconstitution at postprocedure time. Music therapy can be used in

conjunction with (complementary) or as an alternative pharmacological sedation, depending upon the MD order.

For the infant who appears overstimulated and/or is in need of sleep, simple lullabies containing <5 note melodies can provide an aural atmosphere of nurturance. Altering the tempo and meter of the lullaby can help the infant relax and shift gradually into a sleep state.

VI. SELF-REGULATION:

Central to the infant's development is his/her ability to self-regulate. Simple, consistent rhythms and melodies can help the infant organize and acclimate to the environment. Predictable, ordered aspects of music provide structure that assists in the development of self-nurturing behavior, physiological organization, and neurological pathways.

APPENDIX B

MUSIC THERAPY NICU REFERRAL FORM
BETH ISRAEL MEDICAL CENTER[2]

Referrals may be made by the nurse practitioner, case manager, and residents but must have the consent of the attending physician and the parent/caretaker.

The age for referrals is>32 weeks unless approved on a case-by-case basis by the attending physician. If there are any questions or concerns, call Dr. Joanne Loewy at 420-3484 or beeper 15208.

Infant's name_____

Gestational age_____ Chronological age_____

Diagnosis_____

Name of consenting Attending Physician: _____ Beeper_____

Family informed by _____ Beeper_____

REASON FOR REFERRAL
(Check all of the following that apply and write in any comments).

____Bonding: Caretakers and infants who are in need of collaborative experiences. Comments:

____Psychosocial Issues: ACS hold, intrauterine exposure to drugs or alcohol, trauma, stress, violence, family illness, separation/divorce. Specify:

____Respiratory Difficulties:

____Crying/ Irritability:

____Feeding/Sucking/Weight Gain:

____Sedation/Sleep/Pain:

____Difficulty sleeping

____Requires music assistance for sedation during procedure (Date/time:)

_____Self-Regulation

_____   Beeper/extension:_____   Date:_____
Person referring

Please place this form in music therapy referral box located at the nursing station.

APPENDIX C
NICU MUSIC THERAPY ASSESSMENT SUMMARY
2003 D. Hanson-Abromeit

Name_____ Hospital # _____

Referral Date_____ Assessment_____

INFANT BIRTH HISTORY

DOB_____ GA at birth _____

Mode of Delivery_____ Apgars _____ 1 min_____ 5 min _____

Birthweight_____ g LBW   VLBW   ELBW

Length_____cm Head Circumference_____cm

Diagnosis:_____

Complications of birth:_____

Other birth information:_____

Respiratory Assistance:

      □ HVF – settings

      □ CPAP – settings

      □ Nasal Canula – settings

      □ Room Air – settings

      □ Other – settings

Medications:

      □ *Sedatives:* Morphine (MS04)   Ativan Lozepan   Fentanyl   Other

      □ *Diuretics*: Lasix Other

      □ *Anticonvulsants:* Phenobarb   Idilamtin   Other

      □ *Steroids:*   Dexamethosone   Decadron   Other

      □ *Antibiotics:* Ampillician   Gentamyacin   Vancomyocin   Pepracillian   Other

      □ *Other:* Caffeine   Theophylline

FAMILY INFORMATION

Mother's Name _____Mother's Age _____

Father's Name _____Father's Age _____

Sibling _____ Age _____Sibling _____ Age _____

Sibling _____ Age _____Sibling _____ Age _____

Family Availability/Restrictions _____

Date: _____ Location: _____

SOCIAL HISTORY

_____

_____

_____

MATERNAL HISTORY

Grava _____ Para _____

Prenatal Care/Complications _____
_____

Labor and Delivery _____
_____

Medications _____

Other _____

HOSPITAL COURSE

Current Respiratory Support:

       ☐ HVF – settings

       ☐ CPAP – settings

       ☐ Air Canula – settings _____

       ☐ Room Air – settings

       ☐ Other – settings

Current Medications:

       ☐ *Sedatives*: Morphine (MS04)   Ativan Lozepan Fentanyl Other

       ☐ *Diuretics:* Lasix Other

       ☐ *Anticonvulsants:* Phenobarb Idilamtin   Other

       ☐ *Steroids:* Dexamethosone Decadron Other

       ☐ *Antibiotics:* Ampililcian Gentamyacin Vancomyocin Pepracillian Other

       ☐ *Other:* Caffeine Theophylline

Current Feeding/Nutrition:

       Time _____ Type _____

Medical Problems:

       Acidosis (pH<7.3)   Anemia   Apnea

       Bleeding tendency   BPD   Bradycardia

       Desaturations   Feeding difficulty

       Hyperbilirubinemia (lights)   Hydrocephalus

       Hypoglycemia   Hypotension   Hypoxic Events

       IVH grade_____R_____   L   NEC   Osteopenia

       PDA   Pheumothorax   RDS

       Renal   ROP Stage_____R_____L

       Seizures   Sepsis   Tracheostomy

Hearing Screening: Attempt ____ Passed _____

APPENDIX D

MUSIC THERAPY ASSESSMENT[4]
BETH ISRAEL MEDICAL CENTER

Patient_____DOB_____

Average Heart Rate:

    Sleeping: _____bpm

    Awake: _____bpm

    Stress: _____bpm

Respiratory:

    Does infant become tachypeic: _____Yes   _____No

    Define stressors:

Crying/Comfort Sounds:

    Pitch: _____High _____Low _____Average

    Absence of cry: _____Yes _____No

    Colic: _____Yes _____No

    Irritable?   _____Yes _____No

    Feeding Noise:_____

Psychosocial Needs:

    ACS Hold: _____Yes _____No

    Intrauterine exposure to drugs/alcohol: _____Yes _____No

    If yes, specify: _____

    How music therapy can benefit the infant:_____

    _____

    Name of family member who can help the infant benefit:

    _____

Mother's Voice Range (Circle):

    Soprano   Mezzo-Soprano Alto

Family's religious Preference:

Feeding/Intake/Weight Gain/Voiding:

    _____Breast _____Gavage _____Bottle _____ Reflux

Is the infant's suck response in need of assistance?   _____Yes _____No

Is Physical or Occupational Therapy involved?   _____Yes _____No

Can infant self-regulate?   _____Yes _____No

Feed Schedule:

    Sleep:

    Irritable: _____Yes _____No

Stimulation:

    Does baby respond to proprioceptive stimulus? _____Yes _____No

Pain:

    Describe physiological indicators, location, and perceived level (1–10).

    Ongoing procedures that may benefit from music therapy assessment:

Development: Indicate whether infant is organized in:

    Sound: _____Yes _____No

    Touch: _____Yes _____No

    Movement: _____Yes _____No

    Is the infant developing appropriate muscle tone? _____Yes _____No

Sedation:

    Is the infant on a sedative? _____Yes _____No

    Medication(s):_____

    Time(s): _____

Music Therapist_____

Date:_____Extension or beeper:_____

APPENDIX E

PREMATURE INFANT ASSESSMENT AND TREATMENT HISTORY FORM[5]

Birth History

Infant's name:_____   Gender: m f   DOB_____/_____/_____

Birthweight:_____lb_____oz/_____k   Gestational Age––Dubowitz_____wks.

APGARs ____,____,____ Type Delivery:C-section Vaginal Breech Abruption

Family History

Mother's name_____ Age_____ Gravita_____Para____

Father's name_____Phone (H)_____ (W) _____

Address_____

Occupations_____

Related Issues_____ Call/Visit

Admitting Diagnoses:

meconium dusky HMD pneumonia hernias genetic screen   CP screen

Infant's Ongoing NICU Status

Date_____   Date_____   Date_____   Date_____

Age_____days   Age_____days Age_____days Age_____days

AGA_____wks   AGA_____wks   AGA_____wks   AGA_____wks

Wt_____   Wt_____   Wt_____   Wt_____

Bedding: Radiant warmer Incubator Open Crib Co-bedding

Respiration: No Assist. Ventilator CPAP Oxygen hood Nasal Canula Room air

Nutrition: TPN/Lipids NPO G-tube OG/NG PO(bottle/breast) OG/PO PO

# of Weekly Apnea/Bradycardia Episodes: _____ _____ _____ _____

Medical Complications/Surgeries

      UA/UVC   Peripheral IV

      Phototherapy

      Medications:_____

      Intaventricular hemorrhage or Date of normal cranial ultrasound_____

      PDA/murmur   Date of ligation_____

Tested positive for: drugs HIV Staph Pseudomonas

Genetic abnormality _____

Rickets

Tracheostomy

Necrotizing enterocolitis (Date of Colostomy_____)

Eye surgery

Hydrocephalus (Date of shunt _____)

Other_____

Referrals:

PT/OT: tonus/rigidity feeding problems calming   rotation of extremities

MT: Continuous music for: _____ O$_2$Sat _____respiration stability at extubation

   Multimodal stimulation

   PAL for:_____ NNS _____feeding endurance

   Parent training for overstimulation

   Parent counseling

HS WIC CMS Home Monitoring Child and Family Services

Nesting date_____   Discharge date_____

Abbreviations

APGAR APGAR test scores
CMS Children's Medical Services
CP cerebral palsy
CPAP continuous positive airway pressure
DOB date of birth
F female
G-tube gastrostomy device
HIV Human Immunodeficiency Virus
HMD hyaline membrane disease
HS Healthy Start Program
lb pound
m male
MT Music Therapy
No Assist. No respiratory assistance needed by infant
NNS   nonnutritive sucking
NPO nothing by mouth
OG/NG oral or nasogastric tube for feeding
O$_2$ Sat Oxygen saturation level
oz ounce

PAL Pacifier-activated lullaby mechanism
PDA patent ductus arteriosus
PO by mouth, indicating breast or bottle feeding
PT/OT physical and/or occupational therapy for feeding, positioning, muscle development
Staph Staphyllococcus
TPN total parenteral nutrition
UA/UVC umbilical artery or venus catheter
WIC Women & Infants Children food supplement program
Wks Weeksw

Form developed by Jennifer Whipple (2001)
Clinical Music Therapy Program
Tallahassee Memorial Hospital 2001

ENDNOTES

[1]Music Therapy Referral Criteria—Beth Israel Medical Center reprinted by permission of Barcelona Publishers. Taken from J. Loewy (2004), A clinical model of music therapy in the NICU. In M. Nöcker-Ribaupierre (Ed.), *Music Therapy for Premature and Newborn Infants* (pp. 166–167). Gilsum, NH: Barcelona Publishers.

[2]Music Therapy NICU Referral Form—Beth Israel Medical Center reprinted by permission of Barcelona Publishers. Taken from J. Loewy (2004), A clinical model of music therapy in the NICU. In M. Nöcker-Ribaupierre (Ed.), *Music Therapy for Premature and Newborn Infants* (pp. 171–172). Gilsum, NH: Barcelona Publishers.

[3]NICU Music Therapy Assessment Summary reprinted by permission of the American Music Therapy Association. Taken from D. Hanson-Abromeit, H. Shoemark, & J. V. Loewy (2009), Newborn intensive care unit (NICU). In D. Hanson-Abromeit & C. Colwell (Eds.), *Medical Music Therapy for Pediatrics in Hospital Settings* (pp. 15–70). Silver Spring, MD: American Music Therapy Association.

[4]Music Therapy Assessment—Beth Israel Medical Center reprinted by permission of Barcelona Publishers. Taken from J. Loewy (2004), A clinical model of music therapy in the NICU. In M. Nöcker-Ribaupierre (Ed.), *Music Therapy for Premature and Newborn Infants* (pp. 173–175). Gilsum, NH: Barcelona Publishers.

[5]Premature Infant Assessment and Treatment History Form reprinted by permission of the American Music Therapy Association. Taken from J. Standley & D. Walworth (2010), *Music Therapy with Premature Infants. Research and Developmental Interventions* (2nd ed.) (p. 25). Silver Spring, MD: American Music Therapy Association.

ACKNOWLEDGMENTS

The author wants to thank Deanna Hanson-Abromeit, Friederike Haslbeck, Joanne Loewy, Helen Shoemark, Jayne Standley, Kristen Stewart, Jennifer Whipple, Dorothee von Moreau, and Joke Bradt for their valuable support.

Chapter 4

Full-Term Hospitalized Newborns

Helen Shoemark

INTRODUCTION

Most babies are born in the maternity ward of a hospital. Many of these hospitals have a perinatal center called a special care nursery for babies requiring some additional medical support. Only a few of them have specialist care units such as a Neonatal Intensive Care Unit (NICU), which can provide sophisticated care for infants who are born prematurely and have medical issues related to that prematurity. However, if the infant is born with or develops complex medical conditions, they will most likely be transferred to a pediatric center for more significant surgical, diagnostic, or ongoing medical care. They may be cared for in a Neonatal or a Pediatric Intensive Care Unit (PICU). Medically fragile newborn infants may be premature, late premature (now considered a distinct population but not addressed in the music therapy literature yet), and full-term infants. In the life of a newborn baby, each week makes a significant difference to physiological stability, neurological maturity, and emergent social availability. It may seem that all babies should be dealt with as one population; however, the capacities and needs of full-term infants differ from those of preterm infants, and subsequently the interventions we provide and expectations we have also vary. This chapter addresses the needs of the full-term infant with complex medical issues resulting in a long hospital stay. For music therapy with premature infants, the reader can consult Chapter 3 of this volume.

While the research of music therapy for prematurely born infants has grown steadily in the last three decades, research with medically fragile full-term infants has been subjected to very little research, with only a handful of music therapy articles in the literature. Therefore, the evidence for the work is still a hybrid collection drawn from the literature for healthy fetal and infant neurodevelopment, infant mental health, and the auditory experience of the NICU or PICU environment.

When working with medically fragile newborn infants, the music therapist needs to consider the following fundamentals:

1) Music can do harm. If music has sufficient potency to change the physiological and behavioral stability of an infant for the better, then poor use can also make it worse.

2) Less is more: When working with medically fragile newborn infants, the music therapist must understand the potency of each musical element available and maximize them individually or in combination to distill the greatest benefit for the infant.

3) What the music therapist knows about music is as important as what she can do in music. Because the music therapist works in partnership with the family, the ability to impart knowledge and understanding to the parents will be equally if not more important than what the music therapist can do in the moment.

4) Family music is familiar music; familiar music is comforting. The appreciation and use of the family's pre-existing musical preferences honors the family's preferences as a strength.

5) Successful communication with a baby is inherently musical. Interaction is founded in melody, attack, timbre, pulse, and phrasing.

6) Musicality and music are part of the same continuum. The music does not "begin"; it emerges from the musicality of successful interaction.

DIAGNOSTIC INFORMATION

The population of infants in pediatric NICU and PICU includes all infants with complex conditions, whether they were born prematurely, late-preterm, or full-term. This chapter will focus on infants born near or at full-term, but will also encompass the needs of all infants who remain in NICU and PICU after they reach term, and into the first few months of life.

Conditions that keep infants in the hospital postterm are likely to include *congenital heart defects*, lung conditions (e.g., *chronic lung disease*), abdominal wall conditions (e.g., *congenital diaphragmatic hernia*), digestive conditions [e.g., *esophageal atresia* (EA)], brain injuries [e.g., *hypoxic ischemic encephalopathy* (HIE)], and medical issues associated with congenital anomalies and metabolic disorders (e.g., unexplained neurological and circulatory abnormalities). All have the potential to create complications which necessitate long and complex treatment pathways. Some conditions, such as congenital heart defects, are renowned for their association with syndromes such as *Down's Syndrome* (also called Trisomy 21), *22q11 deletion*, *Angelman*, and *Fragile X*.

Long-term developmental outcome may be put at risk from life-saving treatments such as *extracorporeal membrane oxygenation* (known as ECMO), which may save a heart but damage the brain. Conditions such as *gastroschisis* and *omphaloceles* are increasing worldwide possibly due to maternal recreational drug use (Walker, Holland, Winlaw, Sherwood, & Badawi, 2006). Recovery from such conditions is often slow and convoluted as the bowel learns to process food again. Common care patterns for the conditions described above include major surgery, which may be immediate (e.g., day 1 of life for EA infants), delayed while confirming severity of condition (e.g., *Pierre Robin Syndrome*), or a series of surgeries (e.g., *hypoplastic left heart syndrome*). For some, there may be a protracted period of diagnosis (e.g., to identify rare syndromes). While modern neonatal medical treatment advances rapidly, there are still many infants whose conditions cannot be treated and for whom palliative care is offered.

Walker and her colleagues (2006) noted that with improved survival from these major conditions, it is becoming clear that these survivors of major surgical and medical treatment "suffer adverse neurobehavioral and developmental outcomes which resemble those seen in premature infants" (p. 749). These full-term infants need supportive and developmental services from the beginning of their admission. Music therapy can be provided from a variety of theoretical models which will be explored in the following sections.

NEEDS AND RESOURCES

While it can be convenient to classify aspects of infant need by headings such as "developmental" or "psychosocial," the American Academy of Pediatrics has adopted an ecobiodevelopmental framework to address the complex, combined influence of economic, social, and biological markers on infant and child health and development (Shonkoff et al., 2011). The following section considers the infant's developmental, psychological, social, cultural, and contextual needs, which are often enmeshed in music therapy services for hospitalized newborn infants.

The Developing Infant

The hospitalized full-term infant is an emergent social being for whom sensory experiences are the foundation for building relationships with primary carers. For the healthy infant, the first four weeks of life are consumed with sleeping and eating and being cleaned. From weeks four to eight, the infant is still a sensory being who begins to have brief periods of wakefulness and begins to take in more sensory information about his immediate surroundings. Through weeks eight to twelve, the infant emerges as a social being. He recognizes key caregivers and familiar routines and experiences and communicates with gesture, facial expression, and changes in muscle tone. From week 12 to week 16, the infant shows enjoyment through facial expressions and gesture, and positive use of voice begins. While sleep is key for growth and healing in hospitalized infants, the quiet alert state in which the infant begins to interact with his world is vital for all other aspects of neurological development. While it is tempting to think that infants are safest when asleep, being awake and interactive ensures that their neurological development is stimulated in a timely fashion.

Auditory Processing in the Medically Fragile Newborn Infant

While the developmental trajectory of the preterm infant is disrupted by premature birth, the medically fragile full-term infant has benefited from completing his development in his mother's womb. Potentially he has had the opportunity for all his senses and organs and his brain to mature as intended for a human child. Therefore, the music therapist should at the outset consider that the infant can process stimulation just like a healthy baby. However, many of the complex medical conditions may compromise the development and functioning of these more mature capacities. For example, the music therapist should understand those treatments which may negatively impact hearing development. The identified risks to hearing in infancy are low birth weight (< 1500grams), *ototoxic medications* (cause damage to the cochlea and auditory nerve), certain syndromes, and mechanical ventilation for more than five days (Bielecki, Horbulewicz, & Wolan, 2011). Antibiotics such as gentamicin and furosemide used to treat newborn infection can be ototoxic. Whole-body hypothermia treatment for infants with HIE may cause a temporary peripheral hearing loss, which is better than the potential sensorineural hearing loss caused by HIE itself (Mietzsch, Parikh, Williams, Shankaran, & Lasky, 2008). While being mindful of these threats to the baby's auditory development, it is otherwise reasonable to expect that their hearing and auditory processing capabilities are intact.

It may not be possible to confirm a hearing loss, as screening procedures cannot be administered if an infant is ventilated. The music therapist must therefore work hopefully and cautiously, checking for a discernible response to stimuli during assessment. The music therapist may note concerns in the medical record about observation of limited auditory perception.

Inherent Musical Characteristics of Term Infants

It is essential that the music therapist working with newborns understands the developmental progression of auditory processing capabilities to ensure that they prepare suitable stimuli and strategies in treatment plans. Reference is made to the fetal and preterm infant auditory processing pathway because in utero or NICU-based auditory experiences will be significant in planning a starting point for treatment. Further study of the development of hearing and neuroprocessing will be advantageous to the clinician.

Fetal research has revealed that there is a significant change in auditory processing at around 33 weeks in which higher-order processing of stimuli commences, with significant activation to sound in the left temporal lobe (Jardri et al., 2008). This completion of the afferent pathways up into the auditory cortex means that it is after this point that the fetus or preterm infant begins to process the mother's voice as a primary auditory stimulus. Ultimately, this leads to a preference for maternal speech in the full-term newborn infant (Moon, 2011).

Perception and memory for music also develops in utero (Granier-Deferre, Bassereau, Ribeiro, Jacquet, & DeCasper, 2011). By the time a healthy full-term infant is born, variation in his heart rate already indicates he can process auditory intensity, frequency, and some basic variations in tempo (Granier-Deferre et al., 2011).

Context for Patient as Baby

While the medical stability of the hospitalized infant is the primary concern, ongoing neurological and psychological development remains an important pursuit to ensure that critical windows for development are met. The earliest requirement is for the infant to achieve self-regulation, which means that the infant seeks to control his own experience by self-soothing, and, in addition, seeks support from a carer for state control and meeting his physical needs. Treatment is a noncontingent routine in which everything happens at a precise time to ensure that measures are accurate (e.g., physiological signs, blood work). The needs of the infant become secondary to that and as such the infant's own protests are managed as part of that routine rather than responded to as the central issue. Therefore, the infant's loss of power to influence his world leads to a loss of self and mutual regulation (Malloch et al., 2012).

Child-centered practices such as developmental care for preterm infants have had some success in using the infant's cues as a guide for care procedures. However, in the many centers where such a program is not employed, the infant's attempts to self-regulate remain secondary to hospital processes. The infant and his family need interventionists to hold in mind that alongside the medical needs of the infant as *patient,* the infant is a *baby* with psychological and social needs. All interventionists must work with the potential of the *baby* while mindful of the limiting effects of their condition or treatment (Shoemark & Grocke, 2010).

The Newborn Infant as Social Partner

Unlike the prematurely born infant, the full-term infant quickly develops the expected social maturity, which allows him to seek the nurturing care and companionship of his parents. This means that the infant rapidly develops expectations of his world and his sense of agency to effect change. He uses his voice, posture, gesture, and facial expression to inquire, protest, and create partnerships with his carers (Shoemark & Grocke, 2010). The temptation is to keep hospitalized infants in quiet sleep, but once he reaches the age of four weeks (corrected age if born prematurely) or more, he begins to need brief periods of meaningful interaction, and these periods expand with the infant's inevitable maturation.

The availability of the infant for interaction is first dependent on his behavioral state. Thoman (Ingersoll & Thoman, 1999; Thoman, 1990) developed a taxonomy of six overview categories of state which usefully define the shifts from sleep to awake in infants. The Thoman states serve as a core component in determining the availability of the infant for intervention (see Appendix A for the state descriptions).

Infants seek companionship from the earliest moments of life. This need arises as part of the infant's innate strategy to find life-sustaining nourishment. Locating the mother through the familiar sound of her voice, the infant quickly begins to synchronize with his or her mother, communicating at a fundamental level (Crown, Feldstein, Jasnow, Beebe, & Jaffe, 2002; Jaffe, Beebe, Feldstein, Crown, & Jasnow, 2001) and even matching pitch contours with her native language (Mampe, Friederici, Christophe, & Wermke, 2009).

Opportunities for this implicit level of connection may be lost to the hospitalized infant who may be unavailable due to pain, discomfort, and the side effects of medication. These will compromise the infant's capacity to project himself into the world, and he may give parents confusing signs about his willingness or availability for interplay. The music therapist who understands the impact of these external and contextual limitations on the infant and is experienced in infant behavioral cues of engagement and disengagement will be able to help both infant and family to find their way back to each other.

Parents also need support to understand that they provide their baby with vital companionship in which they are the attuned partners in their baby's day. Parents usually know their baby's habits, their cues for fatigue or discomfort, and the strategies that support transition to sleep. This knowledge can be quite implicit, and therefore support to champion their capabilities or bring them into their awareness is valuable in supporting the parent-infant dyad companionship.

The Context of the Lived Experience

The auditory environment of intensive care units (neonatal or pediatric) is renowned for being loud and unpredictable. The critical effects of noise in health care are sleep disturbance, annoyance, and communication interference (Berglund, 1999). During hospitalization, noise in the NICU impinges on the quality of sleep and well-being of infants (Wachman & Lahav, 2010) and therefore quietness is pursued as the optimal environment for NICUs. Increasingly, new hospitals are constructed under strict requirements to minimize noise (White & Consensus Committee on Recommended Design Standards for Advanced Neonatal Care, 2012). The use of single rooms rather than open wards is primarily to control infection, however, also provides the benefit of reduced exposure to secondary noise.

WORKING WITH CAREGIVERS:
THE IMPORTANCE OF FAMILY-CENTERED CARE

Infants with complex conditions often require an extended or "long" admission to the hospital (30 days or more). It is now understood that families need support to ensure that their infant is engaged in a range of activities which enhance neurodevelopment (Laing, 2010). The music therapist can play an important role in this by helping them to develop a repertory of activities which are part of the shared family experience throughout their stay.

We understand that when an infant's development and well-being are put at risk, the key to resilience is to either reduce the risk factors or increase protective factors which ameliorate negative outcomes (Sameroff, Bartko, Baldwin, Baldwin, & Seifer, 1998). While the music therapist can do only a little to change the environment (see the section on Receptive Music Therapy), she can do a great deal to support the family, which serves as the greatest protective factor in a baby's life. Music therapists working in family-centered early intervention have long understood that the efficacy of what they do in sessions is greatly enhanced by the newly acquired skills and knowledge that parents take home and use between sessions (Nicholson, Berthelsen, Abad, Williams, & Bradley, 2008). As such, the music therapist in the NICU should carefully consider how to create an effective partnership with families to expand the role of music in the infant's everyday life.

Renowned psychoanalyst Donald Winnicott noted that "there is no such thing as a baby" (1964, p. 88). He meant that the baby never exists in isolation but is always part of the family of people who created and reflect his existence. The music therapist in the NICU should always be mindful that even when a family is not present, the infant must be considered as a member of that family (Shoemark & Dearn, 2008).

No assumptions should be made about how a family feels about their baby. The arrival of a sick newborn infant may bring joy, pride, fear, or shame, and be influenced by cultural or spiritual background. For instance, families from India may experience some shame, as the sickness may be seen as a punishment from God. They may seek or receive very little support from the community (Edwardraj, Mumtaj, Prasad, Kuruvilla, & Jacob, 2010). In contrast, families from Pacific islands may feel that God sees them as a strong and capable family, and a sick child may be seen as a gift to challenge them.

Alea was born at 36 weeks' gestation with a complex gastrointestinal condition which stopped her from being breastfed or fed through a tube. She received intravenous nutrition to keep her alive while the surgical team made a decision about how to proceed. Babies in this condition often spend long periods crying to protest about being hungry, and nothing will distract them for long. Each morning, Alea's mother Ioana, who came from a Pacific island, would come with a smile and joyful chatter and she would gather Alea into her arms and sing to her for hours. She sang popular songs, and hymns and children's songs. Instead of being upset, Alea spent most of her time settled and safe with her mother's support. When I admired Ioana's joy and singing, she smiled and said "Alea is a gift from God, of course I sing!"

There is now a wealth of literature which acknowledges the pivotal role of the mother in NICU care (Obeidat, Bond, & Callister, 2009), but we are only just beginning to understand that fathers experience the hospitalization of a newborn baby differently from mothers (Fegran, Helseth, Solveig, & Fagermoen, 2008). Fathers often present with a stoic attitude with a focus on their infant's care and the new mother's well-being. They are often unable to address their own needs as they "stay strong" for their family and support the physical, social, and financial needs of the family while they endure this experience. Music therapy may be able to offer the father a unique avenue for self-care (Mondanaro, 2010).

Music is an expected part of parenting in most cultures of the world. Even in this age of receptive music dominance, families do expect to share songs with their babies (Custodero & Johnson-Green, 2008; deVries, 2009). Mothers of hospitalized infants retain a sense that singing is good for them to do with their baby, which may serve as an avenue for the acceptability of music and music therapy in their baby's care (Shoemark, in preparation).

REFERRAL AND ASSESSMENT PROCEDURES

Referral Procedures

Music therapy referrals for full-term infants may encompass similar criteria as those for preterm babies, and also additional reasons. There are two common focal points for music therapy referrals with this population: psychosocial care and developmental care. If the music therapy program is located within the psychosocial or mental health team, the referrals are likely to focus on the immediate experience of hospitalization. Therefore, priority may be given to an infant who is without family support or who is likely to be in the hospital for an extended admission, families who are struggling psychologically with the experience of hospitalization, or families in which there are pre-existing mental health issues.

If the music therapy program is located in a team comprising allied health, such as a developmental care or neurodevelopment team, the referral focus is likely to be the developmental status of infants. This will encompass families who need educational input to support their infant's development. The neurodevelopment team will use their knowledge of typical developmental trajectory to focus on the immediate early intervention needs and also assess the infant for community-based early intervention to commence as early as possible (in particular infants with CDH, HIE, and EA). A music therapist might work within a variety of teams or alone, but in all cases, it is useful to consider the theoretical orientation of the music therapy service to be provided as this will aid in the process of active and appropriate decisions to be made for the broad music therapy program and at the bedside within sessions.

Newborn Music Therapy Model

A theory-based service enables the music therapist to use a theoretical framework to conceptualize infant assessment, prioritization of client caseload, actual session content, and measures for outcomes. This author developed a Newborn Music Therapy Model that encompasses theory, evidence, and current practice for both preterm and full-term infants in two main frameworks, namely the infant-focused framework and the family-centered framework (Shoemark, 2012)

The infant-focused framework is underpinned by the biomedical theory that music can serve as a treatment directly for the infant. The family-centered framework is underpinned by ecological and attachment theories in which music serves as a shared experience. Each framework contains three models of service provision which conceptualize both the infant and the music. The presentation of such frameworks is useful in delineating one's thinking and decision-making about the infant and the service, but in practice, they are enmeshed to meet the evolving needs of infant and family. Fundamental to the decision about which approach is necessary is the understanding of whether music is viewed as a treatment (infant-focused) or a shared experience (family-centered). Further considerations include the maturity of the infant, the constantly emerging evidence, and regulatory requirements of the hospital and further agencies such as the American Academy of Pediatrics. The frameworks are outlined below, but for a full explication, refer to the Rickards and McFerran (2012) text *Lifelong Engagement in Music: Benefits for Mental Health and Well-Being.*

Infant-Focused Framework. The infant-focused framework includes the following three applications:

1) *The infant as patient; music as treatment:* Music is used as an external regulating stimulus for heart rate, respiration, and oxygen saturation (Standley, 2012). Recorded lullaby or otherwise sedative music is dosed to help preterm infants achieve and maintain homeostasis. There is no interpersonal process involved and therefore may be administered by other staff. Recently, the focus of the literature has been on reducing stress responses to critical events such as painful procedures in preterm infants (Butt & Kisilevsky, 2000; Chou, 2003; Keith, 2009; Tramo et al., 2011; Whipple, 2008) but also on ongoing stability (Doheny et al., 2012; Olischar et al., 2011) and weight gain (Cevasco & Grant, 2005; Standley et al., 2010).

2) *The infant as immature dynamic system; music as developmental stimulus:* Music-making is a vehicle for the rehearsal of nonmusical skill development. The music therapist uses singing and associated facial and gestural expression to help late preterm, term and older infants develop age-appropriate social, communication and sometimes motor skills. Evidence for this model is provided by music therapy research (de l'Etoile, 2006; Hanson-Abromeit, 2003; Malloch et al., 2012; Shoemark & Grocke, 2010).

3) *The noxious environment; music as protective agent:* The auditory environment can be very noisy, with frequent peaks of extreme noise which form part of the cumulative trauma of the NICU or PICU experience for infants, families, and staff (Newnham, Inder, & Milgrom, 2009; Philbin, 2000). Music may be provided live by trained and supervised musicians (Shoemark, 2009) or be selected and controlled recorded music. As an aesthetic and cultural experience, the music serves to dissipate the tension and thereby relax and refresh the environment, which in turn changes the experience for the infant.

Family-Centered Framework. The daily lived experience of the hospitalized infants is very focused. Because of his medical condition, the "world" (e.g., all treatments and enrichment) must come to him in his bed. The family-centered framework includes the following models:

1) *The infant as center of his world; music as a shared experience:* Music is an approachable experience which acknowledges the whole family and the relationships within it. The music therapist partners with the family to help them create counterbalancing experiences of joy with their later preterm, full-term or older infant. Drawing on attachment theory, experiences of intersubjectivity build the potential of the family relationships (Shoemark, 1996; Shoemark & Dearn, 2008).

2) *The developing infant; music as therapy:* Music is employed as a vehicle for early intervention. The music therapist views the infant as a dynamic and evolving being (Jaffe et al., 2001; Seifer, 2001) and creates a triadic relationship with the parent and infant to engage in live music-making (Cevasco, 2008; Walworth, 2009), which stimulates an expanded capability (Tronick, 1998).

3) *The mother-infant dyad; music as a vehicle to sustain them:* Music becomes the safe place in which the music therapist uses psychoanalytic and psychotherapy methods with the mother-infant dyad. The parent's preferred music is used as a

basis for in-depth work which requires specialist training for the music therapist (Bargiel, 2004; Nocker-Ribaupierre, 2004; O'Gorman, 2007; Stewart, 2009). This specialist training can be obtained through tertiary programs which focus on psychotherapy.

These frameworks will be used to help theoretically define the methods and assessment procedures as they are outlined below.

Assessment Procedures

After referral, the first step is to gather information and undertake assessment to clarify how the music therapy program may proceed. In information gathering, the intention is to understand all the factors which impact on how the therapist thinks about the infant or the infant and his family, and how the music therapy program will be provided in the immediate time frame. Information gathering usually includes the following information:

1) *Status:* gestational age at birth; age at referral; medical condition; medications which affect availability or hearing; team's treatment plan and priorities; key treatment events that impact on when or how you might commence treatment, such as surgery, extubation, or weaning from sedation; likely admission duration; and discharge or transfer plan.

2) *Demographics:* contact information for family; relevant family characteristics; family availability; key family activity that impacts on how you might interact with them.

3) *Service priority:* reason for referral; priority; need for assessment of specific capability (e.g., auditory processing maturity for recorded music); scheduling; model of service delivery. Priorities may be determined at the team level.

4) *Permissions* from family or medical team may be needed to commence and schedule sessions which include family, or direct service with infant; specific requirements or allowances for holding; authorizations to document the work for further consideration or presentation (audio, video, photography).

After initial information is gathered, the music therapist will consider what kind of music therapy service should be offered to meet the needs of the infant and family. Further assessment of the infant's pretreatment capabilities will be dictated by the decisions about the service selected. The following clinical examples are hypothetical cases:

Charlie was born at 39 weeks gestation with compromised lung function. He is now 42 weeks gestation, medically stable on CPAP (continuous pressure air pathway), and in an open bed. His parents live on a farm two hours away from the hospital and have three other children at home. Charlie has difficulty remaining asleep in the noisy ward. The referral from the bedside nurse is for recorded music to help him sleep.

Using Shoemark's model, the music therapy services for Charlie will be infant-focused. Charlie's need is for external support for state regulation, which means that the service might be framed as "The infant as patient, music as treatment." The assessment must identify Charlie's readiness (ability to tolerate and make use) for recorded music as an external source of regulation. Once readiness is confirmed, the music therapist selects the appropriate music to support Charlie's sleep. However, if the music therapist decides to adopt a family-centered framework for work with Charlie, she might conceptualize this work as "The infant as center of his world; music as a shared experience." After confirming Charlie's readiness for music as a stimulus, the music therapist may talk to the family by telephone to determine if Charlie's mother had listened to music while pregnant and to also understand the family's musical preferences. While his family is not physically present, the music therapist uses their experiences and preferences for music as the basis for selecting the music. A second round of assessment before commencing service may optimize the duration and timing of the music to support Charlie's sleep.

In some cases, the decision may be within one of the frameworks:

Sophie was born full-term, with esophageal atresia, and will need surgery before she is discharged. She is now four weeks old, but still needs to put on weight before the surgery can be scheduled. Her mother Rebecca spends every day with her and actively engages Sophie in a range of age-appropriate activities. She is anxious about Sophie's development and worries that Sophie will miss important milestones while they're "stuck" in the hospital. She self-refers to music therapy.

In this case, music therapy services are family-centered and may focus on "The developing infant; music as therapy: Music is employed as a vehicle for early intervention," in which music therapy supports the family in understanding Sophie's developmental status and how to use musical experiences each day to advance her development. Or it may be "The mother-infant dyad; music as a vehicle to sustain them," if assessment shows that the need is more focused on supporting Rebecca in understanding how she is meeting Sophie's needs. The initial assessment would focus on the family's musical heritage and level of shared experience; the needs of the infant; and the needs of the mother.

Assessment is also shaped by the culture of the unit and the theoretical framework of the wider music therapy program in the hospital. Requirements for assessment are most likely determined at the level of the music therapy team, or, if the music therapist is a sole clinician, in consultation with other team members in the unit. The most readily available assessments focus on infant development. The music therapist can use published data about developmental milestones as a guide for expectation of the infant. The outcomes of standardized developmental assessments conducted by other professionals in the team should be considered. Common tools in Western hospitals include the *Neurological Assessment of the Preterm and Full-Term Infant* (Dubowitz & Dubowitz, 1999), the *Neonatal Behavioral Assessment Scale* (Brazelton & Nugent, 2011), and the *NICU Network Neurobehavioral Assessment* (Lester & Tronick, 2004). If no standardized assessment can be provided by other team members, the music therapist should consider training in the administration of a standardized assessment. This allows the music therapist to independently assess the impact of treatment programs and offer an additional service to the unit.

INTRODUCTION TO MUSIC THERAPY METHODS

Just as referral and assessment are dependent upon the service delivery model, so too are the music therapy methods. It is important to note that the following methods and procedures are not used in isolation, but often in combination, in response to the infant's precarious availability for interplay. There are several foundational aspects of providing music therapy interventions for medically fragile infants presented here before the specific methods are outlined.

Auditory Environment

Medically fragile newborn infants are particularly susceptible to the effects of noise (American Academy of Pediatrics, 1997; Trapanotto et al., 2004). In all applications of music for the hospitalized infant, the music therapist superimposes additional sound (music) onto the existing auditory environment. This brings a responsibility to ensure that the additional stimulation is safe for the infant and does not impinge on staff and family communication.

Music therapists claim that sound (music) can be a source of powerful benefit to clients and, therefore, we must accept that that sound (noise) can also be harmful. It is generally understood by medical and nursing staff that noise is harmful. It is essential that the music therapist understand that she plays a key role in the creation of a safe and meaningful auditory environment. The music therapist should determine if the unit has a committee or team member (usually a nurse or audiologist) who is responsible for monitoring the auditory environment. The music therapist should join the existing monitoring committee to consolidate her role as a key person who understands the potential benefits and disadvantages of sound in the auditory environment. Where there is no existing monitoring program, the music therapist can work with the quality assurance committee to create a suitable monitoring program. In most cases, the quality assurance committee will be grateful that someone is willing to invest the time, and in many cases the music therapist will become their "go-to" person on all things related to the auditory context.

It is strongly recommended that the music therapist become familiar with the use of a basic sound level meter to quantify the environment both without and with the music (Shoemark, 2012). Any NICU or PICU in which music is used should purchase a sound level meter (SLM). These affordable devices can be used for "snapshot" checks (a few minutes) of the environment. For a discussion of safe sound stimulation in the NICU, please consult Gray and Philbin (2000, 2004). Where a sound-level meter is not yet available, the music therapist should make use of smart phone or tablet applications to provide an informal estimation of the environment. The duration of this measurement should be at least the same as the duration of the planned music stimulus to determine if the space is quiet enough for the addition of music. To assess if the environment is sufficiently quiet, the music therapist should consider the level of complex care provided to the infant directly and the impact of "secondary" noise produced by the level of care being provided to other infants in the room and scheduled activities such as medical rounds/nursing hand-over. See Appendix for a basic protocol.

As part of the initial assessment for each patient, the music therapist should assess the ambient auditory environment to ascertain the most likely periods when music can be safely used. This is more relevant for the use of recorded music because when recorded music is played, other activity will continue on around it and the music must be discriminated against that auditory background. During live singing by the family or during a music therapy session, there is a focus on the singing and other people tend to quiet while this occurs. The music therapist should lead by example, by attending to the overall sound level of the unit as a baseline, before adding the additional stimulation of music.

Even on a quiet unit, there is little respite from ongoing noise, whether it be the hiss of oxygen flowing, the motor of the ventilator on standby, or the air-conditioning for the room. To make sound meaningful, we must provide the "space" in which it can be heard. The section above discussed minimizing noise. Nursing staff understand that quiet is needed to support good-quality infant sleep and to enable clear communication. For the family this information is also important in helping them to understand why and how to shape their interaction. When interacting with their baby, the music therapist can encourage parents to also be still and quiet to provide a moment of expectation to which their baby may visibly or vocally respond and initiate communication.

The Music Continuum

An infant, healthy or otherwise, does not have the cognitive or motor capability to make music. However, the infant does have intrinsic musicality at his disposal, and there is no reason to doubt that the medically fragile newborn infant shares this capability. Intrinsic musicality is the musical quality of the infant's expressive communication. It is manifested particularly in the quality of the infant's gesture (hands, feet, arm and leg movements), which may be smooth or jerky (timbre and rhythm) and slow or fast (tempo). Musicality may be present in vocal response (pitch, tonality, attack, timbre, duration, and phrasing), facial expression (timbre and phrasing), and the stilling or cessation of gesture (silence). Models of infant development such as Daniel Stern's "vitality affect" include musicality in the dynamic expressive states of infant expression (2010), while Malloch and Trevarthen's model of Communicative Musicality (2009) exemplifies the musicality of infant communication. As an underpinning for live music-making, the music therapist may consider this musicality as the infant's music-making and use it to stimulate her musical response. In this way, the infant is an active musical partner in the therapeutic relationship.

Safely Working at Threshold

In programs where the work with infants involves a direct relationship between therapist and infant, the music therapist will often work near the infant's threshold for stimulation. This author synthesized Beebe and Lachmann's *Pattern of Expectation* model (2004) to conceptualize the infant's capacity to participate in interplay and the Boston Change Process Study Group's microprocess of change concept to create the *Phases of Interplay* to illuminate within-session therapeutic process (Shoemark, 2008). Interplay may progress smoothly through a series of phases which include observation, assessment, orientation, attunement, fittedness (therapist and client fit together well in the therapeutic dyad), moment of meeting, and closure. However, within each phase, the therapist may need to employ more supportive strategies to accommodate that restricted capability of the infant to cope with stimulation or engage with interplay. The music therapist must learn to recognize the infant's presenting behaviors as they reach or traverse their threshold for stimulation or interplay. If she oversteps the threshold, the therapist must understand how to modify the stimulation or interplay to repair the context and enable the infant to recover. The infant's thresholds may be reached quickly and without warning. White-Traut's Audio Tactile Visual Vestibular multimodal stimulation protocol for preterm infant (Burns et al., 1994) is a useful model of addition and subtraction of stimulation and has been modified with singing for music therapy with preterm infants (Standley, 1998) and full-term infants (Shoemark & Grocke, 2010).

Overview of Music Therapy Methods and Procedures

Improvisational Music Therapy

- Contingent Singing: the therapist's use of infant-directed singing to respond to the immediate interpersonal needs of the infant.
- Live Music to Support State Transition: the use of music synchronized to the infants' physiological and behavioral responses to facilitate self-regulations.

Receptive Music Therapy

- Recorded Music as Contextual Support for State Regulation: the use of recorded music to provide a consistent and predictable external support to improve physiological and behavioral stability.
- Environmental Music Therapy: the use of live music to ameliorate the impact of random noise and to both relax and renew the auditory experiences for everyone in the unit.

Re-creative Music Therapy

- "Songs of Kin:" the use of a family's own music preferences to encourage active engagement.

Compositional Music Therapy

- Lullabies and Play Songs: the use of songwriting to create lullabies and play songs that may become part of the family repertoire with their baby.

Guidelines for Improvisational Music Therapy

It might seem unlikely that music therapy with a newborn infant involves improvisational methods. However the deconstruction of music to fundamental components such as pitch, register, timbre, pulse, and rhythm enables the music therapist to co-construct music which is intrinsically drawn from the infant. The following methods champion the musicality of the infant's rudimentary communication, the innate musicality of the mother-infant relationship, and the timeless traditions of infant-directed singing.

The music therapist can use music-making to acknowledge and promote his capacities to interact with an attuned partner. The therapist attempting this work needs to be mindful that interaction is a demanding task which may easily challenge the infant's capacities. Therefore, the therapist will need to be ready to modify the musical elements in the moment to respond to the rapidly evolving status and capabilities of the infant when thresholds may be crossed (Shoemark, 2008). The therapist may undertake this work directly with infants whose family is not able to be present during wakeful periods; however, it is also vital work in partnership with parents.

Contingent Singing

Overview. Contingent singing is the therapist's use of infant-directed singing to respond to the immediate interpersonal needs of the infant. Contingent singing is indicated when the infant is in a quiet alert state and sufficiently well to engage in interplay. Contingent singing may address goals for basic expressive and receptive communication, developing sense of self, and creating experiences for intersubjectivity. The infant who is sedated or receiving pain medication is unlikely to be an active or aware partner, or may present with altered behavior. Singing to the infant in this state may be defined as a receptive music experience.

Preparation. Scheduling must take advantage of the wakeful periods, often leading into feeding or other periods during which the infant is reliably awake. A quiet environment is needed so that the infant can hear the therapist's voice without the need for increased volume. The infant can remain in his bed to participate. The act of moving from bed to the therapist or parent's arms uses considerable energy and therefore staying in bed may be needed for infants who need to conserve valuable energy. The music therapist new to medically fragile infants should be instructed in any handling procedural requirements. If the infant is older, it may be appropriate to relocate the infant into a rocker or tumble-form seat (usually provided by physical therapy) to promote upright play.

What to observe. At the outset, the music therapist must observe the infant's availability for interplay. The optimal infant state is Quiet Alert, which includes eyes looking for interaction, open and interested facial expression, arms and legs moving smoothly. If the infant is in a fussy state, the music therapist can still commence gentle interaction but will more gently introduce interplay. When the infant looks away, he is regulating the amount of stimulation he is taking in. The music therapist should respect this by waiting for the infant to be ready to re-engage in the interplay. She might gently encourage the infant by singing or calling out his name, but should not pursue the infant by moving into his field of vision. If the infant does not return to the interplay, the music therapist must consider that the infant's threshold for stimulation has been traversed, and she should modify her expectations. In all cases, the music therapist should be ready to give the infant time to process each offering of interaction and make his response before progressing very gently (Shoemark, 2008). If the infant repeatedly self-regulates away from the interaction, the music therapist should keep interaction very modest and support the infant's responses at that level.

Procedures. Contingent singing is led by the infant's availability. The music therapist primarily uses her voice, but also facial expression, posture, and gesture to entice, respond to, or direct the infant. Before 12 weeks of age, the infant will primarily use facial expression, gesture, and posture, and also voice in combinations that are quiet or active, to show that he is or is not available (for a full exposition of these behaviors, see Shoemark & Grocke, 2010). In contingent singing, the key is being able to move along the music continuum using the small steps described below. For many infants, the interplay may take weeks to reach the full involvement of song; however, there is rich work in the orientation and attunement phases (Shoemark 2008). The music therapist must consider the full potential of her voice to support the emergence of the infant into the interplay. She can use her voice or help parents to understand that they can use their voice in the following ways (Shoemark, 2011):

- Silent: includes waiting for a response; listening; breathing in and out
- Half sing: exaggerated patterns when talking—scoops up for a question, dips down to reassure, or keeping a flat line to contain or soothe (infant-directed speech)
- Chant: Repeat a couple of words that sound lovely; a little line of nursery rhyme; the baby's name; an action (e.g., "sleep, sleep, sleep").
- Sing and wait: Sing a line from a song and then give baby time to respond, and then maybe repeat it.
- Sing a whole song: because baby is content or visibly enjoying it; sing it more than once (or the chorus of a song or the favorite part of a song).

If the infant demonstrates availability, the music therapist should use her voice in conjunction with facial expression to entice the infant into interplay. As the infant continues to be interested and answers the therapist, she can develop from highly intonated speech into single line and expanded singing. The therapist continues to modify musical elements such as tempo, volume, timbre, and attack to acknowledge and affirm the infant's efforts. In response to the infant's active partnership with her, the music therapist will reciprocate and promote with brighter and more variable vocal and visual interplay. If the infant becomes fussy or withdraws from the interplay, the music therapist may pause or, dependent on the infant, may conversely become more directive and use a firm timbre and slightly increased volume to contain any escalation. If the infant withdraws from the interplay (looks away), the music therapist will maintain a little "thread" of the vocal stimulus or touch, but will offer more time between the interplay, while waiting for the infant to return. If she determines the infant has had enough interplay, the therapist will gently move into the receptive method of singing more lullaby-like songs while positioning the baby ready for sleep or quiet time. Further information about contingent singing is available from Shoemark (2010, 2011a, 2011b).

Adaptations. If there is deterioration in the infant's physical condition such as sepsis or recovery after surgery, the music therapist can use her knowledge of the "well baby" to provide gentle receptive singing which may support the infant. Rather like the little "thread" when an infant has self-regulated away from interplay, the music therapist creates a modest musical presence which is a quiet and safe version of the infant's preferred musical experience.

While the music therapist may use contingent singing with an infant, she may also facilitate the capacity of parents to sing to their baby. The music therapist may "serve as a facilitator, container, and witness to the contingent interaction of the dyad, affirming the reality of what transpires and confirming or enhancing the mother's judgment of the situation" (Shoemark, 2011, p. 171).

Live Music to Support State Transition

Overview. The music therapist might be called upon to support an infant who is unable to self-regulate his state. The referral may be for an infant who is irritable or has trouble getting to sleep. Using music as synchronization may serve to acknowledge the infant's behavioral state and help him to settle and fall asleep. Some people may consider this to be more a receptive method than improvisational. Working toward state transition is a dynamic process. The music therapist is modifying the music moment by moment to meet the fluctuating state of the infant. This transition is rarely a linear process moving steadily from awake to asleep. The infant may fluctuate between distress and drowsiness, and the music therapist changes the musical elements to acknowledge the state and draw the infant down toward sleep. The constant adjustment of the musical elements is improvised and hence it is included under the method of improvisation.

Accompanying the infant in state transition may be as simple as "singing a baby to sleep", but it may also require the music therapist to accompany the infant and parent through repeated experiences of protracted irritability or even distress. As the therapist takes responsibility for changing this state, she "holds" all the physical and psychological energy of the infant and parent. This can be demanding, and the music therapist should consider receiving supervision.

Preparation. The music therapist should first assess the auditory environment and where possible reduce any noise to both maximize a calm environment and allow the sound of the music to be clearly heard. When the infant is irritable or distressed, or the parent is anxious, it is important that the music therapist prepare herself to provide a calm and soothing presence. Transference of state from client to therapist may hinder the music therapist's capacity to support, and therefore the music therapist should check her own state regularly to ensure she is not taking up the anxious or distressed feeling in her own body or her music.

As Sarah, the music therapist, walked into the unit, she could already hear Javier crying with great force. He had been irritable for the last few days, and now, at noon, Sarah walked in to find the nurse trying to settle him without resorting to sedation yet again. Sarah began his favorite lullaby at a moderately loud level in a key that allowed her voice to be heard below the wail of Javier's cry. She sang slowly with definite attack on the first beat of the bar. For a moment, Javier listened, but he immediately began to cry again. After trying for about 15 minutes, Sarah felt unsure of how to proceed, she felt confused and worried that she could not help Javier. She paused and took stock of herself and realized her muscles were tight, her voice even felt tight, and then she realized she had taken on Javier's distress. He was unable to organize his state and was lost, and now Sarah was feeling it, too. She breathed deeply, knowing that she had the tools to help him. She consciously thought again about the various ways she'd settled him on other days, and began again.

Procedures. The use of music for entrainment, as explained by Loewy (2009), provides useful considerations for undertaking singing to support state transition. Loewy (2009) recommends the use of a familiar song such as a lullaby or song-of-kin (see Re-creative Music Therapy below). The lyrics may be used at the outset to help the parent feel comfortable in singing. The music therapist uses volume and attack to emulate the energy of the infant's presentation and ensure the music is actually discernible to the infant. So if the infant is crying loudly and moving in a jerky, robust manner, the singing will have good volume (maybe *moderate forte*) and definite attack. The tempo, however, will be slow and definite, as this is the starting point for the transition. Loewy suggests that if the infant is crying in rapid bursts, the therapist may use the tonality to produce a vocal accompaniment which is consonant with the pitch of the cry (likely to include the tonic and dominant). This is aligned with the finding that consonance is preferred by newborn infants (Trainor, Tsang, & Cheung, 2002). At the first indication that the infant is aware of the music (e.g., momentary cessation of crying, reduced movements, and/or visual orientation to the music source), the music therapist begins to decrease the energy of the musical elements. As the infant settles further (e.g., crying stopped, muscle tone relaxed, eyelids heavy or closed), the music therapist may remove the lyrics and simplify the intervallic structure of the melody. Generally, a holding meter of 3/4 or 6/8 is considered to be soothing and may be explored, but when parents are participating, it may be more useful to retain the original meter of the song to keep it familiar. As the infant's cry slows, Loewy recommends that the therapist create a more discernible pulse to give a sense of motion for the infant.

This process may be taught in simple form to parents as part of "singing a baby to sleep." When parents are present, they may be encouraged to participate at whatever level is comfortable. If parents are not comfortable with singing, the music therapist can model the purposeful use of singing for state transition. Where parents are accustomed to singing, the music therapist can give direction and encouragement, and possibly use an accompanying instrument to give support. Otherwise, the music therapist can partner with the parents to shape the singing to support the transition, helping them to acknowledge key turning points in their infant's state and respond to them musically.

GUIDELINES FOR RECEPTIVE MUSIC THERAPY

Recorded Music as Contextual Support for State Regulation

Overview. Recorded music is a stable stimulus which provides a consistent and predictable external support to improve physiological and behavioral stability. The use of recorded music to support premature infant's physiological and behavioral state is the traditional application and research base of music in the NICU (see Chapter 3 in this volume). Recorded music for the full-term infant may be employed to meet the needs of the infant who has poor state regulation caused by discomfort or by an unpredictable and intrusive care regime in which the infant is frequently disturbed. The common referral from the bedside nurse may by for irritability or poor sleep. The intention is that the predictable characteristics of the music help to organize the infant's behavior and calm the infant into a quiet alert state or sleep. The full-term infant can learn to recognize the music and build an association between the stimulus and the state (Granier-Deferre et al., 2011). This is the classic example of music medicine (Dileo & Bradt, 2005) in which there is no therapeutic relationship between the therapist and the infant, or Shoemark's music as treatment (see Newborn Music Therapy Framework section).

Some medical treatments are inherently noisy and rhythmic and may preclude the addition of recorded music. Ventilators (or respirators) such as the *High-Frequency Oscillating* or *Jet Ventilation, high-flow Continuous Pressure Air Pathway* (CPAP) and *Extra Corporeal Membrane Oxygenation* (ECMO) all create a level of noise which far exceed the recommended noise levels for a newborn infant (Karam et al., 2008; Surenthiran et al., 2003). Therefore, to be discriminated above the noise, the music would exceed the standards recommended by the Consensus Committee on Recommended Design Standards for Advanced Neonatal Care (White et al., 2012). In this case, the use of recorded music should be deferred until the infant is on less intrusive ventilatory support.

Once the environmental conditions are confirmed, the infant should be observed both with and without music playing to assess the infant's range of physiological stability in both conditions. If the onset of music or the cessation of music causes an increase in negative physiological signs such as increased heart rate or lower oxygen saturation, or stress behavior outside the ranges stipulated by the medical team, then the use of recorded music should be deferred for at least one week to allow for increased maturation or improved medical status.

Preparation. To be effective, the recorded music must be sufficiently loud to stand out against the ambient auditory environment, and discernible without exceeding the recommended sound levels for the intensive care or unit environment. Preparation therefore includes measuring the auditory environment both without and with music (see Guidelines for Music Therapy: Auditory Environment).

After an initial assessment, the use of recorded music occurs most often without the music therapist present, other than in progress evaluation sessions which are necessary to adapt the music according to the infant's maturity and medical progression.

What to observe. In the initial assessment, the music therapist should observe the infant's patterns of response to the ambient environment and then to music. This process is not to determine benefit but safety and suitability. If the infant is awake, he should respond with stilling, and even an attempt to locate the sound source. If he is asleep (because this is the only viable time to conduct the assessment), there should be an orienting response in hear rate where it dips about five beats per minute in response to the stimulus and then returns within the minute to its resting pace. If the introduction of music elicits an increase in bradycardia (irregularity of heartbeat) or apnea (irregularity of breathing) causing the alarm to sound, the music should be discontinued and introduction of the music program deferred for a few days before retesting. If the infant continues to respond negatively to the introduction of music, then it should be considered contraindicated. Both parents and nurses should be advised to contact the music therapist for further evaluation if the infant does not seem to be coping with the music as provided.

Procedures. The program will include two types of sessions. The initial session involves an assessment by the music therapist of the infant's readiness for recorded music as a stimulus. Once the use of recorded music is deemed safe, the music therapist will select appropriately sedative music. While this process could be undertaken by the music therapist, there is merit in discussing musical preferences with the family first. The sedative nature of music is not dictated by the musical style. There is classical, folk, and even gentle rock music which can be classified as sedative. In discussion with the family, the music therapist can validate the family's musical preferences while also applying the requirements for sedative music. Music styles such as heavy metal will provide a narrow opportunity for using family preference, but by discussing musical elements, the music therapist can inform and empower the family's choices while supporting the infant's state.

Johnno was a die-hard ACDC fan. When the music therapist said his sweet baby boy Luke could listen to some music, Johnno was excited for a moment. Perhaps he could bring in his best ACDC playlist. The music therapist asked Johnno what he loved about ACDC, and they chatted about the powerful rhythms, and that really thick texture. The music therapist said she would find some music with good rhythm and a solid texture. She explained it wouldn't be ACDC, but it wouldn't be that classical music either! He hated that stuff. She said that over time as Luke got better, they would introduce music that was more Johnno's style. She came back the next day with a CD of folk music with some cool instruments. It wasn't stuff he knew, but it was okay. The instructions said, "For Johnno to play for Luke in the evenings when they have a cuddle." Johnno played it every night.

It is useful to establish a basic safe presentation protocol based on the unit's infection control, bedside safety requirements, and evidence for safe presentation. This protocol should include decisions about:

- Infection Control: responsibility for ensuring the equipment is regularly cleaned according to hospital requirements.

- Bedside Safety: placement of the playing equipment where it does not interfere with care of the infant and where it cannot be accidentally knocked off the surface.
- Presentation Safety:
  - Location of speakers: about 20 centimeters from the infant's head.
  - Volume: should be 6–10 dBA louder than the ambient environment to be heard by the infant. This should not exceed recommended levels (see Appendix B: Guidelines for Monitoring the Sound Levels in the NICU). The range can be set and marked on the player. The music should be faded in and out over 30 seconds.
  - Frequency and context of presentation: The music can be presented as often as required to meet the intended purpose. This may be negotiated with parents or nursing staff to individualize the application.
  - Duration: There are no firm guidelines for duration for full-term infants, but staff and families should be instructed that the music should not be played continuously as infants will habituate and cease to attend to it as a stimulus.
  - Person responsible for implementing the music program: This will depend on the culture of care in the unit. Where the program is family-centered, the therapist should champion the parents' right to be the ones who use the music as part of the nurturing care. Where the program is infant-focused, frequency will be linked the individual infant's need. For example, if being used for sleep, then the music will be presented each time the infant is settled for sleep.

The therapist should set up the equipment and ensure the bedside nurse understands the protocol. In addition, the music therapist should spend time with the family to teach them the protocol. The program should also be included in the infant's medical record and on a notice on the bed (see an example in Appendix C). The music may become a backdrop for relaxed play or breast-feeding. Siblings can productively be involved in selecting music for their baby.

Further sessions that involve the music therapist will serve to check state of equipment and review suitability and functionality of prepared repertoire with the family. During a long admission, a periodic review of the recordings is required to expand and renew the repertoire made available to the infant and family.

Environmental Music Therapy

Overview. The hospital environment is a 24-hour-per-day, public environment in which infant, family, and staff are subjected to endless noise. To ameliorate the impact of random noise, live music by musicians can serve to both relax and renew the auditory experiences for everyone in the unit (Loewy, 2009; Shoemark, 2009). Musicians may be music therapists, music therapy students, or capable musicians from the community. When musicians are used, the music therapist must educate the musicians to provide appropriate repertoire and supervise the impact of that music on the recipients, including the medical staff. The work is aligned with Shoemark's "Noxious Experience; Music as Protective Agent." The human activity associated with high-level medical care produces high-volume noise. During noisy times, music is likely to interfere with staff communication and contribute to the noisy environment, so it should not be commenced. If the environment quickly changes (for a medical emergency), the music should be ceased, as it may interfere with effective communication among staff. The musicians and all equipment should be removed as quickly as possible. After the crisis, the music may be welcome in the process of everyone's recovery.

Musicians are not skilled in assessing the stress of patients and families and, therefore, should not play directly in front of people. Most people will have little power for enduring an unwelcome experience, but will not want to offend the musicians by asking them to leave if they are not enjoying the music. Performances should be removed to a place (like the corridor or foyer of a unit) where the sounds will easily transmit through the unit and the family can easily locate them to come and enjoy the performance directly if they choose.

Preparation. The music source must be carefully selected. Some instruments cannot be played sufficiently softly to produce a beautiful sound at a safe volume (Shoemark, 2009). Most brass instruments will be too loud, and instruments such as the concert flute should not be played in the unit as the register reflects many of the alarms in the unit and therefore may not be well discriminated or may interfere with nursing care.

The music therapist should liaise with the unit manager or person in charge of the unit for that time. It is important to know what events have taken place up to this point in the day, as it will help determine if the repertoire should focus on relaxing or refreshing (Shoemark, 2009). The music therapist should visit each room to inform staff and families prior to the music commencing and to suggest that their feedback is very welcome. They should be clearly told that they may ask for the music to be stopped at any point.

What to observe. The music therapist observes for visible traits of enjoyment or bother. Recipients enjoying the music will show the customary behaviors such as tapping feet, rocking in time, singing along, and making favorable comments. Bother is sometimes better disguised, as people do not want to criticize efforts to care for them. Therefore, it is important to empower both families and staff to give frank feedback. Nonverbal behavior might include closing the door to a room, turning a back, or pulling curtains around the bed. The therapist should consider moving the musician farther away from that location or instruct the musician to play more quietly or stop altogether.

Procedures. In addition to the above observations, the music therapist must brief and debrief the musicians to ensure they feel well informed in their repertoire choices and style of playing. After the session, the musicians will appreciate feedback as to how their music was received. The music therapist should share any comments or observable impact (Shoemark, 2009).

The following recommendations arose from the *Sweet Melodies* project during which professional musicians from the Melbourne Symphony Orchestra played live in the NICU at The Royal Children's Hospital Melbourne. The musicians should be encouraged to select two types of music: relaxing and refreshing. When only relaxing music was played, staff and families found it to be maudlin and requested a change. Refreshing music was light and joyful, and in the Sweet Melodies project included some folk, children's repertoire, and Disney tunes. A playing period of 20 minutes is sufficient. This 20-minute period may include shorter sets from more than one musician. More than this can become intrusive for staff, and it is taxing for the musicians. Variation is useful and the presence of two musicians can create a sense of shared experience and peer support. Gentle duets make for a nice variation. Variation may be produced through a range of musical instruments, music styles, and the possibility of taking requests from those listening.

GUIDELINES FOR RE-CREATIVE MUSIC THERAPY

Song is the main vehicle for musical interaction between parent and infants. Some mothers may have already begun to sing to their baby when in utero. Such songs will be familiar to her baby at birth and continue to be so for some weeks to come (Granier-Deferre et al., 2011). This information can provide comfort to mothers of hospitalized infants, as it draws something "normal" that they can continue to do in this extraordinary situation. This promotes a sense of doing something "helpful" for their baby at a time when they may feel disempowered. For other mothers, singing may not be something they would think to do, but for many it is acceptable. Along with song, parents will engage in using nursery rhymes and even read to their infants. Each of these modalities can be used by parents, siblings, extended family, and staff to provide the infant with consistent and increasingly familiar joyful interaction. The normality of such activity is important across a long stay in the hospital.

Songs of Kin

Overview. Despite Western society's move toward receptive music, parents are inclined to sing to their babies even in the hospital. Many mothers retain a capacity to use their voice to support their baby. When parents have indicated that they have a capacity and inclination to use music as part of family coping, it may be appropriate to draw on their musical heritage to promote this experience as the continuation of life rather than a contrast to life. Musical heritage may be defined by the parent's own receptive experiences of music to date, including their own experience of being sung to by either or both parents, learning to play a musical instrument, and their own active music-making in choirs or bands and orchestras (Shoemark, in review). Where the parents identify themselves as "musical," the confidence to draw that healthy part of themselves into this current scenario may provide them with an unexpected moment of joy. Loewy and Stewart (2008) champion the significance of "Songs of Kin" which are selected to acknowledge a "caregiver's intentions, ancestry, and/or heritage" (p. 25). "Songs of Kin" include the family's pre-existing valued experience of shared song and draw on the associated positive experiences to strengthen them during this crisis. Infants may recognize "Songs of Kin" more quickly than novel material, thereby optimizing the usefulness of the song when infants are stressed by procedures or recovering from episodes of pain. Songs are portable, and once known are always familiar. They therefore become a shared moment that may enhance attachment between parent and infant.

If the music therapist encounters a family for whom music has no value or appeal, then caution should be exercised. Some gentle education may be offered, but if the family remains uninterested, then it may be that music is not a useful medium and pursuit may cause stress and undermine the parents' own sense of parenting capacity. Nuanced work with parents may be beyond the new music therapy graduate without additional training. New graduates should refer to other psychosocial professionals, including social workers, psychologists, or case managers.

Preparation. It may take some time to gently reveal "Songs of Kin" and therefore the work might occur away from the baby's bedside, during a parent's session with the music therapist.

What to observe. In asking parents to consider previous experiences where music was of personal value, the music therapist may bring the parent into a vulnerable state that should be carefully contained and supported so the parent can return to the bedside intact. For the infant, the impact of song should be carefully monitored for recognition or adverse response.

Procedures. Hospitalization of a newborn infant is a time of stress, and thus the focus should remain on supporting the parents and not unpacking their own history. This does not preclude dealing with deep emotions that arise, but in generating "Songs of Kin", the therapist should be clear that the intention is to collect songs which will offer the family warmth, love, and cherished support.

Once a song or songs are confirmed, the music therapist and parent work as a team to bring the song to the infant. The parent should be encouraged and supported to lead the singing, with the music therapist as backup or providing accompaniment, or simply serving as witness to the interplay. If the parent is not confident enough to sing, he or she can still remain directly in front of the baby to be the key visual person and, while the music therapist sings (and perhaps plays), the parent might rock the baby or jiggle the baby's bedding to create a combined sensory modality experience.

"Songs of Kin" serve as a thread of continuity from home to hospital and back to home upon discharge. They can be the basis for shared singing or conversation in support groups for mothers. Song singing or playing can also be the vehicle for psychotherapy work with fathers which may take place away from the unit to allow them to "tell their story" and derive support from someone outside their family circle (Mondanaro, 2010). Where families have established favorite songs for specific purposes, they can be encouraged to continue this activity to reassure their infant of their continuing presence and nurturing.

There are many ways to extend the usefulness of song. The wider family may have more energy to recall songs that are useful. Grandparents can recall the songs that parents loved as children and help bring these to the parents' recall. Modern songbooks which include recordings within the book can also serve to remind families of songs they love. Such additional material can also enable the parent to "sing along," which offers them support if they are not confident singing. Song serves the infant and family beyond the presence of the music therapist. The purposeful construction of a family songbook provides a vibrant activity which acknowledges the emerging child. In the clinical context, this may be the first item with the baby's name on it that is not medical (Shoemark & Dearn, 2008).

GUIDELINES FOR COMPOSITIONAL MUSIC THERAPY

Lullabies and Play Songs

Overview. Over the course of long admissions, the music therapist can work to stimulate a family's own musicality to create meaningful songs or lyrical melody motifs for shared experience. Drawing on melodic and lyric themes generated during improvisational music-making, the parent may generate new songs which can become part of their family repertoire with their baby. Lyrics reflect their everyday experiences and the songs use simple forms reminiscent of familiar lullabies and play songs. Play songs are songs for interaction with the awake infant who is available for interaction. They might include nursery rhymes or children's songs such as "Old MacDonald," "Wheels on the Bus," "Eensy Weensy Spider," and so on.

Parents who are very vulnerable, are psychologically unavailable to their infant because of distress, or have mental health issues (such as depression) should not be involved in this work, as it may make them more vulnerable.

Preparation. Preparations for live singing at the bedside are guided by the general guidelines for music therapy. Preparations for recording will include availability of recording equipment and the availability of the family. Recording may utilize modern smart phone capability to record voice, or more traditional recording equipment such as microphone and digital recording programs as available. Recording in a quiet room with a good microphone and digital recording program is desirable in producing a good-quality sound. However, if the parent wants to remain at the bedside or does not visit the hospital during work times, the modern smart phone can produce an acceptable recording for the full-term baby. This is not advisable for more fragile infants where strict administration of auditory stimulation is required. For recording at the bedside, the music therapist should confer with the nurse about optimal times for recording (no medical rounds, bedside assessments, etc.) and negotiate for alarms to be silenced for a defined period so that they do not occur during recording.

What to observe. Music therapists should listen for the potential for the parent to create music during initial discussions. A level of comfort with their own voices and a willingness to engage in playful originality may indicate that composition is useful. The music therapist should observe the interplay between infant and parents.

Procedures. Through discussion, the family may be able to recall songs from their own childhood or songs that their own parents sang to them. Using the first line or best-known line from the song, the music therapist can literally give the song "voice" in the NICU or PICU environment to demonstrate the acceptability of the sound and the potential place for the song in this experience. If parents are unable to recall any songs, the music therapist can call on the common childhood repertoire for the most likely songs (e.g., "Twinkle, Twinkle Little Star," "Hush, Little Baby"). Once parents show some acceptance and interest, the songs may be adapted to the current situation using lyrics substitution. For example:

> Emma, Emma little star,
> Oh, we wonder how you are,
> Here we sit and sing to you,
> While you sleep the whole day through,
> When you're ready so are we,
> to take you home to our family.

When families wish to make a recording of songs for their baby, the therapist should begin with the same discussion about repertoire as above. If families are not able to present at the hospital, the music therapist can advise by telephone about how to set up the recording (including advice about recording applications) and also help the family to produce a positive sound for their baby by suggesting they sing happy songs for awake time and gentle lullabies for sleep time. Delivery of the recording may be problematic but can include transfer onto a CD, emailing the digital file, or waiting until they are next visiting the hospital to download the recording from the phone onto another playback format such as CD or MP3 player.

While songwriting may serve as source of therapy for the parent, it would be rare to engage parents in writing original songs during the admission, as it can open the parent to vulnerabilities which they might otherwise keep contained while they try to "stay strong" for their baby.

RESEARCH EVIDENCE

The evidence for music therapy has grown across more than 30 years, and while it is persuasive, only a small number of studies with infants have been completed. The use of instrumental music vs. voice is an ongoing debate in the application of live or recorded music for newborn infants. The selection of the stimulus or medium is dependent upon the intention of the program. Generally, it could be said that if the intention is to modify the immediate environment and decrease arousal, then sedative instrumental music will be a focus of the selection. However, if the intention of the program is to stimulate the infant's neurodevelopment and sense of self, the human voice is a more desirable medium for enticing the infant into dynamic interplay. This debate is worthy of considerable discussion beyond this chapter. In this section, evidence related to the use of music with hospitalized newborn infants is presented.

In their study, del Olmo, Garrido, and Tarrio (2010) used improvised singing to change the physiological parameters of infants (N = 87) up to 6 months old. They compared parent-infant interaction with and without music and found that the addition of music produced a significant decrease in heart rate (mean change = −6.82, *SD* = 14.21, *p* = .02), compared to a minimal change in the no-music group (mean change = −0.19, *SD* = 17.42, *p* = .014). The music was produced by singing with accompaniment from keyboard or guitar and emulated the infant's presenting behaviors, using the infant's cry to indicate tonality and the intensity of the infant and parents' interaction to indicate dynamics of the music.

In a study of hospitalized newborn infants (N = 39), Malloch and colleagues (2012) found that after four weeks of therapist-delivered contingent singing, infants were able to maintain better self-regulation during social interaction, were less irritable and cried less, and were more positive in their response to adult handling than the NICU-based control group who received normal care. Assessed with the Neurobehavioral Assessment of the Preterm Infant, the music therapy group showed a significantly higher overall score than the control group at posttest (*z* = −1.96, *p* = .05). Notably, the music therapy group scored significantly better on irritability (*z* = −3.18, *p* = .001) and crying extent (*z* = −2.51, *p* = .01). These gains are important both in preserving precious weight gain and as prerequisites for social interaction.

This author undertook a micro-analysis of the data from the Malloch et al. study (2012). She subjected a sample of the data (critical events in the therapeutic interplay) to a video-cued narrative analysis (Raingruber, 2003) to generate a taxonomy of adult and infant interplay behaviors (Shoemark & Grocke, 2010). The infant behaviors fell into three categories, namely quiet, active, and unavailable. The therapist's behaviors were defined as enticing, responsive, and directive. When combined, they produce seven markers of the interplay process which guide the therapist in creating the opportunity for interplay, progressing in the interplay and bringing interplay to a close.

Beyond the hospitalized infant population, the capacity of the newborn infant to process recorded music is a topic of great interest to a range of researchers. Granier-Deferre, Bassereau, Ribeiro, Jacquet, and DeCasper (2011) reported that fetuses who heard a descending melody twice per day for three weeks (36 to 38 weeks' gestation) showed a cardiac deceleration upon presentation of that same melody after a six-week retention period. This means that the infant not only recognized the melody he heard in utero, but also was able to recall it after a six-week retention period. This knowledge enables the music therapist to employ recorded music with more certainty about the capacity of the infant to make use of it as a stimulus.

Receptive music has been used with preterm infants to address many issues, including physiological and behavioral homeostasis (Standley & Walworth, 2011) and specific short-term outcomes such as recovery from painful procedures (Keith, Russell, & Weaver, 2009; Tramo, Lense, Van Ness, Kagan, Settle, & Cronin, 2011). For late preterm and full-term infants, the pilot study by Olischar, Shoemark, Holton, Weninger, and Hunt (2011) is relevant. In this study, the impact of music on the quality of sleep in 20 infants was examined by means of an amplitude-integrated electroencephalography. After hearing 20 minutes of a recorded instrumental lullaby (Brahms's "Lullaby"), the duration of quiet sleep and interval between quiet sleep periods got progressively longer in all participants in the intervention group as compared to participants in the control group (no music); however, this difference was not statistically significant ($t = 1.68$, $p = 0.11$).

No research is available yet on the parents of full-term infants using compositional methods. The use of familiar song or "Songs of Kin" is an emergent area of research interest, but at the time of publishing there was no research in the literature. Loewy is best known for articulating the method of this work which honors the intrinsic culture of the family (Hanson-Abromeit, Shoemark, & Loewy, 2008).

Research with older healthy infants is beginning to clarify how we might think about the benefits of re-creative song for postterm infants in hospital. Additional support for the use of known songs may be derived from understanding the listening preferences of healthy infants. Ilari and Sundara (2009) clarified that for infants age five months and older, there is a clear preference for unaccompanied songs. In addition, Tsang and Conrad (2010) determined that six- to seven-month-old infants' preference for pitch is context-dependent. They found that infants preferred low-pitched versions of lullabies and high-pitched versions of play songs. Longhi (2009) characterized the multimodal interaction style of mothers as "songese" (like "motherese") and confirmed that it was effective in providing infants with temporal structure for learning.

Additional insight is gained from understanding the beliefs and attitudes of mothers regarding singing to their babies. In a survey of 100 mothers of infants (age seven to nine months), 92% reported singing to their babies (Ilari, 2005), while in a survey of 60 mothers' spontaneous voice use in the NICU, Shoemark (in review) found that 60% of mothers used singing to interact with their babies. While this was obviously less than the Ilari finding, the infants were all newborns, and singing was still ranked much higher than patterned speech activities (37%) such as nursery rhymes or reading.

Summary and Conclusions

This chapter has offered the reader a point of distinction between prematurely born infants and full-term infants in hospital. The full-term infant seeks the companionship of attuned adults and is therefore available for interplay ranging from an active expectation of partnership to gentle sensory support for sleep. The music therapist can use theory to make decisions about the kind of service that might be provided, whether that be infant-focused or family-centered. Both frameworks will guide the music therapist into thinking about music as a stimulus for treatment or an experience to be shared. Full-term infants are born with the capacities of their healthy counterparts but may be compromised by their serious health conditions or the treatments they receive. Music is an experience that is malleable to their medical status and their behavioral needs. Live singing can be used to soothe the infant to sleep or to stimulate the necessary interaction to maintain health neurological development.

There is a significant need for research about the potential of music for the full-term infant. It is important for this research to be based on theoretical frameworks. Robb, Burns, and Carpenter (2011) provided a seminal article on the need for meticulous explanation of the music itself and the theoretical rationale for those decisions. This supports Shoemark's theory-based framework model (2012). Burns's call for theory-based research (2012) also encourages the music therapist to delineate how music therapy moderates those factors which lead to change in the client. While knowledge from healthy infant development can be utilized, context-specific research is needed to ensure that music is used safely for these infants. There is a particular need to acknowledge the pivotal place of the family in creating and employing their own musicality for their infant. By using music in these earliest experiences, we may support the development of lifelong skills, sense of self, and the use of music as a source of well-being.

GLOSSARY

Based on information provided via National Library of Medicine: http://www.nlm.nih.gov/medlineplus/medlineplus.html

22q11.2 deletion syndrome: A disorder caused by the deletion of a small piece of chromosome 22. Characteristic signs and symptoms include heart defects, an opening in the roof of the mouth (a cleft palate) or other palate defects, mild differences in facial features, recurrent infections caused by problems with the immune system. Some may have complex medical issues requiring significant care.

Angelman syndrome: A genetic disorder that causes developmental delay and neurological problems. Infants may not present with any symptoms at birth but often have feeding problems.

Chronic Lung Disease (CLD) (or Bronchopulmonary Dysplasia): Tissue damage to the lungs which occurs in severely ill infants who have received high levels of oxygen for long periods of time or who have been on mechanical ventilation and supplemental oxygen as treatment for respiratory distress syndrome. It is more common in preterm infants whose lungs were not fully developed at birth.

Congenital Diaphragmatic Hernia (CDH): A birth defect in which there is an abnormal opening in the diaphragm. The opening allows part of the stomach, spleen, liver, and intestines to go up into the chest cavity near the lungs. The lung tissue on the affected side is thus not allowed to completely develop.

Congenital heart defect (CHD): A problem with the structure of the heart that is present at birth. CHDs are the most common type of major birth defect. Structural defects can involve the walls of the heart, the valves of the heart, and the arteries and veins near the heart. Congenital heart defects can disrupt the normal flow of blood through the heart.

Continuous Pressure Air Pathway (CPAP): A device that delivers slightly pressurized air through the nose. CPAP can help keep the airways open and may prevent the need for a ventilator.

Down's Syndrome (also called Trisomy 21): Down's Syndrome is a set of mental and physical symptoms that result from having an extra copy of chromosome 21. Symptoms can range from mild to severe and usually include intellectual impairment, some motor difficulties, health problems which may include heart disease, dementia, hearing problems, and problems with the intestines, eyes, thyroid and skeleton.

Esophageal Atresia: A congenital defect. In most cases, the upper esophagus ends and does not connect with the lower esophagus and stomach.

Extracorporeal Membrane Oxygenation (ECMO): A treatment that uses a pump to circulate blood through an artificial lung back into the bloodstream of a very ill baby. This system provides heart-lung bypass support outside of the baby's body.

Fragile X syndrome: The most common form of inherited intellectual impairment. Caused by a gene mutation which means that the person makes little or none of a protein essential for brain development.

Gastroschisis: A hernia in which the intestine usually protrudes through a hole in the abdominal wall on one side of the umbilical cord. An omphalocele is similar, but the intestines are covered only by a thin layer of tissue and can be easily seen.

Hypoxic Ischemic Encephalopathy (HIE): An injury to the brain which occurs when an infant's brain fails to receive sufficient oxygen or sufficient blood before birth.

Hypoplastic Left Heart Syndrome: A rare congenital condition which occurs when parts of the left side of the heart (mitral valve, left ventricle, aortic valve, and aorta) do not develop completely.

Ototoxic medication: Medication which are used to treat major infections such as sepsis. Medication such as aminoglycosides that damage the inner ear or the auditory nerve.

Pierre Robin Syndrome: A condition present at birth in which the infant has a smaller-than-normal lower jaw, a tongue that falls back in the throat, and difficulty breathing.

Sensorineural hearing loss: A hearing loss that occurs from damage to the inner ear, the auditory nerve, or the brain.

Ventilator (Respirator): A device for assisting or replacing the baby's task of breathing. There are a variety of ventilators which vary the frequency and amount of air delivered.

REFERENCES

American Academy of Pediatrics Committee on Environmental Health. (1997). Noise: A hazard for the fetus and newborn. *Pediatrics, 100,* 724–727.

Bargiel, M. (2004). Lullabies and play songs: Theoretical considerations for an early attachment music therapy intervention through parental singing for developmentally at-risk infants. *Voices: A World Forum for Music Therapy.* Retrieved from http://www.voices.no/mainissues/mi40004000143.html

Beebe, B., & Lachman, F. (1994). Representation and internalization in infancy: Three principles of salience. *Psychoanalytic Psychology, 11,* 127–165.

Berglund, B., Lindvall, T., & Schwela, D. (1999). Guidelines for community noise. World Health Organization. Retrieved from World Health Organization website http://www.who.int/docstore/peh/noise/guidelines2.html

Bielecki, I., Horbulewicz, A., & Wolan, T. (2011). Risk factors associated with hearing loss in infants: An analysis of 5282 referred neonates. *International Journal of Pediatric Otorhinolaryngology, 75,* 925–930.

Brazelton, T. B., & Nugent, K. (2011). *Neonatal behavioral assessment scale* (4th ed.). London: Mac Keith Press.

Burns, D. (2012). Theoretical rationale for music selection in oncology intervention research: An integrative review. *Journal of Music Therapy, 49*(1), 7–22.

Burns, K., Cunningham, N., White-Traut, R., Silvestri, J., & Nelson, M. (1994). Infant stimulation: Modification of an intervention based on physiologic and behavioral cues. *Journal of Gynaecological and Neonatal Nursing, 23*(7), 581–589.

Butt, M. L., & Kisilevsky, B. S. (2000). Music modulates behaviour of premature infants following heel lance. *Canadian Journal of Nursing Research, 31*(4), 17–39.

Cevasco, A. (2008). The effect of mothers' singing on fullterm and preterm infants and maternal emotional responses. *Journal of Music Therapy, 45*(3), 273–306.

Cevasco, A. M., & Grant, R. E. (2005). Effects of the pacifier activated lullaby on weight gain on premature infants. *Journal of Music Therapy, 42*(2), 123–139.

Chou, L., Wang, R., Chen, S., & Pai, L. (2003). Effects of music therapy on oxygen saturation in premature infants receiving endotracheal suctioning. *Journal of Nursing Research, 11*(3), 209–215.

Crown, C., Feldstein, S., Jasnow, M., Beebe, B., & Jaffe, J. (2002). The cross-modal co-ordination of interpersonal timing: Six-week-old infants' gaze with adults' vocal behavior. *Journal of Psycholinguistic Research, 31*(1), 1–23.

Custodero, L. A., & Johnson-Green, E. A. (2008). Caregiving in counterpoint: reciprocal influences in the musical parenting of younger and older infants. *Early Child Development and Care, 178*(1), 15–39.

de l'Etoile, S. (2006). Infant behavioral responses to infant-directed singing and other maternal interactions. *Infant Behavior and Development, 29,* 456–470.

de Vries, P. (2009). Music at home with the under fives: what is happening? *Early Child Development and Care, 179*(4), 395–405. DOI: 10.1080/03004430802691914.

del Olmo, M. J., Rodríguez Garrido, C., & Ruza Tarrío, F. (2010). Music therapy in the PICU: 0- to 6-month-old babies. *Music and Medicine, 2,* 158–166.

Dileo, C., & Bradt, J. (2005). *Medical music therapy: A meta-analysis and agenda for future research.* Cherry Hill, NJ: Jeffrey Books.

Doheny, L., Hurwitz, S., Insoft, R., Ringer, S., & Lahav, A. (2012). Exposure to biological maternal sounds improves cardiorespiratory regulation in extremely preterm infants. *The Journal of Maternal-Fetal and Neonatal Medicine.* Early online 1-4. DOI: 10.3109/14767058.2011.648237.

Dubowitz, L., Dubowitz V., & Mercuri, E. (1999). *Neurological assessment of the preterm and full-term infant.* London: Mac Keith Press.

Edwardraj, S., Mumtaj, K., Prasad, J. H., Kuruvilla, A., & Jacob, K. S. (2010). Perceptions about intellectual disability: a qualitative study from Vellore, South India. *Journal of Intellectual Disability, 54*(8), 736–748.

Fegran, L., Helseth, S., & Solveig Fagermoen, M. (2008). A comparison of mothers' and fathers' experiences of the attachment process in a neonatal intensive care unit. *Journal of Clinical Nursing, 17,* 810–816.

Granier-Deferre, C., Bassereau, S., Ribeiro, A., Jacquet, A-Y., & DeCasper, A. (2011). A melodic contour repeatedly experienced by human near-term fetuses elicits a profound cardiac reaction one month after birth. *PLoS ONE 6*(2): e17304. DOI: 10.1371/journal.pone.0017304.

Gray, L., & Philbin, M. K. (2000). The acoustic environment of hospital nurseries: Measuring sound in hospital nurseries. *Journal of Perinatology, 20,* S99–S103.

Gray, L., & Philbin, M. K. (2004). Effects of the neonatal intensive care unit on auditory attention and distraction. *Clinics in Perinatology, 31,* 243–260.

Hanson-Abromeit, D. (2003). The newborn individualized developmental care and assessment program (NIDCAP) as a model for clinical music therapy interventions with premature infants. *Music Therapy Perspectives, 21,* 60–68.

Hanson-Abromeit, D., Shoemark, H., & Loewy, J. (2008). Music therapy in the newborn intensive and special care nurseries. In D. Hanson-Abromeit & C. Colwell (Eds.), *AMTA monograph series: Medical music therapy for pediatrics in hospital settings: using music to support medical interventions* (pp. 15–69). Silver Spring, MD: American Music Therapy Association.

Ilari, B. (2005). On musical parenting of young children: Musical beliefs and behaviors of mothers and infants. *Early Child Development and Care, 175*(7), 647–660.

Ilari, B., & Sundara, M. (2009). Music listening preferences in early life: Infants' responses to accompanied versus unaccompanied singing. *Journal of Research in Music Education, 56*(4), 357–369.

Ingersoll, E. W., & Thoman, E. B. (1999). Sleep/wake states of preterm infants: Stability, developmental change, diurnal variation, and relation with caregiving activity. *Child Development, 70*(1), 1–10.

Jaffe, J., Beebe, B., Feldstein, S., Crown, C., & Jasnow, M. (2001). Rhythms of dialogue in infancy: Co-ordinated timing in development. *Monographs of the Society for Research in Child Development, 66*(2), vi–131.

Jardri, R., Pins, D., Houfflin-Debarge, V., Chaffiotte, C., Rocourt, N., Pruvo, J. P., & Thomas, P. (2008). Fetal cortical activation to sound at 33 weeks of gestation: A functional MRI study. *NeuroImage, 42* (1), 10–18.

Karam, O., Donatiello, C., Van Lancker, E., Chritin, V., Pfister, R. E., Rimensberger, & P. C. (2008). Noise levels during nCPAP are flow dependent but not device-dependent. *Archives of Disease in Childhood Fetal and Neonatal Edition, 93,* F132–F134.

Keith, D. R., Russell, K., & Weaver, B. S. (2009). The effects of music listening on inconsolable crying in premature infants. *Journal of Music Therapy, 46*(3), 191–203.

Keith, D. R., Weaver, B. S., & Vogel, R. B. (2012). The effect of music-based listening interventions on the volume, fat content, and caloric content of breast milk produced by mothers of premature and critically ill infants. *Advances in Neonatal Care, 12*(2), 112–119.

Laing, S., McMahon, C., Ungerer, J., Taylor, A., Badawi, N., & Spence, K. (2010). Mother-child interaction and child developmental capacities in toddlers with major birth defects requiring newborn surgery. *Early Human Development, 86,* 793–800.

Lester, B. M., & Tronick, E. Z. (2004). *NICU network neurobehavioral scale manual.* Baltimore: Paul H. Brookes.

Loewy, J. (2009). Musical sedation: Mechanisms of breathing entrainment. In R. Azoulay & J. Loewy (Eds.), *Music, the breath and health: Advances in integrative music therapy* (pp. 209–216). New York: Satchnote Press.

Longhi, E. (2009). "Songese": maternal structuring of musical interaction with infants. *Psychology of Music, 37*(2), 195–213.

Malloch, S., Shoemark, H., Newnham, C., Črnčec, R., Paul, C., Prior, M., Coward, S., & Burnham, D. (2012). Music therapy with hospitalised infants—the art and science of intersubjectivity. *Infant Mental Health Journal, 33,* 386–399.

Malloch, S., & Trevarthen, C. (2009). Musicality: Communicating the vitality and interests of life. In S. Malloch & C. Trevarthen (Eds.), *Communicative musicality: Exploring the basis of human companionship.* Oxford: Oxford University Press.

Mampe, B., Friederici, A. D., Christophe, A., & Wermke, K. (2009). Newborns' cry melody is shaped by their native language. *Current Biology, 19,* 1–4.

Mietzsch, U., Parikh, N. A., Williams, A. L., Shankaran, S., & Lasky, R. E. (2008). Effects of hypoxic-ischemic encephalopathy and whole-body hypothermia on neonatal auditory function: A pilot study. *American Journal of Perinatology, 25*(7), 435–441.

Moon, C. (2011). The role of early auditory development in attachment and communication. *Clinics in Perinatology, 38,* 657–669.

Mondanaro, J. (2010, August). *NICU palliative care: Anticipatory grief and bereavement.* International NICU Music Therapy Summit, Beth Israel Medical Center, New York.

Newnham, C., Inder, T., & Milgrom, J. (2009). Measuring cumulative stressors within the NICU: The stressor scale. *Infant Behavior and Development, 85,* 549–555.

Nicholson, J., Berthelsen, D., Abad, V., Williams, K., & Bradley, J. (2008). Impact of music therapy to promote positive parenting and child development. *Journal of Health Psychology, 13*(2), 226–238.

Nocker-Ribaupierre, M. (2004). *Music therapy for premature and newborn infants.* Gilsum, NH: Barcelona Publishers.

Obeidat, H. M., Bond, E. A., & Callister, L. C. (2009). The parental experience of having an infant in the Newborn Intensive Care Unit. *The Journal of Perinatal Education, 18*(3), 23–29.

O'Gorman, S. (2007). Infant-directed singing in neonatal and paediatric intensive care. *Australia & New Zealand Journal of Family Therapy, 28*(2), 100–108.

Olischar, M., Shoemark, H., Holton, T., Weninger, M., & Hunt, R. (2011). The influence of music on EEG activity in neurologically healthy newborns >32 weeks' gestational age. *Acta Paediatrica, 100,* 670–675.

Philbin, M. K. (2000). (Ed.). The influence of auditory experience on the fetus, newborn, and preterm infant: Report of the sound study group of the national resource centre. The physical and developmental environment of the high-risk infant. *Journal of Perinatology, 20*(8), S1–S142.

Philbin, M. K., & Evans, J. B. (2006). Standards for the acoustic environment of the newborn ICU. *Journal of Perinatology, 26,* S27–30.

Raingruber, B. (2003). Video-cued narrative reflection: A research approach for articulating tacit, relational, and embodied understandings. *Qualitative Health Research, 13*(8), 1155–1169.

Rickard, N., & McFerran, K. (Eds.). (2012). *Lifelong engagement in music: Benefits for mental health and well-being.* New York: Nova Science Press.

Robb, S., Burns, D., & Carpenter, J. (2011). Reporting guidelines for music-based interventions. *Journal of Health Psychology, 16*(2), 342–352.

Robertson, A., Kohn, J., Vos, P., & Cooper-Peel, C. (1998). Establishing a noise measurement protocol for neonatal intensive care units, *Journal of Perinatology, 18*(2), 126–130.

Sameroff, A., Bartko, W., Baldwin, A., Baldwin, C., & Seifer, R. (1998). Family and social influences on the development of child competence. *Psychoanalytic Dialogues, 5,* 579–593.

Seifer, R. (2001). Conceptual and methodological basis for understanding development and risk in infants. In L. Twarog Singer & P. Sanford Zeskind (Eds.), *Biobehavioral assessment of the infant* (pp. 18–39). New York: Guilford Press.

Shoemark, H. (1996). Family-centred early intervention: Music therapy in the playgroup program. *Australian Journal of Music Therapy, 7,* 3–15.

Shoemark, H. (2008). Mapping progress within an individual music therapy session with full-term hospitalized infants. *Music Therapy Perspectives, 26,* 39–46.

Shoemark, H. (2009). Sweet melodies: combining the talents and knowledge of music therapy and elite musicianship. *Voices: A World Forum for Music Therapy.* Retrieved from http://www.voices.no/mainissues/mi40009000305.php

Shoemark, H. (2011a). Translating "infant-directed singing" into a strategy for the hospitalised family. In J. Edwards (Ed.), *Music therapy and parent-infant bonding* (pp. 162–178). London: Oxford University Press.

Shoemark, H. (2011b). Contingent singing: The musicality of companionship with the hospitalized newborn infant. In F. Baker & S. Uhlig (Eds.), *Therapeutic voicework in music therapy* (pp. 229–249). Philadelphia, PA: Jessica Kingsley.

Shoemark, H. (2012). Frameworks for using music as a therapeutic agent for hospitalised newborn infants. In N. Rickard & K. McFerran (Eds.), *Lifelong engagement in music: Benefits for mental health and well-being* (pp. 1–20). New York: Nova Science Press.

Shoemark, H. (In review.). A survey of how mothers think about and use their voice with their hospitalized newborn infant.

Shoemark, H., & Dearn, T. (2008). Keeping families at the centre of family-centred music therapy with hospitalised infant. *Australian Journal of Music Therapy, 19,* 3–26.

Shoemark, H., & Grocke, D. (2010). The markers of interplay between the music therapist and the medically fragile newborn infant. *Journal of Music Therapy, 47,* 306–334.

Shonkoff, J. P., Garner, A. S., & the Committee on Psychosocial Aspects of Child And Family Health, Committee on Early Childhood, Adoption, and Dependent Care, and Section on Developmental and Behavioral Pediatrics. (2012). The lifelong effects of childhood adversity and toxic stress. *Pediatrics, 129* (1), e232–e246.

Standley, J. M. (1998). The effect of music and multimodal stimulation on responses of premature infants in neonatal intensive care. *Pediatric Nursing, 24*(96), 532–538.

Standley, J. M. (2012). Music therapy research in the NICU: An updated meta-analysis. *Neonatal Network, 31*(5), 311–316.

Standley, J. M., Cassidy, J., Grant, R., Cevasco, A., Szuch, C., Nguyen, J., & Adams, K. (2010). The effect of music reinforcement for non-nutritive sucking on nipple feeding of premature infants. *Pediatric Nurse, 36*(3), 138–145.

Standley, J. M., & Walworth, D. (2010). *Music therapy with premature infants.* (2nd ed.). Silver Spring, MD: American Music Therapy Association, Inc.

Stern, D. (2010). *Forms of vitality: Exploring dynamic experience in psychology, the arts, psychotherapy and development.* London: Oxford University Press.

Stewart, K. (2009). Dimensions of the voice: The use of voice and breath with infants and caregivers in the NICU. In R. Azoulay & J. Loewy (Eds.), *Music, the breath and health: Advances in integrative music therapy* (pp. 235–250). New York: Satchnote Press.

Surenthiran, S. S., Wilbraham, K., May, J., Chant, T., Emmerson, A., & Newton, V. (2003). Noise levels within the ear and postnasal space in neonates in intensive care. *Archives of Diseases: Child Fetal Neonatal Edition, 88,* F315–F318.

Thoman, E. B. (1990). Sleeping and waking states in infants: A functional perspective. *Neuroscience & Biobehavioral Reviews, 14,* 93–107.

Trainor, L. J., Tsang, C. D., & Cheung, V. W. (2002). Preference for sensory consonance in 2- and 4-month-old infants, *Music Perception, 20*(2), 187–194.

Tramo, M. J., Lense, M., Van Ness, C., Kagan, J., Doyle Settle, M., & Cronin, J. H. (2011). Effects of music on physiological and behavioral indices of acute pain and stress in premature infants: Clinical trial and literature review. *Music and Medicine, 3,* 72–83.

Trapanotto, M., Benini, F., Farina, M., Gobber, D., Magnavita, V., & Zacchello, F. (2004). Behavioral and physiological reactivity to noise in the newborn. *Journal of Paediatric Child Health, 40,* 275–281.

Tronick, E. (1998). Dyadically expanded states of consciousness and the process of therapeutic change. *Infant Mental Health Journal, 19*(3), 290–299.

Tsang, C. D., & Conrad, N. J. (2010). Does the message matter? The effect of song type on infants' pitch preferences for lullabies and playsongs. *Infant Behavior & Development, 33,* 96–100.

Wachman, E. L., & Lahav, A. (2010). The effects of noise on preterm infants in the NICU. *Archives of Disease: Child Fetal Neonatal Edition, 96*(4), F305–F309.

Walker, K., Holland, A., Winlaw, D., Sherwood, M., & Badawi, N. (2006). Neurodevelopmental outcomes and surgery in neonates. *Journal of Paediatrics and Child Health, 42,* 749–751.

Walworth, D. (2009). Effects of developmental music groups for parents and premature or typical infants under two years on parental responsiveness and infant social development. *Journal of Music Therapy, 46*(1), 32–52.

Whipple, J. (2008). The effect of music-reinforced nonnutritive sucking on state of preterm, low birthweight infants experiencing heel prick. *Journal of Music Therapy, 45*(3), 227–272.

White, R., & Consensus Committee on Recommended Design Standards for Advanced Neonatal Care. (2012). Recommended standards for Newborn ICU design. Report of the Eighth Consensus Conference on Newborn ICU Design, Clearwater, FL. Retrieved from http://www.nd.edu/~nicudes/RecommendedNICUStandardsFinal8Aug15.pdf

Williams, A. L., van Drongelen, W., & Lasky, R. E. (2007). Noise in contemporary neonatal intensive care. *Journal of the Acoustical Society of America, 121,* 2681–2690.

APPENDIX A

Thoman's taxonomy of infant states (Thoman, 1990; Ingersoll & Thoman, 1999)

Note: All descriptions are derived from Thoman (1990) unless specified.

1. Alert
   o Eyes— open, bright and shining, and attentive or scanning.
   o Motor activity—typically low (during the first two weeks of life), but infant may be active.

2. Nonalert Waking
   o Eyes—usually open, but dull and unfocused. May be closed during periods of high-level activity.
   o Motor activity—may vary, but typically high.
   o Vocal activity—Isolated fuss vocalizations may occur.

3. Fuss or Cry
   Fuss:
   o Vocalization—Fuss sounds are made continuously or intermittently, at relatively low levels of intensity.
   Cry:
   o Vocal Activity—Intense vocalizations occur either singly or in succession.

4. Drowse, Daze, or Sleep-Wake Transition
   Drowse:
   o Eyes—open but "heavy-lidded" or opening and closing slowly.
   o Motor activity—typically low, but may vary.
   (Note: This state usually occurs when the infant is going from waking to sleep.)
   Daze:
   o Eyes—open but glassy and immobile.
   o Motor activity—typically low.
   (Note: This state typically occurs between episodes of Drowse or Alert.)
   Sleep-Wake Transition:
   o Behaviors of both wakefulness and sleep.
   o Eyes—eyes may be closed, or they may open and close rapidly.
   o Motor activity—generalized activity.
   o Vocal activity—Isolated fuss vocalizations may occur.
   (Note: This state generally occurs when the baby is awakening from sleep.)

5. Active Sleep, or Active-Quiet Transition Sleep
   Active Sleep:
   o Eyes—closed; rapid eye movements (REMs) occur intermittently, ranging from a brief, light flicker of the eyelids to prolonged intense REM storms accompanied by raising of the eyelids and occasional eye opening.
   o Respiration—uneven and primarily costal in nature.

- o   Motor activity—sporadic movements may occur, but muscle tone is low between movements; twitching movements of the extremities. (*Also see vocal activity.*)
- o   Vocal activity—sighs; sigh-sobs; brief, high-pitched cries; "straining" or grunting vocalizations during large stretching movements.
- o   Facial and mouth movements—smiles, frowns, grimaces, mouthing, sucking.

Active-Quiet Transition Sleep:
- o   Eyes—closed.
- o   Motor activity—little.
- o   Respiration—not as regular as Quiet Sleep, but more regular than Active Sleep.
- o   Breathing—may be abdominal or costal or mixed, muscle tone may vary, and isolated REMs may occur.
- o   The baby shows mixed behavioral signs of Active Sleep and Quiet Sleep.
       (N.B. This state typically occurs between periods of Active Sleep and Quiet Sleep.)

6.   Quiet sleep
- o   Eyes—closed.
- o   Motor activity—Tonic level of motor tone is maintained; motor activity usually limited to occasional startles, sigh-sobs, or rhythmic mouthing. Brief periods of limb or body movements may occur (more frequent in preterm infants).
- o   Respiration—relatively slow, regular, and abdominal in nature.

APPENDIX B

GUIDELINES FOR MONITORING THE SOUND LEVELS IN THE NICU

1) Map the physical environment to understand the physical factors which contribute to the additional and abatement of noise. A comprehensive map would include dimensions of the unit, noting the number of beds in the room and where they are located; constructed areas such as nurses' stations; doors and their method of movement (electronic, manual); surfaces of walls, ceiling, and floor; location of the dosimeter; locations of ventilators, pumps, humidifiers, music sources, sinks, trash and linen containers, drawers, and Extra Corporeal Membrane oxygenation patients (Williams, Drongelen, & Lasky, 2007).

2) Determine a standard location for area measurement (Robertson, Kohn, Vos, & Cooper-Peel, 1998). Robertson et al. (1998) determined that central monitoring may provide useful preliminary data, but area measurements are needed for detailed analysis. The standard location might be the farthest point from both the door (or bay opening) and major equipment (ventilation or ECMO).

3) Period of measurement may be determined by the availability of measuring devices. Handheld sound-level meters present a data readout on screen, but do not store data. Monitoring is more likely to be a snapshot measure of a few minutes. A dosimeter can collect data over an extended period which can be downloaded into a computer (software may or may not be included in the purchase). The use of the dosimeter means that data can be collected for a 24-hour period, which offers a comprehensive picture of the full day. The more expensive dosimeters can also include spectral data, allowing a comprehensive picture of loudness and frequency to be captured.

4) Measurements should include (a) equivalent sound level (L_{eq}), (b) maximum sound level (L_{max}), and (c) minimum sound level (L_{min}) for each interval to be measured in A-weighted levels (A weighting gives emphasis to the range heard by the human ear) and slow (which refers to the number of measurements taken in a defined period, usually seconds). Where possible, the peak sound level (L_{peak}) should be measured in dB sound pressure level (SPL) (Williams, Drongelen, & Lasky, 2007).

5) A simple comparison will reveal if the results are above or below the best practice guidelines from the Consensus Committee on Recommended Design Standards for Advanced Neonatal Care (2012). The standards are that the total sound, that is, the combination of continuous sound and operational sound (includes equipment), should not exceed an hourly L_{eq} of 45 dB and an hourly L_{10} of 50 dB, both A-weighted slow. The L_{max} should not exceed 65 dB, A-weighted, slow response.

Appendix C

SAMPLE INSTRUCTIONS FOR RECORDED MUSIC FOR INFANT MEDICAL RECORD OR BEDSIDE

Sunada—Music for state regulation protocol for week beginning 24.05.2013	
Equipment:	MP3 player to be plugged into dry pendant bedside Speakers located <u>at least</u> 20cm from S's head.
Check:	Noisy room / rounds – Do not play. Turn it off if: Sundara does not settle Music interferes with parent-infant communication
Sleep time:	Parents only "Sleep" Playlist (4 tracks; 24 mins.) Start volume 3. Increase till can be heard at bed level. Max. volume 9.
Feed time:	Parents + nursing staff "Quiet Alert" playlist (6 tracks; 20 mins.) Start volume 3. Increase till can be heard at bed level. Max. volume 9.

Document: Please report use in medical record for further assessment.

For review: Contact Helen Shoemark, page 5555

NEVER turn music on and walk away. Please watch baby's response.

Chapter 5

Pediatric Intensive Care

Claire M. Ghetti

INTRODUCTION

Pediatric Intensive Care

Advances in science and medical technology now enable saving the lives of even the most critically ill and injured children and adolescents. Nonetheless, pediatric critical care medicine itself is a relatively new subspecialty. First recognized as a subspecialty in 1985, this area of medicine has experienced rapid growth and development within the past three decades (Odetola, Clark, & Davis, 2006; Rosenberg et al., 2004). There are currently at least 340 pediatric intensive care units (PICUs) in the United States (Odetola, Clark, Freed, Bratton, & Davis, 2005), and they serve infants, children, and adolescents who present a broad range of life-threatening medical, traumatic, and surgical conditions.

Level I PICUs provide the highest degree of specialty and subspecialty care for critically ill children. They require continuous staffing by critical care physicians, nurses, and respiratory therapists, as well as rapid access to a full complement of clinical and surgical pediatric subspecialists (Rosenberg et al., 2004). Intensive levels of continuous monitoring are available in the PICU, including monitoring of heart rate, respiration, *oxygen saturation*, temperature, blood pressure, *intracranial pressure*, *pulmonary arterial pressure, end tidal carbon dioxide levels*, and *arrhythmia* detection (Rosenberg et al., 2004). It is understood that PICUs serve infants, children, adolescents, and in some cases young adults, though for the sake of brevity, "children" will be used throughout the current chapter to represent the conglomerate of these various groups, unless otherwise specified. Due to their medical fragility and intensive requirements for continuous monitoring, children in the PICU typically require a 1:1 or 2:1 patient-to-nurse ratio (Stouffer & Shirk, 2003).

The majority of PICU staff are primarily concerned with medical stabilization and lifesaving efforts. However, there is increasing recognition that the presence and quality of psychosocial support of children in the PICU impacts their ability to cope with this intense environment. Children in the PICU must contend with life-threatening medical conditions, a barrage of medical procedures, lack of consistent sleep, exposure to noise and light, pain and discomfort, impaired communication, and altered or reduced interactions with caregivers (Lee, Chung, Chan, & Chan, 2005). Even common nursing cares such as suctioning of mucous secretions, changing of body positioning, and providing wound care can cause children discomfort and provoke anxiety (Stouffer & Shirk, 2003).

A majority of children who are hospitalized in the PICU remember the experience, especially those who are not mechanically ventilated during the course of their PICU stay and thus do not require ventilation-related sedation (Board, 2005; Playfor, Thomas, & Choonara, 2000). Once children are discharged from the PICU, they tend to maintain neutral attitudes toward their hospitalization although they may have negative recollections of high noise levels, disorientation to time, and discomfort from aspects of treatment such as *nasogastric* or *endotracheal tubes* (Playfor et al., 2000). Children reflecting back upon their PICU hospitalizations identify nurses as providing helpful support during their PICU stay (Board, 2005; Playfor et al., 2000). If children in the PICU are offered music therapy services, this form of therapy and psychosocial support might offer a pragmatic and useful strategy to positively impact children's appraisals of their PICU experience (Board, 2005).

Music Therapy in Pediatric Intensive Care

The pediatric medical and nursing literature falls prey to the same definitional ambiguity as some of the adult literature, where the terms and definitions of music therapy and music medicine are used interchangeably. In such literature, authors commonly cite music therapy research and clinical work, and yet define music therapy as a nursing intervention (e.g., Lee et al., 2005; McDowell, 2005). Other authors attempt to distinguish between the use of "passive music therapy" (i.e., music listening) vs. "active music therapy" (i.e., with therapist involvement) in the PICU, but then also alternate describing it as facilitated by nurses or by music therapists, and interchangeably cite music therapy and nursing literature (e.g., Austin, 2010). Nursing staff in PICU settings have a history of using music listening interventions, and there is a body of nursing researchers and clinicians who view such forms of what they term "music therapy" as a nursing intervention (McDowell, 2005). The expanding body of music therapists working, researching, and writing about music therapy practice in the PICU should help to clarify the beneficial and distinct roles that each discipline can play in meeting the psychosocial needs of children in the PICU.

The clinical practice of music therapy within PICU settings continues to advance. A handful of anecdotal reports and clinical writing informed the early development of clinical practice in this area by describing music therapy during cardiac PICU hospitalization (Dun, 1995) and for the promotion of children's emergence from coma (Kennelly & Edwards, 1997; Rosenfeld & Dun, 1999). Recent developments include a few prospective studies of music therapy in the PICU (del Olmo, Rodríquez Garrido, & Ruza Tarrío, 2010; Stouffer & Shirk, 2003) and a book chapter dedicated to the topic (Ghetti & Hannan, 2008). In a recent survey of music therapists working in pediatric medical settings, of the 40 therapists who reported which units they serviced, 75% stated that they provided services on the PICU (Goforth, 2008). Similarly, in a survey of music therapists working in adult and pediatric medical settings, the most common units receiving music therapy were the "oncology/hematology" unit and "pediatrics/PICU" (Lam, 2007). Music therapy programs are commonly administratively housed within a hospital's child life, mental health (Ferraz, 2003), creative arts therapy, or integrative medicine departments.

DIAGNOSTIC INFORMATION

The American Academy of Pediatrics (AAP) developed guidelines for admission and discharge policies for the PICU in 1999 that remain valid today. The following diagnostic categories are taken from the AAP guidelines, with body systems placed in order of decreasing frequency according to Ruttimann, Patel, and Pollack's (2000) survey of PICU admissions.

- Cardiovascular system (e.g., *congenital heart disease*, *shock*, *postcardiopulmonary resuscitation*, life-threatening *dysrhythmias*)
- Neurologic (e.g., head trauma, seizures, postneurosurgery, progressive neuromuscular dysfunction, *meningitis*, spinal cord compression)
- Respiratory system (e.g., respiratory failure, pneumonia, newly placed *tracheostomy*, airway injury, severe asthma)

- Gastrointestinal system (e.g., severe gastrointestinal bleeding, acute liver failure, emergent removal of foreign bodies from gastrointestinal tract)
- Surgical (e.g., major surgeries, organ transplantation, multiple trauma, major blood loss)
- Multisystem (e.g., drug overdose, toxin ingestion, burn injuries, *multiple organ dysfunction syndrome*)
- Endocrine/Metabolic (e.g., *diabetic ketoacidosis*, severe electrolyte abnormalities)
- Hematologic/Oncologic (e.g., severe complications of *sickle cell anemia*, *exchange transfusions*, *severe anemia* with respiratory compromise, tumors that are compressing important blood vessels or airway)
- Renal System (e.g., *renal failure, renal insufficiency*)

It is important to note that children admitted to the PICU may present with various mental health–related comorbidities, including affective disorders, anxiety disorders, attention-deficit/hyperactivity disorders, pervasive developmental disorders, acute stress disorder, and posttraumatic stress disorder. Thus, the music therapist should be prepared to effectively address a broad spectrum of the child's needs and resources, and will need to consider the child's holistic health and well-being when providing services.

Medical Treatments Specific to the PICU

All children admitted to the PICU receive continuous monitoring, as previously described. Such monitoring may be noninvasive (e.g., heart rate, respiratory rate, oxygen saturation) or invasive in nature (e.g., *continuous arterial pressure, central venous pressure*). Additional aspects of treatment include intravenous therapy that provides fluid replacement; delivery of medication, including chemotherapy; and blood transfusions, by infusing liquids directly into a vein (i.e., an "IV"). Many children will also demonstrate a need for respiratory support through mechanical means, which may be delivered invasively or noninvasively.

Invasive Mechanical Ventilation. Intubation is the process of placing an endotracheal tube (a plastic tube inserted through the mouth or nose into the trachea) to ensure a stable airway, and to allow for the provision of mechanical ventilation and suctioning of secretions. Invasive mechanical ventilation is required when children undergo general anesthesia during major surgery, or it may be required following acute respiratory illness or trauma. Common contributors to respiratory failure in children include pneumonia, asthma, acute respiratory distress syndrome, obstruction of the airway, or neuromuscular impairments (Parker, 2007). Endotracheal tubes cause discomfort, which may necessitate treatment with sedatives (Newth et al., 2009). Too little sedation may render the child in a restless state in which his movements may cause the endotracheal tube to shift and cause damage in the airway (Newth et al., 2009), while heavier sedation can depress respiratory efforts and impede progress toward spontaneous breathing. The endotracheal tube passes through the vocal cords; thus children who are ventilated in this manner will not be able to speak, but may be able to mouth words. Children on mechanical ventilation are not able to eat, and will receive fluids and nutrients intravenously and through nasogastric tubes (via nose and esophagus into stomach) or gastric feeding tubes (via direct input to the stomach). If children require long-term mechanical ventilation, they may undergo a surgical procedure called a tracheotomy in which a surgical incision in the trachea allows for the insertion of a tracheostomy tube directly into the trachea to deliver oxygen to the lungs. Children may receive mechanical ventilation as delivered through a tracheostomy tube over the period of many years, or they may retain the in-dwelling tracheostomy tube and transition to less invasive forms of respiratory support.

Noninvasive Mechanical Ventilation. Children whose respiratory requirement does not necessitate invasive ventilation may receive ventilatory assistance through nasal cannula (pronged, flexible tubing used to deliver oxygen via the nasal passages), face mask, or mouthpiece. Forms of noninvasive ventilation commonly encountered in the PICU include supplemental oxygen delivered via nasal cannula, CPAP *(continuous positive airway pressure)*, and BiPAP *(bilevel positive airway pressure)*, with the latter two delivered through mask.

Suctioning. Children receiving invasive mechanical ventilation, or those who cannot independently manage their secretions, will require periodic suctioning to remove mucous secretions from the lungs. Children will typically experience discomfort during suctioning and may feel anxious due to the temporary inability to breathe.

Sedation. Sedation is used to decrease sensations of pain or discomfort during invasive procedures, or it may be used to ensure that a child can tolerate mechanical ventilation. PICU staff will formally assess a child's behaviors to ascertain the minimal amount of sedation required to enable the child to tolerate mechanical ventilation (Stouffer & Shirk, 2003). Sedation and analgesic medication may result in side effects including changes in heart rate, respiratory depression, nausea, vomiting, and constipation (Stouffer & Shirk, 2003).

NEEDS AND RESOURCES

Individuals in the Intensive Care Unit (ICU) experience a lack of choice and control over elements of their environment, experience limitations in their ability to communicate, and may feel depersonalized due to the invasive and exposing nature of the highly technical environment of care (Chlan & Heiderscheit, 2009). Children in the PICU may experience anxiety and stress related to sleep disturbance, sensory altering medication, or the sensation of being mechanically ventilated (Stouffer & Shirk, 2003). Children who are mechanically ventilated and alert may experience anxiety and agitation due to their inability to speak. Frequent invasive procedures may also cause discomfort and anxiety, and thus are an important focus of music therapy intervention within a PICU setting (Ferraz, 2003; Ghetti, 2012).

Children in the PICU are paradoxically at-risk for both overstimulation and understimulation (Kennelly & Edwards, 1997; Tamplin, 2000). Increased stress and anxiety can cause children to have heightened responses to environmental stimuli, while factors related to their diagnosis or current treatment may interfere with their ability to respond to stimuli or modify the environment to alter sensory input (Mazer, 2010). Children are exposed to noise in the PICU, or "environmental sounds that exist without controls for volume, duration, or cause/effect relations" (Kemper & Danhauer, 2005, p. 283). Common sources of noise in hospital environments include monitoring equipment and their alarms, televisions, overhead paging, beepers, staff voices, and nursing stations (Mazer, 2010). Side effects of continuous exposure to noise include disturbances to sleep patterns, fatigue, hyperalerting, and decreases in appetite (Kemper & Danhauer, 2005). Music therapists must consider if they are unintentionally contributing to noise accumulation for clients, as sounds that cannot be modified by the child or are inappropriate to the child's preferences or situation may be perceived as noise, and weigh benefits to risks accordingly (Mazer, 2010). There is often no acoustical separation between two children in a double room, or four children in a quadruple room, and the therapist should take this into consideration when selecting instruments to bring to a session.

Children in the PICU will benefit from receiving sensory stimulation that corresponds with their ability to process such stimulation, as well as reality orientation when clinically indicated. It is important to develop a system of communication so that the child can make his wants and needs known. Such systems may be rudimentary, including raising thumb up or down for yes or no, use of eye blink to communicate yes or no, picture communication boards, iPads or other assistive communication devices, or enabling a child to write down responses. Some children who are ventilated via an endotracheal tube may mouth words, in which case the music therapist should speak back what the child mouths to ensure accurate comprehension.

Music therapy may play a unique role in humanizing the experience of PICU hospitalization for the child and his caregivers. Live music offers the "introduction of something uniquely human into an otherwise sterile and potentially frightening and painful environment" (Schneider, 2005, p. 221). Music therapy helps acknowledge each person's individuality and dignity (Delabary, 2004), regardless of his age, health status, or level of awareness. For children with even the most devastating neurological impairments, music therapy offers the chance to celebrate the child as a complete human, worthy of celebration and acceptance. By making choices, expressing preferences, and engaging with the music and therapist, the child may reconnect with and exercise his human agency. The flexible, adaptable, and motivating context of music therapy supports the child as he learns ways to act upon and impact his environment.

The needs of a child admitted to the PICU for the first time differ from the needs of a chronically ill child who frequently passes between the PICU and step-down or general inpatient units. The goals of acute PICU care may include minimizing the traumatic impact of a PICU hospitalization by promoting a stable and secure environment along with a way to express related feelings through music (Ferraz, 2003). Children who are chronically ill and experience frequent hospitalizations may benefit from learning how to integrate the hospitalization into their lives, develop their inner resources, and build resilience (Ferraz, 2003).

Luckily, children possess various resources upon which the music therapy process can build. Children tend to demonstrate an innate musicality, and often have not yet adopted inhibitions regarding extemporaneous music-making or use of singing voice. This comfort with "being" in music sets the stage for creatively working through the difficult challenges the child experiences in the PICU. As a child engages in music, especially when partaking in familiar music, he is able to connect with his healthy self, providing a crucial and life-affirming link between his concept of self in home and hospital settings (Ayson, 2008). Likewise, music therapy creates a space where the child can experience joy, relief, success, and achievement (Lindenfelser, Grocke, & McFerran, 2008).

Music therapists should also be mindful of the needs of the child's family. Caregivers experience multiple areas of duress when their child is hospitalized in the PICU. Common stressors include uncertainty regarding their child's prognosis, lack of familiarity with or control over medical treatment, and feelings of fear and grief, all of which are compounded by caregivers' own fatigue (Shoemark & Dearn, 2008). The child's PICU hospitalization also impacts caregivers' current lodging and travel requirements, employment, financial status, social relationships, and other family-related commitments and responsibilities. Among these sources of stress, caregivers report one of the greatest stressors related to a child's intensive care hospitalization is adjusting to alterations in parental role (Melnyk et al., 2004).

Parents need to be re-established as primary caregivers, and given a chance to partake in their child's care to the extent that is desired and feasible. Empowering caregivers to be integral members of the treatment team is a cornerstone of family-centered care. Music therapy can promote a shift toward normalcy in the interactions between caregivers and children. For example, caregivers of infants in the PICU need to experience contingent interaction with their children in order to promote ongoing secure attachment (Shoemark & Dearn, 2008). Music therapy can facilitate nurturing interactions between child and caregiver to promote this attachment. The enjoyment a child may experience when engaging in music therapy may consequently positively impact the caregiver, promoting changes in mood or outlook (Ayson, 2008).

REFERRAL AND ASSESSMENT PROCEDURES

Referral Procedures

Though some hospitals may have electronic referral services in place, verbal referrals remain the most common form of referral among music therapists working in medical settings (Lam, 2007). Music therapists most commonly receive referrals from nurses, child life specialists, physicians, social workers, and rehabilitation staff, including occupational therapists and physical therapists (Lam, 2007). Referral criteria and procedures may vary by facility. An example of a music therapy referral form for the PICU is included in Appendix A.

Assessment Procedures

Assessment and treatment planning are ongoing in the PICU setting, as the child may experience fluctuations in health status or changes in factors such as medication regimen that significantly alter the child's presentation and needs. A music therapist may gather information for an assessment through chart review, interdisciplinary team consultation, talking with family members, and talking with the child or engaging the child in music therapy and noting responses and preferences. Results of initial assessment can be conveyed to the treatment team and placed in the child's medical record in narrative form or by filling in an electronically generated music therapy assessment tool within the child's electronic medical record. An example of a PICU Music Therapy Assessment Form formatted for electronic medical record charting is included in Appendix B. Chlan and Heiderscheit (2009) developed the Music Assessment Tool (MAT) to enable music therapists to determine music preferences of adults receiving mechanical ventilation, in order to inform music-based interventions. Music therapists working in the PICU may find the MAT helpful when designing music listening experiences for older children and adolescents. In addition to these resources, Ghetti and Hannan (2008) provide an example of a paper-based PICU Music Therapy Assessment.

The music therapist completing an assessment of a child in the PICU will consider areas of strength and need in the domains of emotional, social, communicative, physical, cognitive, and sensory functioning. In addition, the music therapist will assess the child and family's cultural perspectives related to health, hospitalization, and treatment as well as their culturally influenced attitudes toward and uses of music. The incorporation of "music of kin" can provide a salient tool with which the music therapist can build a connection with the child and family, enable the child and family to reconnect with their healthy identities and a sense of home, and promote their ability to draw upon previous coping resources (Edwards & Kennelly, 2011; Loewy, Hallan, Friedman, & Martinez, 2005; Loveszy, 1991).

Treatment Planning

Within the field of music therapy, there is a misperception that medical music therapy is restricted to short-term work or is superficial in nature. Though there may be variation in how music therapists practice within this setting, a significant portion of PICU clinical work requires in-depth practice, of which a fair amount is long-term. For example, a music therapist may first work with a teenager in the PICU during the crisis of being newly diagnosed with a rare form of cancer, follow him through years of inpatient stays on the hematology/oncology unit and during health crises requiring PICU hospitalization, and eventually provide support as he grapples with his own mortality during end-of-life care in the PICU. It is not uncommon for children who have been treated for years in inpatient units to experience declines in health that necessitate PICU admission (Lorenzato, 2005). Likewise, neonates who graduate from the NICU will typically be admitted to the PICU for subsequent hospitalizations. Thus, music therapists who also serve inpatient pediatric units and the NICU may follow children across a span of several years, or over the entire length a child's life.

Treatment planning will depend upon the child's specific areas of need in relation to his resources, and how these change over time. The PICU Treatment Prioritization Matrix (Appendix C) may be used to guide the clinician in identifying and prioritizing a child's areas of need that can be addressed through music therapy. The matrix is an expansion of Ghetti and Hannan's (2008, p. 78) PICU music therapy referral criteria. Session frequency and length depend upon a child's needs, but the therapist will attempt to provide a degree of closure at the conclusion of each session in case further sessions are not possible due to discharge or death of the child. Sessions may be as short as 20 minutes or, in cases where a child is engaged in a lengthy medical procedure or is actively dying, sessions may be as long as two hours or more.

Documentation within the child's medical chart of assessment and progress in music therapy is an essential component of providing ethically sound clinical services. Chart notes can convey the music therapist's intentions for therapy, significant outcomes or unusual responses during therapy, and overall progress toward goals. Aside from when other treatment team members witness or take part in a music therapy session, documentation becomes the evidence of the change that is taking place through music therapy. Documenting in the medical chart helps other disciplines gain awareness of the aims and methods of music therapy.

INTRODUCTION TO MUSIC THERAPY METHODS

Although a majority of pediatric music therapists report that the pediatric intensive care unit is among the units that they serve (Goforth, 2008), clinical descriptions of this work remain scant in the literature. The most commonly documented clinical methods with this population are receptive forms of music therapy, including approaches to promote sensory regulation, increase awareness of self and others, provide reality orientation, facilitate nonpharmacological sedation, and support ongoing secure attachment between child and caregiver. Despite the more frequent mention of receptive music therapy methods in the literature on music therapy in the PICU, approaches that are improvisatory, re-creative, and compositional in nature are also valid and beneficial when appropriately matched with the needs and resources of the child. Music therapists should not limit their practice by assuming that children in the PICU are capable only of passive engagement, and instead should take care to draw upon any abilities a child has and develop these into a broad range of active engagement in musical interactions.

For the sake of clarity, the various clinical approaches detailed below are organized into broad categories of receptive, improvisational, re-creative, and compositional interventions. In practice, therapists will likely transcend these categories by combining various approaches within a session, depending upon client needs and the flow of the ongoing therapeutic process. Furthermore, certain intervention areas, such as the use of music therapy as procedural support for invasive or anxiety-provoking medical procedures, may incorporate several of the approaches described below as the procedure unfolds and the client's needs change from moment to moment. Thus, readers should envision the subsections of clinical approaches listed below as possibilities for clinical intervention, and should layer or sequence such approaches in relation to a child and family's ongoing needs and responses. It is also important to note that it is assumed that the professional or student reading this chapter will possess an understanding of child development, and thus will be able to ascertain which approaches are appropriate for certain developmental levels or when approaches require modification to match a child's developmental level.

The utility of some clinical approaches may vary depending upon the treatment context (Ferraz, 2003) and the child's stage of treatment. For example, clinical approaches may vary for a child in the most acute lifesaving stage following a traumatic injury vs. a child who has been moved to the intensive care step-down unit as he recovers from elective surgery. The music therapist will consider the child's stage of treatment and the surrounding context as well as his current needs and resources when deciding which approach will be offered first. Music therapists may find themselves operating on two levels with a child in intensive care: providing ongoing support and an expressive outlet for working through difficult emotions, but also providing acute support for painful or uncomfortable procedures (Ferraz, 2003). Thus, the music therapist remains flexible and responsive to the changing needs of the client.

Because of the nature of this setting and the medically vulnerable state of children in the PICU, music therapy sessions are typically offered individually. However, parents and siblings may be integrated into many of the clinical approaches described below, if doing so would be beneficial for the client (Edwards & Kennelly, 2011). Conversely, the music therapist may choose to extend such services to the parents or siblings separately from the child, in order to allow the family members to have more space to explore their own processes. In cases where a music therapist is functioning as primary therapist for a parent, it is most often contraindicated for that therapist to also work in-depth with the hospitalized child, as this raises issues with appropriate boundaries and dual relationships. However, a music therapist may work in-depth with a child's parent and refer the child to a different therapist or vice versa. More commonly, a music therapist incorporates the family members into the client's course of therapy, in order to provide supportive levels of therapy to the entire family. By demonstrating positive ways to interact with their children, music therapists empower caregivers to take active steps in supporting their children throughout critical care hospitalization.

Music therapists working within the PICU will need to observe the infection control policies of the facility and can work with the epidemiology department to establish guidelines for instrument cleaning, if guidelines do not already exist. Typically, therapists will be able to use nonporous, nonplush instruments and dramatic play props, and will sanitize such items between each use. It is also possible to bring washable or wipeable instruments into *contact isolation, droplet isolation,* or *respiratory isolation* rooms, as long as such items can be sanitized before and after use. The therapist should consider the spatial constraints of the PICU setting when choosing rolling storage carts and larger instruments such as guitars and keyboards.

OVERVIEW OF MUSIC THERAPY METHODS AND PROCEDURES

An overview of music therapy methods and procedures included in this chapter are listed below. The receptive methods and procedures have been sequenced in order of increasing specificity to the individual, whereas the improvisational approaches are presented in order of frequency of use in the PICU. The re-creative and compositional methods and procedures are not presented in a specific order.

Receptive Music Therapy

- Sensory Consultation on the Sound Environment: recommendations for modifications to the PICU sound environment to minimize the negative impact of noise and sensory overstimulation on the patients.
- Environmental Music Therapy: the use of either live music or prerecorded music to promote an atmosphere of calm and mask environmental noises in the PICU.
- Sedative Music Listening: the use of sedative music to decrease arousal, agitation, and anxiety in the child, to improve sleep, or to improve bonding with caregiver.

- Regulated Multisensory Stimulation: multisensory stimulation that begins with simple auditory stimuli and progressively adds musical complexity to help children with disorders of consciousness or severe brain injury to effectively and safely process incoming sensory information.
- Music-assisted Reality Orientation and Awareness: the use of various music listening interventions to promote gradual awareness of oneself, others, and the surrounding environment in children who are emerging from coma or from surgical sedation, or who are experiencing a disorder of consciousness.
- Music Therapy as Procedural Support for Extubation: a sequence of predominantly receptive music therapy approaches to reduce a child's anxiety as he is prepped for extubation, is extubated, and subsequently breathes on his own.
- Music Therapy During or Following Active Dying: the use of vocal improvisation, songs, lullabies, and instrumental improvisation to provide a supportive holding environment for the child transitioning out of life and those who are present for the child.

Improvisational Music Therapy

- Improvised Song/Lullaby: the spontaneous in-the-moment creation of music with lyrics or vocalizations by the child, the therapist, and/or the caregiver that serves expressive purposes.
- Music-facilitated Dramatic Play: an expanded form of improvised song that incorporates play and dramatic action using props and musical instruments to enable the expression of feelings and the symbolic working through of internal conflicts.
- Referential and Nonreferential Improvisation: Referential improvisations are musical improvisations in which the music is used to depict some nonmusical theme, emotion, entity, or experience. Nonreferential improvisations are improvisations in which there is no attempt to represent anything beyond the music itself.

Re-creative Music Therapy

- Developmental Stimulation: an extension of regulated multisensory stimulation in which the therapist promotes a child's increasing levels of engagement and interaction with the music and the therapist to promote developmental gains.
- Music Therapy to Promote Bonding: the use of song and musical interactions to create opportunities for the development of secure attachment between the caregiver and the child.
- Therapeutic Singing: engaging the child in singing for promoting respiratory well-being and for impacting emotional well-being.
- Music-assisted Rehabilitation: the use of a variety of music interventions to impact various areas of neurologic functioning and optimize rehabilitation goals.
- Therapeutic Music Instruction: instrumental instruction in which the child benefits from either the process of playing the instrument itself or from the process of learning an instrument in general.

Compositional Music Therapy

- Songwriting: the creation of songs aimed at communicating content to others, safely expressing a wide range of emotions, and building self-awareness.
- Audio or Video Recording Creation: capturing the outcomes of the creative music process through audio or video recording to enable the child and/or family to retain and re-experience the benefits of that process.

GUIDELINES FOR RECEPTIVE MUSIC THERAPY

Music that is appropriately implemented may impact even the most acutely ill individuals, and thus music offers the potential for therapeutic intervention for children who are not able to actively respond due to injury or advanced illness. Receptive forms of music therapy are used when listening is the child's primary avenue of engaging in an intervention, or when other forms of more active engagement are contraindicated. For example, the music therapist may provide music-assisted relaxation via sedative music listening to promote nonpharmacological sedation while the child is mechanically ventilated, but would not want to use familiar action-song singing with the same child as this might increase alertness and activity to a level that would be detrimental at the moment. Though a child may not be able to demonstrate overt responses to the music, receptive music therapy may enable the individual to experience connection with others and with the world outside of the ICU context (Delabary, 2004). Receptive approaches may be appropriate for children who are not alert, or whose alertness and awareness are emerging. Conversely, receptive techniques may also be indicated for children who are alert, but need modification in their sensory environment.

The following receptive music therapy approaches are presented in order of increasing specificity to the individual. The first two approaches are broad-based, environmental approaches that consider the surrounding sound environment and provide interventions that impact the auditory environment for all those present within a targeted space. Most often, music provided free-field is not appropriate in the pediatric intensive care unit, as specific sensory needs vary greatly from child to child. However, there may be times when environmental approaches to music therapy are beneficial. Music therapists will carefully consider all of the receptive techniques described below, and will determine which approaches provide the most therapeutic benefit, while minimizing any potential undesirable outcomes (e.g., overstimulation, habituation, increased noise). Careful assessment of the child, family, and surrounding environment will help inform the therapist's clinical approach.

Preparation

Prior to initiating receptive music therapy approaches, the therapist will assess client and family needs and preferences to inform the selection of a particular receptive technique, the music to be used, and the method of implementation. The therapist will consider if prerecorded music or live music will best meet the needs of the client and family. Similarly, the therapist will consider which accompanying instrument will be most appropriate based on spatial constraints in the bedside environment, client music preferences, and timbral- and range-related attributes of the instrument. Guitar offers flexibility in positioning, allowing the therapist to move easily from one side of the bed to the other as needed, as well as flexibility in dynamic and melodic range. Portable instruments that provide a long sustain or drone, such as the shruti box (a wooden instrument with bellows that provides a drone from selected tones), can provide a background with which the therapist can sing or tone.

What to Observe

Before beginning a receptive music therapy session, the music therapist will observe the child, including his baseline heart rate, respiratory rate, and oxygen levels as indicated on the bedside monitors. The therapist may also notice the child's breathing patterns and rate as demonstrated by the rise and fall of his chest, and listen for any repetitive sounds in the environment. After commencing music, the therapist will note any changes in physiological parameters or any behavioral indications of pleasure or aversion and adjust the musical qualities as needed. Though infants, children, and adolescents vary in their resting physiological parameters, the music therapist should consider stopping or modifying musical stimuli if a child's heart rate rises significantly, oxygen saturation decreases by several points, or respiratory rate drops in a marked fashion. The client's continuous monitoring system will alarm when physiological parameters exceed client-specific ranges, which will notify the nursing staff. However, it is generally good practice for a music therapist to confer with the client's nurse when physiological parameters exceed normal ranges during music therapy to determine if musical stimuli or interactions should be modified to ensure optimal physiological responses.

Regarding behavioral responses to music therapy, a child's positive responses may include relaxation of facial muscles, positive facial affect, eye opening, visual tracking, vocalizing or speaking, reaching toward musical objects, and various communicative responses. Aversive responses may include grimacing, grinding teeth, startling, averting gaze, closing eyes, very wide eye opening, retracting extremities, moaning, attempting to move away from sounds, or falling asleep.

Sensory Consultation on the Sound Environment

Overview. Sufficient research exists to support the reduction of noise to improve client outcomes in medical settings (Mazer, 2010), yet this is often an undervalued area for intervention. Mazer (2010) strongly supports a critical examination of the sound environment in medical settings, and considers the reduction of noise in such environments as an "evidence-based mandate" (p. 188). Hospital administrators and staff may call upon the music therapist to provide consultations on the sound environment, particularly in the potentially noisy intensive care setting.

Music therapists are trained to consider the sound and sensory environments surrounding their clients, as well as the impact of those sensory environments on their clients. Thus, music therapists are uniquely positioned to act as advocates for a healthy sound and sensory environment for children and families in the PICU. Sensory consultation involves the music therapist assessing the sensory environment and either recommending, or actually making, modifications to that environment to reduce or mask noise or excessive sensory stimuli. The purpose of sensory consultation is to reduce excessive noise, and ensure that environmental stimuli are not compromising children's course of healing or their well-being.

Procedures. When called to provide a sensory consultation for a certain hospital unit or room, or for an individual child, the music therapist will observe noise levels and patterns of sensory stimulation at various points in the day. The therapist may work in tandem with a nurse or member of the hospital's engineering department to measure sound levels using a decibel meter, or may assess noise levels more informally. Anecdotal reports of child and family responses to environmental noise may be compiled, along with lists of noise sources and how often they are present in the environment. The music therapist may offer suggestions for decreasing extraneous noise, and may work in conjunction with nursing staff to limit noises in the overall environment, or reduce sensory stimuli for certain children, depending upon their specific needs.

When a sensory consultation is related to a particular child (e.g., a child who is sedated and mechanically ventilated), the music therapist will assess that child's responses to sound and noise, noting if any environmental sounds cause the child to startle often. The therapist may observe if there are certain timbres of sound or sources of sound that cause the child distress. The therapist furthermore evaluates if there is a tendency to provide too much stimulation at once, or sensory stimulation for such an extended period that the child becomes distressed or habituates to it and fails to respond specifically to it (Wood, 1991). From such an assessment, the therapist may make recommendations to the nursing staff to modify sensory input by decreasing excessive stimulation from overuse of the television, implementing the use of prerecorded music to mask environmental noise, or making attempts to reduce the volume of conversations at bedside.

Environmental Music Therapy

Overview. Related to the concept of sensory consultation to reduce extraneous noise is the practice of environmental music therapy. Music therapists may provide live music, specifically tailored and played free-field in a certain environment, or may suggest prerecorded music to promote an atmosphere of calm and mask environmental noises. The presence of live music may also cue individuals to lower speaking voices, which are a key contributor to noise levels in intensive care settings (Stewart & Schneider, 2000). When a music therapist is providing environmental music therapy, all individuals within that space are considered the recipients of such therapeutic intervention. However, music therapists may incorporate elements that are specific to certain individuals within the targeted environment, such as song preferences or musical styles from cultures of origin (Schneider, 2005).

Environmental music therapy can help humanize the experience of intensive care, by bringing an aesthetic experience into a potentially austere and intimidating environment. The literature describes the development and incorporation of environmental music therapy in neonatal intensive care environments (Schneider, 2005; Stewart & Schneider, 2000), but it also may be relevant and useful at times within pediatric intensive care. Depending upon the physical layout of a hospital's PICU, environmental music therapy may be most appropriately implemented in larger rooms with several patient beds and environments that become noisy due to frequent conversations, alarming of monitors, televisions, and other sounds relating to medical equipment. Furthermore, when used in the PICU, environmental music therapy may be most indicated for children who are not able to engage in more interactive forms of music therapy, or who would benefit from breaks from social interaction.

Under certain circumstances, there may be contraindications for environmental music therapy. Music provided via environmental music therapy is by definition provided to all those in the surrounding environment. Due to its all-encompassing nature, there is the distinct possibility that certain individuals within the sound space will not respond positively to the music provided. The therapist providing environmental music therapy should maintain ongoing dialogue with staff, family members, and children before and after sessions to monitor the impact of such intervention on those who receive it.

Though the music therapist may make every effort to improvise music that is well matched to the environment and is sedative in nature, even very simple levels of musical stimuli may contribute to overstimulation for individuals who are neurologically compromised. The music therapist should exercise caution when implementing environmental music therapy, and may ultimately decide that the broad-spectrum application of music within this approach is contraindicated for certain spaces or for certain individuals within those spaces. In such instances, the music therapist working in the PICU may opt to provide individually tailored sedative music at bedside or use prerecorded music via headphones for children and family members who have more specific needs. See the section on "Sedative Music Listening" for details on this individualized approach.

Preparation. The music therapist can survey staff and families prior to commencing environmental music therapy within a pediatric intensive care unit to ascertain times and areas of peak noise, factors contributing to noise, and musical preferences of those in the environment (Stewart & Schneider, 2000). Information gleaned from such a survey will help the therapist to match intervention more specifically to the needs of those in the target environment. Recommended instruments for providing environmental music therapy include guitar, cello, harp, and hammered dulcimer, the latter of which may be more neutral in association due to its relative novelty (Schneider, 2005). The music therapist will also need to consider where to position herself to avoid interrupting the flow of movement in an area, and to ensure compliance with fire safety codes.

What to observe. Prior to commencing, the therapist will observe people within the environment and will tune in to sounds within the environment. This process of perceiving and adjusting the music accordingly will continue throughout the session of environmental music therapy, so that the sounds occur in relation to the environment, instead of being randomly applied to it. The music therapist should remain willing to discontinue environmental music therapy and change to individualized treatment if any children, family members, or staff demonstrate consistent adverse reactions to the free-field music. Evidence of positive outcomes from environmental music therapy may include less frequent alarming, improvement in children's physiological parameters (e.g., improved oxygen saturation, decreased heart rate), decrease in the volume of staff conversations, and improved positive affect for individuals within the environment (Stewart & Schneider, 2000).

Procedures. The therapist perceives sounds and actions in the environment and uses this information in designing improvised music. For example, the therapist may synchronize her music to the rhythms of ventilators or other medical machinery in the environment or may incorporate tones from the beeps and alarming of monitors on patient care equipment (Schneider, 2005). The purpose of such synchronization is to lessen the impact of these aversive sounds on the clients, families, and staff within that particular environment (Mazer, 2010; Schneider, 2005). Since the music therapist may be partially masking the sound of patient care equipment alarms, the volume of such intervention would need to be such that responsible staff could still hear, and subsequently respond to, such alarms.

Music presented with sedative qualities is the most appropriate choice for environmental music therapy in intensive care settings. Prior to commencing, the therapist should first take steps to determine that all those present in the environment can tolerate auditory stimulation by checking in with the nurses of the patients involved. It is advisable that the therapist also attempt to ascertain if any children or family members have negative associations with the accompanying instrument. For example, some individuals may associate the harp with death (Schneider, 2005), which may cause adverse reactions for a certain recipient within the environment. The therapist may not be able to recognize or address such individual reactions while providing environmental music therapy for the entire room (though if it is brought to her attention, the therapist could certainly follow up with an individual after the session regarding such reactions).

The music therapist can begin a session of environmental music therapy with simple introductory music, such as a series of ascending perfect 5ths (Stewart & Schneider, 2000). The therapist may then provide several extended improvisations, incorporating melodies and motifs from preferred music suggestions from family and staff members. The music therapist will generally avoid dissonance, and thus may improvise using a pentatonic scale (Stewart & Schneider, 2000). Melodies may be set in 3/4 meter (Schneider, 2005) to promote a lulling quality, and, depending upon the age of the children in the room, recognizable lullabies may also be appropriate.

Music therapists may also provide a related form of client/family-centered environmental music therapy while children are in the active dying process. Readers may see the section on "Music Therapy During or Following Active Dying" for more details.

Sedative Music Listening

Overview. Individualized forms of music therapy that incorporate sedative music are indicated for children who would benefit from decreased arousal, decreased agitation, reduced anxiety, improved sleep, or improved bonding with caregivers (Magee et al., 2011; Stouffer & Shirk, 2003; Stouffer, Shirk, & Polomano, 2007). Sedative music listening is indicated for promoting consistent sleep patterns in the ICU environment, and it has been recommended to promote sedation nonpharmacologically by reducing anxiety and agitation (San Diego Patient Safety Council, 2009). Sedative music listening provides a greater level of client- or family-based specificity than environmental music therapy can provide. The music therapist individually tailors intervention to provide live or prerecorded music that addresses child and family needs while taking into consideration their music preferences and cultural values.

Music therapists might prefer to use prerecorded music if the intervention is required at multiple times during the day or at odd times during the night or early morning. In addition to its ease of implementation, using prerecorded music via headphones provides more control over the decibel level of music, reduces ambient sound, presents the music binaurally, and avoids impacting others in the environment (Stouffer et al., 2007). Disadvantages of prerecorded music are that clients, especially young children, may feel isolated from others; the beneficial role of the therapist is minimized; and in-the-moment modifications of the music are not possible. Most frequently, the PICU music therapist will provide live music, as this affords the therapist the opportunity to match musical parameters to the breathing rate of the individual or to synchronize with and mask environmental sounds such as ventilators or other medical equipment. Live implementation also allows the therapist to remain responsive to the changing needs of the child and family, to provide emotional support in real time, to improvise lyrics based on the surroundings, and to incorporate family members into the provision of music.

Prerecorded sedative music listening programs may be useful for children who are having difficulty falling asleep or remaining asleep, for children who must undergo frequent anxiety-producing or painful procedures or nursing cares, or for children who have difficulty regulating their level of arousal through other means. Live sedative music listening may be helpful during painful or anxiety-producing procedures. In addition, live music may be used to provide nonpharmacological sedation, such as when staff desires a child on mechanical ventilation to remain sedated, but does not wish to increase sedatives due to side effects (Stouffer & Shirk, 2003).

In critically ill children, reports of contraindicated effects of music listening, such as seizures that are auditorily evoked, are rare (Zifkin & Andermann, 2001, in Stouffer et al., 2007). There may be instances when the presentation of auditory stimuli, even in simple forms such as voice without accompaniment, may provoke a child and lead to a marked increase in agitation. For example, a child experiencing posttraumatic amnesia following coma may react adversely to any sensory stimulation during a particular time (Magee et al., 2011), and thus music therapy on that particular day may be contraindicated. There may be other rare contexts in which the use of sedative music, in particular, is contraindicated, such as during certain points within extubation trials, when it is desirable for the individual to be calm, yet aroused enough to remain alert and breathing on his own. The music therapist will provide ongoing evaluation of any music therapy approach used in the PICU and will monitor behavioral and physiological responses in order to notice any reactions that would indicate that the use of music should be discontinued and reassessed at a later time. Music therapists should consult with nursing staff regarding the exact interpretation of variations in physiological responses, especially when working with children who are mechanically ventilated (Bradt, Dileo, & Grocke, 2010).

Procedures. Some children will have limited ability to process sensory stimuli, such as those who have experienced neurologic injury, are exhibiting disorders of consciousness, or are neurologically immature. In rare cases, children may experience hyperacusis, or marked sensitivity to sound, due to certain conditions of the central nervous system, including headache, *spina bifida, Lyme disease,* or minor head injury, or following the use of spinal anesthesia (Katzenell & Segal, 2001). The music therapist should proceed with caution when presenting music therapy to any child in the PICU, but will need to start conservatively and progress gradually for any child who demonstrates a sensitivity to sound or difficulty in processing sensory stimuli. Thus, the therapist may begin with a drone or use her voice to tone long, sustained pitches. By doing so, she can ascertain how well the child can tolerate simple sounds before moving to more musical complexity. According to the child's tolerance and responses, the therapist may begin to layer sounds and provide more elaborate accompaniment patterns, as long as they are in the service of promoting a sedating response.

Alternatively, the therapist may begin with a simple ostinato pattern that matches the tempo of the child's breathing or to the pace of the ventilator. The music therapist can then use the principle of entrainment by gradually modifying the tempo to encourage the child's breathing to alter in a desired direction. Bradt (2009) provides clear practice guidelines for entraining a client's breathing pattern.

If live music is used with children who have experienced traumatic brain injury, it should be performed using instruments to which the child responds well, and should include stylistic elements such as steady tempo, descending melodic phrases, repetitive structures, and typical harmonic progressions (Magee et al., 2011). Care must be taken to provide optimal length of music listening. Overuse or prolonged exposure to musical stimuli may prompt the individual to habituate to the stimulus and fail to actively attend to it. Similarly, prolonged exposure to musical stimuli may result in overstimulation and a corresponding decreased ability to selectively attend to and respond to the stimuli.

For children who are in an alert or active state, the therapist may choose to engage the child using familiar music and songs of kin before progressing to more sedative forms of music (Loewy, 2009; Loewy & Stewart, 2005). Once the child is engaged, the therapist may then shift the meter of the familiar melodies into 3/4 or 6/8 meter to provide a "holding" environment (Loewy, 2009, p. 228). The therapist may then reduce stimulation by simplifying the chordal structure to a repetitive V-I harmonic cadence. This lulling harmonic cadence can then fade into increasing periods of silence, concluding with the production of breath tones synchronized to the patient's breathing (Loewy, 2009).

If the use of prerecorded music is indicated, the music therapist can record versions of therapeutic music and songs that the nursing staff or family can use as needed (Stouffer & Shirk, 2003). By recording the desired therapeutic music, the therapist can adjust musical parameters according to client needs and can incorporate client musical preferences, even while adjusting dynamic or metric qualities to promote relaxation or sedation. Thus, the family or nursing staff can play such recordings during or immediately after potentially stressful procedures such as suctioning, bathing, dressing changes, or changes in body positioning, to promote return to a relaxed state (Stouffer & Shirk, 2003). When music is provided via headphones, the volume level should remain between 60 and 80 dB (Stouffer et al., 2007). High-quality recording equipment should be used when creating recordings that will be replayed to clients, and high-fidelity headphones should be used for the playback of any prerecorded music.

Stouffer and Shirk (2003) describe a protocol for providing sedative client-preferred recorded music via headphones to children receiving mechanical ventilation. Parents can add a spoken or sung track onto the recording, to provide additional support and reality orientation. Such client-specific relaxation recordings can be played by nurses when children show mild signs of arousal or agitation while on the ventilator, and they may be used directly after invasive procedures to promote a return to homeostasis and a calm behavioral state (Stouffer & Shirk, 2003).

Regulated Multisensory Stimulation

Overview. Regulated multisensory stimulation follows the sensory regulation approach (Wood, 1991) of selectively and progressively providing sensory stimulation to enable individuals who have experienced severe brain injury to process the information more effectively. The sensory regulation approach assumes that individuals with disorders of consciousness or severe brain injury have a limited ability to process incoming sensory information (Keller, Hulsdunk, & Muller, 2007; Kennelly & Edwards, 1997; Wood, 1991). Due to limited capacity to process sensory information after brain injury, steps are taken to reduce extraneous stimuli and maximize an individual's ability to selectively attend to specific sensory stimuli. This model of sensory stimulation provided within a sensory regulation framework is consistent with the music and multimodal stimulation sequence used with premature, and thus neurologically immature, infants in the neonatal intensive care unit (for more information on music and multimodal stimulation, see Standley & Walworth, 2010, and Chapter 3 of this book).

Regulated multisensory stimulation begins with simple auditory stimuli, such as a drone, or a single sung tone, and progressively layers additional sounds to add musical complexity. As layers of sensory stimuli are added, more demand is placed on the sensory processing pathways, and thus this process is progressive and cumulative in nature. Additional sensory modalities are added as tolerated by the client, such as gentle touch or massage, visual stimulation, and vibroacoustic stimulation. The pacing of increased musical variety and complexity is matched to the child's responses, and thus a perceptive music therapist allows the process to become child-directed. If the therapist is keenly observant of the child's responses, the therapist will modify stimuli as needed and will be able to avoid overstimulating the child or provoking an adverse response (Magee, 2005). Certain children who are sedated are not yet ready to be aroused. The music therapist should confirm with the interdisciplinary team that increased arousal is indicated for a child before commencing with regulated multisensory stimulation.

Preparation. After confirming with the interdisciplinary team that regulated multisensory stimulation is currently indicated for the child, the therapist will try to ascertain if the upcoming session time will be relatively free from interruptions. The therapist will make attempts to minimize any extraneous noise in the environment before starting the session (e.g., will turn off television or radio, close door to hallway, etc.), will minimize unnecessary visual input (e.g., excessive overhead lights, television), and may draw the curtain around the child's bed to do so. The therapist will bring to the session at least one instrument that can provide a sustained sound (e.g., shruti box, Freenotes Wing) to enable gradual layering of auditory stimuli, and will bring a variety of musical instruments that have different timbral aspects to maximize the likelihood that the client will perceive and perhaps respond to some of the musical tones (Kotchoubey et al., 2003).

What to observe. Similar to other forms of music therapy in the PICU, the music therapist will observe the child's physiological parameters at baseline as well as any behavioral indicators of awareness or responsiveness (Magee, 2005). Sudden marked increases in heart rate or respiratory rate or sudden decreases in oxygen saturation may be considered negative responses, and stimulation should be modified or discontinued until the child returns to baseline. As described above, a child's positive responses to sound and stimulation may include relaxation of facial muscles, positive facial affect, eye opening, visual tracking, vocalizing or speaking, reaching toward musical objects, and various communicative responses. The music therapist will attempt to determine if positive behavioral responses are occurring in contingent relation to the sensory stimuli, indicating cognitive mediation is occurring, or if they appear reflexive in nature (Magee, 2007). Aversive responses may include grimacing, grinding teeth, startling, averting gaze, closing eyes, very wide eye opening, retracting extremities, moaning, attempting to move away from sounds, or falling asleep.

Procedures. Once the music therapist has introduced herself to the parent and explained the purpose of her presence, she can make a quick baseline observation of the child and family, including behavioral and physiological states. As in sedative music listening, the music therapist may start with a single, sustained sung pitch or will begin with a sustained drone (e.g., via the shruti box) to assess the child's ability to process auditory stimulation. Singing simple wordless melodies may be an appropriate first step to engaging a child without provoking agitation. If the child tolerates the therapist's singing voice, she may try singing the child's name. The use of voice without accompaniment decreases the level of sensory processing required, and the incorporation of the child's name may promote broader patterns of brain activation (Laureys et al., 2004).

If the child makes no perceptible response to voice alone or to a single drone, or if a child demonstrates a positive response to this minimal stimulation, the therapist will begin to introduce additional timbres (such as adding voice to the drone or vice versa, or playing a pitched tone bar while singing). The therapist should be aware that some sounds will be more stimulative in nature due to their acoustical properties (e.g., plucked instruments, rainstick, triangles, tambourines, solid metal chimes, etc.) and others less stimulating (e.g., shruti box, Freenotes Wing, nylon string guitar). Once the therapist identifies instruments that promote an orienting response, the therapist may alternate playing such instruments on either side of the child's body to determine if the child can localize the sound and track the sound source from side to side (Magee, 2005). The therapist may start with less stimulating instruments and, as the child tolerates stimulation, begin to move to more stimulating sounds and rhythmic patterns, as well as to layering more sounds and adding more musical complexity in accompaniment or rhythmic patterns (Tamplin, 2000).

Once auditory stimulation is well tolerated and the child's engagement with the therapist is expanding, the therapist may choose to add other sensory modalities (Ghetti & Hannan, 2008). The easiest sensory modality to add is visual stimulation, and the music therapist can slowly move colorful instruments from one side of the child to the other to ascertain visual tracking abilities. If the child has difficulty with this task, the therapist may play the instrument while moving across the child's visual field, to encourage the child to track it with his eye gaze. Similarly, a child can be encouraged to watch a captivating instrument as it moves up and down in his visual field, with the therapist assessing the child's ability in this area.

Bass resonator bars or buffalo drums provide a combination of sound and vibration, which provides additional sensory input. Such instruments can be positioned alongside a child's hands or feet to facilitate awareness of oneself in space. Smaller children and infants who can tolerate handling may experience vestibular stimulation as caregivers rock them and sing to them during music therapy sessions. The music therapist may hold a child's hand while singing him his favorite songs to promote an interpersonal connection and provide additional tactile input. During regulated multisensory stimulation, the therapist exercises creativity in presenting the child with novel and humanizing sensory experiences (Tamplin, 2000). The ongoing intent is to gradually promote the child's increasing arousal and awareness to enable a more thorough connection to others and to life around him.

Music-assisted Reality Orientation and Awareness

Overview. For children who are emerging from coma after traumatic brain injury, are being weaned from sedation postsurgery, or who are experiencing a disorder of consciousness, music therapy may be used to provide reality orientation and promote awareness of self and environment. Music-assisted reality orientation and awareness encompasses various techniques that promote gradual awareness of oneself, others, and the surrounding environment. Through the supportive context of music therapy, children receive affirmation and reassurance as they build awareness and responsiveness.

Music offers a particularly effective tool for promoting orientation, as music itself is composed of sound organized through time. The structure and order that is conveyed through music, along with the element of familiarity, can promote awareness and orientation (Kennelly & Edwards, 1997). Furthermore, music stimulates portions of the limbic system associated with emotional memory (Eschrich, Münte, & Altenmüller, 2008), and thus the use of familiar and preferred music can promote higher levels of responsiveness (Baker, 2001). The ultimate goal of music-assisted reality orientation and awareness is that the child gains awareness of himself, reconnects with others, and has some understanding of the meaning of his current situation, and that these improvements are incurred without distress.

As with regulated multisensory stimulation, some children are not appropriate candidates for reality orientation and awareness. The music therapist should confirm with the interdisciplinary team that increased awareness and orientation is indicated for a child before commencing with this approach. As client-preferred music and the singing of one's name can be quite arousing, the music therapist needs to affirm that the child is ready for this level of stimulation and should establish what methods best soothe the child in case nonpharmacological sedation is required during the process.

Preparation. If possible, the music therapist will meet with family members in advance of the session to determine the child's music preferences and experience. The therapist will make attempts to minimize any extraneous noise in the environment before starting the session, as described above. The therapist will bring a variety of novel-sounding instruments to the session, and will include the child's preferred instruments, if possible.

What to observe. The music therapist will monitor physiological parameters and behavioral indicators of awareness and responsiveness prior to and throughout the session, as indicated above. The music therapist will note any sudden changes in physiological parameters or any specific behavioral responses and will attempt to identify relationships between the music and interpersonal interactions and the child's physiological and behavioral responses. In so doing, the music therapist may gain a better understanding of what kinds of music, sounds, and verbal interactions promote increased alertness and responsiveness, and will build off of these accordingly. In addition to the changes in physiological parameters mentioned in previous sections, other positive indicators of responsiveness include vocalizing or verbalizing with communicative intent, using gesture for communication, reaching for or grasping objects, moving in response to music, and following simple requests.

Procedures. Since the music therapist is attempting to ascertain the child's specific responses to sound and to develop upon those responses to promote gradual broadening of awareness, the music therapist will remain alert to the child's subtle responses to sensory stimuli and social interaction. As with regulated multisensory stimulation, the music therapist will begin cautiously, to ensure that the child will not be immediately overstimulated or provoked into reflexive behavior such as startling or withdrawing from the source of sound (Magee, 2005; Tamplin, 2000). The therapist may begin with simple stimuli, such as a drone or a basic guitar or keyboard arpeggiated chord progressions. If the child is receptive to such sound, the therapist may progress by singing a greeting that incorporates the child's name (Magee, 2005). The therapist can then sing improvised lyrics that orient the child to his surroundings, by singing about the day, the session, the weather outside, and the individuals (often family members) present in the room. Lyrics that support reality orientation will vary depending upon the child's developmental level, along with what elements are pertinent and appropriate to reinforce.

Alternatively, the music therapist may sing lyrics that relate to feelings of love and support generating from the child's caregivers. In so doing, the song may act as a musical extension of the feelings caregivers have for the child, and may serve as an additional avenue for support for the child. The music therapist may encourage a caregiver to join the therapist at the child's bedside and contribute ideas or sing lyrics following the therapist's model. Often, caregivers who take part in this process will hold a child's hand during the improvised song, or stroke his hair, and will spontaneously offer additional messages of love and support. In such a case, the music acts as a facilitator and a conduit for this caring interaction.

The music therapist will remain attentive to any communication attempts or movements a child may make during the musical interaction, and will validate these responses and incorporate them into the song (Kennelly & Edwards, 1997). For example, the music therapist may notice that a child demonstrates increased heart rate each time his name is sung, or whenever the name of his sister is sung. The music therapist may acknowledge the child's emerging awareness by singing, "yes, Johnny loves his sister Mary, this we know, Johnny loves his sister Mary, and he lets it show." The music therapist can sing songs that describe what the child is doing or what he has the potential to do, e.g., breathing, hearing, or moving (Kennelly & Edwards, 1997). By acknowledging such communicative and motoric responses, the therapist helps the child build awareness of his selfhood and abilities along with his lasting power to impact and communicate with others. Thus, the interactions within music therapy may facilitate some of the earliest forms of nonverbal communication in heavily impacted populations, such as children who are recovering from acquired brain injury (Rosenfeld & Dun, 1999).

The music therapist may choose to keep certain session elements consistent from session to session in order to facilitate a child's emerging understanding of order and structure within his surroundings. For example, the music therapist may elect to sing the same greeting and closing songs to a child at each session, with modifications in lyrics to reflect themes or incorporate a child's responses on particular days. The songs will serve as a cue for the opening and closing of the session, and will help communicate certain expectations.

The music therapist who desires to foster a child's improved awareness and responsiveness will do well to incorporate a child's familiar and preferred music—information that may be obtained from the child's caregivers, if necessary. Singing familiar songs may promote the highest levels of arousal from a child, which may subsequently contribute to improved awareness of others (Rosenfeld & Dun, 1999). Familiar music may also improve a child's level of orientation and decrease agitation (Baker, 2001). The music therapist may use client-preferred music, adapt lyrics to such music, or create improvised songs to acknowledge and reinforce client responses.

Practicing music therapy in a PICU requires continuous adaptation. The music therapist promoting music-assisted reality orientation and awareness will adapt methods, songs, and music to reflect the child's unfolding responses, current state of being, and the participation levels and needs of family members who are present for the session. Adaptation should be viewed as a consistent process that is integral to any form of treatment and musical interaction.

Music Therapy as Procedural Support for Extubation

Overview. Many children who are mechanically ventilated and begin to show readiness to be removed from mechanical ventilation will not require a complete course of gradual weaning from the ventilator, but instead will be extubated (Newth et al., 2009; Parker, 2007). If a child is able to breathe spontaneously when ventilator settings are reduced, maintain adequate gas exchange, and manage airway secretions, he may be considered a candidate for extubation (Newth et al., 2009). Extubation refers to the procedure of removing the endotracheal tube, though some children will continue to require noninvasive forms of ventilatory assistance following successful extubation (Newth et al., 2009). The use of music therapy for extubation trials is considered a form of music therapy as procedural support (Ghetti, 2012). Chapter 6 of this volume discusses pediatric procedural support in greater detail; however, the use of music therapy as procedural support during extubation will be discussed in the current chapter, as this approach reflects a form of procedural support particular to the intensive care setting.

When music therapy is used as procedural support for extubation, the music therapist provides a sequence of clinical approaches to reduce a child's anxiety as he is prepped for extubation, is extubated, and subsequently breathes on his own. The child will have various emotional and physiological needs during this process, and the music therapist's approaches vary slightly depending upon the child's needs during various phases of the procedure. The research literature outlines the benefits of music therapy for adults weaning from mechanical ventilation (Hunter et al., 2010), but there are currently no controlled research studies evaluating the use of music therapy during endotracheal extubation. However, the methods described below reflect practice wisdom and are consistent with brief clinical accounts described in the literature of music therapy as procedural support for pediatric extubation (Nguyen, Jarred, Walworth, Adams, & Procelli, 2005; Robertson, 2009; Walworth, 2005).

Providing music therapy to support extubation trials is considered an advanced clinical practice within procedural support, and thus may not be recommended for therapists who are new to the intensive care setting. The music therapist hoping to initiate procedural support for extubation needs to gain the trust of the medical team and clearly explain her intention prior to commencing services. Children who are hypersensitive to sound would not be appropriate candidates for music therapy during extubation attempts, as any additional auditory stimuli might provoke anxiety. The music therapist should be prepared to discontinue musical support, if the addition of auditory stimuli provokes intense arousal or overstimulation. Following extubation, encouraging the child to sing may be contraindicated as the endotracheal tube has been placed between the vocal cords, and swelling of the vocal cords is possible. Singing after extubation is most likely contraindicated for children who have been intubated for very long periods of time, or who have experienced edema within the airway.

Preparation. The music therapist should receive a referral or suggest in advance to the physician scheduled for the extubation that music therapy may be indicated for procedural support during the extubation attempt. Advance notification of intent helps ensure that the music therapist has a chance to answer any questions prior to the procedure, and helps increase the likelihood that the music therapist will be paged or otherwise notified at the time of the extubation attempt. In ideal conditions, the music therapist will have met with the child and family in advance of the procedure to build rapport, ascertain music preferences, note child and family coping tendencies, and answer any questions that arise (Robertson, 2009). Developing rapport prior to the first extubation attempt gives the therapist a resource upon which to draw during the trial itself. During the actual extubation trial, the music therapist should position herself so that she is within the child's field of vision, but is positioned out of the way of the medical staff performing the procedure. The therapist should be prepared to shift physical positions as needed, depending upon the positioning of involved medical staff.

What to observe. Before, during, and after the extubation attempt, the music therapist will note the child's physiological signs as displayed on the monitor as well as any behavioral signs of anxiety or discomfort (e.g., grimacing, crying, rapid breathing or heart rate, pulling at tubes). The therapist will use these signs to inform her clinical decisions, providing extra verbal support (sung or spoken) or changing musical parameters (to increase sedative or stimulative properties), as needed.

Procedures. If the child is sufficiently alert, the music therapist may use sessions that occur prior to the extubation trial to determine the child's responses to music and rehearse music-based coping techniques. In some cases, the child will demonstrate mild alertness during these preprocedural sessions, but in many cases, the child will still be heavily under the influence of sedation, and consultations with caregivers will be beneficial.

During the days or hours preceding extubation, ventilatory settings are reduced to assess children's ability to breathe independently. Similarly, children are gradually weaned off of sedation during the time preceding the extubation attempt, as staff will desire them to be alert or easily arousable during the time of extubation. Prerequisites to extubation often involve the ability to breathe on one's own, demonstration of gag reflex and ability to cough, and good management of airway secretions (Newth et al., 2009; Parker, 2007). For successful extubation, the child must be awake enough to allow for spontaneous breathing and following commands (Karmarkar & Varshney, 2008; Newth et al., 2009). Some medical teams will conduct a spontaneous breathing trial prior to extubation, to assess the child's ability to maintain appropriate arterial blood gases while breathing with minimal assistance from the ventilator. The child may demonstrate distress during the trial, in part due to the sensations of the endotracheal tube paired with the reduced ventilator settings (Parker, 2007). The music therapist may provide support during preliminary spontaneous breathing trials to help the child remain calm and promote improved tolerance of the sensations that accompany the trial.

As the medical team continues to reduce ventilator settings and decrease sedation levels in the period prior to extubation, the child may become agitated as he becomes more aware of the sensations related to mechanical ventilation and the presence of the endotracheal tube (Parker, 2007). If the music therapist was not present during spontaneous breathing trials, the therapist will commence support during this time to ascertain the child's responses to sound, establish therapeutic rapport, and gradually begin to use the entrainment principle to gently encourage a more alert, yet calm, state. The music therapist can sing client-preferred music sung in a sedative style to calm the child (Robertson, 2009), and the therapist may interject statements offering support and reassurance. If the child demonstrates agitation or anxiety, the therapist may support positive coping attempts by singing affirmation of the child's responses such as breathing over the ventilator (e.g., "breath-ing, breath-ing, calm and relaxed" in tempo of the child's breathing). During this first stage, which occurs prior to extubation, the therapist continues to adjust musical properties and interpersonal support to promote a calm, alert state. The therapist will need to closely monitor the child's responses, and gently increase stimulative properties of the music if the child appears to relax to the point of drowsing or falling asleep.

The respiratory therapist or medical staff will be assessing parameters such as the child's tidal volume, or amount of air moved with each breath (Parker, 2007). Since the child may naturally entrain to some degree with the tempo of the music provided by the therapist, the therapist should be mindful of such responses and ensure that musical cues are promoting deep, regular breathing, yet are also keeping the child awake and alert. During the second phase of procedural support, the music therapist helps the child prepare for the extubation itself by gently increasing the tempo of music to stimulate an increase in alertness. It is important that the therapist provide a calm and reassuring musical and interpersonal presence, as the pace of interaction with the medical staff may be increasing, and the child's anxiety level and awareness may likewise increase. The therapist will continue to adjust musical qualities as needed during this period, providing gentle stimulation but also reducing complexity of stimuli (such as substituting in wordless singing or single word singing, or simplifying accompaniment) if the child begins to show signs of increasing agitation and fear. The child will require suctioning of the endotracheal tube just prior to extubation, to ensure that he does not aspirate any secretions with his first breath following extubation (Parker, 2007). Suctioning is sensorially unpleasant, and thus the music therapist should aim to decrease stress during and after suctioning, by offering calming musical stimuli and sung or spoken reassurance.

Once the child is extubated, the staff will want him to maintain steady, independent breathing. The music therapist can support this aim by playing music with a clear, steady rhythm, and directly engaging the child in the music-making. If appropriate, the child may be able to join the therapist by playing small musical instruments at this point. Such active engagement gives the child a focal point for attention, while it also promotes ongoing alertness and regular, independent respiration. The medical staff tends to quickly withdraw at this point, and the therapist may remain the main contact with the child as the team continues to periodically monitor the child to ensure adequate oxygenation. The child's coping preferences should be respected during this phase, and if he desires to engage passively, this preference should be respected. If the child begins to demonstrate oxygen desaturation, a gentle increase in the stimulative qualities of the music or cues to increase deep breathing or active engagement in music-making could prompt an advantageous increase in deep, regular breathing. Music therapy may conclude once the child is stable, calm, breathing independently, and able to transition into other supportive activities or interactions.

Some children respond very well to attending to the music as a means of coping with adversity. The music therapist should remain attentive to the child's coping preferences, which may change somewhat during the course of the procedure. If a child calms best by watching the music therapist, or listening to a favorite song, the music therapist can promote this selective use of attention to help the child cope with the discomfort of the extubation process. Thus, provision of sedative, client-preferred music may not be as calming to some children as attention-gaining stimulative forms of their preferred music.

Music Therapy During or Following Active Dying

Overview. Despite the gains made in adult hospice care within the United States, the majority of children who reach end-of-life will do so in the hospital setting, and many of those will die in the PICU (Meyer, Burns, Griffith, & Truog, 2002). Chapter 9 of this volume discusses palliative and end-of-life care for children; however, the use of music therapy within the PICU during withdrawal of life support or active dying will be discussed here.

Music therapy may play a significant role in supporting families as a child is actively dying (Lindenfelser, 2005; Loewy & Stewart, 2005). Various improvisatory and receptive music therapy methods may be used to create an atmosphere that fully supports caregivers' expressions of grief, while it also provides an element of containment. The music therapist will remain responsive to the family members' processing of the event, and will attempt to sensitively pair improvised and re-created forms of music to that evolving process. Live music is advantageous, if the family assents to it, as the therapist can modify musical elements and lyrics as appropriate to the circumstances. Music therapy during or immediately following active dying often consists of the music therapist playing a guitar or harp and singing appropriate songs or singing wordlessly. Use of the voice and lullabies may provide a holding environment that helps lull the child who is transitioning out of life, while also supporting those who are present for the child (Loewy & Stewart, 2005). Other members of the interdisciplinary team may simultaneously be providing services, such as a chaplain praying with the family, a child life specialist helping the caregivers create a keepsake handprint or footprint of the child, and nursing staff continuing to provide comfort care and nursing care at the end-of-life.

Some families will prefer to have privacy during and following active dying. The music therapist can offer recorded music if the family desires. The family's wishes for a child's last moments should take precedence over a therapist's good intentions. If a family does not wish to have music therapy, either live or through recorded music, present during end-of-life, this choice should be respected.

Witnessing and supporting caregivers' grief at the end of their children's lives is emotionally taxing, and leaves the therapist vulnerable to vicarious traumatization and compassion fatigue. It is important that music therapists engaging in this area of practice receive ongoing clinical supervision, and that they possess the emotional maturity to be appropriately present and responsive to caregivers.

Preparation. The music therapist should ascertain which staff member, if not the music therapist, is the main liaison with the parent during the end-of-life phase. Depending upon the facility and the family's preferences, this staff person may be the PICU social worker, the chaplain, the child life specialist, the music therapist, or a favorite nurse or doctor. The music therapist can confer with the staff member who is dialoging with the family during the end-of-life process, to inquire as to the family's receptivity to music therapy. Conversely, if the music therapist has been working with the child prior to active dying, the music therapist might talk directly with the caregivers to determine their preferences regarding music. The music therapist should inquire about preferences for live vs. recorded music, sung vs. instrumental music, sacred vs. secular music, and any desire for particular pieces of music. The therapist should try to ascertain this information concisely, and avoid needlessly burdening family with too many questions or options.

If the family desires live music therapy, the therapist should position herself on the periphery of the family, unless invited by the family to come to the child's bedside. The therapist can position herself relatively close to the door to enable an inconspicuous exit, but should ensure that other staff members will be able to enter the room and approach the bedside as needed. Ideally, the music therapist would have music memorized or load lyric and chord sheets onto an iPad to avoid the need for music stands and songbooks, which might clutter the space.

What to observe. The music therapist will remain observant of and sensitive to the reactions of the family to the music and to the experience of the child's death. The music therapist will use a combination of observation and intuition to select when to change music, when to add words, and when to conclude the music.

Procedures. When live music therapy is used during active dying, the music therapist will enter the space after receiving family assent and will take a moment to assess the atmosphere before commencing music. Family members may already be gathered tightly around the child's bedside, or they may be keeping distance from the child and each other. The therapist will assess whether music should be tailored to the child's immediate needs and responses, and thus synchronized with the breathing of the child, or if it would more beneficial to temper the music to the family's needs. It is generally advisable for the music therapist to begin in a neutral fashion to observe the responses of both child and family to the addition of live music. For example, the therapist may begin by slowly finger-picking a chord progression on guitar. If family members appear receptive to this initial music, the therapist may add wordless singing to the accompaniment, and progress to sedative singing of a requested song or genre of music (Lindenfelser, 2005).

The therapist will balance family and child music preferences with the therapist's own intuitive sense of what those in the room need in the moment, to guide her music selections. Likewise, the music therapist will remain vigilant of the family members' and child's responses, and will modify music accordingly (Loewy & Stewart, 2005). The music therapist should consider including songs of kin to enable connection with the family (Loewy, 2009), and may choose to sing the corresponding song lyrics or omit them, depending upon what is unfolding in the room. If a sedation effect is desired, the therapist may transition into a sedative, musical holding environment by transitioning into 3/4 or 6/8 meter, and reduce the sung phrases into a single relevant mantra that accompanies a grounding and repetitive V-I harmonic cadence (Loewy & Stewart, 2005; Loewy, 2009). If music preferences are not known, or the therapist is not able to provide the family's preferred selections, the therapist may improvise simple lyrics of support and love that might convey the feelings of those in the room, such as "you are loved," "we are here," and/or "you can rest" (Ghetti & Walker, 2008). If the therapist believes complete musical sedation would be desirable, she will then transition into simplifying and ceasing the accompaniment instrument and settling into basic toning in synchronization with the child's breathing. This progressive, sedative musical process may help ease children through the transition from life to death, while supporting both child and family (Loewy & Stewart, 2005).

Music therapy during active dying can take 20 minutes to several hours. When appropriate, the music therapist may also ask family members if they would like to sing or hear any particular selections. Sometimes family members will join the therapist in singing, if the therapist creates a strong musical foundation. At other times, family members will be overwhelmed with emotion and feel that they are unable to sing. The therapist may take leave when there is a natural decline in the tenor of the room, and family members are stabilizing in their experiencing of grief.

In addition to or instead of providing music therapy during active dying, music therapy is also used effectively for the period immediately following a child's death. The therapist can provide a supportive atmosphere that contains the caregivers' grief, or music therapy may be used to create a more nurturing environment as nurses clean the child's body and remove medical equipment from the child after death. Child life specialists may provide an opportunity for family members to create handprints or footprints of the child as a keepsake, and music therapy may be used during this process to create a respectful holding environment for the ritual. The use of music following a child's death will be similar to that used during active dying. Overall, the holding and containing aspects of music therapy impact family and staff alike during the volatile period surrounding end-of-life. For additional description of the use of music therapy at the end-of-life, readers are directed to Ghetti and Walker (2008), Lindenfelser (2005), Loewy (2009), and Loewy and Stewart (2005).

GUIDELINES FOR IMPROVISATIONAL MUSIC THERAPY

Perhaps contrary to popular belief, music therapists practicing in medical settings report regularly using various forms of clinical improvisation. In fact, music therapists working in medical settings report using clinical improvisation approaches more often than behavioral approaches to music therapy (i.e., the use of various techniques to shape behavior) (Lam, 2007). Music therapists working within pediatric intensive care use improvisation in many aspects of clinical practice to ensure that music interactions remain client-centered and responsive to the child's changing needs. This section will discuss clinical approaches that support the child in entering into the improvisation, whether that improvised engagement occurs through singing, playing instruments, or creating dramatic play. The subsections are roughly arranged in order of frequency of use within this setting. The therapist may select to use certain approaches, or may make alterations in certain approaches, depending upon the child's particular needs, resources, and developmental level.

Improvised Song/Lullaby

Overview. The music therapist will often adjust song lyrics to better match the context or a child's current emotional state or situation. The therapist may also attempt to actively engage the child or caregiver in the creation of improvised song in order to deepen their experience of the music and promote emotional expression. Improvised song/lullaby involves the spontaneous creation of music with lyrics or vocalizations that occurs in the moment and serves expressive purposes. Engaging a child in improvised song can empower the child to express his feelings and/or enable a child to work through issues metaphorically, and it may allow for the uncovering of a child's misconceptions about illness or treatment (Ghetti, 2011b; Loewy, MacGregor, Richards, & Rodriguez, 1997; Loewy & Stewart, 2004; Loveszy, 1991; Turry, 1997). Most important, improvised song gives children a voice, and does so in a way that is immediate and open-ended, yet also contained and supportive. A "musical journey" (Loewy et al., 1997) is a form of improvised song wherein the child verbally or musically describes a journey to a chosen destination, which offers the child a means to metaphorically transform his experience of pain or fear. Even children at end-of-life who are losing motor skills and strength may use the natural process of following their imagination through an improvised song to allow them to explore places and themes that are significant to them (Dun, 1995).

When caregivers are encouraged to partake in the development of improvised song or lullaby, they are gently drawn into the expressive experience and reap the same benefits of a supported, nurturing context for expressing their feelings and desires. Through improvised song or lullaby, caregivers may directly convey their feelings to their children, and they may experience a release of tension and anxiety. Caregivers who partake in creating music for their children may experience the empowering feeling of being reinstated in their role of primary caregiver.

Preparation. Spontaneity and sensitivity to the present moment help a music therapist support the unfolding of an impromptu song or lullaby. The therapist "prepares" for such interaction by developing fluid musical skills, including the ability to play various contrasting chord progressions in any key, by learning to accompany the spontaneous singing of others, and by mastering the art of gently prompting others and drawing them into the music. Caregivers and adolescent clients may be more likely to sing when given privacy, and sometimes simply pulling the privacy curtain around the bed can create a contained atmosphere that supports such expression. For children and caregivers who are more reluctant to sing spontaneously, the music therapist may need to model musical structures and provide an initial example, and then fade her singing to encourage a child or caregiver to take the musical lead.

What to observe. If a child is alert and responsive enough to partake in improvised song, he also may be more medically stable, and thus physiological signs will be less important to monitor. Instead, the music therapist will tend to focus on a child's engagement in the music-making, and any signs of discomfort or resistance. These overt behavioral or thematic and symbolic signs of resistance will be important areas of focus for the therapist, as they may be related to underlying conflicts the child is having.

Procedures. Many young children will easily engage in spontaneous creation of songs when they feel comfortable with the music therapist and are given a supportive musical environment (Loewy & Stewart, 2004; Loveszy, 1991). Prior to moving into improvised song, the music therapist may offer the child various rhythm and melodic instruments from which to choose in order to engage him in music-making. When using improvised song, the music therapist may introduce the concept by asking the child if he wants to make a song together, or the therapist may simply build off of a child's musical or verbal responses by spontaneously developing a song without having to introduce the idea first (Turry, 1997). Preschool- and school-age children may need only a transitional statement such as "let's make a story" or "what should our song be about?" As the child states or sings information, the music therapist can musically mirror the verbal content and match tempo, dynamics, harmony, and melodic elements to the child's contributions. Thus, the song may go through several musical shifts in accordance with what the child brings to the song. Younger children may easily and naturally fall into singing spontaneously with the therapist, and may require very minimal prompts to further the action or content of the song. The music therapist becomes an expressive partner and companion as the child journeys through his song (Loewy et al., 1997). Children will often create a natural ending within their song, if given the chance to be self-directed within the improvised song creation. However, if this does not occur, the therapist can sing or speak a closure prompt when appropriate such as "... and how does the story/song end?"

In contrast, an adolescent may start by verbally expressing some emotion, such as frustration, and the music therapist can gently redirect the client into improvised song by saying, "Can we put that into a sound?" The music therapist can then model how words might be sung, rapped, or spoken along with the development of a song that stylistically matches the thoughts and feelings expressed by the client (Turry, 1997). In general, the music therapist will aim to provide a level of structure that supports the client, but that leaves ample space and place for the child's voice to lead the song creation. Thus, the level of structure and musical or verbal prompting (whether it involves mirroring or probing) will vary depending upon the client's comfort with the process, as well as with his expressive contribution.

Depending upon the needs and functioning level of the child, the caregivers may be encouraged to join in the creation of improvised songs or lullabies (Dun, 1995). Caregivers may be more self-conscious about singing in the PICU environment than their children, and thus the music therapist should aim to make them feel at ease and gradually draw them into the song creation. Caregivers might feel most comfortable contributing single words or themes to a song that the music therapist creates in the moment, or they might feel comfortable creating new lyrics for a familiar song or lullaby. The music therapist may sing an initial improvised verse to serve as a model, and may subsequently leave blanks in additional verses to leave space for a caregiver to sing or contribute words.

Some children may enjoy recording their improvised songs to enable themselves or others to listen to them afterward. Recording can be useful, as the process of improvised song/lullaby is often quite significant in the moment, yet recording enables the song to be captured as a permanent creation. After receiving written consent from the guardian and verbal assent from the child for audio recording, the music therapist may record the song through a digital voice recorder or through a computer and microphone into a software program such as GarageBand. Recording improvised song is considered an adaptation, as the simple act of recording the song may impact or impede the improvisatory process, and such an impact should be considered when offering this option.

Music-facilitated Dramatic Play

Overview. Related to the approach of improvised song/lullaby is the concept of music-facilitated dramatic play (Ghetti & Hannan, 2008; Ghetti & Walker, 2008). As in improvised song, a child is given a supportive musical context to extemporaneously express himself, while the therapist mirrors, prompts, and companions the child through the creative journey. Music-facilitated dramatic play takes the process of improvised song a step further by incorporating play and dramatic action using props and musical instruments. The music therapist may provide the child with a variety of washable puppets, musical instruments, and/or medical-related equipment and dolls, to help prompt and further the child's creative process (Fagen, 1982; Froehlich, 1996a).

Music-facilitated dramatic play is appropriate for children who possess enough awareness of themselves and their environment and the cognitive wherewithal to engage in imaginary or cooperative levels of play. Through dramatic play, children may express their feelings, work through internal conflicts, tap into inner resources, and externalize their conceptualizations of their illness or current situation (Fagen, 1982; Ghetti & Walker, 2008; Loewy & Stewart, 2004). Thus, similar to improvised song, music-facilitated dramatic play may provide an avenue for expression, which may allow the music therapist to gain insight into a child's internal experiencing of his critical care hospitalization, and any potential misconceptions. The therapist can then use the dramatic play context to give the child a supportive means of approaching, working through, and resolving fears and conflicts. The musical play provides a nonthreatening opportunity to approach challenging emotions without becoming overwhelmed by them, and thus music therapy may enable the child to cope through emotional-approach (Ghetti, 2011a).

The story song technique was developed in 1988 by music therapist Joanne Loewy (personal communication, January 1, 2013), and is related to the concept of music-facilitated dramatic play. In the story song approach, a nursery rhyme, fairy tale, folktale, or familiar song is orchestrated and re-enacted in order to help individuals resolve their feelings related to a traumatic experience (Loewy & Stewart, 2004; Rubin-Bosco, 2002). Creative use of the elements of "theme, countertheme or conflict, variation, and resolution (and/or recapitulation)" enables a therapeutic process to unfold (Loewy & Stewart, 2004, p. 196). Story songs serve as scripts that can help to elicit and contain the expression of inner conflicts, and allow one to connect with inner resources (Rubin-Bosco, 2002). Children who engage in the process of music-facilitated dramatic play or story song may work through conflicts within the realm of metaphor, and in so doing may experience a "symbolic transformation of perception" (Loewy, 2002, p. 36).

Appropriate use of music-facilitated dramatic play requires that the child have some means of specific expressive communication, so that the therapist can ensure that the therapeutic process unfolds at the child's pace. The child should be able to affirm choices and confirm dramatic action through verbal means or nonverbal communication systems, even if the child's range of communicative response is restricted to "yes" or "no." The music therapist can then seek clarification of a child's dramatic action when needed.

Theoretically, music-facilitated dramatic play may be used on supportive, re-educative, or reconstructive levels. Music therapists who use the technique to elicit interactions on a level more intensive than supportive should have advanced clinical training, as the use of such projective techniques can result in the child delving into deeper intrapersonal conflicts. Furthermore, the music therapist should consider aspects such as the projected length of treatment and the current coping resources of the child before determining if it is appropriate to initiate more intensive levels of therapy. The therapist should ensure that adequate time is available and that the therapist's level of competence is sufficient to support a child engaging in deeper levels of therapy within the intensive care environment. The child may remain in control of the pacing of action in supportive and re-educative levels of therapy, whereas in reconstructive levels, the therapist may choose to be more directive in terms of pacing, with more use of probing. It is recommended that the music therapist working on a re-educative and reconstructive level receive ongoing clinical supervision.

Preparation. The music therapist will make attempts to minimize extraneous stimulation in the environment and provide a suitable level of privacy. If the therapist anticipates that a child will come into contact with significant anxieties during dramatic play, it is advisable to talk with the child's caregivers in advance to discuss the intentions of treatment and what the course of the therapeutic interaction might look like. Once caregivers are informed of the intention of music-facilitated dramatic play (or other expressive interventions like improvised song and songwriting), they may opt to give their child privacy during music therapy, so as to avoid impacting the child's scope of expression. The therapist will need to consider when a dyadic session including both caregiver and child is most indicated, and when a private session with the client might best meet his needs.

Washable puppets such as facial affect puppets (each demonstrating a different emotion), finger puppets, and hand puppets may prove intriguing to the child. Other children may use instruments shaped like people or animals to convey action (e.g., crocodile guiro, duck castanet). Neutral, medical play dolls might be enticing for certain children, while others will want to use stuffed animals or dolls that they have brought from home. It is important that the child select props that are comfortable and meaningful for him, though care should be taken to avoid overwhelming the child with too many choices.

What to observe. Children who are hospitalized may express their fears and concerns more readily through play and puppets than through verbal means (Froehlich, 1996b). The music therapist using music-facilitated dramatic play in the intensive care unit should remain vigilant to the child's emotional and behavioral responses. If the therapist attends carefully to the child's musical, verbal, and nonverbal responses, she can continue to respect and follow the child's pace. When a child trusts a therapist and is given the appropriate expressive means, he will generally express what he is ready to express (Froehlich, 1996b; Loewy & Stewart, 2004). The therapist will take note of what the child says, his action with the props, and his areas of resistance or avoidance, and will use this information to form a clearer picture of what his primary concerns, conflicts, and resources are.

Procedures. Prior to initiating music-facilitated dramatic play, the music therapist may consider engaging the child in less provocative forms of music-making, such as singing a greeting song or exploring novel-sounding instruments. By doing so, the music therapist provides a transition, develops rapport, and has a chance to assess the child in the moment (Froehlich, 1996b). Once a working alliance is formed, the music therapist may suggest that they create a story, or may introduce the puppets/props and then ask the child if he wants to create a story. The dramatic play may take various forms including:

1) The child gives voice to a puppet or prop while the music therapist provides musical mirroring and accompaniment (Fagen, 1982; Ghetti & Walker, 2008; Loewy & Stewart, 2004).

2) The child uses a puppet or prop to create action while the music therapist gives the puppet a voice (spoken or sung) and provides musical accompaniment (Ghetti & Walker, 2008; Loewy & Stewart, 2004).

3) The child uses instruments or voice to create a narrative or accompaniment for the therapist's use of a puppet or prop.

4) The child uses instruments and/or voice to sing or illustrate a story while the therapist provides musical accompaniment and mirroring and/or prompting (Loewy & Stewart, 2004; Rubin-Bosco, 2002).

Children who are comfortable singing will often do so within the musical context, without requiring much prompting. Thus, children's preferences for how they partake in music-facilitated dramatic play are often readily apparent (Fagen, 1982; Loewy & Stewart, 2004). Once a child's preferred method of engaging in dramatic play is ascertained, the therapist can briefly inquire about other simple preferences that will guide the interaction. The therapist can ask the child what instrument the therapist should play, and ask the child for a descriptive word to set the musical tone (e.g., happy, sad, tired, mad, excited, fast, slow), if necessary.

As the action unfolds, the therapist will often musically mirror the action, doing so by altering melody, chord progression, tempo, volume, and accompaniment patterns to match the mood of the action. The therapist might sing lyrics that paraphrase what the child has said, or lyrics that reinforce a child's most salient statements (Ghetti & Walker, 2008; Loewy & Stewart, 2004). The therapist may also sing prompts to further the action or deepen the child's exploration such as "what happened next?," "how did he feel?," "why was he there?," "what was it for?," "what did he think?," etc. The child may work through his own inner struggles by projecting them onto the puppets or props, and may learn and explore new coping resources by having the puppet act them out (Fagen, 1982; Ghetti & Walker, 2008; Loewy & Stewart, 2004; Loveszy, 1991).

Some children will resolve conflicts and bring closure to their narratives without external guidance. Conversely, in particular instances the therapist may need to gently prompt closure and may do so by singing or speaking simple questions such as "... and how does the story end?" The end of a story is a familiar concept for most children, and how the child chooses to end the story can reflect his coping preferences and inner resources.

Depending upon the child's developmental level, the level of therapy used, and the dramatic content revealed, the therapist may employ varying degrees of verbal processing during and after the dramatic process. Verbal processing may be particularly important in the clarification of a child's misconceptions. The music therapist may be able to clarify certain areas of misunderstanding related to illness or treatment, while other areas may be referred to the Child Life Specialist to provide additional follow-up through medical play or medical teaching. Alternatively, the music therapist may use verbal processing to help a child gain awareness of conflicts and identify potential coping strategies.

Some children may be resistant to musically engage in a session and instead prefer to interact verbally or nonverbally with a puppet or prop from the onset. The music therapist allows such a child to direct action and make choices regarding what instruments the therapist plays and how she plays them, in order to match the action of the puppet/prop. Children who receive several music therapy sessions that incorporate music-facilitated dramatic play may always choose to direct their puppets/props and abstain from direct musical engagement. The technique can be just as effective with this approach as with a child who enters into the music-making. Readers interested in additional literature on the implementation of music-facilitated dramatic play are directed to case examples in Fagen (1982), Ghetti and Walker (2008),

Loewy and Stewart (2004), and Rubin-Bosco (2002) or to a task analysis on the subject, which is provided as an appendix to the PICU chapter by Ghetti and Hannan (2008), within Hanson-Abromeit and Colwell (2008).

Referential and Nonreferential Improvisation

Overview. Some children and adolescents will not respond well to musical interactions emphasizing verbal contributions. Perhaps the child has limited or no comprehension of English, or a teenager is withdrawn and does not desire to speak or hear singing. Instrumental improvisation offers a nonverbal expressive outlet, and can create a bridge between client and therapist at times when words are not desired. Furthermore, engaging in instrumental improvisation may help children and adolescents connect with their feelings, and may serve as a conduit for learning more about themselves and their emotional lives.

The therapist and child may decide upon the use of referential improvisation, in which the music is used to depict some nonmusical theme, emotion, entity, or experience (Bruscia, 1998). Conversely, the improvisation may be nonreferential in nature, with no particular intention to represent anything beyond the music itself (Bruscia, 1998). In either case, the goals of partaking in improvisation include building awareness of and expressing various emotions (Turry, 1997), providing a means for interpersonal communication, and promoting constructive use of fine and gross motor skills. Engaging a child or parent/child dyad in clinical improvisation can allow the music therapist to assess interpersonal dynamics and more comprehensively assess a client's full range of responses (Oldfield, 2011).

At times, instrumental improvisation in the PICU environment can become quite loud, especially when louder drums and percussive instruments are offered. Though such free expression might be quite desirable for one child, the sound levels resulting from such expression may be contraindicated for the child's roommate(s). The music therapist must weigh the costs and benefits of any form of music therapy for all those in the environment. For example, the music therapist may feel that one child who is externalizing anger by becoming aggressive toward staff might be able to express his angry feelings through a buffalo drum during an instrumental improvisation. However, the child in the neighboring bed may be at the end of life, with several family members gathered around to pay respects. In order to better meet the needs of both children and their respective families, the music therapist might offer the child who has anger a choice of quieter instruments that he can hit harder, or may use headphones with the child to create a collaborative improvisation using music software on a computer.

Preparation. The music therapist should consider how much structure the client requires to feel secure during improvisation, as well as considering the musical attributes of the instruments offered. Novel-sounding instruments such as the Remo Thunder Tube, ocean drum, kalimba, pentatonic xylophone, rainstick, guiro, vibroslap, cabasa, and kokoriko can pique a child's interest and motivate him to partake in music-making. When offering instrument choices for improvisation, the music therapist should consider the child's ability to independently play various instruments, as well as his ability to tolerate various types of sounds. Children will generally clearly demonstrate their preference for certain instruments, when given several choices. The music therapist should attempt to set up the environment to reduce extraneous stimuli and maximize privacy as previously described.

What to observe. When the music therapist engages in instrumental improvisation with a child, the therapist will note emotional and behavioral responses. The therapist will take note of significant or recurring musical or thematic elements, and may choose to explore these musically or verbally, according to the developmental level of the child.

Procedures. Depending upon what the child's needs and resources are, the music therapist may suggest starting an interaction with improvisation, or may provide an introductory music-making experience beforehand. The child should be offered a range of instruments appropriate for his developmental level and physical abilities (Oldfield, 2011), and options may include adaptive technology that enables music-making, such as an iPad. A therapist using referential improvisation may suggest that the child choose a theme, experience, or feeling, and portray it in sound. Alternatively, as a result of assessing the child prior to the session as well as during the opening portion of the session, the music therapist might identify a theme that is pertinent to the child's current experience and may offer it as an impetus for the improvisation. When using nonreferential improvisation, the therapist will make a broad range of instruments available to the child and will companion the child in the music, as the child desires.

In either referential or nonreferential improvisation, the child may be empowered to choose which instrument the music therapist will play and/or how the therapist will play. In order to assess the child in a variety of roles, a therapist may alternate choice-making with the child throughout the session, offering the child chances to decide the instruments and musical elements, and contrasting those with situations and musical conditions that the therapist creates (Oldfield, 2011). Ensuring that the child has multiple opportunities to make choices helps improve the child's feelings of control and mastery over his environment (Froehlich, 1996b), and may enable him to feel more comfortable within an improvisation experience. During the course of the improvisation, the therapist will musically reflect what the child expresses, engage in a musical dialog with the child, or provide musical grounding and stability for the child's improvisation.

Providing structure is one of the most direct ways to promote grounding and security for children during improvisation experiences (Turry, 1997). Some children will require higher levels of structure within the improvisation in order to feel safe and secure. Children who are experiencing elevated levels of stress, or who are functioning at younger developmental levels will benefit from higher levels of structure and repetition within the music (Turry, 1997). The use of specific musical forms, such as rondo form or 12-bar blues, may provide an effective means for balancing structure with freedom (Froehlich, 1996b). When using a rondo form, the music therapist can introduce a theme or consistent way of playing during the repeating "A" sections, and contrast this with free improvisation by the client during "B" and "C" sections of the ABACA form. As the child develops more comfort within the music context, or for children who can tolerate higher amounts of freedom within the improvisation, the level of structure may be reduced to allow greater freedom of expression. Referential improvisation can provide a level of structure and organization through introduction of themes and concepts (regardless of whether these themes are generated by the client or the therapist).

Verbal processing following improvisation may be indicated for children who are able to reflect upon what they experienced during the improvisation, including discussing feelings and thoughts that were associated with the experience. Translating the child's experience of improvisation into words can enable the child to gain awareness of his emotions and may promote a level of mastery over hospital-related anxieties (Froehlich, 1996b). Verbal processing of an improvisation experience may help the therapist to check her assessment of significant themes or concepts that arose in the music, by contrasting them with the child's verbal description. Unless the child has a private room within the PICU, it may not be possible to ensure privacy for any aspect of a music therapy session, and the therapist should consider how this compromise to privacy might impact the verbal expression of a client. Similarly, some children may have more difficulty identifying their emotions and putting them into words due to their developmental level, their level of comfort with verbal expression, and the quality of rapport developed with the therapist. Thus, the therapist should be mindful that some children will benefit from expressing their emotions through musical means, but should not be forced to translate this expression into verbalization (Froehlich, 1996b).

If consent for audio recording is obtained and the child desires it, the therapist may record the improvisation. Upon listening to the recording, the therapist may ask the child to explain what is happening in the music, or, conversely, the child might create a story that goes along with the improvisation. Either technique may help to facilitate a child's verbal processing related to the improvisation experience.

GUIDELINES FOR RE-CREATIVE MUSIC THERAPY

In the PICU, re-creative approaches to music therapy are often used in combination with other forms of music therapy within a single session. Children may be motivated to engage in the re-creation of favorite songs, either through singing or playing instruments, and the therapist can use this source of motivation to help the child achieve aims in communication, rehabilitation, and emotional expression. The following approaches are briefly described and are not placed in any particular order.

Developmental Stimulation

Overview. Infants and children who experience frequent or prolonged hospitalization are at risk for delays in various developmental domains (Kennelly, 2000). Developmental stimulation through music therapy is an extension of regulated multisensory stimulation, and expands into increasing levels of engaging and interacting with the music and the therapist to promote developmental gains. The therapist may use familiar children's songs to gain a child's attention, cue certain behaviors, motivate him to respond, and promote his exploration of the environment. Musical interchanges between therapist and child can promote social reciprocity and the development of communication systems (Edwards, 2011b). The use of familiar and preferred music may also provide sufficient structure to facilitate parents' active engagement in music-making with their children (Marley, 1996).

Certainly every child who engages in music therapy of any orientation or approach is likely to make gains in various developmental areas. The demarcation of developmental stimulation as a particular clinical approach simply indicates that the main focus of the therapeutic interaction is on the promotion of developmental gains. Developmental stimulation may be appropriate for graduates of the NICU who are subsequently admitted to the PICU when experiencing respiratory distress or other ongoing health challenges. However, developmental stimulation may also be important for older children who spend long periods in the PICU or who have emerged from long periods of sedation.

Preparation. In order to maximize the potential for the child to benefit from a session, the music therapist may confer with the nurse to identify a time when the child is most alert and offer services then. A music therapist using developmental stimulation will offer the child a variety of musical instruments appropriate to the child's developmental level and physical abilities. Developmental stimulation sessions tend to be uplifting and normalizing, and the therapist may make attempts to empower the caregiver to take an active role in music-making with the child.

Procedures. When engaging a child in developmental stimulation, the therapist may begin with a greeting song. During this opening interaction, the music therapist can assess a child's response to musical and social stimulation, and can informally assess a variety of developmental domains. The therapist may use subsequent music interactions and musical structure to provide opportunities for a child to demonstrate various skills, such as making eye contact, visual and auditory tracking, orienting to name, reaching toward and grasping objects, bringing hands to midline, reaching past midline, bringing objects to mouth, demonstrating head and trunk control, engaging in vocal dialog, using gestures or words to communicate, identifying objects, imitating movements or vocalizations, following simple directions, and expressing wants and needs.

Re-creative approaches within developmental stimulation include supporting the child to sing along to familiar songs, imitate rhythms or melodic motifs, or play instruments along with cues (either leading or following), among others (Kennelly, 2000; Marley, 1996). The music therapist will observe the child's abilities and skill areas that are underdeveloped, and will structure the music to prompt a child to explore these new areas. The use of novel and alluring musical instruments may motivate a child to engage actively in the music-making. Similarly, when familiar music is used, it can serve as the impetus for a child to engage and demonstrate a broader scope of skills than the child may display outside of the music therapy context (Edwards & Kennelly, 2011). Readers interested in more detail about particular methods of developmental stimulation appropriate for the PICU may reference the literature regarding hospitalized children within Standley and Walworth's (2010) discussion of infant and early childhood music therapy methods, Kennelly (2000), Kallay (1997), or Marley (1996). Although not specific to hospitalized children, Schwartz (2011) offers a description of music therapy within a developmental framework and describes case examples of such work.

Music Therapy to Promote Bonding

Overview. Just as infants and children are at risk for developmental delays due to frequent or prolonged hospitalization in the PICU, healthy attachment between caregivers and children may also be placed at risk. When music therapy is used to promote bonding, the therapist assists the caregiver in using song and musical interactions to create opportunities for the development and maintenance of secure attachment (Edwards, 2011a).

During music therapy to promote bonding, the caregiver may be supported in engaging in reciprocal vocal exchanges with the child, rocking or holding infant while singing lullabies to the child, or creating audio recordings with the caregiver singing songs or speaking messages of love to the child to be used in the caregiver's absence. The PICU environment often displaces the parent from their role as primary caregiver and nurturer, and this change in role causes significant stress for caregivers (Shoemark & Dearn, 2008). A music therapist using music therapy to promote bonding aims to reinstate the parent in their role as primary caregiver and nurturer. Music therapy serves as a vehicle and a container for the infant and caregiver to encounter each other and develop attachment (Edwards, 2011a).

Reciprocal vocal exchanges between an infant and caregiver are often very musical in nature, and music can both prompt such exchanges and provide a normalizing context within which they may occur. The way that adults tend to talk and verbally interact with infants, known as "parentese" (Standley & Walworth, 2010) or "infant-directed" singing or speech (Edwards, 2011a), often possesses melodious qualities, extended vowel sounds, and the use of rising pitch contour for provoking a stimulating response, and falling pitch contour for calming (Standley & Walworth, 2010). The pairing of music and song with bonding is a natural fit for infants, as infants are responsive to vocally based exchanges and do not necessarily discriminate between speech and music (Edwards, 2011a). Furthermore, positive connections promoted by the music therapy context assist the caregiver in viewing the infant as whole and focusing on abilities and potentials instead of impairments and ailments (Shoemark & Dearn, 2008).

As the ultimate outcome of using music therapy to promote bonding is the development and maintenance of secure attachment between infant and primary caregiver, the use of this technique should be in the service of that singular bond. In cases where the caregiver is regularly present at bedside, the music therapist will encourage and guide the caregiver to take the leading role in bonding with the infant. If the caregiver is not able to be consistently present for the infant, the music therapist will work alongside the interdisciplinary team to ensure that the infant's needs are met, but will also attempt to bring the caregiver's presence to the child's environment through audio recordings and the like. Thus, in such a case, the music therapist may contribute to an infant's secure attachment to others as a nurse might, by being consistently responsive to the infant's distress behavior and providing nurturing physical contact to promote affective regulation (Ainsworth & Bowlby, 1991).

The benefits of maintaining healthy attachment are applicable to children of any age and their caregivers. Potential barriers such as the presence of medical monitoring equipment, limitations to physical positioning, and the influence of sedatives and other medication can create separation between children and caregivers and jeopardize maintenance of a healthy bond. The music therapist may play a unique role in introducing simple ways for caregivers to maintain their roles as nurturers, despite challenges posed by the PICU environment.

Preparation. When the caregiver is present during sessions, the music therapist can attempt to foster an environment that is private and minimizes distractions and interruptions. Some caregivers will feel more comfortable singing if the bedside curtain is drawn, or if there are a minimal number of medical staff persons in the room. For infants and children who lack consistent caregiver support, the music therapist providing intervention will still work to decrease extraneous stimulation and promote a nurturing environment. The music therapist should confirm with the nurse that it is appropriate to hold or reposition the infant.

What to observe. An infant or child who is engaged in infant-directed singing with a caregiver, or who is being held and sung to by a caregiver or music therapist, may display changes in physiological parameters or in behavior state. When caregivers are present, the music therapist will also note the caregiver's emotional and behavioral responses to interacting with the infant, as a sign of the caregiver's own internal experience of the interaction.

Procedures. A variety of reciprocal musical interactions are used during music therapy to promote bonding. The music therapist may encourage the caregiver to use infant-directed speech and singing to promote the infant's awareness of and responsiveness to the caregiver. Caregivers are encouraged to use music of kin and familiar lullabies and children's songs while singing with the infant (Loewy et al., 2005). In order to put caregivers more at ease, the music therapist may model sung interactions with the infant before encouraging the caregiver to take the lead. Alternatively, the music therapist may encourage the caregiver to use familiar children's nursery rhymes or chants, or to begin the interaction with spoken voice and eventually progress to singing.

Similar concepts as those mentioned above can be adapted for older children in the PICU. If the medical staff assents, caregivers may hold the child or sit or lie with the child in his PICU bed to provide nurturing and caring touch. The music therapist may create a soothing musical context in which caregivers may feel more comfortable singing to the child while holding or cuddling with him. Music of kin can provide a familiar, supportive container for this experience of bonding (Loewy, 2009), which may help transcend the barriers to human connection that often arise in intensive care.

The music therapist can work with caregivers to create audio recordings of familiar songs, music of kin, and caregiver's spoken messages to the child, to be played in the caregiver's absence (Hanson-Abromeit, Shoemark, & Loewy, 2008). When creating recordings, the music therapist will work with the caregiver to promote the caregiver's stylistic preferences, while also considering the sensory needs of the child. The finished recording may be used at particular times, such as to soothe the child after distressing nursing cares, to promote sleep, or to stimulate the child when he is awake and alert. Readers seeking more detail on the use of music therapy to promote parent-infant bonding in medical and nonmedical contexts are encouraged to review Edwards (2011b) and Chapter 4 of the current volume.

Therapeutic Singing

Overview. Engaging a client in singing as a primary means of promoting health may be useful for some children within the PICU setting. Therapeutic singing is primarily helpful for promoting respiratory well-being and for impacting emotional well-being (Loveszy, 1991). A common use of therapeutic singing in the PICU environment is to promote deeper respiration and coughing to expel secretions following surgery and sedation. Children are often encouraged to cough at these times, but typically avoid doing so due to associated pain and discomfort. Music may provide motivation for singing, which in turn may lead to deeper inhalations and trigger coughing to expel secretions.

Singing personally salient songs with the music therapist may empower a child and allow him to express more of his inner experience. Singing literally "gives voice" to children who may be disempowered by the intensive care environment. A child's song selections may reveal his fears, hopes, and sources of strength. Songs of kin may be particularly poignant to the child and family within the PICU setting, helping them connect with a sense of familiarity, belonging, and home that in turn can promote therapeutic gains (Edwards & Kennelly, 2011; Loewy et al., 2005; Loveszy, 1991). The music therapist can provide musical accompaniment to support the child as he sings a favorite song and explores and integrates various aspects of himself.

Children who are experiencing complications from pulmonary diseases such as chronic asthma and cystic fibrosis, or severe acute conditions such as acute respiratory distress syndrome, may experience PICU hospitalization. The music therapist should confirm with the physician that singing is currently advisable for any child undergoing significant respiratory compromise.

Preparation. The music therapist will ascertain the child's musical preferences, and may provide musical accompaniment in accordance with those preferences. For example, some teenagers may prefer singing along to rhythmic and harmonic tracks that they create using recording software such as GarageBand.

What to observe. It may be beneficial to monitor any changes in physiological parameters, as improvements in oxygen saturation may be of interest to the treatment team. Songs can also be paired with the child's rate of breathing, and the tempo of songs should enable the child to breathe deeply between phrases.

Procedures. Certain children will be immediately comfortable with singing, even in the intensive environment of the PICU, while others will require much support and mild coaxing. Older children and adolescents may be inspired to sing when given a microphone that feeds into a recording device. Once the child expresses preferences for music to sing, as well as instrumentation for accompaniment, the child can choose to sing alone or have the therapist provide vocal support. As a child is singing, the therapist may subtly change musical qualities, including tempo and meter, to facilitate the child's supported singing of the song. Depending upon the child's preferences, family members may also partake in singing or in providing instrumental accompaniment (Edwards & Kennelly, 2011).

Children may find it particularly reassuring to sing familiar, personally salient songs with the therapist during anxiety-producing procedures such as dressing changes (Edwards & Kennelly, 2011; Loveszy, 1991). Recordings of a child singing these personally inspiring songs can be created for a child's later use during challenging periods of PICU hospitalization. For example, if a child is to undergo repeated painful or anxiety-producing procedures, the music therapist can record the child singing songs with supportive themes. The child can then gain support from this recording during procedures when the therapist is not able to be present.

Music-assisted Rehabilitation

Overview. As children emerge from coma or sedation and gain awareness of the environment around them in the PICU, they may also begin to receive greater levels of rehabilitation therapies. Music therapy is often one of the first forms of rehabilitative and supportive therapy offered to children in the PICU, due to the potential of music to impact children who are emerging from sedation, are unconscious, or are minimally conscious. Thus, the music therapist may have already developed rapport with a child when physical, occupational, or speech therapy services commence in the PICU.

Music-assisted rehabilitation includes a variety of approaches that optimize the use of music to impact various areas of neurologic functioning. The music therapist may cotreat with other rehabilitation therapists during a session, or may work alone during a session, but will incorporate musical techniques that promote rehabilitation goals. Musical elements of rhythm, tempo, meter, melodic contour, harmony, and timbre are drawn upon to stimulate specific responses such as localizing sound, reaching and grasping objects, increasing range of motion, prompting and regulating speech, promoting active cognition and recall, motivating improved head and trunk control, and stabilizing gait patterns (Hurt-Thaut & Johnson, 2003). Children who may be good candidates for music-assisted rehabilitation are those who are highly motivated by music or responsive to auditory stimuli, and have experienced brain injury, have survived multiple traumas, or are deconditioned following long periods of intubation and sedation.

Physicians determine when the initiation of rehabilitative therapies is indicated, including physical, occupational, and speech therapy. The music therapist should ensure that music therapy treatment planning is in alignment with the child's overall rehabilitation plan. The music therapist may need to provide more receptive approaches to music therapy intervention until the team deems that active forms of engagement are indicated. Music-assisted rehabilitation requires constant adaptation to adjust to the child's emerging abilities during the session. The process should be considered stable and unwavering as far as rationale and underlying theory, but fluid and responsive to the needs of the child as it is implemented over time.

Preparation. If cotreating with other disciplines, it behooves the music therapist to briefly meet with the cotherapist prior to the session to discuss each discipline's goals for the session. During the session, the therapists can communicate nonverbally or verbally to suggest to each other next steps to support and challenge the child. When coordinating their treatment efforts in the presence of the child, the therapists should remember to directly address the child, instead of talking about him without acknowledging him.

What to observe. Since physical therapy may include repositioning, such as transitioning to sitting and dangling feet off the side of the bed, the physical therapist will continue to monitor the child's oxygen saturation, heart rate, and respiratory rate to determine if the child is tolerating repositioning (Gutgsell, 2009). Physiological parameters and behavioral responses may be indicators that the child is uncomfortable or in significant pain. The music therapist will also note what instruments and music motivate the child to engage in rehabilitation therapies, and will try to maximize the use of these elements for the child's gain.

Procedures. If the session will focus primarily on physical or occupational therapy, with music therapy supporting the aims of those rehabilitation therapies, the music therapist may offer the child the chance to engage in music while working with rehabilitation therapy (Gutgsell, 2009). The music therapist may proceed with the child as in a typical session, and may offer the child certain instruments that promote movements and positions that are desired by the rehabilitation therapists. With this approach, as the child naturally plays the instrument as it is positioned in space, he engages in movements that are desired by the physical or occupational therapist (Hurt-Thaut & Johnson, 2003). For example, if the child is working on head control, the music therapist can position a novel-sounding instrument slightly above the child's head, so that he must raise his head to see the source of the sound. For a child who is improving neck control, the music therapist may alternate the position of a favorite drum from one side of the child to the other to encourage the child to turn his head to track and target the drum accordingly. The musical accompaniment that the music therapist provides may cue the pacing and direction of the child's movements using rhythmic and melodic cues (Hurt-Thaut & Johnson, 2003).

Musical elements may also support and cue various elements of speech, including pacing, articulation, and prosody. The music therapist will modify tempo, rhythm, melody, and harmony to support particular aspects of speech that are presenting a challenge to the child. Likewise, music may be used to elicit and assess cognitive skills for children undergoing rehabilitation. For example, a music therapist can note whether or not a child varies the tempo of his instrument playing to match the therapist as the therapist modifies this element (Rosenfeld & Dun, 1999).

Live music interaction offers advantages when used during rehabilitation as musical elements, including lyrics, may be adjusted in the moment to match a child's current needs and challenges. Thus, even though familiar and preferred music is frequently used to support the child during rehabilitation, there is also a certain level of improvisation required to optimize the music's therapeutic potential.

The examples provided above are but a few of the ways in which music therapy may be used to promote rehabilitative gains, and are considered representative samples, not an exhaustive listing. Readers desiring to learn more about the use of music therapy to promote rehabilitative gains can reference Ghetti and Hannan (2008), Hurt-Thaut and Johnson (2003), Thaut (2005), and Chapter 10 in this volume for more detailed information.

Therapeutic Music Instruction

Overview. Though used less frequently in the context of the PICU, there may be occasions when teaching a child to play an instrument can be useful for therapeutic reasons. Playing wind instruments may be indicated for children with pulmonary disorders such as asthma and cystic fibrosis, to improve pulmonary functioning and promote clearance of the airway (Griggs-Drane, 2009). As with therapeutic singing, the playing of wind instruments, such as the recorder, can also help children develop deeper respiration following major surgery. School-age children in music programs may have learned the recorder, and the therapist can utilize this pre-existing skill and familiarity to help a child make gains during the long recovery process following brain or cardiac surgery.

In therapeutic music instruction, the child benefits from either the process of playing the instrument itself (e.g., improving pulmonary functioning, developing fine motor skills) (Hannan, 2008) or the process of learning an instrument in general (e.g., improving attention span, increasing self-esteem). It may be both process- and product-oriented, as there are gains from the process as well as benefits derived from the overall outcome (e.g., improved expressive and leisure outlets) (Loveszy, 1991). Therapeutic music instruction may be an avenue for initiating interaction with adolescents and young adults, especially those who are resistant to engage with the therapist otherwise. The use of this approach is more feasible for children who are likely to experience an extended PICU stay, though the music therapist might also give one- or two-session lessons on using music software, playing basic beats on drums, or learning fundamentals about the guitar or keyboard.

Learning a new instrument requires time, ample patience, and good frustration tolerance. Some children will need lots of support to try something new and challenging when they might already be taxed from the stressors of the PICU environment. As the music therapist structures therapeutic music instruction sessions, she should keep in mind the goal of enabling the child to experience some level of success and mastery within each session.

Preparation. The music therapist should ensure that the instruments offered for instruction are viable options for the child to play, and that there are not any positioning-related obstacles to their use. Depending upon the child's developmental level, the music therapist may adapt sheet music or instruments in advance of the session (Loveszy, 1991). Examples of adaptation include the use of colored dots on the keyboard or guitar fingerboard, the use of tape to cover holes on the recorder, and color- or letter-coding on music or lyric sheets.

What to observe. Throughout the instruction, the music therapist will monitor the child's level of frustration and provide subtle modifications as needed to ensure that the child experiences some level of success with the instrument. The music therapist will also monitor the responses of other individuals in the environment, as the therapist should weigh the costs and benefits of equipping a child with a new instrument to practice in the PICU environment, including any annoyances this may cause others.

Procedures. The therapist will make efforts to incorporate the child's music preferences and let the child choose the song to be learned. Some children benefit from watching the music therapist play the instrument at the same time as the child, to model. When doing so, it may be helpful for the therapist to position herself alongside the child, so that the child does not have to correct for a reversed image (as would happen if the therapist sat directly across from the child).

The therapist will modify tempo and simplify music if needed, to ease the learning experience and facilitate mastery. To end the instruction with a sense of accomplishment, the music therapist should conclude the intervention with something that would enable the child to demonstrate what he has successfully learned. Therapeutic music instruction sessions can be videotaped and burned onto DVD(s) so that the child can independently practice on his own.

Infection control procedures for cleaning instruments such as guitars and keyboards before and after individual patient use will follow the guidelines established by the hospital's epidemiology or infection control department for cleaning musical instruments. Certain instruments that trap moisture, such as recorders, may not be approved for use between patients, and thus the therapist may need to provide a new instrument for each child to use and keep. Other instruments, such as the guitar, may be wiped down with hospital-approved disinfectant wipes before and after patient use. The music therapist will need to ensure that clear cleaning policies are in place for the full range of musical instruments and equipment that may be used in a PICU music therapy program.

GUIDELINES FOR COMPOSITIONAL MUSIC THERAPY

Songwriting

Overview. Improvised song was discussed in the improvisation methods section, but more structured forms of songwriting will be discussed here. The creation of songs serves as an avenue to communicate content to others, a forum for safely expressing a wide range of emotions, and a means for building self-awareness (Baker, Kennelly, & Tamplin, 2005b). There are many variations to the compositional approach to songwriting, including substituting lyrics in precomposed songs through fill-in-the-blank or song parody approaches, adding additional verses to precomposed songs, setting words or poetry to music, and creating original music and lyrics. The music therapist should match the songwriting method to the child's developmental level and attention span, for optimal effectiveness. Goals of engaging a child in the songwriting process include facilitating emotional expression, improving cognitive skills, promoting positive self-esteem, increasing coping skills and awareness of inner resources, and promoting social connectivity. Children who have recently experienced traumatic brain injury may benefit from the more heavily structured approaches, such as fill-in-the-blank or song parody (Baker, Kennelly, & Tamplin, 2005a).

Preparation. Depending upon the songwriting method chosen, the music therapist may bring in lyrics sheets with blanks, song lyrics, lead sheets, or various chord progressions. Some children in the PICU will be able to read and work from these sheets, while others may not be able to read or hold a paper, and thus the music therapist will facilitate the child's verbal/vocal engagement in the songwriting process. If the guardian has consented and the child has assented, the music therapist can audio record the songwriting session as a way to document it or create a final product for the child to keep. Conversely, the music therapist can note the child's lyrics, the chords chosen, and any melodic motifs, to later provide the child with a hard copy of the lyrics to keep. Though they may not read music, other children may find it quite significant to receive a transcription of their song, and it may become a source of pride and achievement (Aasgaard, 2005).

What to observe. The music therapist will observe the child's behavioral and emotional responses to the songwriting process and will take note of any significant themes that emerge from the process.

Procedures. In most cases, the child should choose the song's theme. It is important that the child remain in control of the creative expression, and thus the therapist should avoid giving in to the temptation to alter song lyrics or take control of the songwriting (Aasgaard, 2005). The therapist will either choose the amount of structure that would be most helpful to the child, given the child's individual characteristics, or offer the child or adolescent an option of songwriting approaches.

When a music therapist uses a fill-in-the-blank approach, she prompts the child to substitute a portion of new lyrics in place of original ones. Fill-in-the-blank provides the highest level of structure and places the least amount of demand upon the child. In the song parody approach, a child creates a full set of new lyrics but retains the song's original melody and musical structure (Baker et al., 2005a). The music therapist might also offer songwriting with a preset format, such as the AAB structure of the 12-bar blues. For any of these structured approaches, the therapist can sing the original song or a verse as a demonstration; for fill-in-the-blank, she can sing the retained lyrics and pause at the blanks to prompt the child to fill in a word.

Recording software such as GarageBand or Band-in-a-Box allows children and adolescents to specify the genre of music they wish to evoke in their composed song. A wide range of musical styles, including modern R&B, hip-hop, reggae, reggaeton, pop, and country is possible, given such software. Alternatively, many piano keyboards offer chordal accompaniment styles representative of various genres of music. The therapist can offer the child a broad range of musical styles and chord progressions from which to choose for original compositions or to "remix" or alter the sound of precomposed songs for which they are modifying lyrics. The emphasis remains on enabling the child to thoroughly express himself and engage in a creative process to the fullest extent possible.

Some children and adolescents will view the songwriting process as highly private, and will not want to share the final song with anyone other than the therapist (Aasgaard, 2005). This preference for privacy should be respected, and the client should not be pressured into recording or sharing the song with others. Readers seeking more detail on the use of structured songwriting approaches with hospitalized and nonhospitalized children are encouraged to review Baker and Wigram (2005).

There may be occasions when a child desires family members to partake in the songwriting or song recording process. Music therapy provides a normalized and contained context for the exploring and sharing of feelings between family members. The therapist will need to skillfully moderate this process for times when a caregiver becomes overbearing in the creative process. Gentle redirections back to the child's opinions, choices, and input may be required.

Alternatively, a music therapist may decide that a caregiver or sibling could benefit from a deeper, personal expressive process, and may offer a private session in which a caregiver or sibling can write a song to work through their feelings and struggles or to specifically express something to the child. When a child is minimally responsive or aware of his environment, the music therapist may use songwriting with the caregiver to provide an expressive outlet and a means to process the caregiver's experience.

Music therapists may write songs for their clients when they seek specific music to achieve certain aims (Baker & Wigram, 2005). Such songs may be used to help a child understand or work through a hospital-related challenge (such as a particular procedure, a diagnosis, or coping with hospitalization in general) or to support a child's successful engagement in a cognitive, communicative, or motor skill challenge.

Audio or Video Recording Creation

Overview. Capturing the outcomes of the creative music process through audio or video recording enables the child to retain and re-experience the benefits of that process. The recording becomes a resource upon which the child and family can draw during future times of challenge or celebration. A range of recording options are available and are matched to the child's abilities, needs, and length of stay in the PICU.

The recording process and final product offer a number of benefits, including development of an expressive outlet, validation of emotions and self-worth, improved self-esteem, increased choice-making, empowerment, increased attention span, improved follow-through with a long-term goal, and improved social connectivity. Video recordings typically take several sessions for completion, and thus the music therapist offering this approach to a child should ensure that adequate time is available for the child to experience some level of completion with the creative process (Robb & Ebberts, 2003b).

Preparation. In the PICU, it is rare that a child will be stable enough to ambulate or transfer to a separate music therapy room or quiet room for recording, and thus most recording will occur in the child's room. Consequently, the reality of audio or video recording in the PICU is that the recording is likely to inadvertently include environmental sounds such as intravenous pump alarms, overhead paging, and the conversations of medical staff or roommates. Most children will be less bothered by these extraneous sounds on the recording than the therapist will, but the therapist may try to work with staff in the room to temporarily make the space as quiet as possible.

What to observe. The music therapist will observe how comfortable a child is during all phases of the recording process, and will provide support, structure, and encouragement as needed. Emotional responses to the process and final product will serve as indicators of the value of the recording to the child.

Procedures. Composing and audio recording songs may occur within a single session, or may extend across several sessions. Music videos can take several sessions to move through the stages of concept design, storyboarding, song/music selection, video recording, and final editing (Robb & Ebberts, 2003a, 2003b). The music therapist will suggest various approaches to audio and video recording based on the child's anticipated length of stay, developmental level, attention span, stamina, and clinical need. Depending upon the child's wishes, family members or significant hospital staff can be incorporated into the audio or video recording.

Digital voice recorders, MiniDisc recorders, and iPod Touches or iPads (or other tablets) can be used for quick, single-session recordings. These devices tend to be small and easily portable, making them less intimidating to the child and easier to position within the tight quarters of the PICU. For multisession recordings, a music therapist may use a laptop with recording software or an iPad with recording software. Hardware that is battery-powered or bus-powered and minimizes the use of long cables is advantageous in the PICU due to spatial restrictions and the presence of multiple cables related to continuous vital sign and hemodynamic monitoring.

Song composition approaches were discussed in the previous section, and any approach to songwriting (as well as improvised song creation) is valid when creating songs for recording. Some children will actively partake in writing songs, but will want the music therapist to sing on the recording (Aasgaard, 2005). Other children will request to have staff or family members sing or play instruments for the recording. The music therapist will empower the child to actively direct the creation of the recording and take part in all relevant decision-making. Older children and adolescents may be capable of implementing most or all steps of the recording process, given support.

Video may be captured via iPod Touch, iPad, or video camera, and subsequently edited using video editing software on a laptop or desktop computer. Prior to commencing a video project, the music therapist may find it helpful to show the child a sample music video to help elucidate the scope of possibilities for the project (Robb & Ebberts, 2003a). The child may then choose a personally relevant song to use for the project, or choose from a selection of songs that the therapist has identified as being potentially pertinent for the child. If the child's family lives nearby, they can bring photographs or personal items from home that the child would want to include in the video recording (Robb & Ebberts, 2003a). This process of incorporating pictures and items from home may reinforce the connection between the child as he exists outside of the hospital and his current world inside the PICU.

Recordings may be made from songs that caregivers write for their hospitalized children. Such recordings played at the child's bedside may be valuable in promoting alertness and responsiveness to the environment, especially for children regaining consciousness. In such situations, the music therapist can monitor the use of caregiver recordings to ensure that they are functioning to orient and assure the child, and are not confusing the child. Engaging caregivers in the process of creating audio recordings can help provide a safe space for processing mixed emotions and acknowledging and working through doubts and fears. Depending upon the focus of the recording and the caregiver's needs, recordings may take place at the child's bedside or during individual caregiver music therapy sessions in a private location in the unit.

Older children and adolescents who are approaching end-of-life in the PICU may use the songwriting and recording process to express sentiments to significant others and in so doing create a living legacy. The recordings themselves have a life that may surpass that of the child, and they may take on new significance after a child has died (Lindenfelser, 2005). Songs written in music therapy may be played during memorial services (Lindenfelser et al., 2008), or families may use them as a supportive tool to cope with anniversaries and holidays, when the absence of the child is most acutely felt. Readers interested in learning more about the use of audio and video recordings for hospitalized and nonhospitalized children are referred to Aasgaard (2005), Baker and Wigram (2005), and Robb and Ebberts (2003a, 2003b).

RESEARCH EVIDENCE

Outcomes of music therapy with children in the PICU are most commonly described in the literature through anecdotal or case reports (e.g., Dun, 1995; Ghetti & Hannan, 2008; Kennelly & Edwards, 1997; Rosenfeld & Dun, 1999), although a limited number of empirical studies exist (e.g., del Olmo et al., 2010; Hatem, Lira, & Mattos, 2006; Stouffer & Shirk, 2003). Specific outcomes of the few empirical studies of music therapy in the PICU will be described in greater detail within the corresponding music therapy clinical approach sections below.

Meta-analytic reviews of outcomes for hospitalized children may include children in the PICU. A meta-analysis of music-based interventions used during medical treatment of pediatric clients demonstrated an overall mean effect size of .64 (p = .00), indicating a moderate effect (Standley & Whipple, 2003). In particular, children who underwent major invasive procedures, including bone marrow aspiration, wound debridement, and postoperative recovery, demonstrated significantly greater benefits (d = .91) from music intervention than children who underwent minor invasive procedures such as venipuncture and injections (d = .37). Interventions using live music led to greater benefits than those using recorded music (live music d = .82; recorded music d = .55), and results suggested greater therapeutic benefit for adolescents and infants than for children of ages 4 to 12 years (adolescents d = 1.36; infants/children less than 4 years d = .74; children 4 to 12 years d = .43) (Standley & Whipple, 2003).

Authors have identified a lack of music therapy research studies carried out in pediatric intensive care settings to date (Austin, 2010; Ghetti & Hannan, 2008). However, there are several studies of music-based interventions in the PICU not designed or carried out by music therapists that are mislabeled as "music therapy" in the literature. Inconsistencies regarding the definition of music therapy within research studies continue to persist. For example, some systematic reviews examining music therapy in the pediatric healthcare domain define music therapy as involving a therapeutic relationship with a trained therapist (i.e., music therapist), but then include music medicine articles with no music therapist involvement within their reviewed articles (e.g., Mrázová & Celec, 2010; Treurnicht Naylor, Kingsnorth, Lamont, McKeever, & Macarthur, 2011). A systematic analysis of the research literature concluded that studies using a music therapist to implement interventions were found to be more likely to have positive outcomes than music interventions led by a health professional or researcher (Treurnicht Naylor et al., 2011). However, caution must be taken in interpreting the aforementioned conclusion, as the authors were not able to complete meta-analytic statistical analysis due to significant heterogeneity in study interventions, outcomes, and measurement tools (Treurnicht Naylor et al., 2011).

Research studies with adult intensive care clients will be discussed sparingly in the following sections where pediatric studies are nonexistent and the content area remains directly applicable to pediatric populations. It is hoped that future studies targeting the needs and responses of children in the PICU will help elucidate whether children respond to music therapy similarly to adults in intensive care, or whether they stand to uniquely benefit from services in this setting. There were no studies identified that investigated the use of compositional or re-creative forms of music therapy for children or adolescents in the PICU.

Receptive Music Therapy

The most commonly researched clinical application of music therapy with adults or children in intensive care is receptive methods. In a preliminary report, Polomano, Shirk, and Stouffer (2002) described the outcomes of the use of recorded sedative music paired with mother's voice compared to sedative music alone or blank audiotape with 29 children of ages 3 months to 8 years who were receiving mechanical ventilation. Children who listened to sedative music paired with mother's voice demonstrated improved sedation levels (p < .05) on the Sedation-Agitation Scale, with a significant carryover effect at 60 minutes (p < .01) when compared to sedative music listening alone or blank audiotapes (Polomano, Shirk, & Stouffer, 2002). Music audiotapes contained seven to nine songs from the client's preferred music, recorded by the music therapist, who adjusted the songs to emphasize sedative qualities. Primary caregivers were invited to sing along with the songs or to read books with the sedative music in the background of the recording. Tapes were 20 minutes in length and played two times daily at points when nursing staff deemed the ventilated children to be exhibiting signs of agitation (Stouffer & Shirk, 2003).

Hatem et al. (2006) completed a randomized controlled trial with 84 children of ages 1 day to 16 years immediately following cardiac surgery. It is not clear whether the study actually included a music therapist for design or implementation of the "music therapy" intervention, or whether other medical professionals implemented all phases of the research. Children who listened to 30 minutes of researcher-selected classical music with sedative properties demonstrated lower heart rate (p = .04) and respiratory rate (*p* = .02) as well as less observed pain (*p* < .001) than children who listened to a blank CD. The authors acknowledged the importance of musical preference, as two children refused to participate in the study due to its use of classical music.

Research with 51 adults in the ICU suggests other benefits of music therapy that might be applicable to children, though further research is needed to confirm this supposition. Adults who were weaning from mechanical ventilation and received music therapy sessions using client-preferred music as part of receptive, re-creative and compositional approaches demonstrated significant decreases in heart rate (*p* = .026) and respiratory rate (*p* = .000) at the study conclusion, though the study did not include a control group for comparison (Hunter et al., 2010). When providing music therapy, the therapist started services 20 minutes prior to the transition from ventilator to *tracheostomy collar* and continued for approximately 40 minutes into the weaning trial, as anxiety was clinically observed to be highest during this period.

In a crossover design, 22 adults experiencing posttraumatic amnesia received brief music therapy sessions using either live, client-preferred music or recorded versions of the same client-preferred music performed by the original artists. The results indicated significant improvements in orientation on the Westmead PTA Scale (*p* < .001) and reductions in agitation as measured by the Agitated Behavior Scale (*p* < .0001) in the music conditions as compared to the no-music control condition, regardless of whether the music presented was live or recorded (Baker, 2001). The study supports the use of familiar, client-preferred music to promote orientation and reduce agitation, and did not demonstrate a statistically significant difference between the use of live music or recorded music. Importantly, Baker (2001) demonstrated that music therapy and recorded music are not contraindicated for individuals experiencing posttraumatic amnesia, though they caution that such interventions should be systematically and sensitively administered.

Improvisational Music Therapy

One study of 87 infants in the PICU examined the use of live, improvised music (incorporating caregiver's voice if desired) that matched aspects of infant's breathing and vocalizations or crying (del Olmo et al., 2010). The tempo of the improvised music was matched to the infant's rate of breathing and then reduced to 80 or 90 bpm, and the tonality of the music (major vs. minor) was likewise matched to the infant's vocalizations or cries. Heart rate (HR) decreased significantly more (*p* = .014) in infants receiving the live, infant-specific music (mean difference = −6.82, *SD* = 14.21) as compared to infants who were held by caregivers without receiving music (mean difference = 0.19, *SD* = 17.42) (del Olmo et al., 2010). The authors purport that heart rate decreased more (*p* = 0.02) when binary rhythms (mean = 135.00, SD = 18.40) were used, as opposed to when ternary rhythms were used (mean = 138.32; SD = 20.27), which they state is due to heart rate being binary in nature.

Research Conclusions and Implications

The music therapy literature is surprisingly devoid of studies pertaining to pediatric intensive care. The profession would be well-served by targeting this clinical area for quantitative and qualitative investigation. As music therapists partake in research within the PICU setting, they are encouraged to follow recommendations for improving methodological integrity. Researchers should take care to clearly define music therapy, provide sufficient detail in the description of clinical methods to enable replication, and include sufficient sample sizes to ensure adequate statistical power. Music therapists engaging in research are encouraged to review reporting standards for music interventions suggested by Robb, Burns, and Carpenter (2011), and adhere to reporting guidelines for randomized controlled trials (CONSORT

2010) or nonrandomized clinical trials (TREND 2004). Expanding the scope of interdisciplinary research in music therapy may help encourage depth and breadth in the examination of outcomes. Additionally, outcomes from basic science research on the impact of music on the brain may help highlight the ability of music-based interventions to impact neuroplasticity, attention control, and hormonal responses (Mrázová & Celec, 2010).

SUMMARY AND CONCLUSIONS

The description of music therapy clinical approaches discussed within this chapter aims to be comprehensive, though by no means is it exhaustive. There may be additional areas of practice that are valid and indicated for the PICU setting that have not been included here. For example, music therapists who are dual-certified as Certified Child Life Specialists, or those whose job descriptions include portions of this area of practice, may provide medical preparation for procedures and surgery through music therapy approaches. Such individuals may integrate the fields of child life and music therapy, using improvisational music therapy methods to allow children to explore their feelings toward diagnosis or treatment and to convey developmentally appropriate medical teaching when needed (Ghetti, 2011b). What is clear from this review of clinical approaches is that music therapy can be flexibly utilized to provide children in the PICU with opportunities for working through challenges, experiencing growth, and connecting with others. Music therapists who enable these gains to occur within the PICU are ultimately the ones responsible for also engaging in clinical writing and research to bring awareness of the validity of this work to a larger audience.

GLOSSARY

The following definitions are adapted from online versions of the *American Heritage Medical Dictionary* (2007), *Miller-Keane Encyclopedia and Dictionary of Medicine, Nursing, and Allied Health* (2003), and *Mosby's Medical Dictionary* (2009).

Arrhythmias: irregularities in the rhythm or force of the heartbeat.

Bilevel positive airway pressure (BiPAP): a form of invasive or noninvasive ventilation that provides two levels of ventilatory assistance, including a steady flow of air for inhalations and a lower level of positive pressure to make exhalations easier.

Central venous pressure: blood pressure within the large veins of the body.

Congenital heart disease: heart disease that is present at birth and may include arrythmias and structural defects.

Contact isolation: isolating an individual and instituting the use of personal protective equipment (i.e., gown and gloves) for all those who come into contact with that individual to prevent contact transmission of infectious agents.

Continuous arterial pressure: level of stress on the walls of the arteries from circulating blood.

Continuous positive airway pressure (CPAP): a form of invasive or noninvasive ventilation in which a steady flow of air is delivered under constant pressure to increase oxygenation and reduce the work of breathing.

Diabetic ketoacidosis: a potentially life-threatening complication of diabetes mellitus.

Droplet isolation: isolating an individual and instituting the use of personal protective equipment (i.e., gown, gloves, and mask) for all those who come into contact with that individual to prevent droplet transmission of infectious agents.

Dysrhythmia: any irregularity in the rhythm of the heartbeat.

Endotracheal tube: a flexible plastic tube inserted into the trachea to provide a stable airway.

End tidal carbon dioxide levels: the level of carbon dioxide in a person's exhalation.

Exchange transfusion: a treatment wherein an individual's red blood cells or platelets are exchanged and replaced with transfused blood products.

Intracranial pressure: pressure that exists within the cranial cavity.

Lyme disease: a bacterial infection spread through the bite of an infected tick. Symptoms resemble those of the flu. Untreated, Lyme disease can spread to the brain, heart, and joints.

Meningitis: a life-threatening medical condition that may be caused by viruses or bacteria, in which the protective membranes that cover the brain and spinal cord become inflamed.

Multiple organ dysfunction syndrome: occurs in critically ill individuals when two or more organ systems fail due to progressive, interrelated events.

Nasogastric tube: a tube that passes through the nose into the stomach.

Oxygen saturation: a measure of the amount of oxygen that is carried in the blood.

Post–cardiopulmonary resuscitation: the time period following restoration of heart and lung function after cardiac arrest.

Pulmonary arterial pressure: pressure that exists within the pulmonary artery.

Renal insufficiency: partial failure of kidney function.

Renal failure: failure of kidney function, which may be short-term or chronic in nature.

Respiratory isolation: isolating an individual and instituting the use of personal protective equipment (i.e., respirator-type mask) for all those who come into contact with that individual to prevent airborne transmission of infectious agents.

Severe anemia: a marked loss of red blood cell mass that may be fatal if not treated.

Shock: a life-threatening condition that occurs when the body does not get enough blood flow to tissues, which can cause damage to multiple organs.

Sickle-cell anemia: a severe, chronic condition of abnormal red blood cells, which, due to their abnormal shape, may block blood vessels, resulting in pain crises, blood clots, and other issues.

Spina bifida: a birth defect in which the backbone and spinal canal do not close before birth.

Tracheostomy: a surgically created opening in the neck into the trachea through which tubing may be inserted to provide a stable airway.

Tracheostomy collar: a mist collar that attaches over the tracheostomy site to provide moisture.

REFERENCES

Aasgaard, T. (2005). Assisting children with malignant blood disease to create and perform their own songs. In F. Baker & T. Wigram (Eds.), *Songwriting: Methods, techniques and clinical approaches for music therapy clinicians, educators and students* (pp. 154–179). Philadelphia, PA: Jessica Kingsley.

Ainsworth, M. D., & Bowlby, J. (1991). An ethological approach to personality development. *American Psychologist, 46*(4), 333–341.

American Academy of Pediatrics, Committee on Hospital Care and Pediatric Section of the Society of Critical Care Medicine. (1999). Guidelines for developing admission and discharge policies for the pediatric intensive care unit. *Pediatrics, 103*(4), 840–842.

American Heritage Medical Dictionary. (2007). Retrieved from http://medical-dictionary.thefreedictionary.com

Austin, D. (2010). The psychophysiological effects of music therapy in intensive care units. *Paediatric Nursing, 22*(3), 14–20.

Ayson, C. (2008). Child-parent wellbeing in a paediatric ward: The role of music therapy in supporting children and their parents facing the challenge of hospitalisation. *Voices: A World Forum for Music Therapy, 8*(1). Retrieved from https://normt.uib.no/index.php/voices/article/view/449/367

Baker, F. (2001). The effects of live, taped, and no music on people experiencing posttraumatic amnesia. *Journal of Music Therapy, 38*(3), 170–192.

Baker, F., Kennelly, J., & Tamplin, J. (2005a). Songwriting to explore identity change and sense of self-concept following traumatic brain injury. In F. Baker & T. Wigram (Eds.), *Songwriting: Methods, techniques and clinical applications for music therapy clinicians, educators, and students* (pp. 116–133). Philadelphia, PA: Jessica Kingsley.

Baker, F., Kennelly, J., & Tamplin, J. (2005b). Themes within songs written by people with traumatic brain injury: Gender differences. *Journal of Music Therapy, 42*(2), 111–122.

Baker, F., & Wigram, T. (Eds.). (2005). *Songwriting: Methods, techniques and clinical applications for music therapy clinicians, educators, and students.* Philadelphia, PA: Jessica Kingsley.

Board, R. (2005). School-age children's perceptions of their PICU hospitalization. *Pediatric Nursing, 31*(3), 166–175.

Bradt, J. (2009). Music entrainment for breathing regulation. In R. Azoulay & J. V. Loewy (Eds.), *Music, the breath and health: Advances in integrative music therapy* (pp. 11–19). New York: Satchnote Press.

Bradt, J., Dileo, C., & Grocke, D. (2010). Music for anxiety reduction in mechanically ventilated patients. *Cochrane Database of Systematic Reviews, 2010, 12.* Art. no.: CD006902. DOI: 10.1002/14651858.CD006902.pub2.

Bruscia, K. E. (1998). *Defining music therapy* (2nd ed.). Gilsum, NH: Barcelona Publishers.

Chlan, L., & Heiderscheit, A. (2009). A tool for music preference assessment in critically ill patients receiving mechanical ventilation. *Music Therapy Perspectives, 27*(1), 42–47.

del Olmo, M. J., Rodríquez Garrido, C., & Ruza Tarrío, F. (2010). Music therapy in the PICU: 0- to 6-month-old babies. *Music and Medicine, 2*(3), 158–166. DOI: 10.1177/1943862110370462.

Delabary, A. M. L. (2004). Music inside an intensive care unit. *Voices: A World Forum for Music Therapy.* Retrieved from https://normt.uib.no/index.php/voices/article/view/178/137

Dun, B. (1995). A different beat: Music therapy in children's cardiac care. *Music Therapy Perspectives, 13,* 35–39.

Edwards, J. (2011a). The use of music therapy to promote attachment between parents and infants. *The Arts in Psychotherapy, 38,* 190–195.

Edwards, J. (Ed.). (2011b). *Music therapy and parent-infant bonding.* Oxford: Oxford University Press.

Edwards, J., & Kennelly, J. (2011). Music therapy for children in hospital care: A stress and coping framework for practice. In A. Meadows (Ed.), *Developments in music therapy practice: Case study perspectives* (pp. 150–165). Gilsum, NH: Barcelona Publishers.

Eschrich, S., Münte, T. F., & Altenmüller, E. O. (2008). Unforgettable film music: The role of emotion in episodic long-term memory for music. *BioMed Central Neuroscience, 9*(48). Retrieved from http://www.biomedcentral.com/1471-2202/9/48

Fagen, T. S. (1982). Music therapy in the treatment of anxiety and fear in terminal pediatric patients. *Music Therapy, 2*(1), 13–23.

Ferraz, C. (2003). A personal experience in the process of implementing music therapy in a hospital in Brazil. *Voices: A World Forum for Music Therapy, 3*(3). Retrieved from https://normt.uib.no/index.php/voices/article/viewArticle/135/111

Froehlich, M. A. (Ed.). (1996a). *Music therapy with hospitalized children: A creative arts child life approach.* Cherry Hill, NJ: Jeffrey Books.

Froehlich, M. A. (1996b). Orff-Schulwerk music therapy in crisis intervention with hospitalized children. In M. A. Froehlich (Ed.), *Music therapy with hospitalized children: A creative arts child life approach* (pp. 25–36). Cherry Hill, NJ: Jeffrey Books.

Ghetti, C. M. (2011a). Active music engagement with emotional-approach coping to improve well-being in liver and kidney transplant recipients. *Journal of Music Therapy, 48*(4), 463–485.

Ghetti, C. M. (2011b). Clinical practice of dual-certified music therapists/child life specialists: A phenomenological study. *Journal of Music Therapy, 48*(3), 317–345.

Ghetti, C. M. (2012). Music therapy as procedural support for invasive medical procedures: Toward the development of music therapy theory. *Nordic Journal of Music Therapy, 21*(1), 3–35.

Ghetti, C. M., & Hannan, A. (2008). Pediatric intensive care unit (PICU). In D. Hanson-Abromeit & C. Colwell (Eds.), *Effective clinical practice in music therapy: Medical music therapy for pediatrics* (pp. 71–106). Silver Spring, MD: American Music Therapy Association.

Ghetti, C. M., & Walker, J. (2008). Hematology, oncology, and bone-marrow transplant. In D. Hanson-Abromeit & C. Colwell (Eds.), *Effective clinical practice in music therapy: Medical music therapy for pediatrics* (pp. 147–193). Silver Spring, MD: American Music Therapy Association.

Goforth, K. E. (2008). Collaborating goals and interventions to effectively promote psychosocial development of pediatric patients during hospitalization: A survey of music therapists and child life specialists. *Electronic Theses, Treatises and Dissertations* (Paper 4212).

Griggs-Drane, E. (2009). The use of musical wind instruments with patients who have pulmonary diseases: Clinical recommendations for music therapists. In R. Azoulay & J. V. Loewy (Eds.), *Music, the breath and health: Advances in integrative music therapy* (pp. 103–116). New York: Satchnote Press.

Gutgsell, K. J. (2009). Integrative music therapy and physical therapy for patients on mechanical ventilation. In R. Azoulay & J. V. Loewy (Eds.), *Music, the breath and health: Advances in integrative music therapy* (pp. 171–178). New York: Satchnote Press.

Hannan, A. (2008). General pediatrics medical/surgical. In D. Hanson-Abromeit & C. Colwell (Eds.), *Effective clinical practice in music therapy: Medical music therapy for pediatrics* (pp. 107–146). Silver Spring, MD: American Music Therapy Association.

Hanson-Abromeit, D., & Colwell, C. (Eds.). (2008). *Effective clinical practice in music therapy: Medical music therapy for pediatrics in hospital settings.* Silver Spring, MD: American Music Therapy Association.

Hanson-Abromeit, D., Shoemark, H., & Loewy, J. V. (2008). Newborn intensive care unit (NICU). In D. Hanson-Abromeit & C. Colwell (Eds.), *Effective clinical practice in music therapy: Medical music therapy for pediatrics* (pp. 15–69). Silver Spring, MD: American Music Therapy Association.

Hatem, T. P., Lira, P. I., & Mattos, S. S. (2006). The therapeutic effects of music in children following cardiac surgery. *Jornal de pediatria, 82*(3), 186–192. DOI: 10.2223/JPED.1473.

Hunter, B. C., Oliva, R., Sahler, O. J., Gaisser, D., Salipante, D. M., & Arezina, C. H. (2010). Music therapy as an adjunctive treatment in the management of stress for patients being weaned from mechanical ventilation. *Journal of Music Therapy, 47*(3), 198–219.

Hurt-Thaut, C., & Johnson, S. (2003). Neurologic music therapy with children: Scientific foundations and clinical application. In S. L. Robb (Ed.), *Music therapy in pediatric healthcare: Research and evidence-based practice* (pp. 81–100). Silver Spring, MD: American Music Therapy Association, Inc.

Kallay, V. (1997). Music therapy applications in the pediatric medical setting: Child development, pain management and choices. In J. V. Loewy (Ed.), *Music therapy and pediatric pain* (pp. 33–43). Cherry Hill, NJ: Jeffrey Books.

Karmarkar, S., & Varshney, S. (2008). Tracheal extubation. *Continuing Education in Anaesthesia, Critical Care & Pain, 8*(6), 214–220.

Katzenell, U., & Segal, S. (2001). Hyperacusis: Review and clinical guidelines. *Otology & Neurotology, 22,* 321–327.

Keller, I., Hulsdunk, A., & Muller, F. (2007). The influence of acoustic and tactile stimulation on vegetative parameters and eeg in persistent vegetative state. *Functional Neurology, 22*(3), 159–163.

Kemper, K. J., & Danhauer, S. C. (2005). Music as therapy. *Southern Medical Journal, 98*(3), 282–288.

Kennelly, J. (2000). The specialist role of the music therapist in developmental programs for hospitalized children. *Journal of Pediatric Health Care, 14,* 56–69.

Kennelly, J., & Edwards, J. (1997). Providing music therapy to the unconscious child in the paediatric intensive care unit. *The Australian Journal of Music Therapy, 8,* 18–29.

Kotchoubey, B., Lang, S., Herb, E., Maurer, P., Schmalohr, D., Bostanov, V., & Birbaumer, N. (2003). Stimulus complexity enhances auditory discrimination in patients with extremely severe brain injuries. *Neuroscience Letters, 352,* 129–132.

Lam, C.-W. (2007). A survey of music therapists working in medical hospitals. *Electronic Theses, Treatises and Dissertations* (Paper 3308).

Laureys, S., Perrin, F., Faymonville, M.-E., Schnakers, C., Boly, M., Bartsch, V., Majerus, S., Moonen, G., & Maquet, P. (2004). Cerebral processing in the minimally conscious state. *Neurology, 63,* 916–918.

Lee, O. K. A., Chung, Y. F. L., Chan, M. F., & Chan, W. M. (2005). Music and its effect on the physiological responses and anxiety levels of patients receiving mechanical ventilation: A pilot study. *Journal of Clinical Nursing, 14,* 609–620.

Lindenfelser, K. (2005). Parents' voices supporting music therapy within pediatric palliative care. *Voices: A World Forum for Music Therapy, 5*(3). Retrieved from https://normt.uib.no/index.php/voices/article/view/233/177

Lindenfelser, K., Grocke, D. E., & McFerran, K. (2008). Bereaved parents' experiences of music therapy with their terminally ill child. *Journal of Music Therapy, 45*(3), 330–348.

Loewy, J. V. (2002). Song sensitation: How fragile we are. In J. V. Loewy & A. F. Hara (Eds.), *Caring for the caregiver: The use of music and music therapy in grief and trauma* (pp. 33–43). Silver Spring, MD: AMTA.

Loewy, J. V. (2009). Musical sedation: Mechanisms of breathing entrainment. In R. Azoulay and J. V. Loewy (Eds.), *Music, the breath and health: Advances in integrative music therapy* (pp. 223–231). New York: Satchnote Press.

Loewy, J., Hallan, C., Friedman, E., & Martinez, C. (2005). Sleep/sedation in children undergoing EEG testing: A comparison of chloral hydrate and music therapy. *Journal of Perianethesia Nursing, 20*(5), 323–331.

Loewy, J., MacGregor, B., Richards, K., & Rodriguez, J. (1997). Music therapy pediatric pain management: Assessing and attending to the sounds of hurt, fear and anxiety. In J. V. Loewy (Ed.), *Music therapy and pediatric pain* (pp. 45–56). Cherry Hill, NJ: Jeffrey Books.

Loewy, J. V., & Stewart, K. (2004). Music therapy to help traumatized children and caregivers. In N. B. Webb (Ed.), *Mass trauma and violence: Helping families and children cope* (pp. 191–215). New York: The Guilford Press.

Loewy, J. V., & Stewart, A. (2005). The use of lullabies as a transient motif in ending life. In C. Dileo & J. V. Loewy (Eds.), *Music therapy at the end of life* (pp. 141–148). Cherry Hill, NJ: Jeffrey Books.

Lorenzato, K. I. (2005). *Filling a need while making some noise: A music therapist's guide to pediatrics.* Philadelphia, PA: Jessica Kingsley.

Loveszy, R. (1991). The use of latin music, puppetry, and visualization in reducing the physical and emotional pain of a child with severe burns. In K. E. Bruscia (Ed.), *Case studies in music therapy* (pp. 153–161). Gilsum, NH: Barcelona Publishers.

Magee, W. L. (2005). Music therapy with patients in low awareness states: Approaches to assessment and treatment in multidisciplinary care. *Neuropsychological Rehabilitation, 15*(3/4), 522–536.

Magee, W. L. (2007). Music as a diagnostic tool in low awareness states: Considering limbic responses. *Brain Injury, 21*(6), 593–599.

Magee, W. L., Baker, F., Daveson, B., Hitchen, H., Kennelly, J., Leung, M., et al. (2011). Music therapy methods with children, adolescents, and adults with severe neurobehavioral disorders due to brian injury. *Music Therapy Perspectives, 29*(1), 5–13.

Marley, L. (1996). Music therapy with hospitalized infants and toddlers in a child life program. In M. A. Froehlich (Ed.), *Music therapy with hospitalized children: A creative arts child life approach* (pp. 77–86). Cherry Hill, NJ: Jeffrey Books.

Mazer, S. E. (2010). Music, noise, and the environment of care: History, theory, and practice. *Music and Medicine, 2*(3), 182–191. DOI: 10.1177/1943862110372773.

McDowell, B. M. (2005). Nontraditional therapies for the PICU—Part 1. *Journal for Specialists in Pediatric Nursing, 10*(1), 29–32.

Melnyk, B. M., Alpert-Gillis, L., Feinstein, N. F., Crean, H. F., Johnson, J., Fairbanks, E., et al. (2004). Creating opportunities for parent empowerment: Program effects on the mental health/coping outcomes of critically ill young children and their mothers. *Pediatrics, 113*(6), 597–607.

Meyer, E. C., Burns, J. P., Griffith, J. L., & Truog, R. D. (2002). Parental perspectives on end-of-life care in the pediatric intensive care unit. *Critical Care Medicine, 30*(1), 226–231.

Miller-Keane Encyclopedia and Dictionary of Medicine, Nursing, and Allied Health. (2003). Retrieved from http://medical-dictionary.thefreedictionary.com

Mosby's Medical Dictionary. (2009). Retrieved from http://medical-dictionary.thefreedictionary.com

Mrázová, M., & Celec, P. (2010). A systematic review of randomized controlled trials using music therapy for children. *The Journal of Alternative and Complementary Medicine, 16*(10), 1089–1095. DOI: 10.1089/acm.2009.0430.

Newth, C. J. L., Venkataraman, S., Willson, D. F., Meert, K. L., Harrison, R., Dean, M., et al. (2009). Weaning and extubation readiness in pediatric patients. *Pediatric Critical Care Medicine, 10*(1), 1–9.

Nguyen, J., Jarred, J., Walworth, D. D., Adams, K., & Procelli, D. (2005). Music therapy clinical services. In J. M. Standley, D. Gregory, J. Whipple, D. D. Walworth, J. Nguyen, J. Jarred, K. Adams, D. Procelli & A. Cevasco (Eds.), *Medical music therapy: A model program for clinical practice, education, training, and research* (pp. 165–220). Silver Spring, MD: American Music Therapy Association, Inc.

Odetola, F. O., Clark, S. J., & Davis, M. M. (2006). Growth, development, and failure to thrive: Factors that underlie the availability of pediatric critical care facilities in the United States. *Pediatric Critical Care Medicine, 7*(1), 70–73.

Odetola, F. O., Clark, S. J., Freed, G. L., Bratton, S. L., & Davis, M. M. (2005). A national survey of pediatric critical care resources in the United States. *Pediatrics, 115*(4), 382–386. DOI: 10.1542/peds.2004-1920.

Oldfield, A. (2011). Exploring issues of control through interactive, improvised music making: Music therapy diagnostic assessment and short-term treatment with a mother and daughter in a psychiatric unit. In A. Meadows (Ed.), *Developments in music therapy practice: Case study perspectives* (pp. 104–118). Gilsum, NH: Barcelona Publishers.

Parker, M. M. (2007). Tips on extubation in mechanically ventilated children—close observation is the key to successful extubation. *Journal of Respiratory Diseases, 28*(5), 203–207.

Playfor, S., Thomas, D., & Choonara, I. (2000). Recollection of children following intensive care. *Archives of Disease in Childhood, 83*, 445–448.

Polomano, R., Shirk, B., & Stouffer, J. W. (2002). A comparison of music to music with mother's voice on physiological responses and level of sedation with critically ill infants and children [Abstract]. *Eastern Nursing Research Society.* Abstract retrieved from http://www.nursinglibrary.org/vhl/handle/10755/163702

Robb, S. L., Burns, D. S., & Carpenter, J. S. (2011). Reporting guidelines for music-based interventions. *Journal of Health Psychology, 16*(2), 342–352. DOI: 10.1177/1359105310374781.

Robb, S. L., & Ebberts, A. G. (2003a). Songwriting and digital video production interventions for pediatric patients undergoing bone marrow transplantation. Part I: An analysis of depression and anxiety levels according to phase of treatment. *Journal of Pediatric Oncology Nursing, 20*(1), 1–14.

Robb, S. L., & Ebberts, A. G. (2003b). Songwriting and digital video production interventions for pediatric patients undergoing bone marrow transplantation. Part II: An analysis of patient-generated songs & patient perceptions regarding intervention efficacy. *Journal of Pediatric Oncology Nursing, 20*(1), 15–25.

Robertson, A. (2009). *Music, medicine and miracles: How to provide medical music therapy for pediatric patients and get paid for it.* Orlando, FL: Florida Hospital.

Rosenberg, D. I., Moss, M., & the Section on Critical Care and Committee on Hospital Care (2004). Guidelines and levels of care for pediatric intensive care units. *Pediatrics, 114*(4), 1114–1125.

Rosenfeld, J., & Dun, B. (1999). Music therapy in children with severe traumatic brain injury. In R. R. Pratt & D. E. Grocke (Eds.), *Musicmedicine 3: Musicmedicine and music therapy: Expanding horizons* (pp. 35–46). Parkville, Victoria, Australia: The University of Melbourne.

Rubin-Bosco, J. (2002). Resolution vs. re-enactment: A story song approach to working with trauma. In J. V. Loewy & A. F. Hara (Eds.), *Caring for the caregiver: The use of music and music therapy in grief and trauma* (pp. 118–127). Silver Spring, MD: AMTA.

Ruttimann, U. E., Patel, K. M., & Pollack, M. M. (2000). Relevance of diagnostic diversity and patient volumes for quality and length of stay in pediatric intensive care units. *Pediatric Critical Care Medicine, 1*(2), 133–139.

San Diego Patient Safety Council (2009). *ICU sedation guidelines of care.* Retrieved from http://www.chpso.org/meds/sedation.pdf

Schneider, S. (2005). Environmental music therapy, life, death and the ICU. In C. Dileo & J. V. Loewy (Eds.), *Music therapy at the end of life* (pp. 219–229). Cherry Hill, NJ: Jeffrey Books.

Schwartz, E. K. (2011). Growing up in music: A journey through early childhood music development in music therapy. In A. Meadows (Ed.), *Developments in music therapy practice: Case study perspectives* (pp. 70–85). Gilsum, NH: Barcelona Publishers.

Shoemark, H., & Dearn, T. (2008). Keeping parents at the centre of family centered music therapy with hospitalised infants. *Australian Journal of Music Therapy, 19*, 3–24.

Standley, J. M., & Walworth, D. (2010). *Music therapy with premature infants: Research and developmental interventions* (2nd ed.). Silver Spring, MD: American Music Therapy Association.

Standley, J. M., & Whipple, J. (2003). Music therapy with pediatric patients: A meta analysis. In S. L. Robb (Ed.), *Music therapy in pediatric healthcare: Research and evidence-based practice* (pp. 1–18). Silver Spring, MD: American Music Therapy Association.

Stewart, K., & Schneider, S. (2000). The effect of music therapy on the sound environment in the neonatal intensive are unit: A pilot study. In J. V. Loewy (Ed.), *Music therapy in the neonatal intensive care unit* (pp. 85–100). New York: Satchnote Press.

Stouffer, J. W., & Shirk, B. J. (2003). Critical care: Clinical applications of music for children on mechanical ventilation. In S. L. Robb (Ed.), *Music therapy in pediatric healthcare: Research and evidence-based practice* (pp. 49–80). Silver Spring, MD: American Music Therapy Association, Inc.

Stouffer, J. W., Shirk, B. J., & Polomano, R. C. (2007). Practice guidelines for music interventions with hospitalized pediatric patients. *Journal of Pediatric Nursing, 22*(6), 448–456.

Tamplin, J. (2000). Improvisational music therapy approaches to coma arousal. *Australian Journal of Music Therapy, 11*, 38–51.

Thaut, M. H. (2005). *Rhythm, music, and the brain: Scientific foundations and clinical applications.* New York: Routledge.

Treurnicht Naylor, K., Kingsnorth, S., Lamont, A., McKeever, P., & Macarthur, C. (2011). The effectiveness of music in pediatric healthcare: A systematic review of randomized controlled trials. *Evidence-based Complementary and Alternative Medicine,* 1–18. DOI: 10.1155/2011/464759.

Turry, A. (1997). The use of clinical improvisation to alleviate procedural distress in young children. In J. Loewy (Ed.), *Music therapy and pediatric pain* (pp. 89–96). Cherry Hill, NJ: Jeffrey Books.

Walworth, D. D. (2005). Procedural-support music therapy in the healthcare setting: A cost-effectiveness analysis. *Journal of Pediatric Nursing, 20*(4), 276–284.

Wood, R. L. (1991). Critical analysis of the concept of sensory stimulation for patients in vegetative states. *Brain Injury, 5*(4), 401–409.

Appendix A

PICU MUSIC THERAPY REFERRAL FORM

Date of Referral: _____

Place Patient Name Label Here

Reasons for Referral (check all that apply):

o Uncontrolled pain
o Elevated anxiety
o Painful or anxiety-producing procedures

o Requires non-pharmacological sedation
o Weaning from sedation
o Weaning from mechanical ventilation

o Change in functional status
o Alertness/responsiveness desired
o Non-adherent to treatment or rehabilitation

o End-of-life care needed

o Other: _____

o Expressive challenges (e.g., child is
  non-verbal, aggressive, withdrawn)

o Receptive challenges (e.g., due to
  medication or cognitive ability)

o Affective challenges (e.g., child
  appears fearful, depressed, agitated)

o Support for family needed

Pertinent Patient Information:

Name of Referring Clinician:

Signature of Referring Clinician:

Extension/pager number:

Appendix B

PICU MUSIC THERAPY ASSESSMENT FORM FOR ELECTRONIC MEDICAL RECORD

(*Formatted for electronic medical record with patient name, birth date, medical record number, unit, room number, date and time of assessment, and therapist title and signature embedded within entry*)

o Initial assessment   o Re-assessment (specify reason: _____)

Referring Clinician: _____   Date of Referral: _____
Reason for Referral: _____   o No referral obtained

Patient History

  Pertinent Medical History: _____

  Pertinent Social History: _____

Outcomes of Music Therapy Assessment

  Areas of Strength (emotional, social, communicative, physical, cognitive, sensory): _____

  Areas of Need (emotional, social, communicative, physical, cognitive, sensory): _____

  Responses particular to the context of Music Therapy: _____

  Cultural attitudes and preferences regarding music and treatment/hospitalization: _____

Summary and Plan

_____(*Narrative summary of outcomes from music therapy assessment*)
_____

o Recommend physician's orders for music therapy

  Recommended goal areas:

    o (*checklist of possible goal areas, including "other" with narrative area to specify*)

  Recommended music therapy interventions to address goal areas:

    o (*checklist of possible music therapy approaches, including "other" with narrative area to specify*)

o Music therapy not indicated at this time

  o Re-assess under the following conditions: _____

  o Re-assessment not appropriate

o Refer to related therapies

  o (*checklist of related therapies, check all that apply*)

Appendix C

PICU TREATMENT PRIORITIZATION MATRIX

Area of Need	Frequency			Comments
	Persistent	Occasional	Not observed	
Uncontrolled pain				
Anxiety				
Painful or anxiety-producing procedures				
Change in functional abilities				
Expressive challenges (child is non-verbal, aggressive, withdrawn, etc.)				
Receptive challenges (due to medication, cognitive abilities, language abilities)				
Affective challenges (child appears fearful, depressed, overstimulated, agitated)				
Lack of social support				
Family having difficulty adjusting to diagnosis or PICU				
Weaning from mechanical ventilation				
Inadequate sedation				
Weaning from sedation				
Comatose or new onset of disorder of consciousness				
Non-adherence to medical regimen				
Non-adherence to rehabilitation regimen				
Repeated hospitalization or long-term intensive care hospitalization				
Developmental delay				
Approaching end-of-life				
Other:				

1. Check the frequency of each applicable area of need
2. Circle any checked areas of need that are also intense or sudden in nature
3. Prioritize services for any areas of need that receive a circled check within the 'persistent' or 'occasional' categories, with secondary emphasis given to any un-circled 'persistent' or un-circled 'occasional' areas of need

Chapter 6

Surgical and Procedural Support for Children

John F. Mondanaro

INTRODUCTION

Hospitalization due to illness or injury marks a profound interruption in the development of a child regardless of diagnosis, age, gender, cultural background, or socioeconomic status (Bibace & Walsh, 1980; Boey, 1988). Such interruption becomes most poignant when the attempt to normalize through the semblance of routine within the hospitalization is further interrupted by necessary and standard medical procedures, diagnostic testing, and treatment trajectories that can include surgical intervention. The increased recognition of the potential impact of developmental interruption on the psychological safety and resilience of children has resulted in a gradual paradigm shift in health care (Aldwin, 1994; Gaynard et al., 1990; Mondanaro & Needleman, 2011; Orland, 1965; Plank, 1965). Existing literature on the importance of nonpharmacological interventions such as music therapy and other expressive modalities to reinforce coping skills warrants continued movement toward an integrative model of medical treatment. Inclusion of the child and her primary supports within the family as valued members of the treatment team reflects the growing trend toward family-centered care. Family-centered care as an extension of family systems psychology places importance on family relationships, patterns of communication, and the individual roles of each family member in the assessment and treatment of children (Cignacco et al., 2007; Fowler-Kerry & Lander, 1987; Golianu, Krane, Seybold, Almgren, & Anand, 2007; Jeffs, 2007; Pridham, Adelson, & Hanson, 1987; Stephens, Barkey, & Hall, 1999; Windich-Biermeier, Sjoberg, Dale, Eshelman, & Guzzetta, 2007).

Music therapy is uniquely positioned as an effective treatment modality for hospitalized children because of its potential to address body, mind, and spirit integration across a range of consciousness and developmental levels. Its presence along with other creative arts therapies as a natural entry point in the psychosocial and emotional support of children has become increasingly common in pediatric settings (Leeuwenburgh et al., 2007). This chapter will focus on music therapy interventions aimed at supporting children during medical and surgical procedures by offering alternatives to pharmacologic sedation and medical controls or physical restraints previously considered normal protocol (Minnick, Mion, Leipzig, Lamb, & Palmer, 1998).

In spite of this immanent progress in the treatment of children, current medical practice often reflects long-held notions that relegate emotional and psychological well-being to secondary consideration. The simplistic notion that distraction is the sole and primary intervention to support children during procedures still prevails and is unfortunately solidified at the grassroots level in the training programs of most medical disciplines (Mason, Johnson, & Woolley, 1999). The reader should be aware that a preferred and more accurate term is "refocusing," which implies both an intentional use of music therapy and the active choice of the child to engage in the use of music as an external resource for coping. Within the rationale of refocusing strategies, the child becomes an equal participant in the "doing" as opposed to being "done to" as is implied by the word distraction (Leeuwenburgh et al., 2007). This shift in terminology is in keeping with current philosophy of the American Academy of Pediatrics (2006), which supports psychosocial programming in the hospital through its endorsement of Child Life services. Child Life as a profession was founded upon the belief that central to best practice in pediatric care is the preservation of emotional development in children (Gaynard et al., 1990; Orland, 1965; Plank, 1965). This philosophy has continued to thrive with innovative programming in many pediatric hospitals that includes creative arts therapies. It follows that the work of music therapists, besides providing support to children, must also include changing medical culture by understanding the milieu, strong patient advocacy, good interdisciplinary communication, and stringent clinical practice of the myriad of interventions that will be discussed in the Guidelines section of this chapter.

DIAGNOSTIC INFORMATION

Before considering specific terminology related to procedural interventions commonly encountered in pediatric hospitals, it is important to reflect on the implications of the definition of "invasive procedure" in a medical context. An invasive procedure, defined as a "diagnostic or therapeutic technique that requires entry of a body cavity or interruption of normal body functions" (Anderson, 2005), slightly contrasts with an earlier definition that defines "invasive procedure" as an "insertion of an instrument or device into the body through the skin or body orifice" (*Stedman's Medical Dictionary*, 2000). Both definitions emphasize what is being done to the physical body during an intervention as determining criteria for whether a procedure is classified as invasive or noninvasive. Such definitions preclude any reference to the emotional or psychological experience of a child undergoing the procedure, which is incongruous with our understanding of child development (Aldwin, 1994; Bibace & Walsh, 1980; Orland, 1965).

According to Bijttebier and Vertommen (1998), children exposed to the traumatizing impact of repeated medical interventions without adequate emotional support are subject to continued anxiety and distress during subsequent medical treatments. Unresolved conflict around medical treatment parallels the current definition of the post-traumatic stress responses of "intense fear" and "helplessness" (American Psychiatric Association, 2000, p. 463) and may contribute to heightened emotional distress when reactivated.

Hospital admissions from the Emergency Department (ED) to extended stays on an inpatient unit are immanently marked by procedural interventions. During the past several decades, a call to address the unique needs of pediatric patients has grown increasingly strong and explicit (Ali, Dendel, Kircher, & Beno, 2010; Bluemke & Breiter, 2000; Windich-Biermeier, Sjoberg, Dale, Eshelman, & Guzzetta, 2007). According to Rosen (2002), it is clear that "while children may find even the most routine ED procedures terrifying, they historically have received less pain control and anxiolysis than adult patients with similar conditions" (p. 2587). This statement is vague enough to indicate juxtaposition between a presumed greater resilience in children and the possibility that the emotional and psychological needs of children undergoing hospitalization are in fact relegated to secondary consideration. While procedures conducted in the ED follow such protocol due to the need for expediency, there is something richly important that is missing when only the physical impact of a procedure is considered. The lack of acknowledgement of the child as a whole person results in a preclusion of any opportunity to understand existing resources for coping that may exist for the child. Ultimately, this lack of insight can lead to overmedication with anesthesia, which can in turn result in a greater potential for medical error (Bayat, Ramaiah, & Bhananker, 2010; Cote, Karl, Notterman, Weinberg, & McClosky, 2000; Fowler-Kerry & Lander, 1987; Heistein et al., 2005; Pershad, Palmisano, & Nichols, 1999).

Changing hospital culture can only occur from within, and certainly music therapists contributing to the interdisciplinary dialogue share the task of effecting such change. To be an effective partner in such interdisciplinary dialogue, it is suggested that therapists working in a pediatric setting have some familiarity with common procedures.

This recommendation charges the music therapist with the responsibility of synthesizing medical descriptions and rationale with an overarching goal of being able to deconstruct such information when necessary for the child. The provision of psychoeducation about a procedure in accurate but developmentally appropriate language is paramount to the success of such intervention. A foundational understanding of the rationale, sequence of steps (from preparation to completion), and prognostic outcomes of the various procedures and tests to which pediatric patients are likely to be exposed is easily attainable. Such information is best obtained through dialogues with nurses, medical staff, and technologists. This requires music therapists to truly integrate themselves into the care team. It has been the author's experience that many music therapy students and novice therapists tend to be one-dimensional in their wish for acceptance and integration. A commonly heard complaint is that "nobody understands music therapy," but it is equally important for music therapists to understand the work and role of other disciplines with whom they are interfacing. A dialogue about the details of a procedure with a specialist not only delivers pragmatic information that will inform the therapist's work of reinforcing a child's understanding, but also will contribute to a culture of collegiality and mutual respect.

General Medical Procedures

The following is a listing of common medical procedures during which music therapy may provide support for the child.

- Bladder catheterization: hollow, flexible tube inserted into the bladder to allow free release of urine or in some cases to inject fluids for diagnostic testing. Catheters are often placed prior to surgery, and some are placed permanently, as with renal disease.
- Chest tube placement: catheter placed through an opening in the chest where the lungs are located to remove air and/or fluid in order to restore negative pressure in the pleural space of the lungs. Commonly used after chest surgery or lung collapse (Anderson, 2005).
- Endoscopy: used to explore and visualize the interior of organs and cavities in the body.
- Intravenous line placement: Often referred to as an "IV," this tube is placed via venipuncture into a child's vein either to draw blood or to provide medicine, fluids, or nutrition.
- Lumbar puncture (LP, spinal tap): The spinal column is accessed with a hollow needle and syringe to extract cerebrospinal fluid (CSF) for diagnostic testing. The procedure may also be used to inject air or a radiopaque substance for analyzing the pressure of a tumor or to view structures of the spine and brain. Anesthesia is initially injected to numb the pain of the LP, but the child is awake and positioned on one side in fetal position for optimal exposure to the spinal column (Anderson, 2005). Music therapists should understand that procedural support can be tremendously beneficial for the child but may be challenging to negotiate with some medical staff wary of having extra staff in the room. Effective negotiation efforts are generally focused on patient advocacy, exuding confidence, and competence in understanding the procedure and the logistics of the treatment room.
- Nasogastric (NG) tube placement: a tube that is placed through the nose and into the stomach to relieve gas, gastric secretions, or food. Also used to instill medication, fluids,

or food. Used when a child is able to digest food but not eat, most commonly after surgery.

- Paracentesis: A procedure in which fluid is withdrawn from the bladder by way of a small catheter, mainly for the purpose of removing excess fluids from the abdomen. Music therapists should be aware that the preparation of a child for this procedure could be anxiety-provoking for the child due to the sequence of steps required. The bladder must be emptied to reduce the chance of trauma to the organ itself. The child is also assessed with vigilance postprocedurally for adverse reaction such as bruising of the abdominal wall or perforation of the bladder or bowel.
- Renal catheter: catheter placed for the purpose of dialysis.
- Skin puncture biopsy: the removal of a small piece of living tissue for microscopic study to determine or confirm a diagnosis, estimate a prognosis, or follow the course of a disease.
- Suture laceration: commonly known as "stitches." The application is more time-consuming than removal and is preceded with a topical anesthesia.
- Venipuncture: basically any puncture of a vein by a steel needle stylet for the purpose of withdrawing blood, instilling medication, starting a treatment infusion, or injecting a radiopaque substance for X-ray or imaging tests. Sometimes preceded by use of numbing cream (Emla); therapists should know that the cream has a tightening and cool feel on the child's skin when it dries.

The following three procedures generally preclude the presence of a music therapist, but are included here because of the need for preprocedural preparation and psychoeducation to ensure proper compliance. In some cases where strong advocacy is made, the therapist, wearing a protective bibbed apron, may be allowed to accompany a child. In such scenarios, radiology staff exercise justified vigilance toward optimal safety.

- Computed Tomography (CT), formerly known as Computed Axial Tomography (CAT): an X-ray that provides cross-section imaging. The procedure is relatively quick and in some circumstances can be as short as the duration of a held breath (Anderson, 2005).
- Magnetic Resonance Imaging (MRI): a method of choice for imaging a wide range of disease processes because of its lack of ionizing radiation hazards. Therapists should know that patients undergoing MRI are asked to lie completely motionless. The duration of the test can range from 10 minutes to two hours. The time is usually broken into segments.
- X-ray: electromagnetic imaging used to produce images of the bones and other internal structures.

Diagnostic-Specific Medical Procedures

The following represent procedures that are specific to certain illnesses or conditions.

- Chemotherapy infusion: Chemotherapy infusion treatment for children living with a cancer diagnosis involves receiving medicine through an intravenous line (*Stedman's Medical Dictionary*, 2000). Often children are placed in an infusion suite to receive treatment, which can last from two to eight hours, depending on dosage and preliminary setup. The opportunity for children to reap the benefits of peer support and interaction can be richly supported by music therapy group interventions.

- Debridement: Debridement is a procedure that is a regular part of the treatment of burn victims. It involves the medical removal of dead, damaged, or infected tissue to improve the healing potential of the remaining healthy tissue. It is an extremely painful procedure associated with high levels of anticipatory stress (Anderson, 2005).

- Gastrointestinal series (GI-rays): X-rays of the gastrointestinal system include both upper GI (gastrointestinal) series and a lower GI series (barium enema). Before having either of these X-rays, either a child will drink a liquid or it will be introduced into their colon (by way of an enema), which helps the intestine show up on X-ray film. Specific tests called sigmoidoscopy and colonoscopy allow doctors to look inside a child's intestine using a thin tube with a camera called an endoscope. The endoscope is connected to a TV monitor. Colonoscopy looks at the whole colon, while sigmoidoscopy looks only at the lower colon (*Stedman's Medical Dictionary*, 2000). Both tests may be used in the diagnosis and treatment of Crohn's Disease and other irritable bowel (IBD) syndromes. Therapists should know that these illnesses are complicated by psychosocial challenges ensuing from dietary restriction, social acceptance vs. isolation in adolescence, and body image also prevalent in adolescence.

- Hemodialysis: a procedure in which impurities are removed from the blood by way of an external shunt (tube) that transports the blood through the dialyzer and back into the bloodstream (Anderson, 2005). Music therapists should be aware that a multitude of factors could evoke tremendous stress for children receiving the procedure, including clotting and infections in the shunt and erosion of the skin around the shunt entry (port), as well as the prolonged period of immobility, which can be approximately four hours three times a week. Finally, there can be general discomfort prior to, during, and immediately following dialysis.

- Inhalation medication: Inhalation therapies are indicated in the treatment of a wide array of respiratory illnesses, including asthma. They are painless but can be especially challenging for toddlers and preschool children due to the necessity for the child's attendance to the inhaler mask. The treatment is approximately five to 10 minutes, depending on the medication. Music therapy can be effective in refocusing or engaging a child to ease the passing of time (Raskin & Azoulay, 2009).

- Mechanical ventilation: Mechanical ventilation is often a life-saving intervention, but can also be employed on a short-term basis as in surgical procedures. It can also be used in long-term cases of brain injury. The intervention assists or replaces spontaneous breathing by way of a machine called a ventilator (often shortened to "vent"). Two primary types of mechanical ventilation are invasive ventilation and noninvasive ventilation; these types are subdivided into positive pressure ventilation, where air (or another gas mix) is pushed into the trachea, and negative pressure ventilation, where air is essentially sucked into the lungs (Anderson, 2005). Music therapy may be useful as support when weaning a child off of a vent and at other specific junctures of vent care.

- Neonatal life support: "Neonatal life support" is a broad term that may refer to any medical techniques or equipment needed to keep a newborn baby or neonate alive. Neonatal life support can include close observation of the baby's vital signs, temperature control, intravenous or tube-fed nutrition, neonatal resuscitation, and oxygenation. Music therapy can support conservation of energy and self-regulation through the provision of live music entrained to the infant's heart and respiration rates. Goals focus on supporting self-regulation and the conservation of the infant's energy resources needed for neurologic and other organ growth (Loewy, 2000).

- Subdural grid placement: The placement of subdural grids is a surgical procedure in which strips of leads are strategically placed subdurally (under the skull) for the purpose of recording precise information about the origin of seizure activity (Onal, Otsubo, Araki, Chitoku, Ochi, et al., 2003). This phase of seizure monitoring is the intermediary step between VEEG and surgical removal (resection) of the affected part of the brain. Therapists should understand that surgical intervention is indicated for a relatively small percentage of children living with seizures because the seizures need to be focal (localized) enough for surgical intervention to be a viable option. The period of monitoring seizure activity before removing or resecting the affected part of the brain can extend for several weeks. Frequent cleaning of the surgical site and bandage changes to prevent infection are required. Infection control policies can be stringent during these procedures, which may preclude the presence of supporting therapies in spite of the child's needs. Strong advocacy on behalf of the child's emotional needs and adherence to protocol (sterile gown, gloves, and mask) may surmount resistance to the presence of music therapy. Such advocacy is always worth the effort if the child optimally copes when supported.

- Video electroencephalogram (VEEG): VEEG is a first-phase test in seizure diagnosis. It involves the topical placement of 26 electrodes (also called leads) on the child's scalp. The application of the leads can take 30 to 90 minutes, depending on the efficiency of the technologist and compliance of the child. It is not painful but can feel invasive on a sensory level due to the noxious scent of the adhesive and the sound of the air blower used to dry the adhesive. Additionally, there can be prolonged manipulation of the hair and scalp by the technologist as she applies the leads. VEEG is generally scheduled as a 24-hour test but can extend to additional days, which can evoke stress due to loss of routine, social opportunities, school activities, and separation from peers and family in some cases. Additionally, there can be secondary tests used to provoke seizure activity during VEEG testing. Photo stimulation (involving bright light), sleep deprivation, and timed interval hyperventilation are the most common of these tests (Mondanaro, 2008).

- Finally, there should be mention of a state that is often preemptive of diagnostic procedures and surgery in general where anesthesia or sedation is required. NPO pertains to the medical instruction to withhold oral intake of food and fluids from a patient who will be sedated for either a procedure or surgery. NPO, derived from the Latin expression *nil per os,* means "nothing by mouth." It is ordered to diminish the risk of aspiration (choking) due to the presence of undigested food in the system. Music therapists should understand that NPO can be extremely anxiety-producing, especially in busy hospitals where delays in scheduling are frequent. When possible, effort is made to schedule pediatric surgery and procedures early in the morning so that the generally required eight hours of NPO can occur during normal sleeping hours. NPO can be a significant factor to consider when planning any of the various music therapy interventions that will be discussed in the Guidelines section.

The above definitions are intended to impress upon the reader that medical music therapy functions at its most profound level when the music therapist understands the treatment milieu. The therapist should possess a working knowledge of these procedures so as to fully participate in the care of the hospitalized child. Being adept at accurately assessing a child's understanding of her condition and treatment and its impact on coping is an important step in delivering good care.

NEEDS AND RESOURCES

The emotional needs of hospitalized children facing the reality of at least one or more general procedures during their stay can vary depending on their prior experience with hospitalization. A child's experience may be expressed from both a personal perspective and as one that is understood vicariously through others. Factoring in with much importance is the child's stage of development, the cultural beliefs of the immediate family, and the child's relationships with parents, siblings, and even peers. Each of these entities may be considered influential contributors to the child's worldview. The identifying and reinforcing of the child's resources to best handle the external stressors of hospitalization punctuated by procedures is fundamental to the work of the therapist.

Again, it is the child's understanding of the illness and its effects upon the body that will provide the foundation upon which procedures or surgery can be explained. The therapist must also understand that a child's perceptions and overtly expressed feelings about medical care may reflect the beliefs of her primary constellation of caregivers. Working from this place of recognition is rudimentary in forming an approach to treatment that will be most readily accepted by the child and family. Even during adolescence and the beginning of individuation, the therapist must still recognize that while psychoeducation and modeling of adaptive qualities can be helpful, the child will most likely return to the systems that are in existence at home. A thorough assessment of these and other areas prepares the therapist for working most effectively in identifying the child's needs and inner resources.

Music therapy in a medical setting challenges many of the constructs of music therapy literature because the needs of the hospitalized child may present as both physical and psychoemotional simultaneously or as vacillating between the two. The therapist must be astute as to what the clinical focus will be in a given session, and then adjust his approach accordingly. An example of this challenge may lie in the scenario of a child in recovery from neurosurgery with a need for emotional support as well as with significant deficits that will require arduous rehabilitation of both fine and gross motor functioning. Music therapy may be effective in both domains, and it will be the therapist who can delineate the various interventions that will best support the patient in her treatment plan. Presenting the role of music therapy clearly is of paramount importance if the treatment is to be fully understood and supported by both the child's caregivers and medical team.

The child's music history or connection to musical resources at home, school, church, or personally should be viewed as a primary resource of the child and viable entry point for the introduction of music therapy. A child's musical preferences can be accessed by a music therapist by way of live or recorded music and can facilitate meaningful connection with the therapist and care team. Consideration should be given to the family's "Song of Kin" (Loewy et al., 2005). Defined as the music or genre that is identified as significant or sacred to the family, Song of Kin can provide a portal for rich understanding of the culture of both the child and her family. At such times as hospitalization, cultural awareness and respect for a family's heritage may prove to be the initial impetus for receptiveness to music therapy.

Additionally important for a music therapist to know and understand is that there are generally specific policies in place across pediatric settings that support and optimally serve the emotional needs of children. Preserving a child's sense of psychological safety begins with a fundamental valuing of the child's emotional experience. Policies and procedures in place for the efficacy of pediatric care may vary from hospital to hospital but generally include guidelines for the use of a treatment room when possible. Treatment rooms are spaces specifically set up to meet the standard of care that emphasizes the importance of the child's bed and room as "safe zones" (places where the child is free from procedural intervention). Unfortunately, hospital schedules and understaffing often contribute to the breakdown of such policies. Procedures that should occur in the treatment room may often be performed in the child's room due to time constraints. This said, music therapists should understand that policy adherence, while in the best service of the child's psychological well-being, may not always be possible when infection control and/or patient safety are identified concerns.

REFERRAL AND ASSESSMENT PROCEDURES

Referral Procedures

Referrals for music therapy intervention as procedural or surgical support generally ensue from a range of criteria that point to certain catastrophe if unaddressed. Some of these criteria may include a particularly traumatic history of hospitalization experiences; ineffective parental resources in terms of providing important emotional support; significant developmental, behavioral, neurological, or physical challenges; or the reality of an excessively arduous trajectory of medical treatment. The referral itself may come from the medical team, the psychosocial team, patient advocacy representatives, or a parent or caregiver well versed in their understanding of services available to children in hospitals. Such comprehensive care often occurs in specialized institutes or diagnosis-specific consult services. These specialized teams maintain standards of best practice by including therapists specifically focused on the psychosocial well-being of children. Music therapy can be the modality of choice for such teams because of the versatility of interventions and potential to work across a myriad of patient diagnoses and presentations. More commonly, it is the role of the music therapist on staff to solicit from a nurse manager or floor nurse a list of procedures for which support may be needed on any given day. In most scenarios, referrals for procedural and surgical support ensue pragmatically from the details and rationale of the specific medical intervention indicated, and the music therapist's role is to determine the therapeutic approach that can most optimally support the child's ability to effectively cope. As stated before, assessment across a range of criteria is the beginning of a treatment plan.

Assessment Procedures

While most music therapy programs have their own assessment forms that are generated in compliance with hospital regulation, there are general guidelines for inclusion that have become universal. Among these are tenets of family-centered care as described earlier. This philosophy of care identifies the child's illness not as an isolated focus, but rather in the context of the family systems in which she lives. Attention to patterns of communication, roles of family members, and relationships within the family are all factors contributing to the assessment process.

Also richly contributing to the assessment process are criteria for observations that are both clinical and phenomenological, the latter of which pertains to those observations that derive meaning from therapeutic instinct and perception. Phenomenological observations are specifically significant in the assessment of hospitalized children because they emphasize the therapist's synthesis of both observable and historical information with verbal and nonverbal expression of the child's internal and external world. It is of value to note that phenomenological observation can be construed as subjective, so qualification of these statements is necessary. Qualifiers such as "appeared" and "seemed" allow for such statements to have credence based on the therapist's expertise or specialization. Such important observation occurs during the child's interaction with primary caregivers, siblings and peers, medical team members, and psychosocial team members, including the music therapist.

The following tables outline specific areas of clinical and phenomenological observation in regard to developmental and coping style, respectively. They are intended to collectively provide a map by which the therapist can determine and communicate back to the medical team how music therapy can best serve both the child and the family in keeping with family-centered philosophy.

Table 1 references the child's developmental presentation with regard to six domains of functioning. Here the student should understand that delay and regression are vastly different. Developmental delay is primarily defined by underlying pathology, while regression can occur due to internal or external stressors. An example of regression can be found in Mondanaro (2005), in which a six-year-old, developmentally appropriate girl regressed during anticipatory grief work prior to the death of her two-year-old brother. During this work, she regressed to the play of a three-year-old to escape the burden of overwhelming information that her brother was not going to live. The play allowed her refuge from the emotional stress and time to gain mastery over the information that she was receiving. Developmentally on-track children can similarly regress during stressful procedures and medical circumstances. In most cases, the processing time needed for the child to marshal inner resources toward mastery is the greatest point of advocacy by the therapist.

Table 2 focuses on the child's specific mode of coping, with emphasis on the level of the child's communication style, comprehension or understanding, how the child is presenting in terms of stress, and adaptability. The mode of communication, whether direct or indirect, verbal or nonverbal, can reflect directly how the child comprehends the diagnosis, treatment, and ultimately the importance of compliance. The coping style is equally important when planning music therapy as procedural support. The child's desire to visually attend to the procedure or not will determine the role of music therapy, which will be discussed in the Guidelines section of the chapter. The manner in which a child processes stress behaviorally or cognitively will reflect in their interactions with staff and receptiveness to psychoeducation. Finally, the child's adaptability to the circumstances at hand can be reinforced as a resource if positive and modified through teaching if ineffective.

Table 1. Developmental presentation

	Appropriate	*Advanced*	*Delayed*	*Regressed*
Social				
Play				
Cognitive				
Nonverbal expression (arts, music, movement)				
Motor (gross & fine)				
Emotional expression				

Table 2. Mode of coping

Mode of Communication:
    □ Direct (eye contact, engaged)
    □ Nondirect (minimal eye contact, shy)
    □ Verbal
    □ Nonverbal
Level of Understanding
    □ Reason for visit
    □ Illness

           □ Treatment

           □ Need for compliance

Coping Style

           □ Sensitizer (a child who sensitizes to a procedure by watching)

           □ Avoider (a child who avoids watching a procedure in favor of being refocused)

           □ Related to parents' coping style

Stress Presentation

           □ Behavior

           □ Patient's verbal description

           □ Interaction with staff

           □ Investment in process

           □ Anticipation of procedure

Adjustment/Adaptation

           □ Comfort/self-soothe

           □ Ability to separate

           □ Make choices

           □ Relatedness

An additional and important area of assessment is parenting style, which may vary and shift according to the child's response to her hospitalization. This area is of interest because how the parent exercises basic parenting skills, such as nurturance, supportiveness, guidance, limit-setting, and discipline, may obviate the reason for the child's manner of coping during hospitalization. For example, the parent of a child with developmental delay may become overly protective of the child to the detriment of the child gaining mastery through experiences with a therapist. A parent may also project onto the child expectations of how they wish them to be as opposed to what the child can do if empowered to move at her own pace. Contrastingly, a parent of a high-functioning adolescent diagnosed with a chronic condition such as diabetes may demand more responsibility and autonomy from the child than she is capable of managing. This expectation can deny the child the structure and support needed to ensure medical compliance. A child's response to treatment and hospitalization in general can be a reflection of her parenting. Below are several case examples, which further illustrate the importance of this area.

One particular scenario involving a six-year-old boy with significant cognitive and motor delay due to cerebral palsy and his mother illustrates how a parent's expectations may impede the child's natural ability to find success. Numerous photographs of the boy dressed in athletic gear and propped into "normal" poses gave one the sense that this mother was challenged in her reconciliation with her son's condition. The creation of scenarios that symbolized normalcy to her disallowed her ability to see her son's successes on his own terms. This contributed to a cycle of overwhelming expectation of him and of what she perceived to be unmet goals and indifference from the care team. The author's identification of this dynamic in the assessment inspired the negotiation with the mother to take time for herself during music therapy sessions. This separation allowed the boy opportunities to explore by his own volition meaningful connections to the music and instruments. His successes in music therapy began to shift the mother's perspective and level of pride in the reality of her son's unique strengths in spite of his condition.

Another case, involving a four-year-old boy admitted for VEEG testing and his accompanying father, illustrates a common scenario in which a parent's own anxiety about the seriousness of a situation results in downplaying and hindrance in the ability to recognize the child's needs. This loving and well-meaning father projecting his own experience of ease with the test a month prior dismissed his son's fear and the author's offer to prepare the child for what he might expect on a sensory level. The father was unable to rationalize that the emotional experience of his four-year-old would be different from his own as an adult until the child was screaming in terror once the procedure began. The technologist and the author were able to negotiate the needed time to calm and familiarize the child to the materials being used prior to engaging him in music therapy for the completion of the procedure.

WORKING WITH CAREGIVERS

Caregivers, whether parents, other family members, or friends of the family, are often unknowing contributors to the psychological environment in which a procedure is occurring. This contribution may negatively impact the child's ability to cope, and in worst-case scenarios impede the success of the medical intervention. For this reason, it is not uncommon for medical staff to ask that caregivers leave the room in order to ensure success of the procedure. This occurs to the detriment of family-centered care. Even within institutions claiming at the administrative level to endorse a family-centered approach to care, there can be serious breaches of such practice at the clinical level due to time constraints, understaffing, and unchecked assertions about clinical efficiency by ill-informed staff. Music therapists and other psychosocial staff should be aware that parents often feel displaced in their roles as primary caregivers, and much can be done to diffuse tensions that may arise by exclusionary practice. Advocacy for inclusion of family members, when possible, and adherence to the use of treatment-room policies can easily become the responsibility of any member of the psychosocial staff.

Again, it is here that astute assessment from a family-systems approach can be valuable (Kovacs, Bellin, & Fauri, 2006; Shields, Pratt, Davis, & Hunter, 2007). True family-centered care values the integration of emotional and developmental needs into the practice of medicine, by looking at the patient and the illness within the context of the various systems in which they both exist. The identification of the communication patterns, cultural beliefs, and strengths of each family member during assessment is emphasized because the pressures of time and scheduling can result in the relegation and disruption of these systems. Consideration of these factors as well as the impact of the child's illness on the family can inform the therapist's dialogue with medical staff as to how caregivers can be effectively integrated into the procedural support of the patient (Dewees, 2005; Garro, Thurman, Kerwin, & Ducette, 2005).

Contrastingly, well-meant but misguided attempts at supporting a child can be offered by caregivers, who themselves may be challenged by the cacophony of the hospital environment (Ayson, 2008; Mazer, 2010; McDonnell, 1984). The music therapist is uniquely positioned in the care team to empower and support caregiver involvement through the assignment and modeling of role or instrument, respectively. The caregiver's embodying of the music for the patient through hand-holding, stroking, or gentle rhythmic patting supports involvement and closeness that can increase the sense of safety for many children and adolescents. Alternatively, the caregiver's playing of instruments that do not require prior training or expertise, such as the ocean drum, rain stick, pentatonic chimes, or small hand percussion can support the therapist's intervention and contribute to the creation of a generally soothing environment (Mondanaro, 2008). Both scenarios lend themselves to the support of a relaxed state for all involved but may be especially impactful when the caregiver is the child's mother, father, or both. During such scenarios, qualities of synchrony and healthy attachment formed early-on are marshaled in the service of getting through the procedure together. The author has borne witness numerous times across age, gender, and culture to this beautiful phenomenon that is central to the philosophy of family-centered care.

Introduction to Music Therapy Methods

The depth of work that is possible within the definition of music therapy as a form of psychotherapy lends well to the hospital milieu and especially to the specific realm of procedural and surgical preparation and support. While this idea will continue to be central to this chapter, it is also important to state that there are times when the immediate goal is not psychotherapeutic, but rather specifically focused on symptom reduction. A range of interventions will be discussed in the following pages. However the child's needs are assessed, effective therapeutic intervention begins with a conscious valuing of the child's experience during hospitalization and understanding of the negative impact that anxiety and stress can have on coping skills (Boey, 1988; Mondanaro, 2005, 2008; Mondanaro & Needleman, 2011). Brought into fruition thorough education, understanding, and acceptance of the impact on a child's development that occurs during hospitalization, this value invites purposeful intervention at a time when a child has the greatest opportunity to gain mastery in their understanding of their experience. This said, the author maintains that a strong and integrated understanding of child development, developmental psychology, and verbal counseling techniques prepare the music therapist working in medical care for the depth of work that is essential to pediatric care.

Depending on the age of a child, music as a nonthreatening, unexpected, and familiar play arena can provide respite from an environment fraught with unpredictability and uncertainty, which can be the culture of the Emergency Department (ED) as well as the general pediatric unit and intensive care unit (PICU). The very nature of play as a familiar space for the toddler and school-age child can be rendered easily by the therapist's accessing of precomposed music, the child's requests, and/or through improvisation. This space can also be introduced to the adolescent patient but dignified through the use of more sophisticated technology-based instruments such as synthesizers, drum pads, and, more recently, iPads with GarageBand-like applications. The therapist can introduce such intervention as an entry point into the assessment dialogue, and this clarity is recommended so that the initial music intervention delivers valuable assessment information as well as the beginnings of a therapeutic relationship. An important point here that is intended for the novice therapist, and those merely novice to the medical model, is that these first moments with the patient and family are formative of how they will organize their understanding of music therapy and the role of the therapist in the care being rendered. The relegation of music therapy to mere diversion and the therapist to performer is not uncommon in spite of a growing body of research that supports the clinical integrity of the discipline. The culture of awareness is still quite young in hospitals, and the work of establishing a credible presence rests with each clinician's discipline in upholding the clinical rigor of medical music therapy.

Understanding the sequence of steps in the rendering of support for procedures or surgery can be challenging when there are so many factors that seem contingent upon systems beyond the music therapist's direct control. A particularly helpful way the author has found to assist music therapy students and novice clinicians achieve greater clarity in the work within the medical model is to organize the work into three categories of clinical intent: psychoeducation, procedural support, and psychotherapeutic support. These constructs, further delineated according to a child's procedural or surgical needs, can be understood as integral components to supporting coping and compliance with hospitalization and the trajectory of care being provided (Mondanaro, 2008). Deconstructing each component for clarity and clinical rationale will allow the reader to better understand this terminology when referenced throughout the remainder of the chapter.

Psychoeducation

Psychoeducation in the context of medical procedures and surgery is the teaching of pertinent information that will have psychotherapeutic value in terms of a child's mastery of the circumstances of her hospitalization. Psychoeducation also plays an important role in helping the child understand the significance of the procedure or surgery for the treatment of her condition. The music therapist providing interventions at this potentially stressful juncture should be aware of the dynamics that can prevail in the immediate context, including the anxiety of the child as well as that of the parent or caregiver(s), the attending staff, and certainly the environment as well (Mangini, Confessore, Girard, & Spadola, 1995; Mondanaro, 2005, 2008; Mondanaro & Needleman, 2011). Success in this endeavor draws heavily and importantly on the music therapist's own level of confidence and understanding of the procedure or surgery itself. This understanding should include the rationale for the medical intervention; the sequence of events prior to, during, and following the intervention; the sensory aspects that can be experienced; and the child's preferences or choices of support (Mondanaro, 2008).

The domains of psychoeducation and psychosocial assessment fall well within the scope of practice for music therapists, yet they are often delineated as the sole responsibility of other disciplines such as Child Life or Social Work, respectively. While there is a growing number of music therapists earning Child Life certification, the integration of the two disciplines is more commonly found in programs that place the two distinct professions side by side. In such programs, the delineation of roles should be respected with thoughtfulness, as there is no room for territorial mentalities in patient care. While best practice places the patient and family first, such role-crossing can be confusing and challenging to negotiate. Ideally, it is a collaborative approach based on good communication that is most effective (Mondanaro & Needleman, 2011).

Facilitating a dialogue with a child that is meaningful and helpful can vary on an individual basis and will be shaped by the personal information and narrative of the child and family gleaned during the assessment phase. Certainly, information to be addressed by the therapist about the specifics of a procedure or surgery will draw heavily upon the child's present understanding of the illness or injury. Psychoeducation should be delivered using accurate information and terminology at a level that is developmentally appropriate, with the goal of dispelling harmful misconceptions. Such intervention is ideally facilitated in the presence of a parent or primary caregiver, with respectful acknowledgement of the developmental needs of the patient in order to enhance a feeling of control and mastery (Leeuwenburgh et al., 2007; Mondanaro, 2008; Mondanaro & Needleman, 2011).

Finally, psychoeducation can be addressed to the child's parents, caregivers, and even attending staff in advocacy of the use of a treatment room for medical procedures when possible, in order to preserve the child's bed and room as a safe haven within the hospitalization (American Academy of Pediatrics, 2006). Furthermore, the music therapist can advocate for the use of comfort positioning when possible, which generally focuses on the preservation of the child's sense of autonomy and control, through adjustments of how she is placed. Sitting in an upright position as opposed to supine (lying down) is the most common of these adjustments that can optimize the potential for compliance and ultimately successful completion of the procedure. Effective advocacy for such positioning is informed by the therapist's understanding of the procedure and the pressures of scheduling under which the procedural clinician may be working. Again, thoughtful communication and respect for the roles of the other clinicians involved will optimize the potential for the best patient care (Berrios & Jacobwitz, 1998; Cavender, Goff, Hollon, & Guzzetta, 2004; Gaynard et al., 1990; Orland, 1965).

Preprocedural and Presurgical Process

This phase of treatment follows gracefully from the assessment and psychoeducational phases where the therapeutic relationship that has been built burgeons into a therapeutic alliance. Music therapy functions at a deeper level here because time has been given to define and establish the credibility of the therapist as a truly integrated member of the care team. The dialogues that occur at this juncture may focus on determining strategies in which music therapy can be utilized to optimize coping with the stress or pain of the procedure, if any, or defining the roles of not only the patient, but also those caregivers in attendance. Active engagement as a way to reinforce a child's sense of control, or passive participation through listening as a way to refocus the child when the threshold for coping is surpassed, can be determined and communicated to the medical team, thus creating a structure that is manageable for all. Here roles are defined, and a plan that empowers the patient and caregivers in a manner that is truly family-centered is established (Leeuwenburgh et al., 2007; Mondanaro, 2008; Mondanaro & Needleman, 2011).

Again, it is the child's understanding of the illness and its effects upon the body that will provide the foundation upon which procedures or surgery can be explained. The importance of this work cannot be underestimated, as the most common theme encountered is the inattention given to thorough and developmentally appropriate explanation using accurate language (Leeuwenburgh et al., 2007). This, coupled with frequent dismissal of the importance of empowering the child to be an active participant in her care, defines the context of care we are addressing here. The music therapist's attention to these areas is precursory to supporting the child's ability to fully access resources and coping strategies learned before, whatever they may be. Through assessment and dialogue, the child's resources can be first identified and then given purpose within the context of treatment. The therapist can encourage the child's discovery of her own role and power in how she copes with and manages the experience. The therapeutic relationship provides the space in which this self-empowerment can be fostered. Such purposeful application of her own inner resources during stressful and painful procedures is personally empowering and allows not only for better coping, but for another level of mastery as well.

Finally, both procedural and surgical scenarios can involve the added component of "waiting." "Waiting" as a theme of hospitalization is common and actively connects to greater existential themes of uncertainty, loss, separation, and isolation, all of which can be addressed by the music therapist involved.

Procedural Support

Music therapy during actual procedures can range from active engagement when possible to the use of entrainment (as explained in the Guidelines section) when a child is unable to engage for reasons that are emotional, physiological, developmental, or even cultural-religious. The music therapist providing procedural support is working integratively with medical professionals toward the common goal of effective completion of the necessary procedure. The therapist's goal is not psychotherapeutic in this context. The use of music therapy in most procedures is varied and evolves with the therapist's moment-to-moment assessment of how the patient is coping and the progress of the procedure itself. The therapist may shift from the child's precomposed favorite songs to improvisational approaches as determined to be appropriate. Varying sounds and instruments and the nature of interaction with the patient may be indicated as the procedure unfolds.

Shorter interventions such as venipuncture may require the integration of other mind-body strategies, such as breathwork and visualization, that can be supported by the music. More time-consuming interventions such as the placement of electrode leads for electroencephalogram, video-electroencephalogram (VEEG), or respiratory therapy may challenge the music therapist to work malleably as the patient's threshold for coping shifts.

In more long-term procedures, such as dialysis or chemotherapies, which can occur in both outpatient infusion suites and inpatient units, the therapist can move into progressive interventions such as songwriting, story-song creation (Loewy & Stewart, 2004), group improvisation, and interventions that incorporate the therapeutic use of other modalities such as art, dance-movement, drama, and poetry. These other modalities are natural forms of creative expression that may emerge organically in the music therapy process or be intentionally initiated by the therapist to expand the child's experience. Additionally, collaboration and/or consultation with credentialed therapists of other modalities can provide insight for the therapist and diverse experiences for a child undergoing life-sustaining procedures during which the processing of existential themes is immanent (Leeuwenburgh et al., 2007; Turry, 1997).

Postprocedural and Postsurgical Process

Regardless of the procedure or surgical intervention, a child emerges from such an ordeal with a story to tell. The trauma to the body and psyche under such invasion is real to the child, and should be acknowledged as worthy of hearing. Even when prepared and supported by a therapist, parent, favorite nurse, or doctor, the story punctuated by the sequence of events and sensations warrants review and in many cases retelling. Music therapy as a form of psychotherapy finds its greatest poignancy at this juncture of hospitalization. There is need for a forum in which the child's story can be heard, honored, and given aesthetic form and meaning. Most scenarios focus on themes of transition, change, and, again, loss in various forms (control, autonomy, motor skills/strength, speech), all of which can be processed at both verbal and nonverbal levels through music. Improvisation and songwriting serve this process richly by providing the child with the means by which to tell her story literally and in metaphor. This type of process holds importance because the real facts of the procedure or surgery, regardless of the child's understanding, can be threatening for the child to fully contemplate. The therapist can therefore serve to both educate and support through the offering of music therapy interventions that allow the child aesthetic distance from the facts of the procedure or surgery, and a forum that allows the child control of the pace by which information is integrated.

Environmental Awareness: Setting the Stage

The efficacy of the work described thus far and the descriptions of methods to follow are often contingent upon the therapeutic space that is created by the therapist. Attendance to the auditory and sound environment is especially important to the establishment of a therapeutic space in which a procedure is to occur. Overstimulation is common in procedures, and normally tolerated sounds can be provocative to many children, yet the impulse to turn on every light source, television, radio, and sound-making toy available is often acted upon by well-intentioned but ill-informed staff and caregivers. The use of such devices for distraction can be counterintuitive and at times as obtrusive as the ringing of cell phones and disruptive talking. It is often the therapist's task to raise awareness as to the value of minimizing the amount of unnecessary stimulation in favor of the intentional use of music and sound to achieve the desired clinical goal. To this end, the therapist can meet resistance to turning a television or other device off, and this should be processed with the child or caregiver in attendance. Simple and clear explanations, such as explaining that the light activity of the television screen can be disruptive to the therapeutic experience, are often necessary to ensure the optimal effects of the intervention.

Infection Control

Here it is necessary to discuss one of the most basic principles of medical music therapy, namely the rigorous attendance to infection control policies and procedures. The protocol that exists within this domain ranges from those areas for which a music therapist is directly accountable to those that may be administratively imposed in a particular unit, or even hospitalwide.

The former can include specific policies for the use and cleaning of various instruments such as winds or hand percussion. These specific policies can vary from site to site, as they are most commonly generated by music therapy departments in accordance with hospital policy. These departmentally specific policies can include provisional considerations for specific instrument lines that are produced to meet infection control standards. At Beth Israel Medical Center, The Louis and Lucille Armstrong Music Therapy Program maintains a complete line of cleanable instruments produced by the company REMO©. Their Health RHYTHM product line meets most infection control standards put forth within the medical industry, but the therapist should be vigilant to the specific criteria of their hospital to ensure compliance. These instruments can be cleaned with alcohol or bleach-based wipes without compromising the integrity of the instruments' quality. Certainly on a more pragmatic level, therapists can maintain compliance by assigning instruments such as wind instruments (recorder, harmonicas, etc.) for use on an individual basis when possible. This strategy is time- and cost-effective when treatment is extended beyond acute care or in the support of a child receiving treatment such as dialysis or chemotherapy indefinitely or over an extended period of time.

A hospital's Department of Infection Control is primarily responsible for monitoring reported cases of infectious disease in the hospital and for putting forth the required protocol for controlling the spread of such infection. Policy follow-through primarily includes signage generally placed on the doors of patients who are on contact precaution due to either a compromised immune system or a highly contagious virus. Notification is generally posted in yellow, pink, or orange colors for greater visibility and usually requests that a verbal check-in with the nursing station occur before entering the child's room. The requirement of rubber gloves, disposable gowns, and masks may be listed singularly or in combination, depending on the identified infection and requirements of the hospital's Department of Infection Control.

Finally, hospitals, in accordance with state law and standards of public health, may make available to staff such options as an annual influenza (flu) vaccine and hepatitis vaccinations, the latter of which may be especially indicated for staff working clinically with children. Additional protocol includes monitoring of tuberculosis (TB) exposure or infection through skin tests commonly known as PPD (purified protein derivative). Music therapists working in medical settings should know that vaccines for influenza and hepatitis are optional, but PPD is not and may be required as frequently as semiannually.

OVERVIEW OF MUSIC THERAPY METHODS AND PROCEDURES

Music therapy methods and procedures included in this chapter are listed below. They are not listed in any specific order.

Receptive Music Therapy

- Music for Rapport-Building: listening to the patient's music of choice during the rapport-building stage of treatment.
- Music-Facilitated Psychoeducation: the use of music that is familiar or comforting to the child to accommodate the provision of important psychoeducational material.

- Music Listening for Refocusing: listening to music ranging from preselected music by the patient's favorite artist to music improvised by the therapist to refocus a patient's attention during a procedure.
- Music Entrainment: the use of music that initially matches the physiological and emotional presentation of the child and then gradually changes in the desired therapeutic direction.
- Tension Release: the use of music listening to support the release of tension that mounts in the body as a response to pain, stress, and anxiety.
- Soundbath: the creation of an auditory improvised sound space by the music therapist for children who are sedated in postsurgical recovery.
- Music Sedation: listening to a favorite song or a theme-focused improvisation to facilitate a deepened state of relaxation.
- Environmental Music Therapy: the creation of music that meets and modulates the existing sound environment of a given unit from one of mechanical sterility to one of calm and beauty.

Improvisational Music Therapy

- Music Improvisational-Play Opportunities: the use of instrumental improvisation to support creative expression by the child, allowing for expression without editing or abundant rules.
- Soundscape: the creation of a context of sounds that are related thematically and that together may conjure up images of specific places.
- Tension Release through Drumming: the use of rhythm and drumming, often in conjunction with cognitive devices such as counting or rhythmic lyric recitation, to enhance coping.

Re-creative Music Therapy

- Music Therapy for Socialization: the use of shared music experiences, using favorite precomposed songs, to facilitate peer support and normalize the environment.
- Music Alternate Engagement: the use of music to stimulate active engagement of the child in specific, achievable tasks associated with a procedure.

Compositional Music Therapy

- Songwriting and Performance: the organization and reclaiming of pre- and postsurgical time through creative songwriting and further project development into performance opportunities to help the child prepare and transition back into normal life routines.
- Recording and Music Technology: the use of various types of music technology to reinforce agency and control, optimize coping, foster independence and confidence, and offer refuge from overwhelming experiences and feelings.

GUIDELINES FOR RECEPTIVE MUSIC THERAPY

Music for Rapport-Building

Overview. Rapport is the positive, harmonious dynamic between two individuals that serves as the beginning of an effective therapeutic alliance. The discussion of pre-, peri-, and postprocedural support and pre- and postsurgical support must address the importance of rapport and the therapeutic relationship as precursory to any provision of support that is to be effective. Music listening is a natural therapeutic entry point for children because of its propensity to bridge physical, cognitive, emotional, and spiritual domains and its ability to connect at both verbal and nonverbal levels. Listening to the patient's music of choice across genres may serve the rapport-building stage of treatment necessary to establish before engaging the patient in a dialogue focusing on psychoeducation and coping strategy.

Regarding the use of recorded music, it is the author's experience that when introduced initially, it can prematurely define the therapeutic relationship by shaping the child's perception of music therapy. Still, recorded music can serve as a tangible resource for immediate refuge from the hospital environment through the use of headphones. An obvious value of recorded music is that unlike live music therapy, recorded music as a resource is always readily available to the patient. Acknowledging, discussing, and validating this important point during the therapist's initial meeting can prove important to defining the unique role that live music therapy can play in the future relationship. The use of recorded music can also serve as a safe and familiar point of entry into the therapeutic relationship by providing insight into the patient's inner world. This may be most applicable to adolescents for whom music choice becomes an assertion of identity and individuation.

A possible contraindication ensues from the reality that music is not a guaranteed preference for all. Therefore, in such situations where the child is not oriented to music as a comforting resource, it should be thoughtfully explored or respectfully avoided. Additionally, as previously stated, the use of recorded music for rapport-building in the initial stages of meeting a patient and family can also lodge misconceptions as to the clinical rigor of the discipline. The expense of this misconception early in the hospitalization can hinder and even undermine the therapist's credibility as a member of the health care team during the patient's hospitalization.

Preparation. Introducing music as a benign form through which to establish a working rapport is served by a presentation of both familiar and not-so-familiar (non-Western) instruments to encourage exploration. The therapist's invitation to explore as well as his modeling of how to produce sound on the various instruments can foster a sense of trust in the therapist as one with expertise. This approach can reinforce a child's sense of control without the added pressure of having to hold or play instruments directly. The therapist's invitation to the child to give her approval or disapproval of an instrument or its sound can be a first step in restoring the child's sense of herself as an active participant in her care.

What to observe. The therapist's assessment of the moment-to-moment relatedness of the child will provide valuable information about the child's psychosocial well-being. Additionally, the degree to which social referencing with the parent occurs during the therapist's interaction with the child should offer more information about the child's comfort level in the hospital and in the processing of new and potentially threatening information.

Procedures. There are many approaches to introducing services to a child and family. Some therapists may wish to enter a room with their instruments in tow to establish that the service they offer is unique to other disciplines attending to the child. While this messaging can certainly achieve the desired effect, it may in some cases limit the scope of how the service is perceived. First impressions can be lasting, and if one is viewed only as a facilitator of musical experiences, the child and family may have difficulty equating the forum as applicable during times of heightened stress. The author tends to leave instruments outside the room for an introduction of services that is more neutral and focused on establishing identity as an unconditional source of support, whether music is used or not.

Given a range of approaches, the therapist should hone a style of entry that is authentic to himself, and whatever this approach might be, an introduction of services should reference the source of the referral or service, and include identifying information as to who, what, why, when, and where the service is being offered. This dialogue between the therapist, child, and parents or caregivers provides a beginning point from which the use of music therapy to support the child's specific needs can be understood. The therapist's attention to this detail will solidify his role as part of the care team and, in turn, the validity of music therapy as a component of the care being offered. Taking the time to align with the medical team as to how music therapy intervention can support a child through the effective completion of the procedure is obviously precursory to this work. Ultimately, it is the child's understanding and receptiveness to music therapy that is critical if the intervention is to truly have an impact on coping.

The idea of using music must make sense within the child's immediate context. Once the idea of music therapy as a support is accepted, the session will develop naturally and instinctively for both the therapist and the patient. The therapist entering the room can determine much about the music of the child simply by taking a visual assessment of how the room is decorated, or the particular toys or books a child may be holding. Pictures on the wall of family members, pets, or artwork may provide rich opportunity to reflect meaningfully back to the child that you truly see her. To this end, offering "Elmo's Song" to a child surrounded by Sesame Street toys can establish rapport instantly, as can engaging the child verbally about her interests.

Adaptations. The approaches above can be easily adapted to various age groups, again, with much information being gleaned from a visual assessment of the culture that been defined by the child. Adolescents can present as challenging because of the multitude of developmental processes to which they are attending. Authentic acknowledgement by the therapist of the teen's world as it is reflected in her room or personal adornments can provide entry to important connections.

Validating a child of any age by reflecting on the world she has made visible is important, but rapport-building as a goal in and of itself may be superfluous to the process of helping a patient who is already receptive to support and nonpharmacological intervention. As always, it is the value of malleability that will inform the therapist's shift in clinical direction.

Music-Facilitated Psychoeducation

Overview. Music-based approaches to the provision of psychoeducation may be most effective with children of preschool to early-school age, or in the support of children with developmental delays. In these cases, developmentally appropriate music can enhance coping in preprocedural support, postprocedural process, and pre- and postsurgical support. These approaches assist children in their integration of information relevant to a procedure because they offer concrete references compatible to a child's sense of organization.

Psychoeducational approaches focusing on the presentation of medical information may be contraindicated and even futile when developmental delay is assessed or when the child is preverbal. At such times, however, sound and other sensory aspects of the materials used in the procedure can be introduced and explored to familiarize or habituate the child to unfamiliar stimuli. This level of orientation through nonverbal communication can be crucial to ensuring the psychological safety of the developmentally challenged or younger child; such efforts often only ensue from strong patient advocacy.

Preparation. Music therapy interventions are richly informed by the therapist's understanding of comfort positioning (as defined earlier), and its significance to autonomy and control in most children regardless of age, gender, and developmental status. Modeling such positions and advocating for their use in order to maximize the child's ability to actively participate in the procedure are an important part of preparation. Furthermore, advocating for the use of a treatment room whenever possible can provide needed distance from the child's bed or *safe* zone.

What to observe. Referring back to Tables 1 and 2 of the Assessment section of the chapter, the therapist can assess the child's degree of integration and understanding as to the information being imparted and adjust the dialogue and/or music accordingly. Children of any age will give visual cues as to willingness or ability to receive information. Such cues may vary preprocedurally, procedurally, and postprocedurally. The child's response to the actual stress of a procedure can modulate during the course of the procedure and should be monitored by the therapist. As the child's threshold for understanding is surmounted by the sensory experience of the procedure, the therapist can diminish or abandon the goal of psychoeducation to support the child's mastery of the physical environment (materials, instruments, etc.). To this end, the use of tactile material such as a cabassa, shaker egg, or model magic (clay) can serve as an immediate release of tension.

Procedures. Most children cope optimally when given the opportunity to actively participate either in the procedure itself (holding a bandage, clenching a fist, etc.) or in a creative and expressive opportunity through music therapy. Active engagement is therefore the first-line intervention with most children, but the degree of participation may shift as the child's presentation warrants.

Music that is familiar or comforting to the child can be used and modified to accommodate the provision of important psychoeducational material. The cycle of chords in a familiar song or the rhythmic pattern of a nursery rhyme put to music can provide structure and predictability to children. The sequence of events and sensory information specific to the procedure can be integrated into these familiar or improvised songs, which can be mutually played or merely presented by the therapist. Lyrics that emphasize the sequence of events can reinforce a sense of mastery and control during the procedure.

The interventions of the therapist may continue to reinforce the information that was introduced during preprocedural psychoeducation. The referencing and review of procedural details in the real-time events of the procedure can serve as an anchor for a child whose threshold for coping is compromised as the sensory experience increases. An example of this work lies in the scenario of a child undergoing venipuncture. Music-supported review of each stage of the procedure as it is occurring reminds the child of her preprocedural, psychoeducational work with the therapist. The mastery achieved and experienced by the child previously can be referenced both verbally and nonverbally, ensuring greater access to internal and external resources.

Music Listening for Refocusing

Overview. The goal of using music to refocus a patient during a procedure is especially efficacious when the goal is realized mutually (Leeuwenburgh et al., 2007). Such joint effort marks a therapeutic alliance that instills in the patient a sense of active participation in the way she will best cope with the procedure. The music used for the intervention can range from preselected music by the patient's favorite artist to music improvised by the therapist on instruments selected by the patient. Walworth (2005) discusses the use of live music to provide both precomposed and specific styles preferred by the child in a study that is described in the Research Evidence section of this chapter.

Refocusing techniques can be effective during all three areas of procedural and surgical support identified earlier. Preprocedurally and presurgically, both recorded music and live music created by the therapist offer unique points of entry to the therapeutic relationship that can serve the patient's needs. The use of real instruments, especially percussion, can be added to the auditory space established by the recording, which can introduce the possibilities of shared experiences within a therapeutic relationship.

Finally, the value of this intervention to the child, her caregivers, and staff can be undermined by well-intentioned but uninformed comments. As presented in the chapter's introduction, the word "distraction" is often used across a range of disciplines, including music therapy, but is misrepresentative of the clinical rationale that informs this intervention. The word itself implies that the medical intervention is unidirectional and that the most optimal role for the patient is one of ignorance and passivity. Music therapists new to the medical model will often hear the word used and will most likely be challenged to reeducate others about the inaccuracy of the terminology in favor of "refocusing" as previously defined.

Preparation. The music therapist's assessment of and modification and sensitivity to the existing sound environment are critical to the effectiveness of this intervention regardless of whether the music is live or recorded. Vigilance to eliminating unnecessary sounds, such as televisions, electronic games, and radios, can further serve the goal of creating a positive sound environment. The use of music to meet and transform the environment in which the procedure occurs can function profoundly in terms of supporting the patient, caregivers, and even the medical team if attended to with an attention to detail. Ultimately, the therapist's synthesis of the existing sound environment with his own aesthetic sense can lend human quality, order, and beauty to an environment fraught with uncertainty.

What to observe. The therapist should be attuned to the child's nonverbal communication when evaluating music listening as an intervention. The use of music listening, whether recorded or created live by the therapist, can provide invaluable reinforcement to a child's sense of control and purpose in the procedure. Given the dichotomy of feelings that can arise for a child expected to be both passive and compliant, refocusing through listening as an elected strategy can offer important and needed refuge.

Procedures. Preparation in advance as to the patient's musical preference will ensure that the patient's potential to refocus through the music is optimized. The therapist's advocacy for the patient's use of music, whether recorded or live, is essential, as the pace of a hospital unit can relegate such needs to secondary consideration. Communication with medical staff as to the impact that the patient's music may have on coping and compliance is often necessary and welcomed.

In both preprocedural and presurgical scenarios, the therapist's re-creation of familiar music or improvised music across themes that are meaningful to the patient (nature-focused, genre-specific, band- or artist repertoire-focused) can optimize coping. Contributing to this intervention can be the therapist's facilitation of visualization, guided imagery, mind-body awareness through breath exercises, movement, drawing or painting, story writing, and poetry. In one particular case, an 11-year-old boy awaiting an MRI chose to compose animated story-vignettes, accompanied by the author's thematic musical creations on instruments specifically assigned by the patient to each story. Another case, of a 14-year-old girl (who reported being "nonmusical, and more into basketball") awaiting transport to surgery, involved the author's whistling and playing the Harlem Globetrotters' theme on piano, as she shot paper balls into a simulated basketball hoop. Her caregiver had the role of playing a drum roll on the bongos before each throw. Both scenarios illustrate the therapeutic possibilities that can emerge spontaneously to empower a child in reclaiming time as her own.

During actual procedures, the use of listening to refocus the patient may be both a primary and a secondary intervention, depending upon the procedure. For many children from toddler years through preadolescence, preferred active engagement may naturally morph into active listening once thresholds for coping are passed and engagement is no longer possible. Here the therapist can focus on entraining to the child's respiration (see the next intervention guideline), as well as on the creation of a calm environment conducive to the efficient completion of the procedure. The therapist's assessment of the moment-to-moment flow of the procedure is crucial to the timeliness of the transition. During other procedures where lying still is recommended for safety, this approach of facilitating music listening can be appropriately selected by the therapist.

The use of listening to recorded music lends well to procedures that preclude the presence of a therapist due to hospital protocol (see the description of procedures in the Diagnostic section) or when the child has asserted autonomy in selecting her own music and the use of headphones to achieve refuge as a coping strategy. While listening to recorded music through headphones may be effective for the older patient, live music improvised by the therapist allows for in-the-moment modulation according to the changing presentation of the patient's breath, heart rate, and emotional state.

The author recounts the case of a 17-year-old girl receiving a lumbar puncture. Her selection of a preprogrammed groove on a synthesizer, to which the therapist improvised on a string patch and acoustic pentatonic chime, allowed her to cope optimally. The slow electronic groove and string chording provided an auditory anchor of predictability and structure, while the improvised linear melody of the chimes allowed her a vehicle by which to transcend the physical space through her imagination.

The music therapist may need to modify the choice of instruments depending on the space allocation in the treatment room. Much can be achieved with the voice or Native American flute and limited percussion when space is a concern.

Music Entrainment

Overview. Music entrainment (Bradt, 2009, 2010; Rider, 1997) is defined as the creation of music that matches the physiological presentation of an individual, with the goal of affecting a desired change by gradually changing the music. Adapting the definition to the purpose of this chapter, the emotional presentation of the child may also be considered in the process, since for many children emotional expression and physiological responses to stress, anxiety, and pain are inextricably linked.

Music entrainment can be optimally effective for pre-, peri-, and postsurgical support because it can be offered without the use of verbal communication if necessary. As such, it is ideally suited for scenarios where the music therapist's services are requested midway through a procedure or when there has been no opportunity to prepare the child in advance.

The use of entrainment is contraindicated when caregivers and staff have not been educated about the clinical use of music in this way. Misunderstanding can lead to unmet expectations that the therapist's goal is to "entertain" the patient, and when the "entertainment" is deemed ineffective, requests for familiar songs or untimely interruptions can quickly undermine the integrity of the intervention. Clear communication is essential if the therapist's role and clinical knowledge are to be understood.

Preparation. As in any intervention, the therapist should evaluate the logistics of where the intervention is to occur. The type of instruments used will be influenced by this factor. Additionally, the existing sound environment will impact the effectiveness of the intervention. The therapist should be aware of unnecessary sources of stimulation such as televisions or radios. It is a common scenario that in an effort to "distract" the child, every device known to man will be turned on by misguided staff. The misconception that "more is better" can be dispelled through clear communication.

What to observe. During entrainment, the therapist is attending to the child's presentation in order to effectively implement the intervention. Astute observation is necessary and informs the therapist's choices within the rendering of music.

Procedures. The therapist begins this intervention by visually assessing the physical presentation of the child, noting the rhythm of the child's breath, movements, and even the monitored heart rate if available. This visual assessment informs how the parameters for the music intervention are set. The selection of music, be it improvised (Dileo & Bradt, 1999; Rider, 1997) or Song of Kin (Loewy et al., 2005), is determined by criteria that may or may not be foreseeable or controllable by the therapist, such as no prior history with the patient; the therapist is called halfway through a procedure; or when the threshold for engagement has passed. Across a range of scenarios, entrainment can be the best option. Regardless of the nature of the music being offered, instinct, sensitivity, and malleability are required, as the therapist is also rendering the intervention in conditions that may be governed by the pace of the procedure itself. Musically matching both the child's presentation and the energy of the space is a dual task that is charged to the therapist providing entrainment as procedural support. The initial mirroring of both the physical and emotional presentation, specifically respiration, can support the child at a nonverbal level. Once the music is matched to the child, the therapist can begin to gradually employ the principles of entrainment, through the skilled shifting of rhythm and tempo in the direction of the desired change. The intentional use of volume to reinforce the changes in rhythm further deepens the entrainment process.

Music entrainment functions on an auditory and a subliminal level to effect the necessary change needed to optimally support the child. Such intervention can be especially efficacious when a child's threshold for coping is exhausted. Music therapists should be aware that the sound space that is often created when working with the child at this nonverbal level could also support the medical staff administering the procedure. The sense of flow and timelessness that is achieved by the intentional use of the dynamics of music provides a context in which the routine of the procedure becomes ephemeral (Csikszentmihalyi, 1990).

Patient responsiveness, age, culture, logistics, and spatial limitations may require the therapist to adapt the choice of instruments and musical choices in the moment.

Tension Release

Overview. Tension-release interventions (Loewy, Azoulay, Harris, & Rondina, 2009) focus on the use of music therapy to support the release of tension that inevitably mounts in the body as a response to pain, stress, and anxiety. Tension in the body can contribute to general discomfort and, conversely, the physiological responses to discomfort can contribute to mounting tension. Because this cycle can impede effective coping, the resolution of tension through tension-release interventions is indicated pre- and postprocedurally and pre- and postsurgically. The therapeutic possibilities lend well to the abatement of anxiety and stress levels that prevail at these junctures of care.

This intervention differs from refocusing techniques discussed earlier in that the goal is to support the child's active awareness and retrieval of resources, namely the breath, to increase coping ability. The use of music to mirror the cycles of tension that occur in the body can be effective in supporting this type of mind-body connection integral to coping during painful procedures. The effectiveness of tension-release interventions can be contingent upon the therapeutic alliance that is established, however, and the child's role as an active participant is necessary if the music is to serve its purpose.

Tension-release interventions are futile without a therapeutic alliance in place, as the effectiveness ensues from the child's attendance to the breath, visualization, and imagery, and their role as an active participant. Due to this level of awareness and personal investment, the intervention is not suited cognitively to patients with significant developmental delay. Musically, however, the tenets of tension release can be offered through the creation of soundbath, which will be discussed in the next section.

What to observe. The therapist can assess the child's active investment in the process by observing the patient's attendance to deep breathing and effort to focus on the experience as supported by the music.

Procedures. The therapist may begin a tension-release session with brief psychoeducation about the impact of deep breathing on the physiological state. Emphasis on the fact that the breath is an autonomic function controllable by one's mindful attendance can empower the patient in her connection to inner resilience and existing coping strengths.

The child's focus on breathing is well supported by a musical structure that is repetitive and simple enough to support the child's attendance to the task. Complexity demands a certain level of listening that can prove counterintuitive. The definition of cycle in this context is a chord progression that may occur over a four- or eight-bar phrase. The therapist may focus on various musical components (harmonic, tempo, volume, etc.) in the creation of a cycle that supports the patient at a nonverbal level. An example of a harmonically focused cycle would be the use of the propelling motion of the circle of fifths: An introduction of a minor chord would be shifted to the dominant seventh of that chord. The dominant seventh chord harmonically resolves to the sequential fifth. The cycle of minor to dominant seventh, through a partial completion of the circle of fifths, will render the cycle that is to be repeated. When developing this intervention, the therapist should feel free to create progressions according to his own aesthetic standards. A sequence in any given major key would look like: [[:vi, VI$_7$, ii, II$_7$, v, V$_7$, I, :]]. The therapist's entrainment of the cycling music to the child's respiratory cycle further deepens the experience as the therapist shifts the tempo according to the changing respiratory pattern. A harmonic instrument like the guitar or piano is ideally suited for an approach that is centered on the creation of tension-and-release cycles that are harmonically focused. In contrast, drumming and hand percussion can be effective in creating tension release through a cycle of increasing and decreasing tempo and volume.

The voice can also be used to create linear lines that can achieve tension resolution through tonal intervallic synthesis (Loewy, 2011), which uses the harmonic tension created by linear movement across the various degrees of the scale. The building of tension can occur through melodic phrases that are sung or played linearly. The therapist takes liberty with time and breath to create a linear movement that extends and delays resolution of dissonance in the harmonically desired direction. An example in a major scale would follow a cycle of melodic lines such as: [[:I, II//I, III, iii//I, III, iii, IV//I,II,iii, IV//V:]]. This approach can be improvised or adapted to a phrase of a favorite song, the latter of which functions similarly by creating tension by delaying the resolution. As this approach focuses on linear motion, the therapist should explore the use of flute, violin, or recorder as well.

Adaptations. The therapist can adapt to spatial limitation by being well versed in various approaches to facilitating tension release. Beautiful work with this intervention can be done with only the voice. In cases where the child is nonverbal or when music therapy is sought midway through a procedure, the psychoeducational components to tension-release interventions can be bypassed.

Soundbath

Overview. Soundbath, based on the author's work (Mondanaro, 2008; Mondanaro & Needleman, 2011), is an extrapolation of key components from environmental music therapy, entrainment, tension release, soundscape, and other receptive music therapy techniques, for use when a patient is sedated in postsurgical recovery. The technique focuses on the creation of an improvised auditory sound space that can be entrained to both clinical presentation (respiration, nonverbal communication in the face, involuntary movement, etc.) and mechanically monitored information (heart rate, respiratory cycles, etc.).

Ideally, such intervention would be discussed during presurgical sessions so that the music or sounds being created would be integrative of the patient's preferences.

A particular case involving a 13-year-old boy awaiting surgical removal of a benign brain tumor focused on spending presurgical time exploring through improvisation particular sounds and instruments that he wanted used in the therapist's creation of therapeutic soundbaths following his surgery. Postsurgical site cleaning and bandage changing, which were notably agitating to the sedated boy, were markedly eased with the introduction of soundbath as described above. The therapist's entrainment to the clinical responses of the patient during soundbath became integral during the boy's initial days of postsurgical recovery.

Soundbath may require explanation to caregivers and staff who may not otherwise understand the clinical intention of music therapy being rendered for someone who is sedated. The literature on music and the brain (Taylor, 1997; Tramo et al., 2011) provides the necessary rationale for such intervention by establishing that the auditory system remains active even when physical functions are sedated. Music as a form of organized, aesthetic information can provide a point of reference for someone in this state. The ability to connect and be involved in a child's care that this intervention affords parents and caregivers is important on a psychoemotional level. Once explained, the provision of soundbath can elucidate the neurologic value and, perhaps even more importantly, the humanistic intention of such intervention.

Therapists providing postsurgical support must be vigilant to observing not only clinical or observable responses of a child, but also the electronically monitored vital signs as well. Measures for heart rate (HR), oxygen levels (O_2), and respiratory rate (RR) are visible on such monitors and may be indicators of both external and internal stressors to the child. It is realistic that music may prove to be overstimulating at times, as evidenced by sudden or sharp shifts in the readings of heart rate on the electronic monitor. Therapists should communicate observations to the medical team for expertise in interpreting such observations. Many responses may be specific to the moment and/or may be unrelated to music. Still, while some observations can be alarming to the new music therapist, it is important to remember that ongoing involvement in dialogues with the medical team as to such observations is preferred to acting on the inclination to withdraw entirely from the patient's care.

Preparation. The therapist prepares for the provision of postsurgical soundbath with vigilance to spatial consideration, traffic flow for medical staff attending to the patient, and, of course, the indicated preferences of the patient. Both visual and auditory observations of the patient's existing environment are the important precursors to introducing music into the patient's auditory space. Ambient sounds such as an ocean disc or rain stick can bridge the mechanical sounds of hospital equipment with the aesthetic qualities of music.

What to observe. The therapist's vigilance to the clinical and electronically monitored presentation of the patient is essential, as the primary goal is to support coping and regulation of autonomic functions (heart rate, respiration, oxygen levels, etc.). Before introducing the soundbath, it is important that the music therapist observe the child for several minutes. The music can render a range of effects, and the therapist is responsible for communicating to the care team what is observed.

Procedures. Ideally, soundbath should be introduced following a few moments of quiet assessing of the existing environment and the child's presentation. Soundbath is rendered by way of the therapist's synthesis of the existing sound space of the child's immediate environment with his own aesthetic sensibilities. As the goal is not to engage the child or to overly stimulate, the opening music can be an improvised chord progression that meets the existing sound space. It can be developed harmonically by shifting from one tonal space to another: major to the harmonic minor, introducing modal variations of the initial offering, introducing world idioms, etc. An example of how that may be rendered can be as simple as gradually introducing a flatted seventh to transition into a mixolydian mode from the major. The possibilities are endless, and the therapist should strive to free himself from self-editing when creating the soundbath.

There is subjectivity at work here because the intervention is rendered often when interaction with the child is minimized due to postsurgical or medical circumstances that prevent active response. While the goal is not to actively stimulate the child to engage, the therapist can make music references to songs or genres that are preferred by the child.

Soundbath is a continuous piece of music that may express themes and movements. The duration of a soundbath is anywhere from 10 to 30 minutes and is contingent upon the therapist's subjective assessment of the moment-to-moment presentation of the child and music being created.

Ideally, soundbath should be introduced prior to any known procedures, such a bandage changes, bathing, etc., in order to introduce the shift in the auditory sound environment prior to the physical stimuli of medical intervention. Following the procedure, the therapist can assist the regulation of autonomic functioning through the continued provision of familiar sound.

Adaptations. Soundbath as an individual intervention with specific goals can be extended to family members at the bedside, empowering them in something they *can do* for the patient at a time when they may feel otherwise. The use of ocean drums, rain sticks, pentatonic chimes, and other ambient instruments that do not require formal training are recommended as offerings to family members who wish to be involved.

Music Sedation

Overview. The use of music therapy as a form of sedation (Loewy, 2013; Loewy, Hallan, Friedman, & Martinez, 2005) accesses the principles of entrainment to facilitate a deepened state of relaxation. The use of a child's favorite song or an improvisation focusing on a theme can serve this intervention effectively. This intervention has been researched for efficacy, which will be discussed at the end of this chapter.

Preparation. The identification of a song or piece of music that is meaningful to a child is a starting point for this intervention. Furthermore, considerations for the duration of a procedure are pertinent here because the therapist must have a sense of how to effectively time the shift in tempo and volume that will ultimately provide the effects of sedation. Communication with medical staff is necessary in viable cases where music sedation can be considered. In such cases, advocacy for the consideration of an alternative to pharmacological intervention and the many possible side effects is necessary. This is especially important in procedures such as venipuncture and VEEG, where pharmacological intervention is hardly necessary but remains a first-line intervention for staff that may be stressed for time. Observation of infection control policy when indicated and logistical or spatial awareness is mandatory for therapists providing this intervention.

Procedures. The therapist begins music sedation at least five minutes before the procedure begins in order establish a therapeutic space. Focusing the child on the music intervention is more easily accomplished if the therapist is not competing with additional stimuli. The intervention is rendered by creating a piece of music that is meaningful and familiar to the child. Rendering the song in its recognizable form is important because the initial goal is to create a connection that can be sustained through cessation of the procedure. Once the child is engaged, the therapist can gradually modify the various musical components such as rhythm, tempo, volume, and eventually the melody itself in the direction of lulling the child into a restful state. To this end, the lyrics of the song can be gradually simplified to a single phrase or a few words as well, and, in some cases, vowel sounds or syllables can replace the words altogether. Sleep can even occur in the most effective rendering of this intervention, and in optimal circumstances the need for, or the amount of, anesthesia (if any) can be reduced.

Adaptations. The therapist and medical personnel involved in the procedure should maintain a positive rapport and good communication as to the child's process during the procedure. Perceptions of how the child is coping can vary based on clinical and theoretical orientation. An example of the disparate perspectives that can emerge lies in the perception of a child's crying and how it is understood. A music therapist may therapeutically support crying as a healthy expression and release, while another discipline may view crying more narrowly as a sign of distress that must be eradicated. Both perspectives may prove pivotal in the child's process during a procedure, and mutual respect for each discipline's expertise is an absolute requirement for truly integrative care.

Environmental Music Therapy

Overview. Environmental Music Therapy (EMT) (Rosetti & Canga, 2013; Schneider, 2005; Stewart & Schneider, 2000) is the creation of music that meets and modulates the existing sound environment of a given unit, from one of mechanical sterility to one of calm and beauty. EMT can be relevant at any given time to address the environment in which medical interventions occur. The sound toxicity and harmful volume levels within hospital units, from the ED to the ICUs, contributes immensely to the frequency of medical error and heightened stress levels of all. Patients, caregivers, and the attending staff can benefit from the improved sound environment.

There are times when the introduction of music into a busy environment can have an adverse effect of overstimulating both staff and patients alike. Music can calm an environment and those in it, but can also grant license for increased volume and animation in the way people speak and physically move.

Preparation. Positioning and setup of the music therapist and instruments is critical, especially in intensive care units (ICUs) and other busy units where traffic flow must be respected. Setup should be navigated with mutual respect for the medical staff, which is ultimately responsible for procedural and surgical outcomes. The music therapist's awareness and respect for traffic flow and the needs of the staff will distinguish him as an integrated member of the team fulfilling an essential role intelligently. EMT can transform an environment, or it can contribute to a sense of cacophony if the therapist is oblivious to the activity level of the unit.

What to observe. The therapist providing EMT should remain vigilant to the changing environment, be it the shift change for nursing staff or new admissions. Awareness and integration of the surroundings, staff needs, and cultural diversity are what distinguish EMT from mere performance. Additionally, when providing EMT, there may be opportunity to integrate the favorite song or genre of a caregiver or staff member into the music. Astute judgment must be observed at such times in order to preserve the clinical goal.

Procedures. Music therapists providing EMT can work solo or with a small ensemble of preferably no more than four therapists. This is for spatial consideration primarily, but also to dissuade common associations that the intention is for performance. Sessions can range from 20 minutes to an hour, with steadily evolving music or with the inclusion of silence.

The therapist begins EMT by assessing the existing sound environment and activity level of the unit. Once he has a clear sense, the introduction of sound occurs. If the existing noise level is loud or high-pitched, the initial sound may be best served with an ambient instrument–like ocean drum or rain stick or with a low-pitched drone offered by a cello or synthesized string sound. Once entered into the auditory environment, the therapist's choices are infinite. The therapist's synthesis of the existing sound environment, with his own aesthetic sense, can positively shift the context in which postsurgical recovery or any given procedure is experienced. The music may be improvised or it may include precomposed music. However the music is created, the goal is to shift the environment from within, as opposed to attempting to mask or overpower it.

Here it is important to note that the therapist's evaluation of how EMT is impacting patients, caregivers, and staff is continuous within a given session. At all times, the therapist is attentive and responsive to the flow of incoming stimuli from each of these entities, shaping and developing the music accordingly without losing sight of the goal. Notably, challenges to this process can be frequent as onlookers may misinterpret the purpose. To this end, spontaneous applause can be quietly acknowledged and quieted while requests for specific music can be respectfully honored and integrated with subtle nuance so as to stay the intended course of EMT.

EMT can provide support to many children simultaneously without requiring close proximity. It offers possibilities of positively shaping the environment to which many are orienting. Notably, the deft therapist can manipulate the various musical components discussed earlier so as to redirect and reconstitute a semblance of order within an unpredictable environment. In many ways, the principles of entrainment are utilized here, with the unit itself replacing the child in the role of recipient.

The therapist should approach EMT as an invaluable contribution to the environment of care, and thus be aware of his responsibility to ensure quality and relevance in the musical choices made. Whether these are improvised music or precomposed pieces, the therapist's sensitivity, musical skills, and cultural awareness will guide this process. Selecting music that is culturally specific or diverse as needed should be valued in the moment-to-moment flow of an EMT session.

GUIDELINES FOR IMPROVISATIONAL MUSIC THERAPY

Improvisation, as a fundamental aspect of music therapy, holds its place as the crown of interventions (Bruscia, 2001, 1988; Gardstrom, 2003). It offers an unconditional forum in which the patient's experience can be supported, shared, and reflected upon meaningfully with the therapist. Improvisation provides a portal into the verbal and nonverbal aspects of the patient's experience, which may be of additionally profound importance in the support of children with developmental delay. The experience generally afforded during improvisational music therapy is one of empowerment, when the child's sense of control and autonomy is most compromised. Such intervention can be pivotal to the degree of mastery with which the patient is able to marshal through the experience of a procedure or surgery.

Providing voice through various instruments within a milieu controllable by the patient offers opportunities for transformation of roles from one of passivity to one of active participation. Improvised stories and visualization offer opportunities for catharsis and conflict resolution, as a child gathers and organizes important information about a procedure or surgical intervention. During expressive play and improvisation-supported procedures, the therapist's role is to continuously assess and integrate the patient's expression and choices during active engagement. Once a child's threshold for coping has reached cessation, the therapist may shift the focus of improvisation toward synchronization. Here the therapist's skill at following the emotional and physiological presentation through the use of musical components (rhythm, tone, tempo, harmony, etc.) supports the patient on a kinesthetic as opposed to a cognitive, intellectual, or even creative level. The actual procedure is not the time for psychotherapy or any goals of this nature. The goal is to support coping through the completion of the procedure, and to this end it may very well be the trust that ensues from the therapeutic alliance, in conjunction with the phenomenological aspects of music, which offers the best opportunity for success.

As stated earlier in the chapter, music therapy as procedural support may not always be the first-line choice by a medical team, and the therapist should be prepared for less-than-ideal circumstances, such as when the patient's threshold for coping has already been passed or when the therapist is only first meeting the patient, midway through a procedure that is not going well. Again, this is a time when the therapist may transition to receptive techniques, particularly as in an improvised sound space to meet and shift the level of tension exhibited by the patient as well as in the room itself. The introduction of ordered, aesthetic sound or music can provide respite and needed transition from the cacophony of a procedure gone askance of the desired outcome.

Improvisation as a forum for both verbal and nonverbal expression can also encourage a range of emotional experiences for children moving through the vicissitudes of hospitalization. Turry (1997) beautifully describes her use of improvisation in pediatric oncology, bringing emphasis to the effectiveness of improvisation in the here-and-now experience of a child enduring numerous procedures on the trajectory of treatment. Her work with breathing techniques and spontaneous song forms is described in pre- and postprocedural scenarios as well. Across scenarios, care must be taken by therapists to monitor the degree of stimulation experienced by a child during both procedural support and postsurgical recovery.

Overstimulation resulting in noncompliance is contraindicated in the sense of effective integration of music therapy with medical care. The latter scenario may also be contraindicated if the activity level compromises the recovery process. Music therapists are appropriately challenged to be vigilant when introducing this intervention, for in spite of the many benefits of creative expression, hospitalized children are hospitalized for medical reasons, not for music therapy. This truth was pointed out to the author at the beginning of his career by an angry neurosurgeon during interdisciplinary treatment rounds. While the author was mortified at this admonishment, the neurosurgeon was right. This was truly a gift, and the author learned a valuable lesson about what it truly means to be working integratively. Music therapists have to be smart in their collaborations.

Music Improvisational-Play Opportunities

Overview. Music improvisational-play opportunities are facilitated to support creative expression with the use of musical instruments. Here, emphasis is placed on allowance of expression without editing or abundant rules. It is unprecedented in the practice of music therapy because of the potential it offers to children, caregivers, and staff alike to express freely and equally.

Improvisational musical play can be effective during preprocedural rapport-building by allowing opportunities for normalization of the hospital experience. Furthermore, during some procedures where the child's activity level does not impede the completion of the procedure, expressive music play can reinforce a child's sense of control, agency, and autonomy. These qualities can be effectively reinforced during postsurgical recovery not only when the needs are expressive and emotionally oriented, but also when support of fine motor rehabilitation is indicated, as discussed earlier.

Preparation. The therapist must be aware of spatial limitations when preparing for music improvisation. Infusion suites and clinics in which children are treated simultaneously are ideal settings for this intervention because opportunities for invaluable peer support abound. Children can share both their experiences of treatment and their connections to music as a form of expression and creativity.

What to observe. The therapist should be observant of the child's perceptions of expressive freedom offered in improvisation. Structure translates to a feeling of safety and security, and the converse may also be true in some cases. Expression and active engagement may become threatening or scary for some children as the sense of expectation in an area that is unfamiliar becomes overwhelming. Therapists should be sensitive and effective in modifying the degree of structure according the expressed or visible needs of the child.

Procedures. Choice is cardinal to introducing improvisation in a manner that is comfortably paced. Demonstrating and inviting exploration of the various instruments is generally the first phase of improvisational music therapy. Empowering the patient in his choice-making and initiating of sounds, rhythms, and motifs, that can then be supported or mirrored by the therapist marks the movement into the arena of rich improvisational experiences. The initial offerings of a child can be reflected back musically or supported harmonically and rhythmically as she gains comfort and confidence. The therapist's addition of counterpoint harmony or polyrhythmic instrumentation can be provocative of more engagement by the child once a trusting rapport has been achieved. Drumming and percussion initiated by the therapist can provide the child with a naturally nonthreatening entry point into the music. The potential dialogues that can occur through improvised drumming invite a myriad of emotions, which can be interpreted and responded to by the therapist.

Finally, therapists should show consideration of others who are present but not necessarily participatory by remaining aware and sensitive. Overstimulation or themes of exclusion can emerge as points of concern and should be addressed by the therapist proactively by modifying the music as needed. While it is nice to believe that music can benefit everyone, it is a subjective experience, and mindfulness on the part of the therapist will facilitate an environment of care and sensitivity.

Adaptations. The therapist can make active choices as to what instruments should be made available based on spatial limitation, cultural sensitivity, and environmental awareness. Improvisational drumming may not be indicated in an ICU, whereas in the community playroom, such expressive opportunity may be welcomed. Ultimately, the music therapist must use good judgment and make smart decisions without losing the confidence to take risks.

Soundscape

Overview. A soundscape is a context of sounds that are related thematically and that together may conjure up images of specific places. The creation of improvised soundscape provides a rich portal into a patient's inner world while creating connection to the external world as well. Such themes as *garden, city, farm, traffic, playground, beach, etc.,* can activate rich associations and retrieval of memories, and bring to the forefront a gentle reminder that hospitalization and certainly procedures are temporary.

The creation of soundscape offers opportunity for creative expression, socialization, and normalization of the hospital environment. Additionally, the transformative qualities of a created soundscape are rich and expansive of the imagination. Once activated, the imaginative potential of a child can be accessed as a resource when identifying coping strategies throughout the hospital experience.

Soundscape lends well to work in chemotherapy infusion suites and dialysis centers where children internalizing feelings of isolation and separation can be united in a common goal. The potential for meaningful peer support that can be facilitated during shared experiences can last well beyond the music therapy session. Music therapy that provides a forum in which this type of connection can occur may also provide an effective group intervention for therapists who may be overwhelmed with an abundance of referrals.

While the accessing of possible soundscapes to be created requires a certain level of abstract thinking, the intervention can profoundly impact children who are developmentally or neurologically delayed as well. The thematic qualities of soundscape offer refuge from the hospital environment through the same tenets described in Environmental Music Therapy. Notably, the creation of soundscape can be effective with children across a range of developmental issues because of the transformative, metaphysical, and therapeutic aspects of music and sound.

The practicality of soundscape is determined again by the constructs of the given procedure and spatial considerations, and the patient's involvement or degree of attendance.

What to observe. Like other interventions, there may be a noticeable shift in effectiveness as the patient's threshold for attendance shifts. The therapist will make adjustments or incorporate other interventions accordingly.

Procedures. Generally, the therapist will solicit ideas for soundscapes from the children participating and proceed with minimal instruction so as to encourage free expression and creativity. Offering a variety of instruments and encouraging the use of body percussion (clapping, finger-snapping, and chest or leg patting), vocal improvisation, and even whistling contribute to an environment that is fun and innovative.

A rich example often created by the author is a garden theme to contrast the sterility of the hospital setting. While providing a selection of instruments to support the theme is the role of the therapist, supporting the choices of the participants as they embark on the task of creating the theme is important. Rain sticks, ocean drums, and chimes may be used to reference waterfalls, brooks, and rain drops, respectively. Frame drums and bongos can be used to create the sounds of trees creaking in the wind and woodpeckers. Different-size guiros, cabassas, and shakers, all played at different intervals or rhythmic configurations, can render a convincing version of a rich chorus of frogs and insects. Finally, whistled birdcalls and Native American flutes can be added intermittently. The array of sounds can be conducted layer by layer to create a burgeoning garden on a spring morning. A tapestry of synthesized string sounds or guitar picking in a simple two-chord holding [[:I, IV:]] can provide a holding quality as well.

Such intervention can transform an environment and in doing so render a sense of refuge for those in attendance. Soundscapes are fun to create and offer ample opportunities for empowerment. The intervention can be internally validating for a child as her sense of contributing to, and being a part of, an ensemble is acknowledged and honored.

Adaptations. The therapist may easily adapt the intervention of soundscape across areas of the hospital from shared playrooms to bedside with friends and family members, but always in accordance with the child's level of involvement. Other factors that may determine the viability of this intervention include the range of ages that may be represented within an infusion suite and the level of participation exhibited within a group. Understandably, the effects of chemotherapy and other infusion treatments can include nausea, irritability, and exhaustion. Sleeping for one child can be an active choice for coping with a lengthy treatment, but for others it can merely be the physiological response to treatment. Respect for the needs of these children must be shown when creating or encouraging group participation. In any scenario, attentiveness to cessation of the intervention's effectiveness and malleability to introduce other interventions when necessary are essential.

Tension Release through Drumming

Overview. This tension-release intervention uses active drumming (Friedman, 2000; Loewy et al., 1997) and is indicated for use pre-, peri-, and postprocedurally and presurgically, because of the therapeutic benefits of releasing tension related to anxiety and stress levels through active drumming. The use of music to mirror the cycles of tension that occur in the body remains consistent with tension release focusing on more passive participation through visualization. Like the previously discussed tension release interventions, drumming can be equally efficacious in supporting a mind-body connection integral to coping. Here, as in receptive music therapy, the effectiveness of tension release through drumming is somewhat contingent upon the therapeutic alliance that is established. The patient's role as an active participant in the drumming is necessary if the music is to serve its purpose.

Introducing tension release through drumming or percussion will be effective only if the child is receptive to engaging actively with the therapist. Engagement requires the patient to invest creatively and energetically in the session. The patient's ability to do so may be inhibited at any juncture by the overwhelming reality of the physical and emotional impact of the procedure. There may also be distinguishing criteria of the procedure itself that preclude the child's active engagement. Verbal explanation as a preemptive measure may assist the patient in the ability to actively engage in drumming for release.

Preparations. As described in previous discussions, the success of this intervention again requires the therapist to evaluate any spatial considerations and to understand the clinical requirements for the effective completion of the procedure. Good communication with the medical team involved is necessary not only to understand the basic trajectory of the procedure but also to educate about how drumming can function in the service of the child's compliance. Common associations to drumming and its function may pose initial resistance from the medical team, which may see it as loud, disruptive, and too stimulating to the child. The therapist must be able to speak about the importance of release and expression to coping and compliance.

What to observe. Drumming as an embodied form of music therapy can connect to emotional, visceral, and kinesthetic levels of the patient's experience. The sought-after release can be achieved quickly, and the therapist should be aware of the patient's threshold for coping through active engagement, which can be reached sooner than expected.

Procedures. Music therapists can utilize the constructs of rhythm and drumming in conjunction with cognitive devices such as counting or rhythmic lyric recitation toward the development of an additional coping strategy. The therapist may focus the cycle of music on various musical components (harmonic, tempo, volume, etc.) in the creation of a cycle that supports the patient at a nonverbal level. This intervention may also incorporate the patient's favorite song or genre as the context in which the patient can engage in drumming.

The therapist's modeling of a rhythmic pattern on a drum, with either a numeric or a proselike structure, can serve to initiate the child into the shared experience. Following, the therapist and child can create and count cycles of the pattern, giving emphasis to various dynamics like tempo or volume to accentuate the release at the end of each cycle or series. The integration of counting draws the child into an experience that is both creative and concrete in terms of application. The added dimension of deep breathing with mindfulness can further serve the release that is achieved at the end of a given phrase.

Adaptations. Drumming offers immediate gratification, and for developmentally delayed children exhibiting issues with impulse control and attention deficit, such immediate sensory feedback can be overwhelming. Release through smaller hand percussion like cabassa and shakers can be substituted for drums for a more manageable experience.

GUIDELINES FOR RE-CREATIVE MUSIC THERAPY

Music Therapy for Socialization

Overview. The primary goals of music therapy for socialization are to support coping by facilitating peer support and normalizing the environment. Through both of these aims, a child's resources can be reactivated in the sharing of experiences with other children processing similar stress. Gaining mastery within the hospital environment through peer interaction is supported in shared music therapy experiences from re-creating favorite precomposed songs to songwriting, the latter of which will be discussed under Compositional Music Therapy.

Common areas such as inpatient playrooms, rehabilitation centers, and diagnosis-specific treatment centers are all appropriate milieus for socialization through re-creative techniques. Inpatient music therapy groups for children hospitalized for extended diagnostic testing and outpatient clinics such as chemotherapy infusion suites or dialysis centers are prime areas for facilitating peer interaction and building community. Shared experiences of learning to play an instrument or singing favorite songs offer therapeutic benefit in a context where frequency, continuity, and duration of treatment cultivates a community of familiarity and universality. Re-creative music therapy can contribute to this unique culture in which children are able to transcend diagnosis and where normal developmental trajectories can be restarted. Within music therapy experiences focusing on socialization, the long-term goals of creating a strong sense of peer support and community become paramount.

Preparation. Awareness of spatial and time considerations is important in order to set up the ideal circumstances to ensure the child's feelings of success and completion. Involvement of family members and staff can enhance the intervention but can also dilute the clinical intent, especially when the emotional needs of participants other than the patient become evident.

What to observe. A child's ability to organize around re-creative–oriented interventions will vary on an individual basis. Observation will inform the therapist when the child is engaged or not, and the therapist should remain flexible to other techniques as needed.

Procedures. The therapist begins socializing music therapy interventions by initially assessing the age range and receptiveness of the children present. Initiating ideas such as group improvisation, songwriting, or playing of favorite songs provides structure that can feel safe and inviting. This structure is sustained by the therapist's musical presence and maintenance of a tonal center on a melodic instrument around which the participants can organize. The therapist's task of facilitating a safe musical climate continues with the demonstration of the various instruments available. The subsequent distribution of instruments can be an opportunity to match instruments to the assessed abilities and interests of each child.

Younger children can be invited into music participation by distributing small hand percussion such as shakers, cabassas, and hand drums. The provision of structured songs such "Old MacDonald Had a Farm" can invite participation through fill-in-the-blank prompting.

One such scenario the author recalls is that of an Epilepsy Monitoring Unit (EMU), in which eight children undergoing VEEG (described earlier) in separate consecutive rooms were able to extend their monitoring cables to the doorways, where they could see each other playing and engaging in familiar songs. Two music therapists positioned at opposite ends of the corridor synchronized their guitar-playing to provide a cohesive group experience. The isolation of VEEG monitoring was ameliorated by creating such a group experience in less than likely circumstances.

For adolescents, similar scenarios can be created with an emphasis on playing or listening to the favorite songs, artists, or bands identified by each individual. Supporting each participant's voice is important to maintain cohesion and momentum in any direction the experience moves. The creation of an open-ended rap or blues, with space given to the contributions of each participant, can facilitate a spirit of altruism as peer support begins to emerge, first in the context of creating lyrics together and later in the reflection on shared themes.

Adaptations. Re-creative music therapy, requiring a certain conviction from the patient to actively apply or learn musical skills, has specific application in circumstances where the primary goal can include psychoemotional or cognitive motives. Supporting the child's sense of self as it is impacted by illness is an appropriate goal of this type of work.

It should be noted, however, that actual procedural and surgical support may preclude the use of re-creative music therapy techniques. At these times, the child's ego is solely invested in managing the multisensory experience of the procedure itself, and the primary goals of music therapy center on supporting this process through the effective completion of the procedure.

Music Alternate Engagement (MAE)

Overview. This technique focuses on active engagement of the child in specific, achievable tasks associated with a procedure. The use of music or musical components with the therapist provides opportunities for a child to participate in an activity that offers alternate points of focus (Bishop, Christenberry, Robb, & Toombs Rudenberg, 1996). While distraction seems evident in MAE, the therapeutic relationship is central to MAE's effectiveness, which transcends the definition of distraction, as discussed earlier. Here the child is engaged in purposeful creation to refocus her attention or awareness away from unpleasant stimuli. The use of MAE in debridement (Fratianne et al., 2001) allows the therapist to work closely with the child on re-creative tasks within the music to shift awareness from the pain of the procedure.

What to observe. The therapist watches the child's level of attendance to the music stimuli or activity and adjusts accordingly to ensure ongoing effectiveness.

Procedures. The therapist engages the child in the process of music selection in advance of the procedure. Allowance for this time of preparation and planning contributes to the child's sense of control. Carefully assessing the child's musical preferences, with the goal of eventually adapting them to specific points of the procedure, is the preliminary step in this process. Music that is age-appropriate and specific to the child is critical in order to maximize on the therapeutic alliance or partnering with the therapist. The therapist suggests or assigns (depending on the child's degree of engagement) songs to specific phases of the procedure based on his knowledge of the level of stress that is potentially incurred at each juncture. The resulting sequence of songs or verses serves to anchor the child in a familiar space during the procedure. Immediately prior to the procedure, the therapist and child should review the plan.

This intervention is exemplified in the simple scenario of an IV placement. The child chooses a song for the setup of the procedure, which involves sterilizing the skin and placing a rubber tourniquet. A second song is selected for the placement of the IV itself, and a third song is selected for use to mark the completion of the procedure. These markers organize the sequence of events into a manageable form, thus replacing uncertainty with predictability. When indicated, the therapist shifts music components such as tempo or volume within the sequence to maintain the child's attention.

GUIDELINES FOR COMPOSITIONAL MUSIC THERAPY

Songwriting and Performance

Overview. Compositional music therapy in the form of songwriting is best suited as a psychotherapeutic intervention for the patient who is coping effectively with hospitalization and the regimen of procedures or surgical trajectory. The periods of time that can exist pre- and postprocedurally and pre- and postsurgically provide the psychic space in which a patient can make sense of the personal investment and introspection that is marshaled in process-oriented and product-driven creative endeavors. Organization and reclaiming of pre- and postsurgical time through creative songwriting and further project development into performance opportunities offers unique opportunity for preparation and transition back into normal life routines.

The writing of original songs or lyrics at this level, even if simplified or structurally supported by the therapist, requires the patient's psychoemotional investment in the process. Here the patient processes feelings at a deeply introspective level, and existential themes are brought into aesthetic form. The construction of original compositions is not only derived from rich introspective process, but also driven by a desire to create a product that can serve as a marker of time in both concrete and metaphoric terms. The end result of such an investment, be it a song, poem, or free-style rap, can reflect both the here-and-now experience of the child and the hopes associated with the resumption of normal routine.

The particular case of a 17-year-old girl awaiting epilepsy surgery provided the context for such an achievement. The therapist aligned with the patient in a way that provided structure to many weeks of hospitalization punctuated by presurgical testing. The planning and supporting of the patient's delivery of a recital that was missed due to the hospitalization included not only a recapitulation of music she had memorized for the original school function, but also an original piano composition and printed program of the recital pieces she had selected. Through the enactment of a formal recital in the unit, the patient reclaimed lost opportunity and redefined her experience by connecting to the vitality of her own musicality.

Songwriting can take various forms, from spontaneous nonsensical lyric writing to deeply personal and introspective process. In either case, time may be a determining factor, and the therapist should be mindful of the importance of completion when interruption and uncertainty are common experiences.

Contextual factors (emergency procedures, overstimulation, immediate family stress, history of abuse, etc.) should be considered when introducing this intervention. Dismantling defense mechanisms without the time, space, or clinical experience to effectively process emotional trauma is irresponsible and unethical.

Scheduled session times during extended hospitalization is a manageable feat and creates an honored space of sanctuary in which the process can unfold naturally. The only scheduling challenges in this scenario that remain unchanged are the reality that the hospital is an environment of uncertainty and that prearranged individual time can be interrupted by another patient's trauma, unscheduled visits from family and friends, and spontaneously scheduled procedures or tests that will suddenly take precedence. A therapist who understands that this is the context of care in which he is working will learn that adaptability is important to integrate for himself and to model for others. The therapist's countertransference that may be elicited when therapeutic treatment is interrupted may also reflect the child's experience with unpredictability. Awareness of this dynamic will allow the therapist to reconcile the changes in treatment that will best meet the child's needs.

Preparation. Again, prescheduling sessions for this work is recommended so that the process is distinguished as meaningful and significant within the hospital routine. Attention should be given to having adequate resources available so that the process of creating a song, once embarked upon, can continue uninterrupted for the duration of the session. Resources should include instruments that can be used to explore harmonic, melodic, and rhythmic ideas (piano, guitar, synthesizer, Omnichord, percussion); paper; pencils; and a small recording device for playback and review.

Because songwriting can extend over several sessions, provisions for storage or space for safekeeping of unfinished work should also be considered. The therapist's protection of the child's unfinished work is a testament to the value placed upon the child's creativity and personal investment in the process. This value reflects the trust and respect that exists within the therapeutic relationship.

What to observe. The patient's process with creativity may divulge vulnerabilities and misconceptions about self-worth and self-criticism of skill or talent. The therapist can provide a forum in which such feelings can be processed and reconciled or, when necessary, redirected back into the therapeutic intention and purpose of the endeavor.

Procedures. The therapist introduces the idea of songwriting or performance to the child as a means of giving form and structure to her experience. The therapist should be clear about this intention, so that the child is able to invest herself in the process with trust that her creative expression and wishes for the outcome are respected and remain central. To this end, clarity on whether the song is for personal process or to share with others is important to determine. The child's wishes can be especially important to reinforce with caregivers and other staff who may exaggerate or distort the purpose of the songwriting in an attempt to motivate the patient or to simply join in the process. Existing maladaptive patterns of communication may be divulged through these interactions, and the therapist can provide a forum for clarification of the goal and its therapeutic importance to the patient.

Once this preliminary work is completed, the therapist can initiate the process by providing a forum in which the child is comfortable expressing ideas and feelings about the focus of a song. Predictable structures like a 12-bar blues can be offered initially to elicit short phrases specific to a chosen theme. Writing a rap about hospital experiences can offer another point of entry into the songwriting process. Perhaps the poetry that the child has already composed can be the impetus for a song. Therapists should know that committing thoughts to a written form requires the child to become specific about her thoughts and ideas, and this can be intimidating. The therapist creatively introduces musical forms that comfortably invite expression while respecting the child's pace. Charlton (2013) utilizes songwriting and Rap to support healthy creative expression in teenagers living with Sickle Cell disease. Giving creative form to the anger and frustration felt by some patients provides for more authentic communication between patients, the medical team, and caregivers.

Working with school-age and adolescent siblings of infants who had succumbed to Sudden Infant Death Syndrome (S.I.D.S.), the author found the use of groove and instrumental breaks effective in eliciting expression. The children and adolescents respectively created developmentally appropriate rhythmic patterns that were supported harmonically on guitar by the therapist. Further development of the music by way of each individual's participation on various instruments solidified a form that could be rendered with intermittent breaks intended for verbal expression of complicated feelings. The author introduced harmonic cadence to prepare the children for the break, which could be taken by anyone wishing to express a remembrance or thought about their loss. Following the shared thought, the therapist would resume the groove, continuing to the next cadence and break. This form, effective in the described setting, has proven impactful during pre- and postsurgical phases for many patients as well. It is a form that offers structure and freedom, opportunities for both verbal and nonverbal expression, and refuge into the music when words are simply too much.

Finally, a more formalized approach to songwriting can be introduced once comfort and momentum have been established. The therapist can assist in organizing the child's expression of ideas around the structure of *verses* that explore themes, a *chorus* that provides emphasis of an overall theme, and of course a *bridge* and recapitulation to create diversity within the song.

Adaptations. Group songwriting in outpatient infusion suites, dialysis centers, and other long-term contexts can offer a similar forum, as described under Re-creative Music Therapy.

Recording and Music Technology

Overview. Recording and music technology is an exciting area of music therapy intervention that merges the creative process with technical aptitude and skill. By the very nature of this integration, a child or adolescent is empowered in a way unlike other areas of music therapy. While the recording milieu can offer the means to display expression and process, it also allows for editing and refinement of what is to be shared. Recording technology allows an individual to show what she desires to show the world, be it authentic or idealized. This latter point becomes central to the therapy process as the therapist supports the child's informed choice to use recording as a means of escaping or transcending an experience, or as a forum for authentic sharing. Encouraging integration and reconciliation of the losses sustained during illness and hospitalization takes on a whole new meaning when the magical process of recording is accessed. Barry and colleagues (2010) outline a specific use of recording integratively to ease stress and anxiety before radiation treatment. Their work is described in the Research Evidence section of the chapter.

The areas of indication for this type of intervention are again those junctures in the hospital experience where time is afforded, as in pre- and postprocedurally and pre- and postsurgically. The specific and advanced goals of this work lend themselves well to the periods of waiting and transition inherent to extended illness as well. Here the introduction of various types of music technology can reinforce agency and control, which can in turn optimize coping. The patient is provided with an opportunity to master a skill directly, but with aesthetic distance not necessarily attributable to the process of songwriting. Aesthetic distance (Landy, 1993) pertains to the comfortable balance of one's subjective and objective attachment to a subject. The recording process endows the child or adolescent with concrete tools by which to share her experience, while still inviting creative expression.

Creating grooves, loops, and arrangements of musical ideas with the use of technology can offer an additional point of focus for a child overwhelmed with hospitalization. Recording as a unique forum of creative process may allow a child refuge from direct interaction with others and temporary refuge from inner feelings that may be overwhelming. Such distance and space can be especially appreciated during adolescence. At the other end of this spectrum is the possibility of magnifying one's creative expression in songwriting through the use of production technology. Again, the creation of a tangible object, as in a recording or music video, not only marks the hospital experience as a time of mastery, but also provides a way of reclaiming time itself through the creation of something meaningful on multiple levels.

Compositional approaches to music therapy can foster independence and confidence within the safety of the unconditional therapeutic relationship. Role definition is important here to ensure that the therapeutic relationship is strong enough to be enacted at times when technology cannot sufficiently support the immediate needs of the child experiencing the stress of a traumatic procedure.

The introduction of technology challenges the therapeutic relationship by casting the object of technology to center stage of the process. The use of recording technology is seductive to most children because of the implied power and control. It is not ironic that these themes are activated in the hospital setting, yet it is the therapist's responsibility to provide presence and witness to the child's experience. Presence through witnessing is operative here because the potential for isolation and reclusivness exists when a child is solely focused on the medium.

Preparation. The music therapist must be familiar with technology and equipment, especially the current innovations in computer software and programs created for recording. Some of these resources are Finale, GarageBand,™ Pro-Tools, Band in a Box, and other recording studio and track management programs. It is also recommended that the therapist create an acoustically optimal space where the possibilities of interruption are minimized.

The recording process can incur moments of heightened frustration when the limitations of technology infringe upon the organic process of creating music. The therapist integrating technology should be adept at trouble-shooting, as this will affect the therapist's credibility and competence. Authenticity about one's level of understanding when introducing technology is again the best policy, and will also invite a shared experience in the work. Collaboration can provide another entry point into a therapeutic relationship that is strong enough to provide support when technology fails to do so.

Procedures. The idea of a recording studio as a resource within a music therapy program is a luxury considering that in most hospitals space is an issue. Fortunately, the rapid development in technology has rendered a range of home studio resources that can be utilized across a range of settings. As a result, recording sessions can be held at bedside if needed.

The first step toward embarking upon a recording project is to solidify the goals and expectations, discussing with the child her interests in sharing her recordings with others and the therapeutic aim of the recording process and the recording itself.

An important conversation to be had in preparation for recording focuses on the arrangement of the song to be recorded: Is there a chorus? A bridge? How many verses will there be? The child is empowered to take artistic control in asserting her preferences and aesthetic standards here, and in doing so makes a personal investment in the project.

On the day of recording, the therapist should solidify the time and space, with clear messaging to outside parties that "recording is in session." Attention to this small detail can prevent unnecessary interruptions from occurring and ensure that valuable time is not lost.

The sequence of steps in the actual recording process is determined by the arrangement and vision of how the song should sound in terms of instrumentation. Generally, the rhythm section (drum and bass) tracks are recorded first, followed by the placement of harmonic instruments such as piano, guitar, and synthesizer. Next in line are melodic instruments such as string or wind instruments, and instrumental solos. While the vocals are typically recorded last, a rough vocal track known as a "scratch vocal" is often recorded early-on to serve as a point of reference for instrumental tracks and vocal harmonies or background vocals. Once the lead vocal track is finished, the entire recording may be taken through a mixing and mastering process in which special effects can be applied.

Considering that most recording projects take more than a few sessions to complete, the therapist should be sure to safely preserve the completed work. When working with computer programs, saving and backing up any work is sufficient. When working with live-to-digital recording devices, burning a compact disc (CD) of the work not only saves what has been completed, but also provides a work-in-progress recording that can be reviewed. A sense of pride is often attached to the physical object that the patient can take away from the session.

The finished product can hold tremendous value for a child, as it is truly a personal accomplishment that can be seen, heard, and felt. It additionally serves as a testament to the therapeutic relationship, a marker of time, and a legacy for the child's family. Like songwriting, the recording process is highly creative and the therapist's role can be supportive and encouraging from start to finish. Schreck (2013) presents beautiful examples of his work with terminally ill children, who while moving through the vicissitudes of treatment, create such legacies through their songwriting and recording.

Adaptations. The use of recording technology can become overstimulating for children exhibiting poor impulse control, attention deficit, or symptoms on the autistic spectrum, but simplification and strong therapeutic presence can provide the necessary constructs through which to introduce the medium to this population. Certainly, technology can offer creative and expressive opportunities for developmentally delayed children at these same junctures of hospitalization, and this detail can be found in Chapters 10 and 12.

RESEARCH EVIDENCE

Research literature on the use of music for procedural and surgical support includes music therapy interventions as well as music medicine interventions. It is important to make a clear distinction between these two practices.

Music medicine involves the use of prerecorded music for symptom management by non–music therapy medical professionals. Research in music medicine generally reports on the effects of listening to recorded music on various physical and physiological responses (e.g., heart rate, blood pressure). Whereas research on listening to prerecorded music in medical patients certainly has reported beneficial results, it lacks the important therapeutic alliance that is central to music therapy.

Music therapy focuses on the use of music within a therapeutic relationship by a music therapist to address a range of goals from cognitive, behavioral, psychoemotional, social and existential to needs that are physiological or physical in origin. The therapeutic relationship and the individualized use of music interventions to meet each patient's unique needs are necessary in order to go beyond symptom management and, instead, address psychosocial and psychotherapeutic needs of patients and their families. Notably, however, the abundance of music medicine research has increased curiosity and understanding within the medical community as to the use of music as a nonpharmacological agent in medical treatment. The result of this stimulus has appropriately charged the music therapy community with the task of generating research on music therapy itself.

Dileo and Bradt (2005) encourage such research efforts by defining 12 specific goals of inquiry ranging from the need to distinguish music medicine from music therapy to isolating the effects of specific musical components (tone, rhythm, harmony, etc.) on targeted physical symptoms. The emphasis on utilizing various research methods, including randomized controlled trials, integrative of quantitative and qualitative approaches (as in mixed methods research) is made to a divided audience of music therapy scholars and clinicians. The main issue with research efforts in a field like music therapy is that there are obvious challenges when attempting to study and quantify the aspects of music therapy as a therapeutic process that lie beyond definition. Music therapy as an art form within the helping profession can be compromised when research methodology infringes upon the integrity of the therapeutic work. Ghetti (2012) acknowledges this dilemma in substantiating the need for an indigenous model of music therapy. In her qualitative analysis of the existing literature on the use of music therapy for procedural support, Ghetti suggests an organization of current methodology and clinical practice into three general areas. These categories include music engagement (use of music to actively engage the child to optimize coping), integrative approaches (focusing on the child's sensory integration and understanding), and music-assisted relaxation techniques. Ghetti (2012) also extrapolated from her review the following major categories that were found to be congruent across practitioners:

> assessment, preparation, modification of the environment, level of patient engagement, focus of attention, type of music used, role of therapist, role of the music, role of the patient, sense of control/empowerment, issues impacting coping, individualized nature of procedural support, issues related to pain perception, and limitations to effectiveness. (p. 17)

The themes identified by Ghetti provide insight into the underpinning philosophy of music therapy as a helping profession. That the shared beliefs across theoretical orientations have allowed the profession to thrive and develop in spite of the absence of research gives testament to the validity of music therapy in medical treatment. It is understandable that therapists working specifically within the domains of procedural and surgical support have relied upon existing methodology to forge the work. It is worth recognizing the development of this important context of care as it has occurred thus far while also discussing legitimate research models that have contributed to the methods discussed here.

Research methods that potentially infringe upon patient care are challenging to implement, especially at such high-stress points of hospitalization as procedural and surgical intervention, yet the literature is expanding. Efforts to conduct randomized controlled trials (Caprilli, Anastasi, Grotto, Scollo-Abeti, & Messeri, 2007; Kain et al., 2004; Loewy, Hallan, Friedman, & Martinez, 2005; Yu, Liu, Li, & Ma, 2009) are rendering compelling findings that substantiate the existing body of anecdotal findings. The attention given to this standard of research (Bradt, 2012) and systematic review efforts (Klassen, Liang, Tjosvold, Klassen, & Hartling, 2008; Treurnicht Naylor, Kingsnorth, Lamont, McKeever, & Macarthur, 2010) are generating needed visibility for this movement within the profession. Clearly more research will further substantiate the existing body of anecdotal reporting and methodological development that has occurred in the last 60 years.

The culture of medical care is a contributing factor to the successful implementation of music therapy studies that can be rendered simultaneously to quality patient care. Driven by the increasing pressure to compete for business, hospital administrations are becoming increasingly dedicated to patient satisfaction surveys such as the Hospital Consumer Assessment of Healthcare Providers and Systems (HCAHPS). It is therefore recommended to use research protocols that place emphasis upon findings that can translate into goals that meet the interests of hospital administrators. To this end, this author examined the impact of a psychosocial care model inclusive of psychoeducation, procedural support, and psychotherapeutic support over a four-year period on children's coping with epilepsy testing procedures and surgery in a pediatric neuroscience institute (Mondanaro, 2008). The treatment model integrated music therapy and Child Life philosophy and was administered by a clinician who was dually certified in music therapy and Child Life. Qualitative data gleaned from patient surveys, unsolicited written feedback from families, and daily epilepsy-monitoring unit (EMU) journal entries were gathered on 835 children from the ages of one through 21 who received epilepsy treatment according to the standards of care defined in this chapter. The data indicated optimal levels of coping with procedural and surgical treatment of epilepsy without the use of anesthesia or restrains, resulting in positive implications of cost effectiveness. The results from this study illustrate the effectiveness of integrative care (Leeuwenburgh et al., 2007).

Efficacy research specific to procedural and surgical support is sparse. This author has chosen to present the few studies that he feels to be relevant, while also organizing other pertinent literature according to diagnosis- or procedure-specific criteria for the reader's independent inquiry.

Receptive Music Therapy

A study by Loewy and colleagues (2005) that compared the use of live music as a relaxation technique to chloral hydrate (a form of anesthesia) was conducted with 60 children, ages one month to five years, who were undergoing EEG testing. A first-of-its-kind study, the results were significant for illustrating that music therapy as a nonpharmacological treatment was effective in supporting coping by facilitating a sleep state in 97% of the children during an EEG as opposed to the 50% receiving chloral hydrate. This study is historically significant because it implicates music therapy as a risk-free intervention. The research also indicated that the recovery time from chloral hydrate was substantially greater than when music was used, which additionally suggests both time- and cost-effectiveness.

Another study (Fratianne et al., 2001) tested the efficacy of music-based imagery and musical alternate engagement in assisting burn patients in managing their pain and anxiety during debridement. Twenty-five patients, seven years of age and older, were randomly divided into two groups. Members of group A received music therapy during their first dressing change, while members of group B did not receive music therapy until their second dressing change the following day. Measurements of pulse, patients' self-report of pain and anxiety, and the nurse's observation of patients' tension indicated significant reductions in self-reported pain in those who received music therapy for their first dressing change in contrast to those who did not receive music therapy ($p < .03$). The conclusion was that music therapy is a valuable noninvasive intervention for the treatment of pain during debridement.

Walworth (2005) looked at the impact of music therapy–assisted computerized tomography scans (N = 57), echocardiograms (N = 92), and other procedures (N = 17) in pediatric patients ages six months to seven years. Music therapists began the live-music intervention in the waiting room and continued into the treatment area, where the child's favorite song or genre was provided along a continuum of music offerings. The results of the study showed a decrease in the number of staff members needed to be present, a reduction in procedural time, and the elimination of patient sedation. Walworth's study indicates again that cost- and time-effectiveness are valuable outcomes of the use of music therapy for procedural support.

Finally, of particular interest is a study by Caprilli and colleagues (2007) focusing on the use of live music rendered by professional musicians, not necessarily music therapists, in the context of venipuncture being administered to a group of 108 children ages four through 13. Two randomly assigned groups of 54 children each were compared and evaluated for levels of distress experienced before, during, and after the procedure. Children in the first group went through the procedure while interacting with the musicians in the presence of a parent, while children of the second group received the procedure without the interaction of the musician, but still in the presence of a parent. Treatment effects were measured by means of the Wong-Baker FACES Pain Rating Scale® and the Amended Form of the Observation Scale of Behavioral Distress. Results indicated that distress ($p < .001$) and pain intensity ($p < .05$) were lower in the music group compared to the control group. This study is interesting because the use of live music interaction is a form of receptive music therapy, and the indication is positive for the use of music therapy with venipuncture. Also significant here, while unmeasured, is the presence of a parent in both scenarios. Clearly, a family-centered approach to care was practiced.

The following categorization of articles utilizing receptive techniques includes both music therapy and music medicine literature and is provided as a convenient guide to the reader. These articles span a range of medical milieu including work in dentistry (Aitken, Wilson, Coury, & Moursey, 2002), pediatric oncology units (Barry et al., 2010; Pfaff, Smith, & Gowan, 1989; Shabanloei, Golchin, Esfahani, Dolatkhah, & Rasoulian, 2010), and epilepsy monitoring units (Loewy et al., 2005; Mondanaro, 2008). Additional diagnosis-specific reports include cerebral palsy (Yu et al., 2009) and epilepsy (Mondanaro, 2008).

Findings targeted on specific medical interventions include general procedural support (Walworth, 2005); presurgical distress (Chetta, 1981); postsurgical care (Allred, Byers, & Sole, 2008); various types of venipuncture (Berlin, 1998; Caprilli et al., 2007; Fowler-Kerry & Lander, 1987; Malone, 1996; Noguchi, 2006; Tamhankar & Chennuri, 2010; Windich-Biermeier et al., 2007); EEG (Loewy et al., 2005; Mondanaro, 2008); dressing change, burn wound care, and debridement (Bishop, Christenberry, Robb & Toombs-Rudenberg, 1996; Daveson, 1999; Fratianne et al., 2001; Neugerbauer & Neugebauer, 2003; Protacio, 2010; Whitehead-Pleaux, Baryza, & Sheridan, 2006); bone marrow transplant and aspiration (Pfaff, Smith, & Gowan, 1989; Shabanloei, Golchin, Esfahani, Dolatkhah, & Rasoulian, 2010); and radiation therapy (Barry et al., 2010).

Finally, there is a report on integrative treatment combining music with acupuncture (Yu et al., 2009).

Improvisational Music Therapy

The literature available on the specific use of improvisation during procedures is integrative of receptive approaches, supporting the commonly held philosophy that the therapist should remain adaptive to the shifting presentation of the patient. Research studies that specifically target the use of live music improvisation in procedural and surgical support are sparse but compelling nevertheless (Kain et al., 2004; Loewy et al., 2005; Malone, 1996; Mondanaro, 2008; Walworth, 2003). The results of most of these studies have already been presented under Receptive Music Therapy.

Kain and colleagues (2004) investigated the impact of interactive music therapy, including improvisational and re-creative music therapy interventions, compared to oral midazolam and a control group on the perioperative anxiety of 123 pediatric patients. The results suggested that anxiety reduction was the greatest in the midazolam group ($p < .01$). Of interest is the fact that the music therapy interventions were provided by two music therapists; the results clearly indicated a therapist effect (i.e., one therapist was more effective in helping children reduce their anxiety than the other). However, even after controlling for therapist effect, the children in the midazolam group were the least anxious.

Re-creative Music Therapy

Barry and colleagues (2010) designed a mixed methods research study to investigate the effects of an interactive music therapy intervention by way of a music therapy CD (MTCD) creation with 11 children, ages 6 to 13, diagnosed with various types of cancer and undergoing radiation therapy for the first time. The participants were randomly assigned to a MTCD group or a standard care control group. The children as well as the parents and treatment staff were asked to fill out questionnaires related to the child's distress and coping during radiation therapy treatment. These questionnaires contained closed-ended as well as open-ended questions. The music therapy intervention involved children creating a music CD with the use of computer-based music software with the support of the therapist. The study found that 67% of the children in the control group used social withdrawal as a coping strategy, compared to none of the children in the music therapy group. The qualitative data provided more strong support for stress-reducing effects of the music therapy intervention. The conclusion was that MTCD offered children a developmentally appropriate and creative forum that contributed to optimizing coping and autonomy prior to initial radiation treatment.

Compositional Music Therapy

The author has not identified research evidence for the use of compositional-based interventions.

SUMMARY AND CONCLUSION

The emotional and psychological impact of hospitalization, and specifically procedures on pediatric patients, is undeniable. Music therapy as an integrative therapy does much to ensure optimal coping of pediatric patients in medical settings by attending diligently to their needs through thorough assessment, a therapeutic relationship, and individualized treatment. These points of focus are cardinal to the work of music therapists across theoretical orientations. The growth of the profession is steadily moving toward becoming fundamental to programming in pediatric hospitals, and, optimally speaking, music therapy is uniquely positioned in health care because of the range of therapeutic possibilities it offers.

Music therapists are challenged, however, to provide evidence of efficacy necessary to secure appropriate positioning with the medical industry. Research on music therapy as procedural and surgical support is highly indicated because efficacy in these areas leads to reportable cost-effectiveness (Walworth, 2005), reduced medical error (Cote et al., 2000), higher patient satisfaction scores (Loewy et al., 2005), and ultimately an investment in the future of our children by supporting them during potentially traumatic events.

Advocacy for the patient's emotional and psychological safety should not be limited to scenarios defined as invasive or even noninvasive, especially given that these current definitions are based purely on physical criteria. When we reflect on the survival rates of hospitalized children even 60 years ago (Plank, 1965), and acknowledge the increasing appearance of programming aimed at the needs of children (Leeuwenburgh et al., 2007), it is clear that the value placed on the emotional and psychological health of hospitalized children has shifted positively. It is reasonable to believe that this shift has contributed to the paradigm in which we now practice and that today, more than ever, music therapists can join the treatment dialogue with confidence and a commitment to patient advocacy.

REFERENCES

Aitken, J., Wilson, S., Coury, D., & Moursi, A. (2002). The effect of music distraction on pain, anxiety and behavior in pediatric dental patients. *Pediatric Dentistry, 24*(2), 114–118.

Aldwin, C. (1994). *Stress, coping and development: An integrative perspective.* New York: Guilford.

Ali, S., Drendel, A., Kircher, J., & Beno, S. (2010). Pain management of musculoskeletal injuries in children: Current state and future directions. *Pediatric Emergency Care, 26*(7), 518–524.

Allred, K., Byers, J., & Sole, M. (2008). The effect of music on postoperative pain and anxiety. *Pain Management Nursing March, 11*(1), 15–25.

American Academy of Pediatrics. (2006). Child life services. *Pediatrics, 118*(4), 1757–1763.

American Psychiatric Association (APA). (2000). *Diagnostic and statistical manual of mental disorders—Text revision* (4th ed.). (DSM-IV-TR). Arlington, VA: Author

Anderson, D. (2005). *Mosby's medical, nursing, & allied health dictionary* (6th ed.). St. Louis, MO: Mosby.

Arts, S., Abu-Saad, H., Champion, G., Crawford, M., Fisher, R., Juniper, K., & Ziegler, J. (1994). Age-related response to lidocaine-prilocaine (EMLA) emulsion and effect of music distraction on the pain of intravenous cannulation. *Pediatrics, 93*(5), 797–801.

Ayson, C. (2008). Child-parent well-being in a pediatric ward: The role of music therapy in supporting children and their parents facing the challenge of hospitalization. *Voices: A World Forum for Music Therapy, 8*(1). Retrieved June 29, 2011, from https://normt.uib.no/index.php/voices/article/viewArticle/449

Balan, R., Bavdekar, S., & Jadhav, S. (2009). Can Indian classical instrumental music reduce pain felt during venipuncture? *Indian Journal of Pediatrics, 76*(5), 469–473.

Barry, P., O'Callaghan, C., Wheeler, G., & Grocke, D. (2010). Music therapy CD creation for initial pediatric radiation therapy: A mixed methods analysis. *Journal of Music Therapy, 47*(3), 233–263.

Bayat, A., Ramaiah, R., & Bhananker, S. (2010). Analgesia and sedation for children undergoing burn wound care. *Expert Review of Neurotherapeutics, 10*(11), 1747–1759.

Berlin, B. (1998). Music therapy with children during invasive procedures: Our emergency department's experience. *Journal of Emergency Nursing, 24*(6), 607–608.

Berrios, C., & Jacobowitz, W. (1998). Therapeutic holding: Outcomes of a pilot study. *Journal of Nursing, 36*(8), 14–19.

Bibace, R., & Walsh, M. (1980). Development of children's concepts of illness. *Pediatrics, 66*(6), 912–917.

Bishop, B., Christenberry, A., Robb, S., & Toombs Rudenberg, M. (1996). Music therapy and child life interventions with pediatric burn patients. In M. A. Froelich (Ed.), *Music therapy with hospitalized children: A creative arts child life approach* (pp. 87–108). Cherry Hill, NJ: Jeffrey Books.

Bijttebier, P., & Vertommen, H. (1998). The impact of previous experience on children's reactions to venipunctures. *Journal of Health Psychology, 3*, 39–46.

Blount, R. L., Bachanas, P. J., Powers, S. W., Cotter, M. C., Franklin, A., Chaplin, W., Mayfield, J., Henderson, M., & Blount, S. D. (1992). Training children to cope and parents to coach them during routine immunizations: Effects on child, parent, and staff behaviors. *Behavior Therapy, 23*, 689–705.

Bluemke D., & Breiter, S. (2000). Sedation procedures in MR imaging: Safety, effectiveness, and nursing effect on examinations. *Radiology, 216*(3), 633–644.

Boey, K.W. (1988). The measurement of stress associated with hospitalization. *Singapore Medical Journal, 20*, 586–588.

Bradt, J. (2009). Music entrainment for breathing regulation. In R. Azoulay & J. Loewy (Eds.), *Music, the breath and health: Advances in integrative music therapy.* (pp. 11–19). New York: Satchnote Press.

Bradt, J. (2010). The effects of music entrainment on postoperative pain perception in pediatric patients. *Music and Medicine, 2*(2), 150–157.

Bradt, J. (2012). Randomized controlled trials in music therapy: Guidelines for design and implementation. *Journal of Music Therapy, 49*(2), 120–150.

Bruscia, K. (1988). A survey of treatment procedures in improvisational music therapy. *Psychology of Music, 16*, 1–24.

Bruscia, K. E. (2001). A qualitative method of analyzing client improvisations. *Music Therapy Perspectives, 19*(1), 7–21.

Caprilli, S., Anastasi, F., Grotto, R., Scollo-Abeti, M., & Messeri, A. (2007). Interactive music as a treatment for pain and stress in children during venipuncture: A randomized prospective study. *Journal of Developmental and Behavioral Pediatrics, 28*(5), 399–403.

Cavender, K., Goff, M., Hollon, E., & Guzzetta, C. (2004). Parents' positioning and distracting children during venipuncture: Effects on children's pain, fear, and distress. *Journal of Holistic Nursing, 22*(1), 32–56.

Charlton, M. (2013). Hear my song: Giving voice to adolescents with sickle cell disease. In J. Mondanaro & G. Sara (Eds.), *Music and medicine: Integrative models in the treatment of pain.* (pp. 335–346). New York NY: Satchnote Press.

Chetta, H. (1981). The effect of music and desensitization on preoperative anxiety in children. *Journal of Music Therapy, 18*(2), 74–87.

Cignacco, E., Hamers, J., Stoffel, L., van Lingen, R., Gessler, P., McDougall, J., & Nelle, M. (2007). The efficacy of nonpharmacological interventions in the management of procedural pain in preterm and term neonates. A systematic literature review. *European Journal of Pain, 11*(2), 139–152.

Cote, C., Karl, H., Notterman, D., Weinberg, J., & McCloskey, C. (2000). Adverse sedation events in pediatrics: Analysis of medications used for sedation. *Pediatrics, 106*(4), 633–644.

Csikszentmihalyi, M. (1990). *Flow: The psychology of optimal experience.* New York: Harper & Row.

Daveson, B. (1999). A model of response: Coping mechanisms and music therapy techniques during debridement. *Music Therapy Perspectives, 9,* 32–38.

Dewees, M. (2005). Postmodern social work in interdisciplinary contexts. *Social Work in Health Care, 39*(3), 343–360.

Dileo, C., & Bradt, J. (1999). Entrainment, resonance, and pain-related suffering. In C. Dileo (Ed.), *Music therapy & medicine: Theoretical and clinical applications* (pp. 181–188). Silver Spring, MD: The American Music Therapy Association.

Dileo, C., & Bradt, J. (2005). *Medical music therapy: A meta-analysis & agenda for future research.* Cherry Hill, NJ: Jeffrey Books.

Fowler-Kerry, S., & Lander, J. (1987). Management of injection pain in children. *Pain, 30*(2), 169–175.

Fratianne, R., Prensner, J., Huston, M., Super, D., Yowler, C., & Standley, J. (2001). The effect of music-based imagery and musical alternate engagement on the burn debridement process. *The Journal of Burn Care & Rehabilitation, 22*(1), 47–53.

Friedman, R. L. (2000). *The healing power of the drum: A psychotherapist explores the healing power of rhythm.* Reno, NV: White Cliffs Media.

Gardstrom, S. C. (2003). An investigation of meaning in clinical music improvisation with troubled adolescents. Unpublished doctoral dissertation. Michigan State University.

Garro, A., Thurman, K., Kerwin, M., & Ducette, J. (2005). Parent/caregiver stress during pediatric hospitalization for chronic feeding problems. *Journal of Pediatric Nursing, 20*(4), 268–275.

Gaynard, K. E., Wolfer, J., Goldberger, J., Thompson, R., Redburn, L., & Laidley, L. (1990). *Psychosocial care of children in hospitals: A clinical manual from ACCH child life research project.* Mount Royal, NJ: ACCH.

Ghetti, C. M. (2012). Music therapy as procedural support for invasive medical procedures: Toward the development of music therapy theory. *Nordic Journal of Music Therapy, 21*(1), 3–35. DOI: 10.1080/08098131.2011.571278.

Golianu, B., Krane, E., Seybold, J., Almgren, C., & Anand, K. (2007). Nonpharmacological techniques for pain management in neonates. *Seminars in Perinatology, 31*(5), 318–322.

Heistein, L., Ramaciotti, C., Scott, W., Coursey, M., Sheeran, P., & Lemler, M. (2005). Chloral hydrate sedation for pediatric echocardiography: Physiologic responses, adverse events, and risk factors. Retrieved February 22, 2006, from http//pediatrics.aappublications.org/cgi/content/abstract/peds.2005-1445v1

Jeffs, D. (2007). A pilot study of distraction for adolescents during allergy testing. *Journal for Specialists in Pediatric Nursing, 12*(3), 170–185.

Kain, Z. N., Caldwell-Andrews, A. A., Krivutza, D. M., Weinberg, M. E., Gaal, D., Wang, S., & Mayes, L. C. (2004). Interactive music therapy as a treatment for preoperative anxiety in children: A randomized controlled trial. *Anesthesia & Analgesia, 98*(5), 1260–1266.

Klassen, J., Liang, Y., Tjosvold, L., Klassen, T., & Hartling, L. (2008). Music for pain and anxiety in children undergoing medical procedures: A systematic review of randomized controlled trials. *Ambulatory Pediatrics: The Official Journal of the Ambulatory Pediatric Association, 8*(2), 117–128.

Kovacs, P. J., Bellin, M. H., & Fauri, D. (2006). Family-centered care: A resource for social work in end-of-life and palliative care. *Journal of Social Work in End-of-Life and Palliative Care, 2*(1), 13–27.

Landy, R. J. (1993). *Persona and performance: The meaning of role in drama, therapy, and everyday life*. New York: Guilford Press.

Leeuwenburgh, E., Goldring, E., Fogel, A., Kanazawa, M., Lynch, T., & Mondanaro, J. (2007). Creative arts therapies. In S. Chisolm (Ed.), *The health professions: Trends and opportunities in U. S. health care* (pp. 397–424). Sudbury, MA: Jones and Bartlett.

Loewy, J. V. (2013). Music sedation and pain. In J. Mondanaro & G. Sara (Eds.), *Music and medicine: Integrative models in the treatment of pain* (pp. 95–104). New York NY: Satchnote Press.

Loewy, J. (2011). Tonal intervallic synthesis as integration in medical music therapy. In S. Baker & S. Uhlig (Eds.), *Voicework in music therapy: Research and practice* (pp. 252–268). Philadelphia, PA: Jessica Kingsley.

Loewy, J., Azoulay, R., Harris, B., & Rondina, E. (2009). Clinical improvisation with winds: Enhancing breath in music therapy. In R. Azoulay & J. Loewy (Eds.), *Music, the breath and health: Advances in integrative music therapy* (pp. 87–102). New York: Satchnote Press.

Loewy, J., Hallan, C., Friedman, E., & Martinez, C. (2005). Sleep/Sedation in children undergoing EEG testing: A comparison of chloral hydrate and music therapy. *Journal of Perianesthesia Nursing, 20*(5), 323–332.

Loewy, J., & Stewart, K. (2004). Music therapy to help traumatized children and caregivers. In N. Boyde Webb (Ed.) *Mass trauma and violence: Helping families and children cope.* (pp. 191-215). New York: Guilford Publications, Inc.

Loewy, J. (2000). *Music therapy in the neonatal intensive care unit*. New York: Satchnote Press.

Loewy, J., MacGregor, B., Richards, K., & Rodriguez, J. (1997). Music therapy pediatric pain management: Assessing and attending to the sounds of hurt, fear and anxiety. In J. Loewy (Ed.), *Music therapy and pediatric pain* (pp. 45–56). Cherry Hill, NJ: Jeffrey Books.

Malone, A. B. (1996). The effects of live music on the distress of pediatric patients receiving intravenous starts, venipunctures, injections, and heel sticks. *Journal of Music Therapy, 33*(1), 19–33.

Mangini, L., Confessore, M.T., Girard, P., & Spadola, T. (1995). Pediatric trauma support program: Supporting children and families in emotional crisis. *Critical Care Nursing Clinics of North America, 7*(3), 557–567.

Marx, J. A., Hockberger, R. S., Walls, R. M., & Adams, J. (2002). *Rosen's Emergency Medicine: Concepts and Clinical Practice* (5th ed., vol. 3). St. Louis, MO: Mosby.

Mason, S., Johnson, M. H., & Woolley, C. (1999). A comparison of distractors for controlling distress in young children during medical procedures. *Journal of Clinical Psychology in Medical Settings, 6*, 239–248.

Mazer, S. (2010). Music, noise, and the environment of care: History, theory, and practice. *Music and Medicine, 2*(3), 1–10.

McDonnell, L. (1984). Music therapy with trauma patients and their families on a pediatric service. *Music Therapy, 4*(1), 55–63.

Minnick, A., Mion, L., Leipzig, R., Lamb, K., & Palmer, R. (1998). Prevalence and patterns of physical restraint use in the acute care setting. *Journal of Nursing Administration, 28*(11), 19–24.

Mondanaro, J. (2005). Interfacing music therapy with other creative arts modalities to address anticipatory grief and bereavement in pediatrics. In C. Dileo & J. Loewy (Eds.), *Music therapy at the end of life* (pp. 25–32). Cherry Hill, NJ: Jeffrey Books.

Mondanaro, J. (2008). Music therapy in the psychosocial care of pediatric patients with epilepsy. *Music Therapy Perspectives, 26*(2), 102–109.

Mondanaro, J., & Needleman, S. (2011). Social Work and Creative Arts Therapy Services. In T. Altilio & S. Otis-Green (Eds.), *The Oxford Textbook of Palliative Social Work.* (pp.465-469). New York: Oxford University Press.

Neugebauer, C. T., & Neugebauer, V. (2003). Music therapy in pediatric burn care. In S. L. Robb (Ed.), *Music therapy in pediatric healthcare: Research and evidenced-based practice* (pp. 31–48). Silver Spring, MD: AMTA.

Noguchi, L. K. (2006). The effect of music versus nonmusic on behavioral signs of distress and self-report of pain in pediatric injection patients. *Journal of Music Therapy, 43*(1), 16–38.

Onal, C., Otsubo, H., Araki, T., Chitoku, S., Ochi, A., Weiss, S., Elliott, I., Snead, O.C. 3rd, Rutka, J.T., & Logan, W. (2003). Complications of invasive subdural grid monitoring in children with epilepsy. *Journal of Neurosurgery, 98*(5), 1017–1026.

Orland, E. (1965). *Protecting the emotional development of the ill child: The essence of the child life profession.* Connecticut: Psych Social Press.

Pershad, J., Palmisano, P., & Nichols, M. (1999). Chloral hydrate: The good and the bad. *Pediatric Emergency Care, 15*(6), 432–435.

Pfaff, V. K., Smith, K. E., & Gowan, D. (1989). The effects of music-assisted relaxation on the distress of pediatric cancer patients undergoing bone marrow aspirations. *Child Health Care, 18*(4), 232–236.

Plank, E. (1965). *Working with children in hospitals: A professional guide.* Chicago: Year Book Medical Publishers.

Pridham, K., Adelson, F., & Hanson, M. (1987). Helping children deal with procedures in a clinic setting: A developmental approach. *Journal of Pediatric Nursing, 2*(1), 13–22.

Protacio, J. (2010). Patient-directed music therapy as an adjunct during burn wound care. *Critical Care Nurse, 30*(2), 74–76.

Raskin, J., & Azoulay, R. (2009), Music therapy and integrative pulmonary care. In R. Azoulay & J. Loewy (Eds.), *Music, the breath, and health: Advances in integrative music therapy* (pp. 69–86). New York: Satchnote Press.

Rider, M. (1997). Entrainment music, healing imagery, and the rhythmic language of health and disease. In J. Loewy (Ed.), *Music therapy and pediatric pain* (pp. 81–88). Cherry Hill, NJ: Jeffrey Books.

Rosen's Emergency Medicine: Concepts and Clinical Practice (5th ed., vol. 3). (2002). St. Louis, MO: Mosby.

Rossetti, A., & Canga, B. (2013). Environmental music therapy: Rationale for multi-individual music psychotherapy for modulation of the pain experience. In J. Mondanaro & G. Sara (Eds.), *Music and medicine: Integrative models in the treatment of pain* (pp. 275–294). New York NY: Satchnote Press.

Schneider, S. (2005). Environmental music therapy: Life, death, and the ICU. In C. Dileo & J. Loewy (Eds.), *Music therapy at the end of life* (pp. 219–229). Cherry Hill, NJ: Jeffrey Books.

Shabanloei, R., Golchin, M., Esfahani, A., Dolatkhah, R., & Rasoulian, M. (2010). Effects of music therapy on pain and anxiety in patients undergoing bone marrow biopsy and aspiration. *AORN Journal, 91*(6), 746–751.

Schreck, B. (2013). A symphony of life: Harvesting emotions by preserving legacy & honoring pain. In J. Mondanaro & G. Sara (Eds.), *Music and medicine: Integrative models in the treatment of pain.* (pp. 237–252). New York NY: Satchnote Press.

Shields, L., Pratt, J., Davis, L., & Hunter, J. (2007). Family-centered care for children in hospital. *Cochrane Database of Systemic Reviews.* Issue 1. Art. No.: CD004811. DOI: 10.1002/14651858.CD004811.pub2.

Stedman's Medical Dictionary (27th ed.) (2000). Philadelphia: Lippincott Williams & Wilkins.

Stephens, M., Barkey, M., & Hall, H. (1999). Techniques to comfort children during stressful procedures. *Advances in Mind-Body Medicine, 15,* 49–60.

Stewart, K., & Schneider, S. (2000). The effects of music therapy on the sound environment in the NICU: A pilot study. In J. V. Loewy (Ed.), *Music therapy in the neonatal intensive care unit* (pp. 85–100). New York : Satchnote Press.

Tamhankar, P.M., & Chennuri, V.S. (2010). Can Indian classical instrumental music reduce pain felt during venipuncture? *Indian Journal of Pediatrics, 77*(7), 821–822.

Taylor, D. (1997). *Biomedical foundations of music therapy.* St. Louis, MO: MMB Music.

Tramo, M., Lense, M., Van Ness, C., Kagan, J., Doyle Settle, M., & Cronin, J. H. (2011). *Effects of music on physiological and behavioral indices of acute pain and stress in premature infants: Clinical trial and literature review.* Music and Medicine, *3(2), 72–83.*

Treurnicht Naylor, K., Kingsnorth, S., Lamont, A., McKeever, P., & Macarthur, C. (2010). The effectiveness of music in pediatric healthcare: A systematic review of randomized controlled trials. *Evidence Based Complementary and Alternative Medicine,* 2011. DOI: 10.1155/2011.

Turry, A. (1997). The use of clinical improvisation to alleviate procedural distress in young children. In J. Loewy (Ed.), *Music therapy and pediatric pain* (pp. 89–96). Cherry Hill, NJ: Jeffrey Books.

Walworth, D. D. (2005). Procedural-support music therapy in the healthcare setting: A cost-effectiveness analysis. *Journal of Pediatric Nursing, 20*(4), 276–284.

Whitehead-Pleaux, A. M., Baryza, M. J., & Sheridan, R. L. (2006). The effects of music therapy on pediatric patients' pain and anxiety during donor site dressing change. *Journal of Music Therapy, 43*(2), 136–153.

Windich-Biermeier, A., Sjoberg, I., Dale, J., Eshelman, D., & Guzzetta, C. (2007). Effects of distraction on pain, fear, and distress during venous port access and venipuncture in children and adolescents with cancer. *Journal of Pediatric Oncology Nursing: Official Journal of the Association of Pediatric Oncology Nurses, 24*(1), 8–19.

Wolf, P. (2005). Determinants of outcome in childhood epilepsy. *Acta Neurologica Scandinavica, Supplementum, 182,* 5–8.

Yu, H., Liu, Y., Li, S., & Ma, X. (2009). Effects of music on anxiety and pain in children with cerebral palsy receiving acupuncture: a randomized controlled trial. *International Journal of Nursing Studies, 46*(11), 1423–1430.

Chapter 7

Burn Care for Children

Annette Whitehead-Pleaux

INTRODUCTION

In the late 1970s, Christenberry was the first music therapist to write about treating burn patients with music therapy. She described providing interventions to address a variety of the needs of this population, including sensory stimulation, contractures, respiratory issues, anxiety, pain, social issues, and adjustment. Her initial description of music therapy treatment for burn patients remains true to this day. At this time, music therapy is applied through all three phases of burn care, namely acute, rehabilitative, and reconstructive. Since those early days of music therapy in burn care, music therapists in the United States and Australia have explored the effects of music therapy interventions on both pediatric and adult burn survivors. However, given the very small numbers of music therapists working in this subspecialty, the amount of evidence to support the application of music therapy is quite limited. It is the hope of the author that over time more music therapists will work in burn centers and burn units and provide much needed services and conduct research to support these services for this population.

DIAGNOSTIC INFORMATION

Etiology of Burns

Burn injuries are common. In the United States of America, of the approximately 2 million people injured by burns, "80,000 are hospitalized, and 6,500 die from burns" (Sheridan, 2012, p. 8). There are seven different causes of burn injuries: chemical, contact, electrical, flame, flash, radiation, and scald. Chemical burns results from an acid or alkali coming into contact with the skin. Chemicals will continue to burn until the chemical is flushed away by water or some other agent. Contact burns are caused by touching a hot surface like a stove burner. Electrical burns result from electricity traveling through a body and heating the tissues. Electric burns can cause damage both internally and externally. When people come into contact with fire, they sustain a flame burn. This differs from a flash burn, which is a burn injury caused by an explosion. Radiation burns are caused by exposure to radiant energy. The most common type of burns is scalding, an injury caused by hot liquids or steam.

Physiology of Burns

The severity of burns is determined by the depth of damage to the skin and tissues. Burn depth is rated by degrees. A first-degree burn (superficial burn) affects only the epidermis, the top layer of the skin. The skin is red, swollen, and painful. This burn heals on its own in a few days and leaves no scars. A second-degree burn affects not only the epidermis but also the *dermis*. It is also called a deep partial, which indicates that the dermis is injured. Depending on the severity of the injury to the dermis, this type of burn may heal on its own in two to three weeks. If the dermis is severely injured, this degree of burn may need surgical intervention to heal. A third-degree burn denotes a burn injury that affects both layers of the skin and extends into the subcutaneous tissue. It is also called a full thickness burn. Burns of this depth can heal only with surgical intervention. Finally, fourth-degree burns extend beyond the skin and affect the muscle and/or bone tissue. These burns require surgical intervention and can be very debilitating. Total burn site area (TBSA) is an estimation of the percentage of the body's surface area that is affected by the burn (Pham, Gibran, & Heimbach, 2007; Sheridan, 2012).

Skin is the largest organ, and damage to it affects many of its functions. These functions include but are not limited to maintaining the fluid and electrolyte balance of the body, temperature regulation, providing the brain with sensory information, and protecting the body from infection (Pham et al., 2007; Sheridan, 2012). Without the skin's protection, the body is at greater risk of infection from bacteria, viruses, and fungi. Preventing and managing infections is a large part of burn care and can include a number of different agents, either topical or internal. Often infectious agents are tested for sensitivity to medications in order to directly target the infections with the most effective medication and guard against creating drug-resistant strains of the infectious agent.

In addition to the skin, the *pulmonary* system may be injured. If the individual breathes in hot gases, steam, or hot liquids, the *larynx, trachea, bronchus,* and lungs may be burned (Sheridan, 2012). These injuries can be life-threatening, as the body and brain may not receive the necessary amount of oxygen to survive. The pulmonary system may also be affected by the inhalation of dangerous gases (Traber, Herndon, Enkhbaatar, Maybauer, & Maybauer, 2007). When inhaled, carbon monoxide limits the red blood cells' ability to carry oxygen to the body. If noxious or toxic gases are released by the materials involved in a fire, the individual may be exposed to these. The effects of these gases are dependent on the properties of the specific chemical makeup as well as the length of exposure to the gases. Exposure to these dangerous gases can result in greater injury to the lungs and anoxic brain injury. With both types of inhalation injuries, life-saving measures are initiated quickly; these often include intubating the patient to protect the airway from closing. Recovery from inhalation injuries often includes the use of breathing exercises to enhance the function of the lungs (Carrougher, 1998).

Burn injuries affect not only the tissues that are injured. Burn shock is a physiological state that occurs in burn patients. The exact biology for burn shock is not known as of yet; however, the symptoms are well understood (Warden, 2007). Burn shock is characterized by a hypodynamic *state* that is followed by a hyperdynamic phase. During the hypodynamic state, the child has a below normal amount of fluid within his body and the burn team works to provide fluid resuscitation to help maintain the body systems while reducing edema. When in the hyperdynamic state, the body develops a hypermetabolic response that includes "near doubling of the cardiac output and resting energy expenditure" (Sheridan, 2012, p. 12), an increase in the body temperature by 1 to 2 degrees Celsius, and an increase in protein breakdown. Burn shock and hyperdynamic state both affect many body systems and can create serious and potentially fatal complications to the burn injury.

The Basics of Burn Care

Burn care is provided by a multidisciplinary team. Burn teams are often composed of burn surgeons, nurses, anesthesiologists, physical and occupational therapists, social workers, psychologists, psychiatrists, child life specialists (in pediatric units), recreation therapists, and other mental health professionals (Sheridan, 2012). The team's focus is not only on the child's wounds but also on the individual's psychosocial adjustment to the injury, changes in appearance and ability, and losses. The combination of short-term and long-term outcomes is key to quality burn care. Music therapists are a valued member of the burn team. However, many burn centers across the United States do not employ music therapists at this time.

The treatment options for a burn depend upon its depth and whether the skin can heal within the first two to three weeks. If the burn is partial thickness, with some of the dermis intact, the wound will most likely heal on its own. For these wounds, bandages with antimicrobial agents like bacitracin are applied daily to every three days (Bessey, 2007). If the wound is full thickness, the damage to the dermis is too great for the skin to regenerate on its own. These wounds require surgical intervention (Bessey, 2007). The basic surgery to cover a wound is called excision and grafting (Muller, Gahankari, & Herndon, 2007). This procedure requires the surgeon to excise or remove the eschar (dead tissue) from the wound and then graft skin over the wound. Skin is obtained from a donor site, an area of the body from which skin is taken to cover the wound. Most commonly, the skin removed from the donor site is the epidermal layer. The donor site is then dressed with a bandage that will remain in place for up to two weeks. The skin graft is sewn to the healthy skin that surrounds the wound and a dressing called a stent is placed over the graft to hold it in place. This dressing will remain on the wound for one to two weeks. Once the stent is removed, the surgeon will evaluate the success of the graft and decide when to start rehabilitation and compression therapy.

Phases of Burn Care

Burn care has four distinct phases. The length that each individual spends in the various phases depends upon the TBSA as well as the complexity of the injury. The first phase is the initial evaluation and resuscitation, which starts immediately and can last up to 72 hours. In this phase, the burn team works to identify all injuries, perform fluid resuscitation, and decrease the edema (swelling) in the torso and extremities (Sheridan, 2012). Physical and occupational therapies (rehabilitation) focus on positioning and splinting to keep the extremities in positions that will allow for the greatest functional movement postburn.

As a member of the burn team, the music therapist is able to begin work with a child when the patient arrives at the hospital. The music therapy interventions focus on pain and anxiety management during wound evaluation and dressing changes as well as outside of procedures. The music therapist may also focus on providing music therapy interventions to normalize and aid in the adjustment to the hospital environment, decrease agitation, increase relaxation response, and provide or reduce stimulation in the room. In addition, providing support to the child and family regarding the initial shock of the injury and trauma can be accomplished by a music therapist outside of procedural care.

The next phase, initial excision and biologic closure, occurs for the first one to seven days. The burn team identifies which wounds require surgery and creates an initial surgical plan, excises much of the eschar, and temporarily or definitively closes the wounds (Sheridan, 2012). Rehabilitation continues to focus on positioning and splinting. Depending on the wound depth and location, the physical and occupational therapists may add range of motion interventions for different joints.

During this phase, the music therapist maintains the interventions that focus on procedural support, pain and anxiety management, normalization, and adjustment to the hospitalization. In addition, the music therapist can provide anxiety management preoperatively as well as pain and anxiety management postoperatively. The music therapist may cotreat with physical and occupational therapy to provide pain and anxiety management during the rehabilitation sessions and alternative motivations for movement.

Definitive wound closure is the third phase and can occur from weeks one through six. During this phase, the surgical team focuses on closing wounds with permanent coverage and begins to separate the child from intensive care support (Sheridan, 2012). Rehabilitation concentrates on positioning, splinting, and range of motion but will begin to add strengthening exercises. Music therapy continues to focus on pain and anxiety management, procedural support, preoperative anxiety management, postoperative pain and anxiety management, and cotreating with rehabilitation. Based on the severity of the patient's wounds and complications from the burn injury, the patient may start to require music therapy interventions for grief, loss, *Acute Stress Disorder* (ASD), *Post-Traumatic Stress Disorder* (PTSD), and concerns about appearance and function.

The final phase is rehabilitation and reconstruction. This phase can be broken into two subphases. The first, rehabilitation, occurs as the child's wounds are closed and rehabilitation takes the lead in the child's care (Sheridan, 2012). Rehabilitation concentrates on range of motion, strengthening, functional movement, and scar management. The entire burn team turns its attention to the child's reentry to the community. Music therapists will scale back the focus on procedural support as the child has learned ways to cope and the wounds have essentially healed. If ASD or PTSD symptoms are present, the music therapist addresses those symptoms. Grief, loss, disfigurement, function, and self-identity postburn may become more present in this phase as the survivor begins the process of community reintegration. Music therapy is well suited to work in conjunction with the efforts of the entire burn team to address these areas of need.

The second subphase is reconstruction. During this phase, the surgical team focuses on improving function and appearance (Sheridan, 2012). Rehabilitation works with the surgical team to support and enhance function through splinting, stretching, and exercises while working on appearance through pressure garments, massage, and reconstructive make-up. During this phase, the music therapist continues to work with the child on the immediate issues of surgical procedures including preoperative anxiety, postoperative pain and anxiety management, procedural support, and rehabilitation support. In addition, music therapy focuses on physical function, disfigurement, identity, and community reintegration.

Additional Disorders and Conditions

Given the nature of burn injuries, there exist a number of complications that are common in patients with serious burns. These disorders and conditions can be broken down by the body systems: neurologic, psychiatric, cardiovascular, pulmonary, hematologic, otolaryngologic, enteric, ophthalmic, renal, endocrine, genitourinary, and musculoskeletal (Sheridan, 2012). For this chapter, the focus will be on the complications that directly impact the treatment planning and interventions of music therapists. These conditions are delirium, nerve and spinal cord injuries, ASD/PTSD, and the musculoskeletal conditions of heterotopic ossification, muscle loss, and hypertrophic scar formation.

Neurologic conditions can include transient delirium, seizures, peripheral nerve injuries, and spinal cord deficits (Sheridan, 2012). Delirium is a state of altered sensory experiences that may lead to agitation and disorientation. It can be caused by the *metabolic state, hypoxia,* brain injury, and *opioid medication* (Ilechukwu, 2002). With supportive medical interventions, this delirium can be resolved. Delirium limits the child's ability to interact in a meaningful way with staff, family, and the environment. Peripheral nerve injuries can result from the burn injury or from compartment syndrome, a syndrome that is caused by the compression of the nerves or circulatory system for a part of the body often caused by edema in burn survivors (Sheridan, 2012). Electrical burns can result in neural injury that develops weeks postburn due to conditions such as compartment syndrome (Sheridan, 2012). Both peripheral nerve and spinal cord injuries can result in limited movement in affected portions of the burn survivor's body.

The main psychiatric complication seen in burns is trauma, as burn injuries are often caused by traumatic events. The APA describes the individual's experience of events that cause trauma as "intense fear, helplessness, or horror" (2004, p. 428). Often, the events that lead to a burn injury can meet the criteria for a traumatic experience, and approximately 30% of burn survivors develop PTSD (Sheridan, 2012). In addition, burn care can lead to the development of ASD or PTSD when adequate pain and anxiety medications are not available to the burn survivor. Aside from ASD or PTSD from the burn injury or the burn care, the burn survivor may have a trauma history premorbid to the burn of which the survivor may or may not be aware. The trauma symptoms may not be present initially as the individual may be in shock, experiencing delirium, in intense pain, or medicated. However, over time, the symptoms of trauma will become apparent and require the burn team to address these additional needs of the burn survivor.

Children and adults experience or express some of the symptoms of ASD and PTSD differently. Adults often respond to stimuli that are specific to the trauma. Children may respond to stimuli that may or may not be directly related to the trauma. One example is in adults, when in re-experiencing the trauma through dreams, the dream content directly relates to the trauma. With children, the dreams can generalize to monsters, rescuing others, threats to self or others, or frightening without recognizable content. Children's developmental stages will impact the way children express the symptoms of trauma. For example, children may not have the language skills or the higher brain functions to subjectively report on such symptoms. Instead, young children may present as mute or withdrawn as a symptom of avoidance. Adolescents who have PTSD may have symptoms that differ from those of adults, such as invasive images, restlessness and aggression, difficulty sleeping, difficulty concentrating, loss of interest in previously enjoyed activities, withdrawal from family and peers, and significant changes in life attitude. To safely care for individuals with ASD or PTSD, the music therapist needs to seek additional training in the area of trauma.

Heterotropic ossification (HO) is the formation of bone outside the skeleton. In burn survivors, HO will most frequently form in the elbow, knee, and hip joints. HO can occur in individuals with burn injuries and spinal cord injuries. The exact etiology of this condition is unknown at this time. In individuals with burns, the condition occurs weeks postburn. It can be deeply painful for the burn survivor to move the joint. HO can result in decreased movement to no movement in a joint (Sheridan, 2012). HO is treated with physical therapy and surgical interventions. When working with burn survivors who have or are suspected of having HO, music therapists need to adapt the music experiences to accommodate the child's abilities. Consultation with the physical or occupational therapist about the indications or contraindications for movement in the affected joint(s) is recommended.

As with peripheral nerve injuries, muscle loss due to the burn injury or compartment syndrome can result in limited motor function in an affected limb or part of the body. The music therapist may need to adapt the interventions to meet the burn survivor's abilities, recognizing that this condition may be permanent. Music therapy may focus on learning new ways to adapt to this limitation in the burn survivor's abilities.

Hypertropic scar formation is a condition that affects many burn survivors. Not only does this affect the individual's appearance, but also hypertrophic scars can decrease the individual's physical abilities. Scars are treated in a variety of ways, from massage to compression garments and surgical interventions (Sheridan, 2012). Scars can create a variety of physical and psychological issues that can be addressed in music therapy. Physically, scars can create physical limitations. First, the scar may be thick and reduce the child's mobility and function. Next, as scars form, the skin contracts, which limits the child's ability to move. Psychologically, scars change the child's appearance. Depending on the location of the scar, these disfigurements can have a significant psychological impact upon the child. One mitigating factor is the child's developmental stage. Generally, younger children adapt to scars and changes in their bodies with greater ease than adolescents. This has a great deal to do with the developmental stages the adolescent has passed through and is currently in, as well as the solidification of his identity. Additionally, itch is a major condition suffered by a majority of burn survivors. Itch can extend beyond the healing process and scar formation for many years. Its etiology and effective treatment continues to be point of research in the burn community. Music therapists must be aware of the burn survivor's itch and how it affects the individual's ability to focus, tolerate frustration and pain, and sleep.

It is important for music therapists to realize that burns affect the entire population of children, from typically functioning to those with developmental and intellectual disabilities, to children with physical disabilities, to children with mental illness. Although the main focus for the burn team is on the burn injury and its many complicating factors, premorbid conditions, including ADHD, autism, developmental and intellectual disabilities, mental illness, and genetic disorders, can impact the burn team's approach to the burn survivor and his needs. In addition, approximately 20% of pediatric burn injuries result from abuse or neglect (Sheridan, 2012). Both premorbid conditions and child abuse lead to complex burn care treatment that focuses not only on the burn injury but also on the needs (physical or psychological) of the other condition/abuse history. In addition to the having knowledge about burns, music therapists working in pediatric burn units need to be knowledgeable in a wide variety of interventions and needs for children with intellectual and developmental disorders, neurologic disorders, physical disabilities, mental illnesses, and trauma histories.

NEEDS AND RESOURCES

Although each burn survivor's needs and resources vary greatly based on the extent of the injury, associated conditions, coping strategies, stress responses, and many other factors, there are general needs that many burn survivors may have. The needs of pediatric burn survivors can be broken down to seven general areas: physical, cognitive, emotional, social, communication, family, and medical.

Physical Needs

Individuals with burn injuries have many physical needs, the largest being pain management. Pain management is nearly a universal need for burn survivors. The injury of a burn is mainly in the skin, where pain receptors (nociceptors) reside. Pain management is not only a need for burn survivors when they have open wounds but can be a result of stretching tight or scarred skin, exercises, and movement. Pain remains a significant consideration as burn survivors enter into the reconstructive phase of treatment. With each subsequent surgery, pain management becomes a need as the body heals as well as new rehabilitation exercises are introduced. In addition, remembering previous admissions for the burn injury and the pain felt can affect a burn survivor's interpretation of pain from the current medical procedure, at times increasing the amount of pain the individual feels.

Physical function, which includes gross and fine motor skills, is another large goal area for many individuals who are affected by burn injuries. If the burn is over a joint or caused injury to the muscle tissue or motor neurons, physical function may be affected. Physical and occupational therapists aim to address the burn survivor's physical functioning goals. Music therapists, working in collaboration with the physical and occupational therapists, can help burn survivors address a variety of goals in this area, including to increase fine and gross motor skills, increase motivation for movement, improve gait, and enhance the function of the oral musculature.

Burn injuries can involve the pulmonary system as well as the skin. In addition, the lungs may be affected by pneumonia and other infections while the burn survivor is in the ICU. This, combined with the general deconditioning of the individual's body, can result in reduced pulmonary function. Burn survivors may need interventions that increase pulmonary function.

A final area of physical needs is that of relaxation. As burn survivors are in postoperative recovery, they may need interventions to help with this process, easing agitation or pain and enhancing relaxation. These needs extend beyond the postoperative period and can continue through the entire hospitalization. At times, sleep is disrupted by pain, anxiety, medical interventions, and many other reasons. As a result, burn survivors may need assistance with sleep inducement.

Cognitive Needs

During the acute recovery from burn injuries, burn survivors may present with different cognitive needs. These can range from decreasing hallucinations associated with medications or delirium to improving orientation and neurological function. This is especially true for burn survivors who have sustained a neural impairment due to an *anoxic injury,* brain injury from the burn, stroke, or severe infection.

A subcategory of cognitive needs for pediatric burn survivors is developmental needs. A child's developmental age will mitigate how the child interprets and responds to a burn injury and changes in his body as well as their needs. A three-year-old has different needs compared to a 17-year-old, despite having the exact same burn injury. The three-year-old's needs during a dressing change are pain management, safety, and opportunities for mastery and control, while the 17-year-old's needs are to learn self-coping strategies, education about the medical procedure, support about the changes to his body and identity, and pain management. Children may regress in their developmental stages when presented with a significant injury and hospital stay. For example, a seven-year-old may start calling the mother "Mommy" and demand the parents feed him, despite having the skills to do so. In addition, children need support to maintain their current level of functioning as well as to continue to progress in their development throughout the hospital stay. As burn injuries, if extensive, can take months to heal, children in burn units are especially in need of developmental support.

Psychological Needs

Pediatric burn survivors have many psychological needs. One of the greatest needs is anxiety management. Like pain management, anxiety management is nearly universal for burn survivors. Anxiety can stem from a variety of sources, such as pain, the incident that caused the injury, fear of medical procedures, external locus of control, concerns about family members/home/friends, preoperative anxiety, and concerns about postburn abilities and appearance, to name a few. It is important for the music therapist to take into consideration the child's developmental level and source of the anxiety in planning which intervention(s) to use to manage the child's anxiety.

Agitation management is an important need within the pediatric burn population. Agitation may result from pain, anxiety, medication, separation from family, reduction in physical function, and delirium. Agitation can be damaging to the child's healing process in three main ways. First, due to the hypermetabolic state created by the burn injury, the energy expended in agitation can decrease the energy available for the body to invest in healing. If there is not enough energy for healing and to maintain the hypermetabolic state, the body will start to draw energy from muscle tissues. It is important to limit the loss of muscle tissues to aid in the patient's physical rehabilitation later. The second way that agitation can be damaging to the child's healing process is the potential that the child can reinjure surgical sites or remove important devices (*IVs, NG tubes,* breathing tubes, etc.). Finally, the emotional state and resulting endocrine/immune reaction to that emotional state can decrease healing. If agitation can be managed nonpharmacologically, the burn survivor benefits. Pharmacological interventions for agitation, although effective, all carry a risk. If music therapy can help to reduce the amount of medication needed, the child will be exposed to fewer of the side effects of the medications.

The hospital environment at times may not allow for the burn survivors to fully express their emotions and thoughts related to the injury and treatment. The focus is often on what treatment is best and how the individual's body is responding to the treatment. There may not be time or trained individuals available to give the burn survivor the time and space to express freely.

Hospitalization can be filled with stress for child and adult burn survivors. When working with children, the parents and family members are a key component of their care. Parents usually play a very important role in to the child's ability to cope. Children and family members may need support to increase the use of or to learn new coping skills. These can range from ways to constructively use downtime in the hospital to ways to manage medical procedure and deal with difficult news. Children can base their reactions to medical procedures based on their parents' reactions. For most parents, seeing their child with a burn injury is quite overwhelming and distressing. A parent's role is to care for their child and protect her/him from any pain or suffering. Many of the medical procedures associated with burn care can be painful and scary to the child, thus distressing to the parent. Added to that, the parent's role as primary caregiver to the child has been temporarily taken over by the hospital staff. The parent is in a new environment, unable to provide the usual care to their child, and seeing their child undergo very distressing procedures. It often falls to the music therapist to assist the parent in finding ways to be comforting to their child through the procedure and beyond. At times, the injury is so great that the parent is not able to be an effective support for the child during dressing changes or other procedures. With children, engaging in stress management conducted in a developmentally appropriate manner can help with their need for stress reduction. Opportunities to increase relaxation can help with stress management as well as facilitate the healing process. It then becomes the music therapist's job to take on the comforting presence that would be the parent until the parent is able to be present to support the child.

One area within coping that can be a distinct need within burn survivors is in regard to faith and religion. The connection to faith can bring much needed hope, patience, and support. However, it is important to note that faith and religious beliefs can be challenged when devastating injuries occur. Questions like "Why did this happen to me?," "Why does God let this happen?," etc., are common from patients and family members. Prior to introducing religious/faith-based music to the session, the music therapist must assess if the child and/or family are ready. Knowing if the music will be received as supportive or a reminder of the faith crisis is key to knowing how and when to apply religious/faith-based music.

Children may not have much experience with or understanding of hospitalization prior to a burn injury. Therefore, one area of need is that of education about the medical experiences. Children may need basic information, such as orientation to the hospital and the personnel who work there. Specific education about medical procedures may be aimed at increasing understanding, enhancing mastery over the procedures, or decreasing anxiety for the procedure. Mastery may include allowing the child to express his experience with medical interventions in a creative manner.

Burn survivors are often faced with changes in their appearance and function. Learning to accept these changes is often a challenge facing these individuals. The developmental level of the child when he was injured as well as where he is at the point to treatment will influence the degree to which appearance and function are the child's needs. Along with these changes, burn survivors may be in need of enhancement of self-image and self-esteem.

Communication Needs

When in the burn unit, children may require support in their communication skills. One area of need may be to improve the child's language skills, improving his ability to express his experience, learn the words to better communicate, and continue on his development of language skills. Burn care often requires the patient to communicate with the caregivers about pain, fear, and other difficulties. For pain, children often are asked the exact location, the type of pain, and the level of pain. Younger children often have not developed these language skills to adequately communicate with the team. With coaching, the child, depending on his developmental level, may learn these skills. There are times when a child is unable to communicate orally. This is most often due to the child being *intubated* but awake, having a *tracheotomy*, or having surgery on or around the mouth. In these instances, the child will need to learn alternative ways to communicate his thoughts and emotions.

Social Needs

The social needs of children with burns can be related to medical isolation due to infections, isolation due to the distance between the burn unit and the child's home, and insulation from the community because of discomfort with appearance or abilities. Increased opportunities for appropriate interaction with peers and others are a definite need for those who are isolating themselves from society.

Pediatric health care has moved from a traditional medical model to a family-centered care model, in which the medical team not only focuses on the needs of the child in the hospital but also looks at the needs of the family as they care for the child who is hospitalized. Family members can include parents, guardians, grandparents, aunts and uncles, and siblings. Families of burn survivors often are in need of support as they cope with the injuries the child has sustained as well as the medical procedures the child has to undergo. Some families may be in need of support to develop healthy family systems for coping with stress or ways to interact in an adaptive and constructive manner. Sometimes family members and burn survivors do not engage in honest communication about their experiences and may need support from the burn team to achieve more open and effective communication.

Finally, finding ways to normalize the hospital setting for the child and family is a basic need. This may include providing recorded music in the room that is familiar to the child, assisting the child and family to resume a schedule similar to the schedule at home, or facilitating connections with loved ones and friends whom the child is unable to see during hospitalization.

Multicultural Sensitivity

When working with people, music therapists must assess each child's and family's culture to provide quality and meaningful treatment. It is important to consider not only the child's culture of heritage, but also his culture of religion, culture of generation, culture of location, and culture of identity (Whitehead-Pleaux & Clark, 2009). Music is a vital component of many of these cultures. It is quite common for patients to identify with multiple cultures at one time. Additionally, it is not uncommon for these differing cultures to create discord within the family and the patient. While conducting the assessment, the music therapist must explore how the child identifies with the various cultures that influence his life, focusing on how and if they express these cultures musically.

Along with assessing the child's culture, it is just as important for the music therapist to conduct self-exploration of the cultures and biases. These cultural influences and biases can cloud a music therapist's understanding of a child's needs or expressions. With this clouded vision, the therapeutic relationship and process can be jeopardized. Through self-exploration, the music therapist can become a blank slate for each client's cultural expression.

Whitehead-Pleaux (2009) explored the impact of culture on a patient and family member's music therapy treatment through an acute admission. The author describes the use of multicultural music therapy techniques to modify the music analgesia interventions during dressing changes as well as other aspects of the patient's care. In addition, the author describes the process of self-exploration, which allows for more effective multicultural music therapy treatment. Along with exploring how different cultures can be incorporated into music therapy practice, this case study offers an interesting view into the daily work within a burn unit.

Strengths and Resources

Within the burn survivor population, each child and family is different and yet may have some similar resources or strengths. It is important to keep in mind that burn survivors are a population that contains people with all ranges of abilities and disabilities that are related to the burn, premorbid to the burn injury, and post–burn injury. Three key strengths of the pediatric burn survivor population are creativity, family support, and resilience. Children's creativity is vital to a child's expression about the trauma, the burn care, and their fears and experiences. Children engage their creativity in play as well as through the creative arts for expression of these thoughts and emotions. In addition, a child's creativity is a vital resource when working on adaptations to physical limitations. The author has seen children learn to play instruments in unusual ways, play video games with their feet, paint by holding a paintbrush in their mouths, and even suck their toes when their hands are injured.

Family support is key to a child's emotional and physical recovery from a burn injury. The presence of a trusted loved one, parent, or other caring adult has such a strong effect on children. This adult can provide comfort, boundaries, support, understanding, and education to the child. People who have been exposed to traumatic events are less likely to develop PTSD if they have family support (Brewin, Andrews, & Valentine, 2000). Most pediatric burn teams recognize the importance of the presence of a parent and work to embody the principles of family-centered care to foster family support.

One interesting difference between pediatric burn population and the adult burn population is children's internal drive to resume play and life. Depending on the child's developmental stage, children may not have a set body image and may be able to adjust easier to changes in appearance and ability. Adults and older teens may have more difficulty adjusting to the changes in their body, which can inhibit their resumption of daily activities and recreational pursuits. Younger children often are not hampered by these difficulties, as their development has not reached the point of having these more abstract thoughts. Younger children tend to be more easily motivated to return to play, education, and social interaction. However, as these young burn survivors grow up, they may continue to process the burn injury, trauma, and changes in their appearance and function in relation to the developmental stage they have entered. When working with pediatric burn survivors who are in the reconstructive phase of care, it is important to continue to assess the children periodically about coping, peer relationships, self-image, and risky behavior.

REFERRAL AND ASSESSMENT PROCEDURES

Referral Procedures

The referral process for pediatric burn units is similar to the referral process for all hospitals. There is variation in the way this process is conducted from facility to facility, based on the hospital's policies and regulations. For some, the music therapist may assess and provide treatment to a patient or family member only when a physician orders music therapy services. In other hospitals, specific staff can make referrals to music therapy. These professions may include but are not limited to social workers, psychologists, psychiatrists, nurses, physical therapists, occupational therapists, and pastoral counselors. Yet at other facilities, all staff (including the music therapist), patients, and family members may make referrals for music therapy. Finally, some hospitals do not require referrals for music therapy services.

The music therapist must work with the managers of the hospital or unit when implementing a music therapy program to be in alliance with the hospital policies and procedures.

Assessment Procedures

Once a referral is made to music therapy, the music therapist often will have a specified period of time, usually 72 hours, within which to conduct the assessment of the child or family member. As with all populations that music therapists serve in the United States, the assessment is to be based on the American Music Therapy Association's (AMTA) Standards of Clinical Practice. The assessment will explore the "categories of psychological, cognitive, communicative, social, and physiological functioning focused on the client's needs and strengths" (AMTA, 2011). When conducting the assessment, the music therapist will want to focus on the patient's level of pain, coping, splinting requirements and movement limitations, body image and self-esteem, attitudes about and understanding of medical interventions, developmental level, and mental status. It is also important for the music therapist to note the family dynamics and the family's ability to cope.

As music therapists assess the child's pain, noting the pain level at rest as well as the pain level during procedures is key. Having an understanding of the physical and psychological components of pain will help the music therapist to devise interventions that are fully effective with the child both in and out of the medical procedures.

Coping varies from individual to individual. A child may cope on a range from active to passive. Some children cope better with parental support (based on the parent's ability to provide support) or not. The patient's style of coping and coping needs may vary upon different situations. Knowing how the child copes can help the music therapist to create interventions that best serve the child. As a patient heals and adjusts to the hospitalization, the coping strategies he uses may change. Music therapists need to be aware of these changes and adapt the interventions to incorporate these changes.

Splinting requirements and movement restrictions are critical to include in the assessment. Knowing what the client can accomplish physically impacts the type of intervention the music therapist plans to use. If necessary, the music therapist can work with the members of the treatment team, mainly the surgeons, physical therapists, and occupational therapists, to work out ways to treat the patient with the best possible outcomes for all. Splinting requirements and movement restrictions change throughout the hospitalization and treatment. The music therapist needs to stay apprised of these changes and adjust the treatment plan accordingly.

Children may have a limited understanding of medical procedures and treatments. By assessing the child's understanding and attitudes, the music therapist can develop interventions that help the child to understand the medical treatments on a developmentally appropriate level as well as explore further the child's attitudes and help him to move through any attitudes that inhibit investment in the treatment and wellness.

The music therapist must assess for the child's developmental level, not relying upon the child's age. Patient's developmental level can be affected by the child's response to the trauma and/or medical treatment or premorbid to the child's injury. When children are under great stress, like hospitalization or after experiencing a traumatic event, they can experience regression in their development. For example, a child who had attained the developmental milestone of potty training may regress to soiling himself; a teen who had been independent of his parents may demand that his mother attend to his every need. Premorbid developmental delay may be present in patients. It can have many sources, including environmental factors and intellectual disability. Music therapists need to take the child's developmental level into account when planning treatment and interventions.

Finally, mental status is important to ascertain before treatment planning. Mental status can be affected by medication, disorientation due to isolation, and brain injury (often in burns from anoxic injury). Mental status is one area that can fluctuate and may need regular assessment. By designing the treatment plan and interventions to meet the child's mental status, needs, and abilities, the music therapist can design treatment that is effective and does not overstimulate the child.

When working with children and teens, it is important to treat not only the patient but also the entire family. Therefore, it is recommended that the therapist assess not just the patient but also the family members who are present. There are many factors to take into account when working with families; the author will focus on two. It is important to note the family dynamics. Is the child in the role of a child or parentified? Is the parent in the role of a parent? Did this dynamic exist before the burn injury or has the family dynamic changed since the injury? Similarly, the music therapist needs to assess the coping of the family members present. Are the parents able to cope with the child's injury and treatment? Will the mother or father be able to be present during procedures and support the child or are they limited in their ability to cope at this time? Is the parent experiencing guilt over the child's burn? Is the team suspicious of the burn being an intentional injury? Are there prior reports of abuse or neglect? These are important questions for the music therapist to consider as she creates treatment plans and interventions. Other team members, mainly the social workers or care coordinators, will explore many of these questions with the family members. The music therapist can gain much of this information from the patient's chart.

A thorough music therapy assessment is difficult in the early days of an acute admission. A child may not be able to talk about his experiences. Parents may be very focused on the injury and on whether the child will live. In addition, they may be overwhelmed by the hospital experience. This may prevent them from accurately reporting on the variety of questions within a medical music therapy assessment. Therefore, the initial assessment may be quick and focus on the main issues of pain, coping, and basic music likes and dislikes. But the assessment does not happen only in that initial session; it should continue through each session. As the medical status stabilizes and/or improves, the patient and family will speak more about the patient, his experiences prior to the injury, family dynamics, and music interests and experiences. Assessment is an ongoing process within pediatric burn care during which the music therapist's understanding of the child and family gradually evolves.

Introduction to Music Therapy Methods

In 1979, Christenberry wrote the first journal article about the use of music therapy in burn care. This article focused on a clinical practice model for music therapy with burn patients. Christenberry described the needs of burn patients (decreased sensory stimulation, contractures, respiratory issues, anxiety, pain, social issues, and adjustment) and the ways music therapy can address these needs.

Since this seminal article, other authors have described clinical practice models for music therapy in pediatric burn units. Rudenberg and Royka (1989) described how music therapy can be incorporated into child life departments to address the psychosocial and rehabilitation goals.

Similarly, Bishop, Christenberry, Robb, and Toombs Rudenberg (1996) continued to explore the integration of music therapy within a child life department. In 2005, Edwards broke from the previous model of music therapy integration with child life to describe a stand-alone model of music therapy in a pediatric hospital that focuses on pain management and psychological stress. Despite the significance of exploring the different models of music therapy application in a pediatric hospital that treats burn patients, these articles offer no evidence to support the use of music therapy interventions with this population.

Neugebauer (2008) described a music therapy program at a pediatric hospital. The program was broken down into the three phases of burn care: acute, rehabilitation, and reconstructive. Within each phase, Neugebauer describes the needs of the populations, music therapy treatment, and evidence supporting these treatments. This, by far, is the most detailed description of a music therapy program in a pediatric burn hospital. Based on these articles and chapters about music therapy programs in burn units, a variety of designs for music therapy programs are presented.

A majority of the music therapy sessions are individual sessions. As music therapists are often addressing pain and anxiety management during medical procedures as well as cotreating during physical and occupational therapy sessions, the sessions are with one patient at a time. In addition, with the emotional nature of the pain, anxiety, and body changes, individual sessions provide the space for an individual child to express the difficult emotions, thoughts, and memories he has.

With some patients, there is a need to conduct family sessions. This often helps the parent or sibling to provide support for the patient. Parents may be overwhelmed by the dressing changes and not know how to support their child. By working with the parent and the child simultaneously in a family session, the music therapist can help support the child while helping the parent to learn new ways to support his child. Family sessions can also be used to address communication or family dynamic issues.

Dyads and group sessions are possible within burn units as well. Many hospitals have rooms where two patients stay. If the two patients are of similar age or have similar needs, the music therapist can conduct dyad sessions with the pair. Additionally, if two patients are in PT/OT at the same time with similar music tastes and needs, the music therapist can work with both in a dyad during the PT/OT session. Groups are possible when the unit or outpatient populations are homogeneous enough (age, developmental level, language, etc.) to conduct a group session.

This portion of the chapter will focus on the music therapy interventions used in pediatric burn care. It is important for the reader to note that given the dynamic nature of pediatric burn care, a vast number of music therapy interventions may be used, based on the specific needs and strengths of each patient. In addition, even the specific interventions listed here are modified to meet the patient's abilities, the environmental factors, and the goals of the cotreaters.

OVERVIEW OF MUSIC THERAPY METHODS AND PROCEDURES

An overview of music therapy methods and procedures included in this chapter is presented below. They are not listed in any particular order. As with any population, burn survivors are individuals, each with their specific injury, pre-existing needs and strengths, supports, and music therapy needs. Therefore, each treatment plan is created specifically for each patient. The interventions listed in this chapter are not the only music therapy interventions used with pediatric burn survivors, but just the most common.

Receptive Music Therapy

- Music Analgesia: the use of live music during medical procedures to decrease agitation, anxiety, duration of distress, and pain perception; to increase relaxation response; and to learn and utilize pain management techniques and coping strategies.
- Music Relaxation: the use of music-guided relaxation with children who are in distress, have low levels of pain, experience hypertension, and have high muscle tone due to stress.
- Stimulative Listening for Children Who Are Sedated: the use of live music to facilitate alertness and orientation to reality in children who are sedated but need to be roused.

- Stimulative Listening During Joint PT/OT Services: the use of live music during physical and occupational therapy sessions with children who exhibit noncompliance with and anxiety during PT/OT, and anxiety and pain with movement.

Improvisational Music Therapy

- Instrumental Nonreferential and Referential Improvisation: the use of instrumental improvisations to facilitate the expression of thoughts or emotions regarding the hospitalization, injury, or accident; improve stress and pain management; increase self-esteem; increase acceptance; and increase fine and/or gross motor skills.
- Song Improvisation: the intentional expression of a concept, idea, or feeling in song format in the moment to increase verbal communication; reduce anxiety and agitation; increase the use of adaptive coping strategies; share the experience of pain; increase the expression of thoughts or emotions regarding the hospitalization, injury, or accident; increase pulmonary function; and address oral musculature needs.

Compositional Music Therapy

- Fill-in-the-Blank Songwriting: the use of a structured songwriting format to help the child to express emotions or thoughts related to the injury, accident, and future; to develop attention; to address educational goals; to improve fine motor skills through lyric writing; and to express thoughts and emotions related to the intersection of spiritual beliefs and accident.
- Songwriting: the use of a free-form songwriting process to address the goals as listed in the fill-in-the-blank songwriting intervention.
- Music Collages: the creation of a collage of sounds and samples to enable the child to tell his story and explore difficult feelings or experiences.

Re-creative Music Therapy

- Music Instruction: teaching a child to play an instrument to build self-esteem, enhance self-image, enhance coping with hospitalization and/or loss, improve physical function, and facilitate expression of thoughts and emotions.
- Singing Familiar Songs: singing familiar songs with the patient (and his family) to address communication, psychosocial, cognitive, and physical goals.
- Lyric Analysis: listening to a recorded or live version of a song followed by analysis of the lyrics to address communication, psychosocial, and cognitive goals.

GUIDELINES FOR RECEPTIVE MUSIC THERAPY

Within pediatric burns, receptive music therapy interventions are used to help the burn survivor attain a variety of goals and objectives. These interventions can include music analgesia, music relaxation, stimulative listening, eurhythmic listening, action listening, music appreciation activities, song communication, song lyric discussion, imaginative listening, and self-listening.

Many of the receptive music therapy interventions explored in this chapter have similar contraindications. The contraindications for these interventions are as follows. First, if the burn survivor has significant hearing loss and is unable to hear these music therapy interventions, the intervention is not appropriate. Next, if the child is experiencing delirium, hallucinations, or delusions from burn delirium, septic delirium, and/or medication withdrawal, it is important for the music therapist to assess the child prior to the medical intervention for the appropriateness of the music therapy intervention. If the child is unable to attend to the music stimuli due to psychological disturbance or becomes agitated by the music stimuli, the intervention is not indicated. Third, some individuals do not find music to be an effective coping strategy. If this is the case, music therapy is contraindicated. Finally, receptive music therapy interventions are not indicated if it is not culturally appropriate for the burn survivor to engage in music.

Music Analgesia

Overview. One of the main music therapy interventions used in pediatric burn care is music analgesia. This intervention is indicated with the child is undergoing a medical procedure and requires support. Support is a broad term to include pain management, anxiety and agitation reduction, teaching and increasing use of effective coping strategies, and increasing the relaxation response. The medical procedures where music analgesia can be applied can include procedures such as dressing changes, rehabilitation, IV starts, suture removal, staple removal, *PICC line placement,* and many other procedures. This intervention is used with a variety of different goals, including to decrease agitation, anxiety, duration of distress, and pain perception; to increase relaxation response; and to learn and utilize pain management techniques and coping strategies.

Edwards (1995) wrote a case study of a single session with a patient in which she cotreated with nursing during a debridement bath. In this case, Edwards illustrates the music analgesia intervention with clarity and eloquence. The outcome from this one session was a decrease in the child's anxiety, which allowed the child to cope effectively with subsequent debriding baths without the music analgesia intervention. Although this is a great example of the intervention, it does not provide evidence of efficacy. Prensner, Yowler, Smith, Steele, and Fratianne (2001) presented the theories and clinical practice model for music analgesia and music relaxation interventions for pain and anxiety management in burn patients during painful medical procedures. In their examination of electronic music technologies (EMTs) in music therapy practice in a pediatric medical hospital, Whitehead-Pleaux, Clark, and Spall (2011) described indications and contraindications for EMTs with pain management. EMTs, including listening to MP3 files and songwriting, were recommended for mild to moderate pain but not during medical procedures or when a patient was experiencing moderate to severe pain. In these instances, the authors recommended traditional acoustic music analgesia interventions.

Music analgesia can play a supportive role in that the music therapist is providing support by playing music for the child. In these sessions, most of the verbal interactions between the music therapist and the patient focus on the ways the patient can cope with the procedure. Through this work, the child learns new ways to self-manage his pain through music and explores the changes in his body. At times, this intervention can become transformative, helping the child to transform significantly. An example of this is when the session turns from support to helping the child develop a new identity, integrating the one from before the burn with the changes in his body and his new experiences postburn.

Preparation. In preparing for a session in which the music therapist is going to use music analgesia intervention during a procedure, the music therapist must prepare musically. It is important for the music therapist to know the child's preferred music prior to the session. This can be learned through asking the child and/or his family members. If the music therapist is unable to ascertain this information prior to the session, general assumptions can be made based on the child's age, where he lives, and the current music scene. It is important to give the child the power to say he does not like a certain song to avoid reducing the effectiveness of the intervention.

In addition to preparing musically for the session, the music therapist must communicate with the professional with whom she will be cotreating. This can be a nurse, physician, anesthesiologist, physical therapist, or occupational therapist. The music therapist must understand the procedure and the plan for the day. This allows the music therapist to plan musically and therapeutically for the parts of the procedure that are more difficult, frightening, or painful. Timing the end of songs with the end of a part of the procedure helps to create a musical environment that remains supportive and present in the most difficult parts. The more the music therapist is familiar with the medical staff with whom she is cotreating, the better. With cotreating in difficult medical procedures, often the only possible communication between staff is meaningful eye contact or a few words. Having a good relationship with the staff member allows for better-quality work and a seamless delivery of the services by all involved. By communicating with treatment team members prior to the session, the music therapist can better anticipate the child's music therapy needs and adapt the music interventions to the process of the medical procedure.

Finally, it is important for the music therapist to know the child's coping style. Does the child use active or avoidant coping strategies? Does the child cope better when he can be involved in or at least watch the procedure? Or does seeing the procedure create more anxiety for the child? Or does the child use a combination of these strategies? The planning for music analgesia interventions requires the music therapist to construct the music therapy intervention in such a way that it embraces the style of coping in which the child engages. For the child who engages in avoidant coping strategies, the music therapist can create an environment that limits the child's vision of the procedure and/or prompt the child to focus on the music therapy intervention. If the child engages in active coping strategies, designing the intervention to allow the child to split his attention between the procedure and the music therapy intervention will increase the child's successful coping. Whether a child employs active or avoidant coping strategies, preparation and narration of the steps of the procedure are needed to aid in the child's coping.

When providing music analgesia during medical procedures, music therapists often have very little control over the environment. It is important to turn off or down all TVs, movies, games, and recorded music prior to starting the session. The music therapist needs to be next to the child's head or in his line of sight but needs to be prepared to move quickly and be flexible in location during the session.

What to observe. During this intervention, it is vital for the music therapist to attend to the child, hospital staff, family member(s), support people, and environment. The music therapist must be aware at all times of the child's responses to the music and the medical procedure, his fears, and his reactions to the environment. These responses can be expressed physically, physiologically, behaviorally, or verbally. The music therapist can modify the music by varying the tempo, timbre, voicing, arrangement, style, and song in an instant to meet the patient's current needs. This is a fluid process that changes sometimes moment-to-moment, and it is vital for the music therapist to be flexible in his musical skills and to be able to make these modifications with little effort so that his focus can remain on the child, procedure, staff, and family members.

Procedures. As the procedural support session begins, the music therapist can once again explain to the child how listening to music or singing along can help him to feel less pain and anxiety and feel more relaxed. This is presented in a manner congruent with the child's developmental level.

As stated above, the music therapist stands near or by the patient's head, or in his line of sight if possible. This allows for a few key factors in the music analgesia intervention. First, the music therapist can see the child's facial expressions and gear the music intervention to decrease anxiety, increase relaxation, and decrease pain perception or duration. Next, if the child is able to watch the therapist play, it adds more sensory information to the music therapy intervention, which helps to create a more compelling experience for the child. Third, proximity allows the music therapist to engage in alternative forms of music analgesia, including singing quietly next to the patient's ear, adding therapeutic touch to the music, and holding the child's hand for comfort. Fourth, it allows the music therapist to communicate directly with the child. The music therapist, if appropriate, can ask the child what song he wants to hear, what tempo, and what emotion in the music (happy or sad song), or ask questions about the songs. This keeps the child engaged actively or passively in the music analgesia intervention.

A key principle that influences the intervention of music analgesia is the Iso principle. Briefly, the Iso principle states that music can alter a person's emotional state through the process of carefully matching the person's mood in the music and then gradually changing the mood within the music (Altshuler, 1948). This musical shift happens through the manipulations of the basic foundations of music, which can include rhythm, melody, scale, mode, timbre, texture, instrumentation, volume, and lyrics. Within music analgesia in burn care, it is possible to help a patient to change his emotional state to something better than before, but it is rare that music can create a shift that removes the pain or anxiety completely. The music therapist can use pre-existing music or improvise music to meet the child's emotional state via the music. Nearly any song can be modified to express a myriad of emotions, so the song choice is often not as important as the other music elements. Once the child hears that the music therapist understands his mood in the music, there is a shift in the child's expression. Sometimes the child begins to relax. Other times, the child will begin to vocalize the emotional state in time with the music or in the same key as the music. Sometimes the child will modify the "melody" of his vocalizations to reflect the melody that the music therapist is singing. When the music therapist hears or sees these changes, she can begin to gradually modify the music elements to change the child's emotional state. As medical procedures are very dynamic events with many different steps, this principle is used many times throughout the intervention. Each time the pain or level of fear increases, the music therapist modifies the music elements to match the child's mood. Once the mood is met and the child calms some, the music therapist can then begin to alter the musical elements to guide the individual's emotional state to one that is less distressing.

It is imperative for the music therapist to remain cognizant of the physical surroundings in the room. Often in medical procedures, the medical staff has to change positions, adjust monitors, attend to IVs, and fetch equipment. The music therapist needs to be aware of where the other staff is, where they may move next, where the equipment is, and where the parent is. This awareness coupled with the ability to keep playing as the music therapist moves from spot to spot is key to providing music analgesia.

The music therapist needs to continue the intervention until the medical procedure is completed if possible. Depending on how the session is ending, it is recommended that the music therapist continue to sing a song or two to help decrease the child's association of the music therapist with the painful procedure. This can also help to continue to de-escalate the child and family member from the medical procedure. If the child is exhibiting an association of the music therapist with pain, the music therapist may need to provide sessions outside of medical procedures to continue to reduce this association.

Adaptations. The first adaptation to this intervention is increasing the range of interaction from the child. Usually initiated by the music therapist, this intervention can work with a patient who is unresponsive to patients who actively participate. Active participation can include making song choices, singing, vocalizing, making choices within a song, playing instruments, spontaneous song creation, and improvisation. These changes can then expand the intervention from the supportive music therapy level to vocal and instrumental re-creative interventions.

Another adaptation that can be made to the music analgesia intervention is to invite a family member who is present during the medical procedure to participate in the music-making. One way is to invite the family member to join in singing with the child and the music therapist if it is appropriate within the session. The music therapist continues to control the music tempo and texture as needed to meet the child's needs and current mood. If the parent is reluctant or unable to sing, the music therapist can include the parent in directing the song choice as appropriate.

One final adaptation is to include the other hospital staff in singing. This adaptation can help to create a stronger musical container to hold the child. It can serve to reduce the child's fear of the staff member. It can help to enhance positive associations with the staff member for the child. And not least is that it can help the staff member to relax and reduce his stress about the procedure. All of these benefits can positively affect a child's ability to cope with the procedure as well as the rest of the hospitalization and possible future hospitalizations.

Music Relaxation

Overview. Music relaxation is another common intervention used in pediatric burn care. This intervention is indicated for children who are anxious, agitated, and/or in distress; have low levels of pain; have high levels of stress; experience hypertension; and have high muscle tone due to stress. The goals of music relaxation are similar to those mentioned for music analgesia, namely to decrease agitation, anxiety duration of distress, and perception of pain; increase relaxation response; learn and utilize pain management techniques and coping strategies; and facilitate sleep.

Different levels of practice and training come into play in this area of music therapy practice. Specific situations exist where advanced skills are needed for the music therapist to assess if music relaxation interventions are appropriate for patients who are experiencing altered states of consciousness due to medication and *dissociative symptoms*. Additional training in medications and withdrawal, dissociative symptoms/trauma, and creating altered states of consciousness with music are necessary to conduct these sessions in a manner that will do no harm to the patient. This education needs to include fieldwork as well as trainings.

Many medications used for pain and anxiety loosen the patient's hold on reality. Some of the main medications that cause this side effect are opioids, *benzodiazepines,* and *ketamine*. If a patient is on significant doses of one or more of these that alter one's perception of reality, the music therapist must evaluate the child to see if music helps to ground the patient or loosens the patient's connection to reality. Similarly, if a child is undergoing withdrawal from medications, the child may experience hallucinations and delusions. In these instances, the music therapist must evaluate the child to see if he is having difficulty connecting reality with music relaxation interventions and if the child is able to attend to the music and directions. If the child is able to be grounded by the music relaxation intervention, it is then indicated, but the music therapist must take specific precautions and continually observe the child for increased psychotic symptoms. If the child cannot be grounded in music, this intervention is not indicated at this time.

The other situation that must be evaluated by the music therapist is the presence of significant dissociative symptoms of trauma. Dissociative symptoms can be present both in Acute Stress Disorder and in Post-Traumatic Stress Disorder. Prior to conducting a music relaxation intervention, the music therapist must fully assess the child's trauma symptoms and responses to music. The music therapist needs to know about the etiology of the trauma symptoms. Are they a result from the burn injury? Were they caused by medical care? Were they premorbid to the burn injury? Could they result from child abuse? Does this child have a history of abuse or neglect? The answers to these questions will help to direct the music therapy intervention. Next, the music therapist needs to evaluate the child to see which music relaxation interventions will decrease the symptoms and which may activate the symptoms. For example, if the child is experiencing frequent dissociative symptoms, a relaxation intervention that features open guided imagery is contraindicated. If the child was abused by a female, recorded relaxation music with a female voice may be contraindicated. The music therapist must remain cognizant of the music choices and the elements within music in relation to the child and his experiences. Similarly, very careful evaluation of the music must be made to know which music helps to ground the patient and which will activate the dissociative symptoms. It is best to avoid extramusical sounds, music recordings with nonmusic sounds, with patients who are experiencing dissociative symptoms. Some examples of these are a rain storm, waves on the shore, a rowboat on the water, rainforest sounds, and forest sounds. These sounds, although pleasant and relaxing to many of us, may be similar to sounds the dissociating patient heard prior to or during the traumatic incident. The extramusical sound may be completely benign and unrelated to the trauma, but the patient, when in an altered state of consciousness, may interpret it as a trigger to the trauma memories. An example is that a patient who was raped found the sound of gentle waves in the music to remind her of the sound of the assailant breathing. By eliminating the use of music with these extramusical sounds, patients who have experienced trauma will not be at risk for triggering of the trauma symptoms.

Preparation. To prepare for a music relaxation intervention, the music therapist has to do work outside of the actual session. Music selection is key, and the music therapist needs to weigh many different factors. First, the music must be appropriate for the child's needs. It needs to be culturally and age-appropriate. Attention must be paid to the timbre, orchestration, tempo, and presence of voices. The music therapist must evaluate the rhythm, melody, and harmony for complexity. Some people find simple music relaxing, while others find complex music relaxing. The music therapist must also evaluate the music for novelty vs. repetitiveness. Different patients have different needs for these various factors. A thorough assessment of the child's needs prior to the session will help the music therapist make these choices. This intervention can be used for a variety of sessions. It can be used in individual, family, dyads, and group sessions. When working with more than one person, the music therapist must balance the different personal tastes of each of the group members and find a music selection that all the members will agree is relaxing.

The music therapist will need to find a physical space that suits her needs. The location can be in the child's room or in a different room. It is best if the music therapist can create an environment that is quiet and a place where the session will not be disturbed. Patient rooms can be used but do present some challenges, which can include noise from roommates, staff intrusions, and proximity to phone. The physical space needs become more pressing with a dyad or group. By working with the patient's nurses and other staff, some of these disturbances can be minimized. The space needs to be a comfortable temperature and with comfortable chairs or beds that support the patient's wounded areas, splints, and infection control needs.

What to observe. During music relaxation sessions, the music therapist needs to remain vigilant, watching the child and the environment. When observing the child's responses, the music therapist needs to be mindful of physiological, physical, and behavioral changes. If the child is hooked up to monitors, viewing the physiological responses is quite easy. Without a monitor, the music therapist needs to be aware of the child's rate and depth of breathing, skin color, muscle tightness, facial expression, and comfort. The music therapist must be aware of any changes in the environment as well, such as changes in sound level, presence of others in the room, and time constraints.

Procedures. To conduct a music relaxation intervention, the first step is to make sure the child is in a comfortable position. The music therapist must make sure all the child's extremities are comfortably positioned and the child is warm enough. The music therapist needs to test the music's volume to ensure that it is comfortable for the child. Once these steps are completed, the music therapist can begin to lead the child through the induction. An induction is at the beginning of the relaxation intervention and helps the child to draw his focus to the music and the music therapist and begin the relaxation process. There are many different inductions available that can include breathing exercises, grounding experiences, and imagery. One example of an induction is to prompt the child to imagine that he is placing all of his worries and concerns into a box, securing the box, and placing it outside himself so he does not have to think about these concerns throughout the relaxation intervention. The induction can include music or not. The music therapist makes these decisions based on the child's developmental level, needs, and abilities. Once the induction is complete, the music therapist can then engage the child in a variety of music relaxation interventions, including autogenic training, progressive muscle relaxation, and/or music-guided imagery. The music therapist can use a combination of multiple methods in succession. The session can be directive or unstructured. An example of a directive session is one where the music therapist speaks much of the time, directing what the child sees and experiences, and what body part he focuses on. An unstructured relaxation intervention allows for the child to have more input from his imagination into the experience. Instead of directing a child to imagery of a beach, the music therapist would encourage him to imagine a place where he feels safe. As the intervention finishes, the music therapist must then bring the child back to reality. This can be done in a variety of ways that are developmentally appropriate for the child, ranging from counting backward to increasing the awareness of bodily sensations and the room environment. It is important to take time to help the child transition from his altered state of consciousness to this reality to ensure that the child is grounded and centered.

Adaptations. There are countless ways to adapt the music relaxation intervention. The adaptations can include making changes to the recorded or improvised music, using different relaxation scripts, standing or walking relaxation experiences (these are meditative movement experiences that include walking in place or walking, where grounding is attained through the repetitive movement in walking as well as the connection to the Earth/ground/floor), and beyond. Music relaxation interventions allow for great creativity by the music therapist.

Stimulative Listening for Patients Who Are Sedated

Overview. In burn care, there are times when patients are sedated to help with pain management, energy consumption, and healing. Music therapy still has a vital role to play with these patients. Stimulative listening for patients who are sedated is one such intervention. This intervention is indicated for patients who are sedated but need to be roused. The goals for music therapy are to facilitate alertness and to orient to reality.

If the child is agitated by sound or music, this intervention is not appropriate. Agitation is not a state that is helpful to the child at this point in his recovery from his burn injury.

Preparation. To prepare for the session, the music therapist must first find out what music the child prefers. Once the genre and bands/artists are known, the music therapist can research and rehearse the music to prepare for the session. This sort of intervention is one for which a music therapist can bring music and lyrics to the session. However, the music therapist must have enough mastery over the songs to focus her main attention upon the child. The child's physical, physiological, and behavioral responses to the music must be noted. The music therapist can manipulate different elements of the music to note the burn survivor's responses.

What to observe. With a close eye on both the child and the monitors, the music therapist can note any changes in the child's physiological measures and behavior. If the heart rate, breathing rate, mean arterial pressure, or movements increase in the patient, the music therapist will need to modify the music. These modifications can include changing the song, tempo (faster or slower), volume, accompaniment style, and voicing.

Procedures. To conduct this intervention, the music therapist will want to work with the medical staff to choose a time that will be fairly free of interruptions. When the music therapist enters the room, she is to introduce herself and explain the purpose of the intervention to the child in terms that are developmentally appropriate and fairly simple. It is important that the music therapist speak directly to the child despite the patient being sedated. Sitting or standing near to the patient's head, with a clear view of the monitors, the music therapist will then begin to sing familiar songs to the patient. Often the impulse for a session such as this is to play music that is soft and quiet. However, it is important to consider the sounds within the room over which the music therapist will need to play. These can include the ventilation machine, monitors, bed, and other devices. The music therapist will need to play and sing over these sounds, but not overly loudly so. It is best to start with a song that has a slow to moderate tempo. Song lyrics can contain positive messages or other emotions. It is best to avoid songs with dark lyrics or images at this point in the child's care. There is no one type of music or tempo that works for all patients.

An example is a five-year-old with whom the author worked. He was agitated frequently, and the best music that helped to calm him was a Latin American folksong, "Los Pollitos" (the Baby Chicks), played at 50 bpm (beats per minute). In stark contrast, a two-year-old relaxed only when any upbeat song was played between 100 and 120 bpm. A third example was a 17-year-old whose breathing rate decreased and volumes increased (indicating a relaxed state) when the music therapist played reggae.

Patient preference plays a large role in the most effective music for this intervention. However, the music therapist is unable to ask the child which songs he would prefer, so she must resort to careful observation to find the music that will work best for these interventions.

Adaptations. This intervention can be adapted in many ways. First, the music therapist can bring in a variety of recorded music that is the child's preferred genre. It is possible that the original recording of the song by the child's favorite artist may stimulate more memories and associations than live versions by the music therapist. However, a drawback of using prerecorded music is that one cannot modify the various music elements nor change songs as quickly as on a live instrument. A second adaptation is to involve the family members in singing to the patient. This adaptation can help provide additional stimulation as the parent's voice will stimulate memories and associations that are not possible by the music therapist's voice only. Finally, if the family members are not able to be present, the music therapist can record the parents singing and speaking to the child. This recording can be left in the room for the nursing staff to use as appropriate. This adaptation may bring significant benefit to the family members as well as the child. Oftentimes, when patients are sedated and just waking up, the family members do not have an active role in caring for them. By giving the family members a job and a way to connect to the child, the family members can feel more connected to the child and their role as a caregiver.

Stimulative Listening During Joint PT/OT Services

Overview. The final receptive music therapy intervention used in pediatric burn care is stimulative listening during joint physical and occupational therapists services (PT/OT). This intervention is applied during physical and occupational therapy sessions that are focusing on physical rehabilitation and the attainment of range of motion, function, and strength to function independently after hospitalization. The indications for this intervention include noncompliance with PT/OT, anxiety during PT/OT, and anxiety and pain with movement. The goals for this intervention typically are to increase fine and/or gross motor functioning, increase motivation to move, and decrease anxiety, pain perception, and duration of distress.

Preparation. The best way to prepare for this sort of session is to meet with the cotherapist and the child prior to the session. In the meeting with the cotherapist, the music therapist needs to learn the PT/OT goals, familiarize herself with the interventions the PT/OT is planning to use, and discuss how the music therapist he can be of help to aid the PT/OT in attaining these goals. The music therapist can offer ideas and work with the PT/OT to come up with a feasible session plan. In addition to meeting with the cotherapist, the music therapist must also meet with the patient to develop a plan with him. Learning what has been the child's experience in PT/OT and really listening to the emotional content the child shares is very important. The music therapist needs to find out what music the child prefers and is interested in listening to during the session.

What to observe. When conducting a stimulative listening session in cotreatment with PT/OT, the music therapist will want to monitor the patient's physical, psychological, and behavioral responses to the interventions, both PT/OT and music therapy. What is the child's facial expression? How is he breathing? What are his vocalizations? Additionally, the music therapist needs to observe how the child is participating in the PT/OT interventions. Is he resisting the exercise or engaging in it? Is the relationship between the PT/OT and child positive or tense? Is the child expressing fear, pain, or anxiety before or during the exercise? Finally, the music therapist needs to observe the PT/OT's current intervention, communicate with the PT/OT, and plan ahead for the next exercise in order to be ready to modify the music therapy intervention to best meet the child's needs and help him be successful in his PT/OT goals.

Procedures. To conduct this intervention, the music therapist places herself in close proximity to the patient. As with other cotreating session, it is vital that the music therapist be able to change locations as the PT/OT moves to perform the various interventions. The music therapy intervention must be focused on supporting the work of the PT/OT at all times. If the child has significant anger or frustration at the PT/OT, this session is not the time to process those emotions. This session's main goal is to help the child to attain his PT/OT goals in a positive manner. As with other interventions, the music therapist chooses music based upon the child's preferred genres. The music therapist can then manipulate the musical elements of the songs to meet the child's emotional and physical needs. This type of session can rely heavily upon the Iso principle, using the music to match the patient's mood and then helping to modulate his mood to something better or more conducive to completing the exercises in the PT/OT session. In addition, the music therapist can manipulate the song elements to match the physical movements of the PT/OT session. By changing the style of accompaniment from staccato to legato, the music therapist can support musically the type of movement needed at that time. Similarly, changing the tempo to match the tempo of the exercise can help the child to structure his movements. Finally, the music therapist can use the cadences in the songs or the end of the song to signify the end of an exercise or series of repetitions. This requires careful planning in the moment and some improvisation within the song to extend or shorten the song to match the exercise. Throughout the session, the music therapist plays and sings the child's preferred songs, adjusting the musical elements to meet the child's needs.

Adaptations. This type of intervention can be modified in a variety of ways. First, this sort of supportive session can be used not just with PTs/OTs but with other professionals, including nurses, anesthesiologists, and physicians at the hospital. The main goal continues to be providing support to the child to complete the goals of the cotreater(s). A second way to adapt this intervention is to expand it to include vocal re-creative and instrumental re-creative aspects. Finally, the intervention can be modified to include action listening, as discussed next.

Action listening is using musical elements to elicit behavior or movement in a patient. The music therapist must design the intervention to support the PT/OT's goals and session plans as well as select musical styles that are familiar to the child. The action listening intervention centers on spontaneous song creation. These songs describe the movements for the exercise the child is currently doing or the patient's emotional state. The lyrics, melody, and rhythm provide either the directions for the exercise or match the child's emotional state. Songs about the exercise can be a simple counting song for stretches or repetitions of the exercise. An example of this could be leg lifts. When the child needs to lift the leg up, the music therapist could improvise a song with lyrics that say "up" or "lift your leg to the sky" and then sing "down" or "bring your leg back to the bed" for the second half of the leg lift. The melody of the song reflects the direction of the child's movements, ascending as the child is to lift his leg and descending as he brings his leg back to the bed. When exercises are rhythmic in nature or the child is having trouble structuring his movements, creating a song that is more rhythmic, emphasizing the beat, can help the child to structure his movements. This form of song creation is quite beneficial, as it helps to provide the prompts for the child in a nonthreatening manner as well as increases the potential for more repetitions because the child is focused on the music and benefiting from the pain and anxiety reduction benefits of music. In the moment, the music therapist can choose the music that either supports the mood of the child or helps to change the mood of the child. The music should also be chosen with the child's reactions to music in mind. Finally, the music selection needs to keep in mind the type of movement the PT/OT is requesting the child make. As the exercise commences, the music therapist will need to modify the tempo to meet the tempo of the exercise. This may fluctuate through the repetitions, based on familiarity with the exercise, increased comfort or pain with movement, and fatigue.

If multiple patients are receiving PT/OT at the same time and all benefit from music therapy, it is possible to conduct a dyad/group session using these techniques. The main modification is to help the children take turns. The music therapist must work to balance the needs of each patient, providing the additional focus to the patient who is experiencing pain or anxiety, or is distressed.

GUIDELINES FOR IMPROVISATIONAL MUSIC THERAPY

Creative music therapy interventions are frequently used in pediatric burn care. These interventions can include instrumental nonreferential improvisation, instrumental referential improvisation, song improvisation, and instrumental mixed media improvisation. In 1998, Edwards described the clinical rationale for creative and compositional methods with pediatric burn patients. She included several case examples of song improvisation, fill-in-the-blank songwriting, and songwriting. This clinical practice article is an important step in creating an evidence base to demonstrate the efficacy of creative music therapy interventions. This section will explore these four interventions.

The contraindications for these interventions include significant hearing loss, if music is not an effective coping style, if the patient is agitated with music, if instrument playing is not culturally appropriate, or if the patient has physical limitations that do not allow for playing the instrument.

When the child is improvising about intense topics that are related to the initial trauma or subsequent traumas associated with the burn injury, it is vital that the music therapist be observing the child's emotional shifts as he improvises. In addition, if the child is focusing on physical goals like grasp, range of motion, or endurance, the music therapist must watch the child's movements for correct grasp, correct movement, indications of pain, and tiring. Depending on the child and his needs, pain and tiring may not indicate it is time to stop the intervention. As with all interventions where the music therapist may be addressing multiple goals in one intervention, it is key for the music therapist to remain focused on all areas she is addressing with the child.

Instrumental Nonreferential and Referential Improvisation

Overview. Both instrumental nonreferential and referential improvisation interventions can be used for a large variety of goals in pediatric burn care. Nonreferential improvisation is the process of improvising freely with no specific theme, idea, or task assigned by the therapist. Referential improvisation is to improvise with a reference, an idea, theme, or task, essentially expressing the thoughts, essence, and feelings about the idea, theme, or task through the improvisation. These interventions are indicated when the child needs to express himself, has anxiety, is agitated, has gross and/or fine motor needs, or is unwilling/unable to communicate verbally. The goal areas for these interventions include physical, cognitive, emotional, and social. Within physical goals, the music therapist may focus on pain management, increasing fine and/or gross motor skills, or increasing pulmonary function. This is accomplished by specific instrument choice that will address the patient's specific physical needs.

Within the area of cognition, the music therapist may use instrumental nonreferential interventions to improve orientation, reduce developmental regression, or improve neurological function. With these types of interventions, the music therapist will choose instruments and music styles that address the patient's needs both developmentally and neurologically.

Examples of the emotional/psychological goals that this intervention may address are anxiety management; decreasing agitation; increasing use of adaptive coping strategies; increasing the expression of thoughts or emotions regarding the hospitalization, injury, or accident; improving stress management; increasing self-esteem; and increasing acceptance. When addressing emotional/psychological goals, the music therapist must have a variety of instruments present to allow for the greatest freedom of expression for the child.

Finally, the social goals that may be addressed can include decreasing isolation, facilitating resumption of leisure activities, increased interaction with family/loved ones/peers, and supporting healthy family systems. Again, bringing in a variety of instruments allows for the greatest interaction and expression.

Preparation. The music therapist must have a certain level of proficiency in improvising a variety of different styles, scales, and modes to provide this intervention in a quality fashion. This requires study and practice of styles, scales, and modes until the music therapist is sufficiently proficient that she can improvise with the client, not for the client, while remaining observant with a therapist's eye. Prior to the start of the session, the music therapist should inventory her instruments and choose a variety of potential instruments the child may want to use. Careful consideration for the child's physical abilities as well as infection control status must be made when selecting potential instruments. The instruments used can include traditional acoustic instruments as well as electronic music technologies (EMTs) such as a keyboard, QChord, iPad, or iPod Touch. Devices such as the iPad or iPod Touch are small and easy to use and can contain apps that represent a variety of instruments all in one small package. With patients who have strict infection control status, these devices can give both the music therapist and the patient a variety of instruments to choose from without jeopardizing the child's health. The music therapist can often choose the scale and key for the melodic instrument apps, which can create a more successful experience for the patient and allow for greater musical expression by him.

The music therapist, if possible, should arrange the space so that the patient is facing her. If possible, the music therapist may want to sit so she is at an eye level similar to that of the patient. Allowing the patient to choose an instrument(s) is important, as it helps the patient to have the experience of mastery and control in an environment that is totally out of his control.

What to observe. The music therapist needs to observe many different things during these sessions, depending upon the goals she is addressing with the patient. These can range from physical function to emotional expression to facial expression to energy level. Musically, the music therapist needs to attend to what the child is playing. What are the motifs? Is it organized (keeping developmental level in mind)? Are there repeated themes? How does the child react when the music therapist mirrors or echoes the motifs or themes? Is the child repeating the same theme or rhythm over and over throughout the song? How does he respond when the music therapist changes the rhythm, tempo, style? Is the child aware of the music therapist's music? Is he interacting with the music therapist?

Procedures. To conduct this intervention as a nonreferential improvisation, the music therapist may give the child a choice of instruments. If a specific physical goal is being addressed, the music therapist can limit the choices of instruments to those that address the specific physical goal. For example, if a child needs to extend and flex his elbow, the music therapist can limit the child's choices to ones with which the child must extend and flex his elbow (drums, tambourine, xylophone, marimba, etc.). Once an instrument is chosen, the music therapist can choose what instrument she will play or allow the child to make that choice. Depending on the patient, either the music therapist or the patient will start the improvisation. When using nonreferential improvisations, the improvisation is not influenced by questions or ideas for the patient to ponder. Instead, the music is created from each individual's current state of being.

When using referential improvisation, this intervention may be a thoughtful part of the session planning or organically develop from previous interventions in the session. If it is a planned intervention, the music therapist may want to either allow the child to choose a topic/emotion or recommend one for the child to improvise about. Once the topic is chosen, the child may be given options of which instrument the music therapist will play. If a specific physical goal is being addressed along with the emotional, social, and/or communication goals, the music therapist can limit the choices of instruments to those that address the specific physical goal. Once an instrument is chosen, the music therapist can choose which instrument she will play or allow the child to make that choice. Depending on the patient, either the music therapist or the patient will start the improvisation. The music therapist may improvise with the patient. In this improvisation, the music therapist may take a more supportive role within the music, creating a container that holds the patient's music. Or, if appropriate, the music therapist can echo the patient's motifs. If the patient is repeating the same motif over and over, the music therapist, depending on the situation and the goals, may want to challenge the patient musically to step beyond a repeated pattern and explore their resistance to change. This type of challenge needs to be used only with careful consideration of the myriad needs and strengths of the patient as well as the patient's culture.

Adaptations. This intervention can be modified in a variety of ways. Vocalizations or singing can be added to the improvisation. The improvisation may develop into a songwriting experience. Additionally, the improvisation may morph into a conductive improvisation with the child directing or cuing the music therapist's improvisation. This intervention can be used not only with individual sessions but also with family, dyad, and group sessions. Once the intervention is complete, the child may begin to talk about the emotions or ideas he was improvising about. It can be paired with nearly any other music therapy interventions.

Song Improvisation

Overview. The next type of improvisatory intervention used is song improvisation. This intervention consists of the patient expressing intentionally a concept, idea, or feeling in song format in the moment. It can address a variety of goals in pediatric burn care. Song improvisation is indicated when the patient needs to express himself, has anxiety, is agitated, has pulmonary function needs, is unwilling/unable to communicate verbally, or has an interest in music. The goal areas for this intervention include communication, emotional, physical, cognitive, and social goals. First, the communication goals often focus on increasing verbal communication. Next, the emotional goals can include anxiety management; decreasing agitation; increasing use of adaptive coping strategies; sharing experience of pain; increasing the expression of thoughts or emotions regarding the hospitalization, injury, or accident; increasing self-esteem; and increasing acceptance. Within physical goals, the music therapist may focus on increasing pulmonary function and addressing oral musculature needs. Within the area of cognitive goals, the music therapist may work with patients to improve orientation, reduce developmental regression, or improve neurological function. Finally, the social goals that may be addressed can include decreasing isolation, increased interaction with family/loved ones/peers, and supporting healthy family systems. Additional contraindications for this intervention are extreme anxiety with expression about trauma or hospitalization and having physical limitations that do not allow vocalizing.

Preparation. As with instrumental improvisations, the music therapist must have a certain level of proficiency in improvising a variety of different styles and in a variety of different scales/modes to conduct the song improvisation. Prior to the start of the session, the music therapist should review the genres of music the child prefers. Choosing instruments or EMTs that allow the music therapist to provide musical accompaniment that reflects the child's preferred music may aid in the child's success with improvising his ideas, emotions, or experiences.

If possible, the music therapist may want to arrange the space so the patient is facing the music therapist. With adolescents, this configuration may be too direct or intimate. The music therapist may want to consider placing herself to the side, perpendicular to the patient. If possible, the music therapist may want to sit so that she is at an eye level similar to that of the patient.

What to observe. The music therapist needs to observe many different things during these sessions, depending upon the goals she is addressing with the patient. Musically, the music therapist needs to attend to the patient's melody, tempo, volume, and lyrics. This observation is similar to the previous intervention.

Procedures. To conduct this intervention, the music therapist may want to either allow the child to choose a topic/emotion or recommend one for the child to improvise about. The music therapist can start by posing an open question for the child, asking what he would like to sing about. If the child is not able to identify a topic, the music therapist will then offer a variety of topics. These topics can range from benign (hospital food) to issues that the child is currently facing. The topic may also be generated organically from the session. If the child does not suggest or pick a topic, the music therapist can tease one out of the discussion, the events going on, or the child's body language. In this improvisation, the music therapist may take a more supportive role within the music, creating a container that holds the patient's music, or take an active role in creating the melody and lyrics. As the music starts, if the child does not start the vocalizations, the music therapist can start with singing about the topic or what she is observing or just make vocal sounds to match the topic/mood. With body language, eye contact, and verbal encouragement, the music therapist prompts the child to join in the improvisation vocally, creating the song. The music therapist can also sing a phrase, leaving out a word for the child to fill in, pausing at the point with an expectant look upon her face. An example of this is, "Today, Hester is feeling _____." If there is instrumental music, continue to play but add music elements that promote the feeling of anticipation, like the 7th of the chord. The music therapist can then repeat what the child said, then repeat the line. This repetition allows the child to know the music therapist heard him and that his input is valued. As the song continues, it is hoped that the child will start taking a larger role in the song improvisation, creating lyrics and melodies. However, even if the child sticks to only adding phrases when prompted, the intervention continues to have great value.

It is important for the music therapist to keep the form of a song in mind, with repeated melodies for the verses, chorus, and bridge sections. Coming back to the chorus can help the child to emphasize a key idea within the song and bring unity to the experience. The familiar form of the song will help to provide a container for the child's expression as well as a feeling of familiarity that he may need.

Adaptations. This intervention can be modified in a variety of ways. The child can accompany himself. If the child desires, the intervention can morph into a conducted intervention, one that allows him to cue or direct the improvisers. Similarly, it can be modified to become a mixed media improvisation, one in which the child not only uses his voice but also instruments or other sources of sound/music. This intervention can be modified to be used with a dyad or group to spontaneously create a song that has a common theme shared by multiple patients. Next, it can be paired with nearly any other improvisatory, music listening, or lyric analysis music therapy interventions. Finally, if the child wants to or the music therapist feels there is therapeutic value to record the song improvisation, the music therapist and child can document the song through writing the lyrics, melody, and harmony; recording the initial improvisation; rehearsing the song and perfecting the melody, accompaniment, and lyric (based on child's desires); and recording it for the child's keeping.

GUIDELINES FOR COMPOSITIONAL MUSIC THERAPY

Within pediatric burn care, there is often great therapeutic benefit from a variety of composition interventions. The most frequently used interventions in this category are fill-in-the-blank songwriting, songwriting, and music collages. Within the article by Magee, Bertolami, Kubicek, LaJoie, Martino, Sankowski, Townsend, Whitehead-Pleaux, and Zigo (2011), a case study explores a single session where the music therapist used the intervention of songwriting on GarageBand to help a patient connect to her sister and mother, who are also hospitalized. The music therapist facilitated a songwriting intervention as well as created individualized CDs to address a school-age girl's anxiety regarding the hospitalization of herself, her mother, and her sister for burns.

Similarly, Whitehead-Pleaux, Clark, and Spall (2011) outline a few case vignettes which use songwriting with EMTs when working with pediatric burn patients. Indications and contraindications are explored for this intervention.

Whitehead-Pleaux and Spall (in press) continued to explore ways to incorporate EMTs into creative music therapy interventions. One case explores using a songwriting intervention with GarageBand with two school-age kids awaiting surgery. Another case explores the use of GarageBand to create a music collage with a school-age boy. The patient has severe needle phobia and must undergo repeated weekly needle sticks. The music collage allowed the patient to express his experience in greater detail than he could via language. This section will explore these interventions.

Fill-in-the-Blank Songwriting

Overview. One way to introduce children to songwriting is to use fill-in-the-blank songwriting. The indications for this intervention are the ability to communicate, the need to express/discuss a specific topic, anxiety, low levels of pain, distress with medical care, and desire to share a message with another. Fill-in-the-blank songwriting can address a variety of emotional/psychological, cognitive, physical, and spiritual goals. The main emotional/psychological goal is expressing emotions or thoughts related to the injury, accident, and future of the patient. Next, cognitive goals can include sequencing ideas, attention development, and educational goals. Physical goals can include fine motor (writing with a pencil or typing lyrics on a computer) and pulmonary function. Finally, spiritual goals can include increasing connection to the hope base as well as expressing thoughts and emotions related to the intersection of spiritual beliefs and accident. Contraindications can include diminished cognitive function due to medication, medication wean, brain injury, septic delirium, trauma symptoms, inability to discuss emotions without triggering trauma symptoms, and cultural restrictions on songwriting.

Preparation. To be ready to facilitate this intervention, the music therapist must first prepare the song. The first step is to choose a song that either targets the specific topic or is of a genre that the child enjoys. Next, the music therapist needs to remove key words or phrases, which will allow the child to express his ideas in the song. Finally, the music therapist must learn the melody and the accompaniment for the song. As the music therapist prepares the song, she must keep in mind the child's cognitive functioning and developmental level. The task needs to be balanced to where it is not too easy but not too complex, designed in a way that meets the child's goals while remaining aesthetically pleasing and successful for the patient.

When facilitating this intervention, the music therapist will want to sit in proximity to the patient, either facing him or sitting to the side. The music therapist will need to bring the song sheet and a writing instrument or the electronic file on a device that allows for the patient to write his ideas. The music therapist may need to write the ideas of the patient if the patient is unable to write due to physical limitations or illiteracy. Finally, the music therapist will need to bring the instrument on which she is accompanying the patient or the music file to which the patient will be singing.

What to observe. The music therapist will need to observe the patient's progress toward the goals specified in the treatment plan. In addition, the music therapist needs to keep an eye out for increased frustration with the tasks within the songwriting intervention. If the tasks become too difficult or abstract for the patient, the music therapist will need to step in to aid the patient in completing the tasks. It is important to remember with this and almost every music therapy intervention that the quality of the music product does not matter nearly as much as the process of creating the music product. In addition, it is important for the music therapist to create a space in which the patient can express himself in his music cultural style free of judgment or influence from the therapist.

Procedures. Fill-in-the-blank songwriting can happen in one session or over a number of sessions, depending on the patient's tolerance for the cognitive tasks, physical expenditure, and emotional state. When working in burns or in a hospital with children who are injured or ill, a music therapist needs to be aware that their energy level, tolerance, and focus may be limited by the illness or injury. If the child can read and write, the music therapist can give the song sheet to the child to fill out. The music therapist can help the patient by prompts, examples, and clarifications. Often, as each section of a song is completed, the music therapist will sing the completed sections as reinforcement for the child's work as well as a musical review of the lyrics to continue the creative process of the child. Once the song is completed, the music therapist asks the patient to sing along if appropriate. If the child is unable or reluctant to sing the song, the music therapist can sing the song to the child. It is often a good idea to type the lyrics on a sheet for the patient to retain as a reminder of the therapeutic gains made in this intervention. In addition, the music therapist can rehearse the song with the child and make a recording for the child to keep.

Adaptations. This intervention can be adapted in a variety of ways. First, once the song is written, the child can play an instrument or instruments to add to the accompaniment. Next, after recording the fill-in-the-blank song, the music therapist and child can create a music video to further expand upon the ideas or emotions of the song. A third adaptation is to incorporate this intervention into a medical procedure or PT/OT session. In these sessions, the child will write a song that relates to the experience in the procedure or PT/OT session. Finally, this intervention can be modified to be a family, dyad, or group intervention. When this is used with more than one individual, the music therapist needs to incorporate the experiences and words of all the participants, while keeping the song cohesive and related to the theme.

Songwriting

Overview. Songwriting is another common composition intervention employed in pediatric burn centers. This intervention is indicated for children who are able to communicate, the need to express/discuss their experiences, anxiety, low levels of pain, distress with medical care, and desire to share a message with another. The goals and contraindications for this intervention are similar to those listed in the fill-in-the-blank intervention.

Preparation. To be ready to facilitate this intervention, there is very little preparation to do prior to the session(s).

What to observe. The recommendations for observations to be made by the therapist are similar as the ones for the previous intervention.

Procedures. Songwriting is an intervention that can take place in one session or over a series of sessions. This is often dictated by the patient's expected length of stay, developmental age, cognitive functioning, ability to focus and tolerate the difficult multistep process, physical expenditure, and flow of ideas. If the child can read and write, the music therapist can let the child write the words to the song. Songwriting can be a daunting task for many kids. One way to help kids to break down the tasks is to first come up with the theme of the song. Second, ask if the child wants to compose the music or lyrics first. If it is the lyrics, the next task is to ask the child to brainstorm different ideas, not worrying about phrasing. The music therapist or patient writes the ideas down. Together, the patient and music therapist look for the important message within the ideas and decide where that message should be: the first verse, the chorus, the last verse? From that bit of structure, the music therapist can help the child to identify which ideas go together and the sequence of the ideas. Together, they craft the verses and chorus. The music therapist can help the patient by prompts, examples, and clarifications. If building on a brainstormed idea, the music therapist can even offer options of how to phrase the child's ideas to fit the structure of the stanza.

Regardless of whether the child wants to compose the music first or second, determine if acoustic instruments or EMTs are best to compose the music for the song. If you determine that acoustic instruments will best meet the patient's plan for how the song is to sound, choose the instruments that best match his ability to direct the composition. With children who are younger or developmentally at an earlier stage, the music therapist may have to take a greater role in the composition. For children with more limited abilities in composition, the music therapist can facilitate the composition process by giving the child choices like fast, medium, or slow tempo; choices of scale or mode; choices in meter; does the melody go up or down here?, etc. If EMTs will better meet the patient's abilities and musical stylings, there are a myriad of apps and programs that are designed for music composition. These range in difficulty and genres of music. Choose one that matches your child's developmental and intellectual abilities as well as the child's chosen genre for the song. Some apps and programs assemble songs through samples. Others allow the user to choose notes in the melody or accompaniment. It is important that the music therapist be quite familiar with the app or program in order to easily navigate its features.

Once the song lyrics are written and the music composed, the music therapist and patient can then put the two together. If it is not a single-session songwriting, the two can rehearse and fine-tune the song over a number of sessions prior to recording it. If it is a single session, a quick rehearsal before recording is about all that will be possible. It is good to give the patient not only a typed copy of the lyrics but also the song file on a CD so that he can remember it and his accomplishment.

Adaptations. Adaptations similar to those discussed for the fill-in-the-blank songwriting intervention can be used.

Music Collages

Overview. Music collages are an interesting form of composition to use with children—especially children who are undergoing difficult medical procedures and who have experienced trauma and rejection by their peers because of appearance. Children do not always have the ability to talk about concepts and emotions in an abstract way, as their brain has not fully developed these skills. However, telling the story about an experience solely through sounds and samples allows the child to bring his inner experience to the music therapist in a way that captures the emotional content and the thoughts of the child. This intervention is indicated for children who are in a place in their life where they are feeling secure and safe enough to explore difficult feelings or experiences. The patient must have a way to either indicate his choice for the sound/sample choices or be able to manipulate the instruments or EMTs by himself. The goals for this intervention focus solely on expression of emotions and thoughts, as well as anxiety reduction. This intervention is contraindicated when the child is not oriented to time, place, and person and/or is experiencing active hallucinations or trauma symptoms, if music is not a preferred method for coping, and if music is not culturally appropriate. This is an intervention that should be carefully applied to someone who is recently injured or who has just undergone a significant surgery. Outpatients are well suited to this intervention.

Preparation. To prepare for this session, the music therapist should have familiarity with either the chosen EMT device or the array of instruments to be used. With EMT devices, a program that allows the user to assemble different samples to create a composition is well suited for this intervention. Examples of these programs are GarageBand, Audacity, and Fruity Loops. Due to infection control procedures and small spaces within a hospital, using an EMT device can allow the music therapist to bring a myriad of sounds and samples to a patient in one small device.

What to observe. The music therapist will need to observe for signs of distress. If the emotional content or memories are becoming too overwhelming or too anxiety-provoking, it is important for the music therapist to find a way to help the child tolerate these feelings or to set aside the work for another day, accomplishing the completed song collage over a series of sessions.

Procedures. When meeting with the child, the first task is to discuss on a developmentally appropriate level the experience/emotion upon which he will be basing the song collage. The music therapist may want to take notes while the child shares in order to help the child break down the sequence to the parts which he will pair with sounds or samples. If using acoustic instruments, help the child explore the instruments' sounds and start matching the sounds to the different parts. Similarly, the music therapist can help the child explore the different sound files and samples in the program, finding the one that matches each part of the sequence laid out earlier. Samples and loops can be created by the child by recording his voice (singing, talking, vocalizing, etc.), him playing an instrument, or other ambient sounds. These sound files can be modified via the features on the EMTs and then incorporated into the music collage. Once the sounds and samples are figured out and sequenced, with the instruments, the child can perform the song collage with or without help from the music therapist. If the song collage is created on the EMT, there is not a chance to perform it, but it can easily be burned to a CD for the patient to keep. In addition, in subsequent sessions, the music therapist and patient can continue to work with the sounds/parts of the collage to process difficult information/emotions.

Adaptations. Adaptations of this intervention are many. One adaptation is to then compose a song via songwriting that is related to the song collage. Then these compositions could be combined into one composition, which further tells the patient's story. Another adaptation is to create a video to accompany the song collage. Finally, over time, the patient could create a response to the song collage that illustrates the solution, changes, or growth from the earlier song collage.

GUIDELINES FOR RE-CREATIVE MUSIC THERAPY

The final types of music therapy intervention that are used in pediatric burn care are categorized under re-creative music therapy and include instrumental re-creation and vocal re-creation. This section will explore each of these interventions. The contraindications for these interventions include significant hearing loss, if music is not an effective coping style, if the patient is agitated with music, if singing or playing an instrument is not culturally appropriate, or if the patient has physical limitations that do not allow vocalizing or the movements needed to play an instrument.

If possible, the music therapist may want to arrange the space so that the patient is facing the music therapist for these interventions. With adolescents, this configuration may be too direct or intimate. The music therapist may want to consider placing herself to the side, perpendicular to the patient. If possible, the music therapist may want to sit so that she is at an eye level similar to that of the patient.

Music Instruction

Overview. A great intervention to use with kids who will be hospitalized for a significant amount of time or are hospitalized repeatedly for multiple surgeries that span over a few months is music instruction. Children's interest usually centers on learning to play the guitar, drums, or piano. This intervention is indicated if the child has an interest in learning to play an instrument and has the cognitive ability to stick with a task that might be frustrating. For instrumental instruction, the child must have some mobility in his upper or lower extremities. For vocal instruction, the child must have the ability to create sound with his voice. Although the child may believe that the sessions are mainly aimed at learning to play an instrument, the music therapist understands that important underlying goals include building self-esteem, enhancing self-image, coping with hospitalization and/or loss, improving physical function, and facilitating expression of thoughts and emotions.

Preparation. To prepare for this type of intervention, the music therapist needs to assess the child's physical needs and limitations. With vocal instruction, the music therapist needs to assess the patient for the ability to produce sound safely vocally. If need be, the music therapist should consult with the nurse, respiratory therapist, or surgeon for clearance to sing. With instrumental instruction, the music therapist must meet with the child to learn what instrument he is interested in learning. Then the music therapist must do a thorough assessment of the functioning of the child's hands, wrists, elbows, and shoulders, as contractures and deep burn injuries can limit movement and flexibility. If the child expresses interest in playing an instrument that is inaccessible based on physical limitations, the music therapist should consider ways to adapt the instrument to accommodate for the child's abilities. If accommodation of the instrument to meet the child's limited motor abilities is not feasible, the music therapist should consider other related instruments that accommodate the child's abilities and are agreeable to the patient as a suitable substitution. The guitar is an excellent example of this process. The guitar requires significant flexibility in the wrist of the hand that fingers the chords as well as finger flexibility and strength. If a patient is unable to flex his fingers due to contractures or fused joints, an adaptive device like a guitar barre or a slide may provide an accommodation that allows the child to learn the guitar. If this adaptation still does not meet the child's abilities, the music therapist could suggest a Strumstick, dobro, or mountain dulcimer. It is important that the music therapist is upfront with the patient, explaining why the instrument of their choice is not a viable option, and then discusses the options available. Involving the patient as the decision-maker in this process is important, for he must be invested in learning the instrument.

What to observe. During the music instruction sessions, the music therapist must observe for physical and emotional signs of tiring. Vocally, if a patient is recovering from an airway injury, the music therapist must be vigilant to not strain the healing voice. With instrumental lessons, if the patient is playing with a portion of his body that was burned, the music therapist needs to be mindful of fatigue and skin condition (especially with stringed instruments). If the child is becoming frustrated or overwhelmed by the curriculum of the session, the music therapist needs to modify the session plan to provide success experiences.

Procedures. When providing music instruction, it is important for the music therapist to meet with the child regularly for a set amount of time. In these sessions, depending on the child's skill level and interest, the music learned can vary from traditional curriculum to songs of the child's preferred genre. The music therapist needs to balance the patient's skills, abilities, and desire to learn technique with success and the objectives for the intervention. If a child wants to play a song that has many complex chords, it is the job of the music therapist to modify the harmonies to make the song accessible to the patient's abilities if possible. It is important to keep in mind that the music product (in this case, the patient's music skills) is not the focus of music therapy. Instead, it is the process within the sessions. In essence, the music skills developed by the patient are secondary to the therapeutic goals of the session/series of sessions. For example, the patient may not emerge from a series of music instruction interventions as an amazing pianist, but his goals of increased self-esteem, improved fine motor skills, and stimulation of cognitive development will be met.

Adaptations. The main adaptations are few. First, instrumental and vocal instruction can be combined when a patient is learning an instrument like the guitar or piano as well as learning to sing. Another adaptation is to combine these interventions with songwriting. The patient learns to play his own song on his instrument or to sing it. As the patient gains skills, the sessions can be combined with improvisational interventions as well.

Singing Familiar Songs

Overview. This intervention consists of singing familiar songs with the patient. It is indicated when a child needs to express himself, has anxiety, is agitated, has pulmonary function needs, is unwilling/unable to communicate verbally, or has an interest in music. The goal areas for this intervention include communication, emotional, physical, cognitive, and social goals. First, the communication goals often focus on increasing verbal communication and to gain clarity in speech. Next, the emotional goals can include anxiety management; decreasing agitation; increasing the use of adaptive coping strategies; increasing the expression of thoughts or emotions regarding the hospitalization, injury, or accident; and increasing self-esteem. Within physical goals, the music therapist may focus on increasing pulmonary function and addressing oral musculature needs. Within the area of cognitive goals, the music therapist may work with patients to improve orientation, reduce developmental regression, or improve neurological function. Finally, the social goals that may be addressed can include decreasing isolation, increased interaction with family/loved ones/peers, and supporting healthy family systems.

Preparation. The music therapist must have a certain level of proficiency in playing the songs and genres that the child prefers. This requires some study and practice outside of the session, becoming proficient at playing and singing the songs. Prior to the start of the session, the music therapist should review which genres of music the patient prefers. Choosing instruments or EMTs that allow the music therapist to provide musical accompaniment that reflects the patient's preferred music may aid in the patient's success.

Procedures. To conduct this intervention, the music therapist can allow for the selection of music in a variety of ways. First, the music therapist can choose the songs based on the child's preference. Next, the music therapist can give the patient a limited number of songs from which to choose. Finally, the music therapist can allow the child to choose the songs. Songbooks of songs the music therapist knows can be given to the patient to choose songs from.

Adaptations. This intervention can be modified in a variety of ways. The child can not only sing but also play instruments with the song. This intervention can be modified for use with a dyad or group to spontaneously create a song that has a common theme shared by multiple patients. Next, it can be paired with music listening or lyric analysis music therapy interventions. Finally, if the child wants to or the music therapist feels that there is therapeutic value in recording the child singing the song, the music therapist and child can help with rehearsing the song and perfecting the melody and accompaniment, and record it for the child's keeping.

Lyric Analysis

Overview. The final type of intervention used is lyric analysis. This intervention consists of the patient and music therapist listening to a recording of a song or the music therapist singing a song and the patient analyzing the lyrics. It can address a variety of goals in pediatric burn care. Lyric analysis is indicated when the child needs to express himself, has anxiety, is agitated, is unwilling to explore feelings/thoughts/issues via traditional talk modalities, or has an interest in music. The goal areas for this intervention include communication, emotional, physical, cognitive, and social goals. First, the communication goals often focus on increasing verbal communication. Next, the emotional goals can include anxiety management; decreasing agitation; increasing use of adaptive coping strategies; sharing experience of pain; increasing the expression of thoughts or emotions regarding the hospitalization, injury, or accident; increasing self-esteem; and increasing acceptance. Within physical goals, the music therapist may focus on increasing pulmonary function and addressing oral musculature needs. Within the area of cognitive goals, the music therapist may work with patients to improve orientation, reduce developmental regression, or improve neurological function. Finally, the social goals that may be addressed can include decreasing isolation, increasing interaction with family/loved ones/peers, and supporting healthy family systems.

Preparation. To prepare for this intervention, the music therapist needs to have a variety of song sheets available for the child to read. These allow the child to first read the correct words rather than have misconceptions about the song content, and, second, it allows the child to focus on phrases and themes of the song, referring to specific sections in the discussion phase of the intervention. The music therapist needs to possess the song file or be proficient in playing the song live in the session.

Procedures. To conduct this intervention, the music therapist may want to either allow the child to choose a song(s) or bring specific song(s) for listening. The music therapist can start the intervention by asking which song should be used or introducing the song. Then, when listening to the song, the music therapist sits quietly, making periodic eye contact with the child. Once the song has finished, the music therapist can start the discussion by posing open questions about the music. When the child is ready, the music therapist can turn the discussion to the content of the song lyrics, asking open questions of the child. It is important for the music therapist to allow the patient the space to project his feelings upon the songwriter. This projection allows the patient to talk about topics or feelings that may be too sensitive for the patient to own yet. Additionally, it is important for the music therapist to avoid yes/no questions, for these can lead to dead ends in the conversation. When interpreting the child's expression, it is important to view it not from the music therapist's cultural lenses, but through the child's cultural lenses.

Adaptations. There are a variety of ways to modify this intervention. The patient may not just listen to the song, but also sing the lyrics. Another way to modify it is to invite the child to bring a song to the session that describes how he is feeling or something that is important to him. This intervention can be modified for use with a dyad or group to analyze a song that has a common theme shared by multiple patients. Next, it can be paired with music listening or song-singing music therapy interventions. Finally, the intervention can be paired with fill-in-the-blank songwriting. By modifying either the song used in the lyric analysis or a related song, the music therapist can help the patient to continue to work on the issues within the song and move forward in wellness.

RESEARCH EVIDENCE

Although several publications regarding music therapy for pediatric burn care exist, the research on the use of music therapy with this population is very limited. The majority of the music therapy research in burns focuses on music analgesia, which reflects the biggest need of this patient population: pain management. Clinical music therapists spend much of their time in the burn unit working alongside nurses, PTs, OTs, physicians, and other medical professionals in concert to ease the sufferings of the burn patient. It follows that the bulk of the research into the effects of music therapy with burn patients focuses on music analgesia. The research and clinical practice articles on creative methods with pediatric burn patients has yet to be fully explored for efficacy. At the time of the writing of this chapter, there exists no research about the use of creative or compositional methods with pediatric burn patients. However, one can find case studies and clinical practice guidelines for the use of creative and composition music therapy interventions. As more music therapists work with pediatric burn patients, it is hoped that these clinicians will add to the knowledge base.

In their examination of music-assisted relaxation interventions into preoperative anxiety, Robb, Nicholas, Rutan, Bishop, and Parker (1995) conducted a randomized clinical trial with 20 pediatric burn patients. Anxiety was measured using the State Trait Anxiety Index for Children. Patients were randomly assigned to either an experimental group (receiving music-assisted relaxation interventions) or a control group (receiving only the standard of practice). The results indicated that the experimental group reported significantly less anxiety at posttest (M = 27.9, SD not reported), compared to the control group (M = 34.4, SD not reported)(p = .04). Finally, the physiological measures did not yield any statistically significant results. In addition, the patients and staff reported favorably about the intervention.

In 2001, Fratianne, Prensner, Hutson, Super, Yowler, and Standley tested how effective music-based imagery and music alternative engagement interventions were for the pain and anxiety of burn patients undergoing debridement. The researchers employed a repeated-measures design. The 25 pediatric and adult participants were randomly assigned to two groups. Measures, including pulse, self-reported pain, self-reported anxiety, and the nurses' observations of patient tension, were taken at four different times (prior to the debridement, during the debridement, directly after the debridement, and when the patient returned to his room). The first group received debridement with music therapy support on the first day; on the second day, they underwent debridement procedures without music therapy. The second group received this sequence in reverse order. The authors found a greater reduction (p = .004) in the patients' report of pain perception in the music therapy condition (mean change score = −2.18), compared to the no-music condition (mean change score = −0.06).

Whitehead-Pleaux, Baryza, and Sheridan (2006) explored the use of music analgesia with 14 pediatric burn patients ages 6 to 16 undergoing a painful medical procedure. The children were randomly assigned to either a music analgesia group or a standard care control group. The results of this study found no difference between the music analgesia conditions and the control in regard to self-reported anxiety, self-reported pain, behavioral distress, heart rate, and respiration rate. However, the authors remarked that the patients' anecdotal reports did not match the quantitative data collected, which led the authors to wonder whether the tools they used to measure the patient's pain (Wong-Baker FACES Scale and Nursing Assessment of Pain Intensity (NAPI)) and anxiety (Fear Thermometer) were appropriate to accurately measure the impact of this intervention. First, the patients were noted to not accurately reflect upon the amount of pain they experienced (exhibiting a very high pain rating on the behavioral distress scale (NAPI), but reporting a low score on the FACES Scale). In addition, the icon of the thermometer in the Fear Thermometer was not an image with which a majority of the children were familiar. Finally, the NAPI was found to be an effective tool, but the application of it once during the session did not capture the data the authors were seeking. The authors recommended changes to increase the effectiveness of this line of research, which included time sampling for heart rate, blood oxygenation, behavioral distress, and level of engagement in the music therapy intervention for more effective measurement of the effects of music therapy on pain and anxiety.

In 2007, Whitehead-Pleaux, Baryza, Zebrowski, and Sheridan conducted an exploratory study that combined qualitative and quantitative research methods to further explore the effects of music therapy on nine pediatric burn patients undergoing medical procedures. In this study, the patients completed quantitative measures and also participated in a structured interview. In addition, parents, nurses, and the music therapist participated in structured interviews about the application of music therapy in the medical procedure. The data from this study indicated that music analgesia appeared to decrease behavioral distress when the patient was engaged either actively or passively in the music analgesia intervention ($p < .0001$). There was no statistical difference between active and passive engagement and behavioral distress ($p = .104$). When behavioral distress was analyzed over time with age factored in, the results indicated that children who were older benefitted more from the music analgesia intervention. The physiological measures yielded no significant differences. The interview data indicated that participants experienced decreased pain and anxiety, improved mood, enhanced relaxation, and increased compliance. The interviews of the parents and nurses illustrated that music therapy had a calming effect upon the parents and the nurses.

In 2009, Whitehead-Pleaux, Baryza, and Sheridan presented the results of phase two of this study, a randomized controlled trial. In this study, 41 children, ages 6 to 18, were randomly assigned to the three conditions: music therapy support, verbal support, and control. The authors measured behavioral distress (NAPI), heart rate, and level of engagement every two minutes of the procedure while anxiety (using the Multidimensional Anxiety Scale for Children) and mood (Visual Analog Mood Scale) were measured after the procedure. When exploring the difference between the three conditions in regard to behavioral distress, the authors found a significant difference between the music therapy condition and control ($p = 0.03$) and verbal support and control ($p = 0.03$), while there was no difference between the music therapy and verbal support conditions ($p = 0.54$). Although not significant, trends in self-reported mood measures suggested that the patients who received music analgesia felt happier, more energetic, more relaxed, and less anxious than the control. The trends also indicated that patients who received verbal support were less confused, sad, and angry, and happier than patients in the control group.

Finally, in a randomized prospective crossover trial, Tan, Yowler, Super, and Fratianne (2010) compared music conditions with a standard care control during dressing changes in 29 burn patients ranging from 8 to 71 years of age. The study found that patients who received the music analgesia intervention and music relaxation interventions experienced significantly less pain than the control group during ($p < .05$) and after ($p < .025$) the dressing changes. In addition, the music therapy condition resulted in less anxiety and muscle tension during the dressing change than the control condition ($p < .05$). The small, heterogeneous sample of this study is of course problematic.

SUMMARY AND CONCLUSION

The application of music therapy in pediatric burns is a wonderfully dynamic corner of our field. The needs of the population are very diverse and demanding. Therefore, the music therapy programs include a wide range of individualized interventions. These challenges offer a vibrant environment for creativity. Music therapy offers great potential for change and for easing a child and family's time through one of the most horrific events of their lives. Working both in acute care and reconstructive care phases with patients allows the music therapist to establish long-term relationships with the patient. This combination of acute work and long-term care allows the music therapist to address the issues of body image, bullying, and assuming adult roles.

Burn care is a field within medical music therapy that has yet to be fully explored, and research is quite limited. With few music therapists working with this population, it has been challenging to conduct research in this area. It is hoped that over time, more music therapists will find employment in pediatric and adult burn care and that these music therapists will conduct or stimulate the clinical research needed to expand the evidence base of the current music therapy practice. This research is much needed so that music therapists will learn about best practices for serving pediatric burn patients, easing their suffering, reconnecting them with life, and aiding in their transition back home.

Despite the fact that Christenberry first described the population in 1979, this population remains greatly underserved and underresearched in the United States. Very few burn units and hospitals employ music therapists full-time. Some music therapists are employed part-time or on a contract basis. It is the hope of the author that music therapists will seek out positions in burn units and hospitals. With a greater population of music therapists working in burn units, a greater number of patients and families will receive the benefits of music therapy.

GLOSSARY

Acute Stress Disorder (ASD): a disorder in which anxiety, dissociative, and re-experiencing symptoms develop within one month of exposure to a traumatic event.

Anoxic injury: a brain injury caused by lack of oxygen in the brain.

Benzodiazepines: a class of medications used to address anxiety and other symptoms.

Bronchus: the part of the respiratory system that conducts air into the lungs.

Dissociative symptoms: a variety of symptoms from mild detachment to more severe detachment from immediate surroundings, physical, and emotional experience.

Dermis: the layer of skin under the epidermis.

Endocrine: pertaining to the system of glands that produces secretions that help to control metabolic activity.

Enteric: pertaining to the intestinal system.

Genitourinary system: the system that includes the reproductive and urinary organs.

Hematologic: pertaining to the blood and its components.

Hypermetabolic: increased metabolic activity.

Hypertropic scar: a scar that is raised.

Hypoxia: a state in which a body or a portion of the body is deprived of oxygen.

Intubated: having a flexible plastic tube inserted in the trachea to maintain an airway.

Intravenous therapy (IV): a tube inserted in a vein for delivering medications and fluids.

Ketamine: a medication used for anesthesia, often used for conscious sedation.

Larynx: the "voice box."

Metabolic state: the status of a range of biochemical processes that occur within the body.

Musculoskeletal system: the muscle and bone systems.

Nasogastric tube (NG tube): a flexible tube that is used for medication and nutrition that extends from the nose to the gastric system.

Ophthalmic: pertaining to the eye.

Opioid medication: narcotic medication used to treat pain.

Otolaryngologic: pertaining to the ear, nose, and throat.

PICC line (Peripherally Inserted Central Catheter): a long, slender, small, flexible tube that is inserted into a peripheral vein but extends to a large vein in the chest near the heart.

Post-Traumatic Stress Disorder (PTSD): a disorder in which anxiety, dissociative, and re-experiencing symptoms develop one month or more after exposure to a traumatic event.

Pulmonary: pertaining to the lungs.

Renal: pertaining to the kidneys.

Trachea: internal structure used for breathing.

Tracheotomy: a surgical procedure that creates an opening in the neck through one wall of the trachea to create a way for air to get to the lungs.

REFERENCES

Altshuler, I. M. (1948). A psychiatrist's experience with music as a therapeutic agent. In D. M. Schullian & M. Schoen (Eds.), *Music and Medicine.* New York: Henry Schuman.

American Music Therapy Association. (2011). Standards of Clinical Practice. (Online). 11/5/12. http://musictherapy.org/standards.html

Bessey, P. Q. (2007). Wound care. In D. Herndon (Ed.), *Total burn care* (3rd ed., pp. 127–135). Philadelphia: Saunders Elsevier.

Bishop, B., Christenberry, A., Robb, S., & Toombs Rudenberg, M. (1996). Music therapy and child life interventions with pediatric burn patients. In M. A. Froehlich (Ed.), *Music therapy with hospitalized children: A creative arts child life approach* (pp. 87–108). Cherry Hill, NJ: Jeffrey Books.

Brewin, C. R., Andrews, B., & Valentine, J. D. (2000). Meta-analysis of risk factors for posttraumatic stress disorder in trauma-exposed adults. *Journal of Consulting and Clinical Psychology, 68*(5), 748–766.

Carrougher, G. (1998). *Burn care and therapy.* St. Louis, MO: Mosby.

Christenberry, E. B. (1979). The use of music therapy with burn patients. *The Journal of Music Therapy, 16*(3), 138–148.

Daveson, B. A. (1999). A model of response: Coping mechanisms and music therapy techniques during debridement. *Music Therapy Perspectives, 17*(2), 92–98.

Edwards, J. (1995). "You are singing beautifully": Music therapy and the debridement bath. *The Arts in Psychotherapy, 22*(1), 53–55.

Edwards, J. (1998). Music therapy for children with severe burn injury. *Music Therapy Perspectives, 15*(1), 21–26.

Edwards, J. (1999). Anxiety management in pediatric music therapy. In C. Dileo (Ed.), *Music therapy and medicine: Theoretical and clinical approaches* (pp. 69–76). Silver Spring, MD: American Music Therapy Association.

Edwards, J. (2005). A reflection on the music therapist's role in developing a program in a children's hospital. *Music Therapy Perspectives, 23,* 36–44.

Fratianne, R. B., Prensner, J. D., Hutson, M. J., Super, D. M., Yowler, C. J., & Standley, J. M. (2001). The effect of music-based imagery and music alternative engagement on the burn debridement process. *Journal of Burn Care and Rehabilitation, 22*(1), 47–53.

Ilechukwu, S. T. (2002). Psychiatry of the medically ill in the burn unit. *The Psychiatric Clinics of North America, 25*(1), 129–147.

Magee, W. L., Bertolami, M., Kubicek, L., LaJoie, M., Martino, L., Sankowski, A., Townsend, J., Whitehead-Pleaux, A.M., & Zigo, J. (2011). Using music technology in music therapy with populations across the life span in medical and educational programs. *Music and Medicine, 3*(3), 146–153.

Muller, M., Gahankari, D., & Herndon, D. N. (2007). Operative wound management. In D. Herndon (Ed.), *Total burn care* (3rd ed., pp. 177–195). Philadelphia: Saunders Elsevier.

Neugebauer, C. T. (2008). Pediatric burn recovery: Acute care, rehabilitation, and reconstruction. In D. Hanson-Abromeit & C. Colwell (Eds.), *Medical music therapy for pediatrics in hospital settings: Using music to support medical interventions* (pp. 195–230). Silver Spring, MD: American Music Therapy Association.

Neugebauer, C. T., & Neugebauer, V. (2003). Music therapy in pediatric burn care. In S. L. Robb (Ed.), *Music therapy in pediatric healthcare: Research and evidence-based practice* (pp. 31–48). Silver Spring, MD: American Music Therapy Association.

Pham, T. N., Gibran, N. S., & Heimbach, D. M. (2007). Evaluation of the burn wound: Management decisions. In D. M. Herndon (Ed.), *Total burn care* (3rd ed., pp. 119–126). Philadelphia: Saunders Elsevier.

Prensner, J. D., Yowler, C. J., Smith, L. F., Steele, A. L., & Fratianne, R. B. (2001). Music therapy for assistance with pain and anxiety management in burn treatment. *The Journal of Burn Care Rehabilitation*. Retrieved from http://www.ncbi.nlm.nih.gov/pubmed/11227691

Robb, S., Rutan, R., Bishop, B., & Parker, J. (1995). The effects of music-assisted relaxation on preoperative anxiety. *Journal of Music Therapy, 32*(1), 2–21.

Sheridan, R. (2012). *Burns: A Practical approach*. London: Mason Publishing.

Tan, X., Yowler, C. J., Super, D. M., & Fratianne, R. B. (2010). The efficacy of music therapy protocols for decreasing pain, anxiety, and muscle tension levels during burn dressing changes: A prospective randomized crossover trial. *Journal of burn care & research, 31*(4), 590–597. DOI:10.1097/BCR.0b013e3181e4d71b.

Whitehead-Pleaux, A. (2009). Ismaee il musika—listen to the music. *Voices, 9*(3). Retrieved from http://www.voices.no/mainissues/mi4000999049.php

Whitehead-Pleaux, A., Baryza, M. J., & Sheridan, R. (2006). The effects of music therapy on pediatric pain and anxiety during a donor site dressing change. *Journal of Music Therapy, 43*(2), 136–153.

Whitehead-Pleaux, A., Baryza, M. J., & Sheridan, R. (2009). Exploring the effects of music therapy on pediatric pain: Phase 2. *Journal of Burn Care and Rehabilitation, 30*(2), s81.

Whitehead-Pleaux, A., & Clark, S. (2009, November). *Changing Keys: Moving from Ethnocentrism to Multiculturalism*. American Music Therapy Association Conference, San Diego, CA.

Whitehead-Pleaux, A., Clark, S. L., & Spall, L. (2011). Indications and counter-indications of music technology in a pediatric medical setting. *Music and Medicine, 3*(3), 154–162.

Whitehead-Pleaux, A., & Spall, L. (in press). Innovations in medical music therapy: The use of electronic music technologies in a pediatric burn hospital. In W. Magee (Ed.), *Music technology in health settings*. Philadelphia, PA: Jessica Kingsley.

Whitehead-Pleaux, A. M., Zebrowski, N., Baryza, M. J., & Sheridan, R. (2007). Exploring the effects of music therapy on pediatric pain: Phase 1. *Journal of Music Therapy, 44*(3), 217–241.

Chapter 8

Children with Cancer

Beth Dun

INTRODUCTION

Children with cancer and their families talk about the experience of being diagnosed and treated for cancer as a "roller-coaster ride." A diagnosis of cancer usually denotes the start of a long and uncertain journey with many stages. The experience of the journey varies for each individual child and their family, and is dependent on a wide variety of variables. There are many aspects to the treatment of cancer for children and adolescents, and the application of music therapy with this population is required to be flexible and varied (Dun, 2007).

DIAGNOSTIC INFORMATION

Children's cancers are rare. Cancer incidence among children and adolescents is a small fraction— about 2% of all cancer cases in the US (Kline, 2008). Due to significant developments in treatment over the last few decades, the cure rates and *remission* rates for childhood cancer have improved (Stewart, 2003). Overall, survival is now estimated at 80%, although survival rates vary according to the type of cancer (Kline, 2008). The types of cancers that occur in children vary greatly from those seen in adults, and while any cancer in a child is considered very serious, it is worth noting that cure rates for children's cancers are higher than those for adults.

Types of Childhood Cancer

Each type of cancer has its own name, treatment, and prognosis. Cancer in children can be generally divided into leukemias, lymphomas, and solid tumors such as brain tumors or tumors of the other organs and tissues in the body (Murphy, 2011).

   Leukemia. Leukemia is a cancer of the early blood-forming cells. Most often, leukemia is a cancer of the white blood cells, but some leukemias start in other blood cell types. Leukemia is often described as being either acute (growing quickly) or chronic (growing slowly); almost all childhood leukemia is acute. Leukemia starts in the bone marrow or the soft inner part of certain bones, where new blood cells are made. In most cases, the leukemia invades the blood fairly quickly. From there it can spread to other parts of the body such as the lymph nodes, spleen, liver, central nervous system (i.e., the brain and spinal cord), testicles, or other organs (Kline, 2008).

   There are two main types of acute leukemia. Acute lymphocytic (lymphoblastic) leukemia (ALL) is the most common form of childhood leukemia. This leukemia starts in the bone marrow from the lymphoid cells, also known as lymphocytes, which are a type of white blood cells (Kline, 2008). Acute myelogenous leukemia (AML) is a less common form of childhood leukemia. This type of leukemia, also called acute myeloid leukemia, acute myelocytic leukemia, or acute non-lymphocytic leukemia (ANLL), starts from the myeloid cells that form white blood cells (other than lymphocytes), red blood cells, or platelets (Kline, 2008).

Lymphoma. Lymphoma is a tumor of the lymphatic tissue. This tissue can be found throughout the body, and is an important part of the body's immune system. The two most common lymphomas in children are Hodgkin's disease and non-Hodgkin's lymphoma. Hodgkin's disease often presents as swollen lymph glands of the neck or upper body. There are two common types of non-Hodgkin's lymphoma (NHL). B-cell NHL usually involves the lymph nodes of the head, neck, and throat, or abdomen; T-cell NHL affects lymph nodes in the chest (Kline, 2008).

Solid tumors. Solid tumors occurring in children present as an abnormal mass of tissue that usually does not contain cysts or liquid areas. Solid tumors may be benign. Different types of solid tumors are named for the organ or type of cells that form them. The more common types of solid tumors in children include blastomas and sarcomas.

Blastoma is commonly used as part of the name for a tumor, as in glioblastoma and medulloblastoma (types of brain tumors), hepatoblastoma (a liver tumor), nephroblastoma (a Wilms tumor of the kidney), neuroblastoma (a childhood tumor of neural origin), osteoblastoma (a bone tumor), and retinoblastoma (a tumor of the retina in the eye).

Sarcomas are solid tumors that are formed from young cells that normally become bone, muscle, and other soft tissues, such as ligaments and joints. Sarcomas begin when a change or mutation occurs in one of these young cells, allowing the cell to grow uncontrollably and form cancerous tumors. There are many types of sarcomas that occur during childhood, including rhabdomyosarcoma (cancer of the muscle cells) and osteosarcoma and Ewing sarcomas (both cancer of the bone). About 12 in every 100 children with cancer have a sarcoma (Murphy, 2011).

Brain tumors. A brain tumor is the most common type of solid tumor in children and is characterized by the growth of abnormal cells in the tissues of the brain. Brain tumors can be benign (noncancerous) or malignant (cancerous). Although brain tumors rarely spread to other parts of the body, most of them can spread through the brain tissue. Even so-called benign tumors can, as they grow, press on or invade normal brain tissues, causing damage that is often disabling and can sometimes cause death. The major differences between benign and malignant brain tumors are how readily they spread through the rest of the brain and whether they can be removed and not come back. But both types can potentially be life-threatening. Brain tumors are different in adults and children. They often form in different places, develop from different cell types, and may have a different treatment and prognosis (Kline, 2008). Even though survival rates for some childhood brain tumors have increased over the past 30 years, survivors often suffer lifelong side effects from treatments such as surgery, radiation, and chemotherapy (Taylor et al., 2007).

Cancer Treatments

The type of cancer treatment depends on the type and severity of cancer and the child's age. Treatment of childhood cancer can include chemotherapy, radiotherapy, and surgery. Typically, these take place in a center that specializes in treating childhood cancers. Once a child's diagnosis is confirmed, a protocol or treatment plan is decided by the oncology doctors. The protocol is a "recipe" of treatment which determines the doses and the timing of drugs and other treatments and is often divided into blocks, phases, or cycles.

Chemotherapy. Chemotherapy is the term given to the treatment of cancer using strong drugs called cytotoxics (i.e., cell poisons). These drugs injure or kill cancer cells but will also affect some normal cells and can cause side effects. Chemotherapy can be given in many ways. In children, it is usually given by tablets or by injection into the blood, tissue, or spinal fluid. The drugs enter the bloodstream and work to kill cancer in parts of the body to which the cancer has spread. The duration of chemotherapy treatment and the type of drugs used depend on the type of cancer the child has and his response to the drugs. Chemotherapy is often given in cycles. A cycle is a period of chemotherapy treatment followed by a period of rest. The rest period allows time for the body to build healthy new cells before the next treatment. Every child's treatment cycle differs, so a child may receive daily, weekly, or monthly chemotherapy treatments (Murphy, 2011).

Phases of chemotherapy treatment. The goal of the first phase of treatment is to kill the leukemia cells in the blood and bone marrow. This puts the leukemia into remission. This is also called the remission induction phase. The second phase is consolidation, which begins once the leukemia is in remission. The goal of consolidation/intensification therapy is to kill any remaining leukemia cells that may not be active but could begin to regrow and cause a relapse. Maintenance is the third phase of treatment. The goal in this phase is to kill any remaining leukemia cells that may regrow and cause a relapse. Often the cancer treatments are given in lower doses than those used for induction and consolidation/intensification therapy. This is also called the continuation therapy phase (Kline, 2008).

Chemotherapy side effects. Many of the drugs used in chemotherapy carry the risk of both short-term and long-term problems. Short-term side effects include nausea, vomiting, fatigue, anemia, hair loss, abnormal bleeding, and kidney damage. Longer-term effects can include infertility, growth problems, organ damage, or increased risk of other cancers. Other medications may be prescribed to counteract as many of the side effects as possible (Kline, 2008). Chemotherapy can suppress the immune system, leaving children at risk of contracting infections. These immune-suppressed children may be placed in isolation in their rooms and need to stay away from crowds until their immune function improves (Ghetti & Walker, 2009; Walker, 2008; Walker, 2009). However, at other times during treatment, the child usually manages normal routines and may go back to child care, school, or preschool.

Radiotherapy. Radiotherapy is a treatment using exact, carefully measured doses of high-energy radiation. It is painless and similar to having an X-ray taken. The radiation rays penetrate deep within the body and are able to destroy abnormal tumor cells and prevent them from reforming. Radiotherapy is used alone, or in combination with chemotherapy or surgery. Pediatric patients who require radiotherapy will usually receive radiation therapy treatment each day for five days a week over a period of four to six weeks (Kline, 2008).

Before radiation therapy treatment commences, patients undergo a stage of planning and simulation so that the exact target area of the cells to receive the radiation can be established and immobilization devices can be constructed. Radiation therapy requires a fixed patient position for daily treatment and, therefore, requires the use of individualized devices such as casts for immobilizing the patient, molds for stabilization, and shields for protection of normal tissue regions from radiation exposure (Barry, O'Callaghan, Wheeler, & Grocke, 2007). Radiation treatment is rarely given to children less than three years of age because of the significant effects of radiotherapy on an infant's developing brain. Children less than three years of age will usually instead receive high-dose chemotherapy immediately following surgery, with the aim to delay or avoid the need for radiation treatment (Kline, 2008).

Surgery. Treatment for childhood solid tumors usually begins with surgery, where all attempts are made at achieving complete removal of the tumor, with minimal harm to the surrounding tissue. Following surgery for most but not all tumors, treatment usually consists of chemotherapy and/or radiotherapy. This is often necessary to kill the microscopic tumor cells that may remain after surgery (Murphy, 2011).

Different types of surgery are used to treat cancer. Primary surgery removes all or most of the tumor at the time of diagnosis. Second-look surgery is sometimes performed after treatment with chemotherapy and/or *radiation* to see how well treatments have worked in killing the cancer cells, and any remaining tumor may be removed. Supportive care surgery is done to help the child through their cancer treatment. Most children have a *central venous line* (catheter) placed to make it easier to deliver *intravenous* fluid and medicine as well as draw blood for testing. Often treatment makes it difficult for the child to eat, so a feeding tube may be placed in the child's stomach or digestive tract until they are able to take enough nutrition by mouth (Murphy, 2011).

*Hematopoietic Stem Cell Transplant (*HSCT). Children with certain types of cancer may receive a hematopoietic stem cell transplant (commonly referred to as a bone marrow transplant). This is a procedure carried out to replace defective bone marrow stem cells with healthy cells. Bone marrow is a spongy tissue inside certain bones of the body that produces blood cells. If a child has a type of cancer that affects the function of blood cells, an HSCT (in conjunction with chemotherapy to kill the defective cells) may allow new, healthy cells to grow. An HSCT may also be used to treat cancer that does not involve blood cells because it allows higher doses of chemotherapy to be used than would otherwise be tolerated (Murphy, 2011). Over the past 20 years, HSCTs have become established procedures for treating children with a range of cancers and other conditions (Hirst, 2009a).

There are different types of HSCTs. An Autologous HSCT is a type of transplant only used for children with solid tumors such as brain tumors and neuroblastomas. The child's own stem cells are collected prior to the child being given high-dose chemotherapy, after which the stem cells are reinfused to facilitate recovery. An Allogeneic stem cell transplant I is a type of transplant undertaken for children with a range of conditions in which the child's bone marrow is affected. This includes leukemias, bone marrow failure, and a range of genetic and immunological conditions. An Allogeneic HSCT requires identifying a related or unrelated donor who is an acceptable match with the recipient. Donors may be matched siblings, other partially matched relatives, unrelated marrow donors, or unrelated umbilical cord bloods. The unrelated donors and cord bloods are identified through national or international bone marrow registries or cord blood banks (Hirst, 2009a). Allogeneic HSCT requires a conditioning course of therapy which may include chemotherapy, radiation therapy, or a combination thereof. This conditioning is aimed at suppressing the child's bone marrow and immune system in order to allow engraftment of the donor cells. Numerous complications from this treatment may need to be addressed, including Graft vs. Host Disease (GVHD), infection, mucositis, and gastrointestinal issues.

An HSCT is a particularly aggressive treatment. The aim is to kill all the cancer cells, but in the process the immune system is destroyed. Therefore, immediately after the transplant, there is an acute treatment phase where the child must be placed in sterilized isolation for one to three months, given antibiotics in anticipation of infection, and receive blood transfusions because the chemotherapy has attacked not only the white blood cells but also platelets and red blood cells (Hirst, 2009a).

Other procedures. Children diagnosed with cancer experience repeated invasive and possibly distressing medical procedures. These include chemotherapy by venipuncture, line access, lumbar punctures, biopsies, audiograms, blood cultures, bone marrow aspirate, bone scan, CT Scan, echocardiogram, electrocardiogram, gallium scan, glomerular filtration rate (GFR), magnetic resonance imaging (MRI) scan, PET scan, ultrasound scan, X-ray, central line, insuflon and nasogastric insertions.

Treatment-related pain is experienced by about 50% of patients in pediatric oncology care, whereas disease-related pain is reported by only 25% of pediatric oncology patients (Blount et al., 2006). Pain associated with medical procedures is often viewed as one of the worst experiences in children with cancer (Hedstrom, Haglund, Skolin, & von Essen, 2003). Pain and distress does not necessarily decrease with repeated procedures and may worsen if pain is not adequately managed (Hockenberry, 1988).

Regular lumbar punctures and bone marrow aspirates are important in the successful management of patients with leukemia and lymphoma. These procedures are usually the most painful and distressing procedures associated with cancer treatment (Jacob et al., 2007). As children do not habituate to these painful procedures, deep sedation or general anesthesia is often used for lumbar punctures and bone marrow aspirates. Sedation is often used to promote cooperation and to reduce anxiety during these procedures, and multiple procedures can be performed under the same anesthetic (Barnes et al., 2002). However, some children can undergo these procedures without sedation. These are usually children who can lie exceptionally still for the procedures and have successful coping management strategies in place.

For more information related to pain perception, pain theories, and pain management, please consult Chapter 2 in this book.

Hematology

The focus of this chapter is primarily related to pediatric cancers. However, in some hospitals, children with hematological conditions are treated in the same unit as those with cancer; therefore, definitions of some hematological conditions will be outlined here.

Hematology is concerned with the study, diagnosis, and treatment of diseases of the blood while oncology refers to the study, diagnosis, and treatment of cancer. These include children with conditions such as sickle cell disease, aplastic anemia, and hemophilia.

Sickle cell anemia is the most common form of sickle cell disease (SCD). SCD is a serious disorder in which the body makes sickle shaped red blood cells. "Sickle shaped" means that the red blood cells are shaped like a crescent. Normal red blood cells are disc-shaped and move easily through blood vessels. These cells contain an iron-rich protein called hemoglobin which carries oxygen from the lungs to the rest of the body. Sickle cells contain abnormal hemoglobin called sickle hemoglobin or hemoglobin S. Sickle hemoglobin causes the cells to develop a sickle, or crescent, shape. Sickle cells are stiff and sticky. They tend to block blood flow in the blood vessels of the limbs and organs. Blocked blood flow can cause pain and organ damage and increase the risk of infection (Baggott, 2011).

Aplastic anemia is a type of anemia. The term "anemia" usually refers to a condition in which the blood has a lower-than-normal number of red blood cells. Anemia also can occur if the red blood cells don't contain enough hemoglobin. In people who have aplastic anemia, the body doesn't make enough red blood cells, white blood cells, and platelets. This is because the bone marrow's stem cells are damaged (Baggott, 2011).

Hemophilia is an inherited medical condition where the blood does not clot properly due to a lack of a protein in the blood called a "clotting factor" that works with platelets to stop bleeding at the site of an injury. People with hemophilia tend to bleed for longer periods of time after an injury, and they are more susceptible to internal bleeding (Kline, 2008).

NEEDS AND RESOURCES

A diagnosis of cancer usually heralds the start of a long and uncertain journey with many stages. There is the initial stage of diagnosis, usually followed by a period of treatment, which, depending on the diagnosis, could be short and intense or long and complex, leading to the end of treatment, and the extended long-term follow-up stage. Along the way, there may be significant turns of events that impact and change the direction of the journey. The experience of individual children and their families at each stage is different and dependent on a number of variables, including age, developmental level, specific diagnosis and responses to treatment, and cultural and /or psychosocial issues that pre-existed prior to diagnosis.

Treatment

A child diagnosed with cancer is confronted with a multitude of stresses and challenges, not least of which is coming to terms with and understanding the ramifications of treatment. Young children, particularly, may have difficulty understanding the diagnosis, adjusting to treatment and side effects, and coping with unfamiliar medical procedures and separation from normal routines (Hadley, 1996). An adolescent, who is already going through a challenging period of uncertainty and physiological and psychological changes, often finds the diagnosis of cancer overwhelming (Abad, 2003).

Initial hospitalization can be tense and confusing for both the child and the family. Children who are admitted to the oncology unit for the first time are often bewildered, confused, and/or frightened (Dun, 1999). Parents coming to terms with the impact of diagnosis may feel overwhelmed and unable to provide the full support needed for their child (Robb, 2003b). A small subset of families has pre-existing vulnerabilities or difficulties that may be aggravated by the diagnosis of cancer, resulting in increased risk for clinically significant levels of distress and deterioration of functioning (Kazak et al., 2007). These can include marriage difficulties, unemployment, and/or mental illness.

In the initial stage, the needs of the child and adolescent include reduction of anxiety and adjustment to diagnosis and the hospital environment. Parents also need support in managing their own anxiety and strategies to help them deal/cope with their child's anxiety. At this point, families are faced with many uncertainties of what may lie ahead for their child, including, realistically or not, a fear of death.

As treatment commences, often beginning with a hospital admission, the child and family are confronted with a strange and unfamiliar environment over which they have very little control. Hospital environments often limit children's freedom to make choices about daily activities, sleep and meal schedules, visitors, and medical treatment (Robb, 2003). Responses to treatment and hospitalization vary widely across the age span. Infants, for example, may experience attachment issues and delays in development. In addition, they may need constant attention to keep them from pulling out tubes and other medical equipment (Ghetti & Walker, 2009). Toddlers who have just begun to walk and are developing some independence and do not have the comprehension to understand what is happening may find it frustrating to be restricted by being attached to an intravenous line and may be fearful of hospital staff. Preschoolers may also be fearful of hospital staff and procedures and, due to their developing yet still imprecise ability to verbally communicate, may become irritable. The lack of routine is a source of stress for all younger age groups in particular (Ghetti & Walker, 2009). School-age children may be concerned with appearing different because of their hair loss or other effects of illness or medication and may miss family, school friends, and normal situations of everyday life. Adolescents, for whom peer acceptance and body image are significant issues, may find the impact and side effects of treatment, such as loss of hair and the inability to engage in normal social activities with their peers, distressing. In addition, this is a time of establishing their independence and identity, and cancer treatment increases their dependence on parents (Abad, 2003; Kennelly, 2001; Ledger, 2001). For children and adolescents of any age, regression to behaviors of a younger age or difficult behavior as a reaction to the stress of hospitalization may occur.

For the family, as the treatment protocol begins, it generally results in a change in lifestyle, family roles, and responsibilities (Hadley, 1996). Families report that initially they are completely consumed by their sick children. Life revolves around treatment regimens, hospital admissions and appointments, and caring for their child, while other aspects of life fade into the background (Degraves & Aranda, 2008). Family difficulties may arise at this time due to the time and attention a child with a severe illness may receive. For example, siblings and spouses may feel jealous or excluded. Adults often try to protect children by not communicating with them about the illness, leaving the child in need of emotional support that may or may not be available from medical staff (Robb, 2003). Kupst (1992) found that children's ability to cope with the stresses of the disease was significantly related to the adequacy of the parents' coping.

Allogeneic transplant (HSCT) is a specialized treatment and has its own cluster of effects on children of all ages. During transplant, the child spends time in an isolation room where everyone who enters the room must wear a gown and mask. The child is not allowed out of the room, and visitors are restricted. The room is environmentally controlled and therefore sensory-limited, and there is separation from normal life experiences. The child does not have his own physical or psychological space, and movement is inhibited.

Children who are hospitalized for lengthy periods after their transplantation may experience delay and regression in reaching developmental milestones. Physical impairment from pain, medications, and poor nutrition may lead to an inability to process information and a greater amount of uncertainty (Degraves & Aranda, 2008). The psychosocial impact of an HSCT can be significant on the child, the parents, siblings, and other family relatives and can have a long-term impact on children and families. The highest levels of parental stress are reported both in the pre-transplant period and during the acute phase immediately after the transplant, although for some parents stress levels remain high for an extended period. Those parents who display the greatest anxiety during the acute phase are most at risk of higher stress in the longer term (Hirst, 2009a).

Children and adolescents in the acute treatment stage need interventions that diminish the negative effects of hospitalization, provide supportive environments that encourage normalization, and focus on the pre-existing "healthy" aspects of self. They need creative and age-appropriate opportunities to help to maintain or attain developmental milestones. The need to manage anxiety continues in this stage, often in relation to managing pain and procedures. Social and emotional needs may arise from having a life-threatening illness, including the need to manage depression and opportunities for self-expression. Some may see other patients who have become their friends at the hospital decline in health and, sometimes, die (Robb, 2003b). Long-term patients who have been bedbound for an extended period and have weakened muscles, or children recovering from brain tumor removal, may need rehabilitation. For more information related to rehabilitation, please consult Chapter 10 in this book.

Most adolescents place greater emphasis on the immediate demands of the present than on future concerns such as good health or death. This can result in compliance to treatment regimens being challenging for adolescents, especially if it results in loss of autonomy, and particularly when the possibility of death is less prominent for the young person than for their parents or health professionals (Thomas et al., 2006).

The ability to develop coping strategies is a significant aspect of the adjustment to hospitalization for a serious illness, such as cancer. A motivational theory of coping, developed by Skinner and Wellborn (1994), offers a theoretical framework for examining how unique characteristics of children and their environment interact during times of stress (Robb, 2003). According to this theory of coping, children who remain engaged with their environment generally cope with stress in an active, flexible, and positive manner. Therefore, there is a need for clinical interventions that promote active engagement and encourage independence.

Establishing some sense of normality has been reported as helping families manage the everyday ups and downs of their child's condition (Degraves & Aranda, 2008). Once a child and their family become accustomed to the routines and settings of treatment, initial feelings of not understanding, not knowing what will happen when, and not being sure of what things mean gradually give way to a sense of life as ordinary and cancer and its treatment as routine (Stewart, 2003). Over the past 20 years, studies have indicated that most families with a child with cancer are competent and able to cope and adjust well over time despite initial or recurrent periods of extreme distress (Kazak et al., 2007).

Significant and Unexpected Events

Treatment for childhood cancer is unpredictable, and there can be unanticipated events, symptoms that are not easily interpreted, and reminders of the life threat inherent in a cancer diagnosis (Stewart, 2003). The peak and trough–like trajectory of childhood cancer means that patients can be close to death at times and, at others, healthy and responding well to treatment. Significant turns of events may happen along the way, including unexpected and unplanned hospital admissions for infections, other illnesses, relapse, or because of unsuccessful treatment. Severe reactions to treatment may mean the child is admitted to the Intensive Care Unit (ICU) in a serious condition for some time, and may take a long time to recover, possibly requiring rehabilitation. Any or all of these events can challenge the family's coping, especially if they had been progressing well. During these unexpected events, extra support that is individually tailored is usually needed.

One of the uncertainties with which families are faced is the threat of treatment failure or recurrence. Relapse is experienced as a constant interchange between hope and fear in the context of uncertainty. Research shows relapse to be more distressing than diagnosis because of the increased awareness of the threat of death and greater doubt surrounding the child's ultimate survival (Degraves & Aranda, 2008). When a child relapses, families manage the tensions between the states of fear of death, and the desire to remain positive and hopeful. However, the difference between relapse and diagnosis is that at relapse, families often specifically express a desire for cancer not to control their lives. Two main coping strategies have been found to help families to achieve this: "maintaining normality" and "living in the moment" (Degraves & Aranda, 2008).

End of Treatment

The outcome for any individual child is unpredictable and can include cure, relapse, sustained remission, long-term toxicities, or death from the illness or treatment. The improvement in outcome for most, but not all, children with cancer has thus created a powerful paradox of increased optimism accompanied by uncertainty (Stewart, 2003). This uncertainty continues on even after treatment is completed.

After prolonged absences from school life and other social and physical activities, children and adolescents may have difficulty adjusting to a normal life. This is not only because of school absence but also because healthy peers commonly find it hard to empathize with the experiences of young people as patients. Other delayed and long-term effects of chemotherapy and treatments include sterilization, sexual issues, reduced capabilities (e.g., limb loss), reliance on others, and low self-esteem (McCaffrey, 2006).

While long-term effects may follow for any child treated for cancer, there is strong evidence that bone marrow transplant places the child at higher risk of a wide range of long-term effects. These may include physical, psychosocial, developmental, and cognitive problems, some of which may appear many years after the transplant.

Multicultural Issues

Attending to the needs of children and adolescents with cancer and their families from culturally and linguistically diverse backgrounds (CALD) may be challenging to health care professionals. Behaviors based on cultural beliefs and values become more obvious as people draw on their cultural values in order to conceptualize and explain the illness (Munet-Vilaro, 2004). The family's cultural context may directly influence how they define and manage their child's cancer. Knowing and being aware of this dynamic can guide health professionals in delivering holistic, culturally competent care (Thibodeaux & Deatrick, 2007).

Differences exist in cultural attitudes toward the disclosure of a cancer diagnosis to patients. In countries such as the USA, universal disclosure is practiced, but in countries such as Italy, Egypt, and Japan, being truthful about a patient's diagnosis is seen by many as a cruel and untactful act (Navon, 1999). A study by Martinson and colleagues (1994, as cited in Thibodeaux & Deatrick, 2007) found that in China there was a belief that bad news or sadness should not be discussed with children or extended family. Understanding such cultural beliefs and family structures may help health professionals provide culturally competent interventions to address fear, anxiety, and support concerns (Thibodeaux & Deatrick, 2007). Furthermore, there has been some research which shows that in certain communities, no words for "cancer" exist, while in others, uttering any "bad words" is believed to negatively affect patient outcomes (Levy, 1997, as cited in Surbone, 2008). With Greek parents of children with cancer, Patistea and colleagues (2000, as cited in Munet-Vilaro, 2004) found that communication between parents and the healthy siblings was a difficult process during the diagnostic stage of a child with cancer. Parents were not amenable to establishing an open communication pattern with the healthy siblings and wanted to be the ones deciding the content and amount of information disclosed. The stigma associated with cancer for families from some cultural groups may result in a level of secrecy about the child's illness and increasing isolation of the family within their own community.

The level of interaction that other staff (e.g., allied health providers) may have with the CALD child or their family may be dependent on a variety of factors. For example, given that "music is a common language," the music therapists may be able to engage CALD children quite readily in music therapy sessions. For other providers, language differences and limited resources available in other languages to support general and specific conversations create significant barriers to working with CALD families. While therapies such as art and music therapy are "universal languages," a lack of understanding of the therapeutic role (rather than as play/entertainment) of these approaches may mean that some CALD families reject services, particularly when children are very ill (Hirst, 2009b).

REFERRAL AND ASSESSMENT

Referral Procedures

Referrals for music therapy may come from a variety of professionals involved in the multidisciplinary care of the pediatric cancer patient. Referral processes differ depending on the facility, and in some settings, music therapy services can only be obtained through a physician's order (Ghetti & Walker, 2009). Referrals may consist of a completed written form that is forwarded to the music therapist, a referral note entered in a patient's chart, or an emailed, online, or verbal referral (Ghetti & Walker, 2009). In some centers, self-referrals are possible from patients and their families. This can be important for reinstating the children's and families' choice and control over their lives (O'Neill & Pavlicevic, 2003).

Assessment Procedures

A careful and thorough assessment process can help the music therapist identify the needs of the child, develop rapport, and identify positive coping strategies (Lane, 1996). Through assessment, the music therapist ascertains musical preferences and experiences and determines appropriate goals and techniques, in order to develop the most appropriate music therapy program (Ledger, 2001).

Assessment tools. Music therapists working in this area use many different strategies for assessment. Ghetti & Walker (2009) emphasize that a variety of sources should contribute to the assessment of children with cancer in medical settings. They recommend that music therapists employ "a combination of methods, including observation of patient and family during both the presence and absence of musical interaction, chart review to assess medical and social history and treatment progress, and patient and/or family interview. Due to variation in patient health status depending on treatment phase and response to treatment, frequent reassessment of patient needs and strengths will be required to assure appropriate goal and intervention planning" (p. 159).

Assessment domains. Several areas of assessment are specific to children being treated for cancer. These areas are outlined below.

1) Diagnosis information: specific diagnosis, time since initial diagnosis, any relapses, and whether the patient is in remission.

2) Patient's treatment protocol: documents the type of treatment the child is receiving, including surgery, chemotherapy, and radiotherapy.

3) Treatment phase: whether the child has commenced treatment, and if so, at what phase he is in his treatment.

4) Treatment side effects: Side effects that a child may be experiencing or has experienced in the past which may impact on participation in music therapy sessions should be noted. These may include mucositus, sore throat, nausea, vomiting, diarrhea, constipation, hair loss, tender skin at the radiation site, and possible side effects from medications that may influence compliance or attention (such as side effects from steroids).

5) Specific physical and environmental requirements/special precautions: Any physical and environmental precautions, including infection control precautions, should be noted. It is important to note if the child must remain in isolation and/or immobilized in bed (e.g., post–spinal surgery for a removal of spinal tumor) and observe any medical equipment precautions.

6) Pain and anxiety: Levels of pain and anxiety are regularly assessed. The reader should consult Chapter 2 for guidelines regarding pain assessment.

7) Current coping strategies: Coping strategies displayed by the child and the family are important to record in the assessment, including attitude toward medical procedures. It is useful to identify both positive and negative coping tendencies to serve as a baseline against which adaptive strategies developed during the course of music therapy interventions may be compared (Ghetti & Walker, 2009). Main support networks for the child, as well as their current availability, should be appraised.

8) Functioning in psychological, cognitive, physical, communicative and social domains: As with any hospitalized child, the level of functioning in these domains needs to be taken into account. This includes any developmental delays or disabilities, and hearing and visual impairments (Douglass, 2006). The chapter on general pediatric inpatients in this book expands upon this assessment need.

9) Patient's music history, preferences, and responses to music: This includes instruments learned, music experienced at school or preschool, and any likes or dislikes of certain music or types of music, including any preferences for specific bands.

10) Specific cultural and linguistic needs: This includes identification of their first language spoken at home and an assessment of their English language skills.

INTRODUCTION TO MUSIC THERAPY METHODS

Music therapy with this population needs to be flexible to take into account the child's current condition, energy, and needs, which vary across the course of treatment (Dun, 2007, 2011). Music therapists working with this population will be aware of the importance of following infection control precautions, which include strict hand hygiene protocols.

An overview of music therapy methods and procedures included in this chapter is listed below.

Receptive Music Therapy

- Music Listening for Relaxation: the use of familiar live or prerecorded music to settle and calm a child who may be stressed or fearful of going to sleep.
- Music-Assisted Imagery: the use of music-assisted imagery in actively engaging the child who may be too weak to actively participate in music-making, to aid relaxation, reduce anxiety, and facilitate self-expression.
- Music for Stimulation and Comfort: the use of familiar songs to offer gentle stimulation and comfort for children who are unable to actively or physically participate.
- Song Lyric Discussion: playing a favorite song and inviting the adolescent to reflect on the lyrical content of the song with the option of discussion about feelings around his diagnosis, hospitalization, and treatment.

Improvisational Music Therapy

- Dramatic Play Free-Flowing Improvisation: the use of dramatic play in combination with interactive improvisation to help the child extend the boundaries of his restricted environment, explore feelings, and make sense of the world and what is happening to him.
- Instrumental Improvisation: the use of instrumental improvisation to facilitate nonverbal expression of emotions, musical interaction with family and/or music therapist, and a sense of control and mastery.
- Song Improvisation: the use of the element of lyrics added to improvisation to become aware of, explore, and express thoughts and feelings.

Re-creative Music Therapy

- Group Music-Making for Normalization: the use of regularly scheduled music therapy groups in the cancer unit to enhance normalization and offer opportunities for socialization for cancer patients and their families.
- Instrumental Instruction: teaching a child to play an instrument to stimulate cognitive development, enhance mastery and empowerment, and facilitate self-expression.

Compositional Music Therapy

- Songwriting: the use of a variety of songwriting formats to offer the child opportunities for expression and communication of thoughts and feelings.

- Music Artifacts: the creation of music artifacts such as CDs, videos, or other recordings of the child to assist in decreasing anxiety and increasing positive coping while also creating mementos for family members.

GUIDELINES FOR RECEPTIVE MUSIC THERAPY

The use of receptive music therapy can be planned as a segment of a music therapy session or as an entire session (Grocke & Wigram, 2007). A receptive experience could be spontaneously offered if the child is tense or showing signs of being agitated, distressed, worried, or having difficulties sleeping.

Regardless of whether the receptive experience takes place as an entire session or part of one, it is important to prepare the space as much as possible. The music therapist reduces stimulation; turns off or turns down lights; turns off any sound devices, such as television, radio, and music players; closes doors; draw curtains if possible; and limits any interruptions where possible. After the music therapist has confirmed that the child is comfortable, she positions herself in a comfortable position.

Music Listening for Relaxation

Overview. Young children who have difficulty settling may find it easier to relax by having live familiar music played to them in a way that initially matches their mood and energy (Sahler et al., 2003), followed by less engaging music that gradually becomes slower in tempo, with more consistent dynamics, accompaniment style, and key. The main goal is to settle and calm a child who may be stressed or fearful of going to sleep. It could also be helpful to reduce pain, reduce distress prior to procedures, regulate breathing, provide mental escape from the hospital environment, and reduce anxiety (Grocke & Wigram, 2007).

What to observe. Initially, the music therapist will observe the child's energy levels and mood, make sure the child continues to be comfortable and settled, and, as the experience progresses, will keep monitoring the child, looking for changes in body language that might indicate the child is not comfortable or unsettled, and check in with the child about whether he is okay. The music therapist will observe breathing patterns and body movement to adjust singing and accompaniment when necessary to calm and settle.

Procedures. Once the child is in a comfortable position, the music therapist sings a quiet, engaging song to attract the child's attention away from any stressful thoughts or feelings. This song will be engaging but also quiet enough not to excite the child too much. The quality of voice, pitch, and tempo of the song will engender a sense of safety: A high voice might convey sense of insecurity or inexperience; a low voice might sound too gruff (Grocke & Wigram, 2007). The music is not fast, though if a child is anxious and wriggling, it may need to start at a faster pace to match the energy level of the child, and then gradually slow down. The music therapist will encourage the child to focus on his breathing by asking the child to breathe in and out with the music, making sure the rhythm of the music initially matches the child's breathing, and then will incrementally slow down the tempo, continuing to maintain a steady rhythm (Sahler et al., 2003). The music therapist may use improvised music or song, or a familiar song, depending on the age of the child. Helping a child to regulate his breathing is an important strategy for managing pain or anxiety. Often the breathing is shallow, and sometimes the child instinctively holds his breath when in pain (Snyder Cowan, 1997). Maintaining a regulated breathing pattern that encourages the releasing of held breath will assist in managing pain and anxiety (Grocke & Wigram, 2007). The following example demonstrates the application of the intervention with a two-year-old with Acute Lymphocytic Leukemia.

Sally had had a long hospital admission due to complications related to treatment. Her mother was an anxious person who often appeared overwhelmed with the situation for her only child and sometimes had difficulty providing the emotional support that was needed for Sally. The mother stated to the music therapist that Sally had difficulty getting to sleep and often didn't stay asleep for very long. Recorded music had been suggested and trialed but was reported not to have had any effect, as Sally appeared irritated by it, becoming distressed, and asked for it to be turned off. Sally always seemed to engage readily and happily in active music therapy, choosing familiar songs, playing instruments, and interacting actively with the music therapist. The music therapist planned to finish each music therapy session with some receptive music to encourage Sally to relax and settle to a deep, relaxed sleep. Usually at sleep times, her mother or grandmother would "pat" Sally gently to help her sleep, and if they stopped, Sally would prompt them to continue to "pat pat." So during the music therapy session, when Sally showed signs of fatigue, the music therapist suggested she lie down in her bed for some "pat pat" songs. Sally readily complied, snuggling into her pillow and blankets, and, while her mother patted her, the music therapist at first sang familiar songs in an engaging, yet gentle manner, accompanied by quiet guitar-playing. As Sally's breathing slowed, the music therapist slowed the singing and playing, continuing with familiar songs, until Sally appeared to almost be asleep, as indicated by regular breathing and closed eyes. The music therapist maintained guitar accompaniment while changing from singing to humming and then to guitar accompaniment only, until her mother indicated that Sally was fast asleep. Her mother reported that her transition to sleep was much quicker than without the music and that after this session, Sally appeared to be in a deeper sleep and stayed asleep for a longer period than usual. In subsequent sessions, when Sally was distressed or agitated or feeling particularly unwell and indicated that she did not want to participate in active music therapy, she would sometimes initiate a request for "pat pat" songs and then readily settle to sleep.

Adaptations. Relaxation for a school-age child may use songs sung to the child, but the child might prefer a relaxation script accompanied by either improvised guitar accompaniment or recorded music. The child is often given the choice, to engender a sense of being in control.

Music therapists providing relaxation for an adolescent can both facilitate relaxation and/or teach adolescents relaxation techniques (Davis, Gfeller, & Thaut, 2008). This can create the potential for adolescents to continue to manage independently some of their own pain and anxiety when there is no music therapist present.

Music-Assisted Imagery

Overview. Music and imagery experiences are particularly useful for children with little energy for physical activity and yet who are still cognitively active and needing to engage, such as children who want to be involved in activity but are too weak or fatigued to get out of bed or sit up. For children who have been in hospital for a long period of time and may be identifying with being a sick patient, it can be effective in encouraging them to imagine themselves outside of hospital as a healthy person in a more attractive setting. It can also be used for relaxation (Sahler et al., 2003), anxiety reduction, and expression of feelings.

This intervention is not suitable for a child or adolescent in an altered state of consciousness (e.g., under any type of sedation), as cognitive function may be impaired. This kind of experience is offered to the child as an option, as they need to fully engage with it to make the most of it. If a child is not interested or not engaged, they may feel uncomfortable or awkward in the experience and not respond.

What to observe. Changes in posture or body language or wriggling might indicate that the child is not comfortable, and certain facial expressions (frowning) may also indicate that the child is uncomfortable.

Procedures. The music therapist will discuss and prepare the session with the child beforehand (Sahler et al., 2003). The music therapist might introduce the concept of music and imagery by describing it as a "dream while awake," or making up a story to music. Preparation will include what music will be used, and time might be spent listening to different types of music with the child to determine what music will be used. The music therapist will provide several choices based on the child's preferences, and one piece will be chosen for the session. Sometimes the child will not be capable of making a decision about the music or may not care or mind what music is used, in which case the music therapist will choose on the child's behalf. The piece of music will be short in length—possibly only 5 to 7 minutes. It will be instrumental (not containing words) and may be classical or light classical. For example, George Winston, *Forest* (Windmill 0193411157-2), and Mozart, *Adagio* (from Clarinet Concerto in A major, K. 622: II) (Grocke & Wigram, 2007).

Once the music has been chosen and the space prepared, and the child is comfortable, a short induction lasting two to three minutes will be used. Types of inductions used include encouraging the child to focus on his breathing or a progressive muscle relaxation. A transition image will be suggested to the child based on the discussion during preparation, such as a favorite place, holiday destination, room at home, or other place (Grocke & Wigram, 2007).

The music is started, and the music therapist gently guides the child's imagery by encouraging the child to describe what is happening in/to the music. She will use prompts such as "What is happening now?" and "Can you see anything in your dream/story?"

When the music has ended, the music therapist will allow the child to complete any imagery or narrative. She may make a statement that the child can revisit that imagery any time in their mind or dreams. She will gently bring the child's attention back to his breathing, the room, and any noises that can be heard. Depending on the age of the child, the music therapist will lead a discussion with the child about the experience and how it might be used in the future to help him.

Mark was a 10-year-old boy undergoing a bone marrow transplant (HSCT) following relapse of Acute Lymphocytic Leukemia (ALL). He had experienced a lot of treatments over a number of years, and was realistically fearful of what lay ahead. Mark liked to play around on keyboard and guitar and kept a guitar in his room throughout his hospital admissions. By week 2 of isolation for his HSCT, he was feeling unwell and lay in bed most of the day, sleeping or watching television, unwilling to sit up and actively be involved in any activities. The music therapist suggested that he might like to try some music and imagery, where he didn't have to sit up, but could lie still, close his eyes if he wished, and use his imagination to make up stories to some special music. He seemed willing to give this idea a go, and so a time for the session was arranged when there would be only a few interruptions.

The music therapist used a relaxation induction to help Mark settle and relax, and then put on a short piece of classical music (four minutes). She encouraged Mark to narrate what was happening in the music. Mark told a story of a boy going on a long walk up a mountain. It was a long way to get to the top, but when he finally arrived at the top, he could see forever. When the music was over, the music therapist and Mark reflected on his story. Mark shared how he and his family went camping in the mountains, and the mountain in his story was that mountain. At the end of the session, Mark said that he enjoyed the experience and would like to do it again. It was something he felt he could do without a lot of concentration or energy, and it took him to a place in his imagination where he was healthy and out of the hospital, and also a place where he felt positive and hopeful.

Adaptations. Music and imagery can be used with a younger child (under five) less formally. The preparation will not be as extensive, the child will not be asked to choose the music, and the piece of music will be much shorter (two to three minutes). The music therapist may simply ask the child to tell a story to the music, with the therapist asking prompting questions.

Music and imagery can also be utilized during a procedure. School-age children and adolescents who can visualize an enjoyable experience or pleasant memory can be encouraged to describe the event in detail as they visualize it during the procedure (Hockenberry, 1988). Music can be played to reinforce the experience. The music therapist encourages the young person to listen to the music and describe the pleasurable event during the procedure. A previous music and imagery experience may be revisited during a procedure, especially if the imagery was strong and the experience positive.

Music for Stimulation and Comfort

Overview. Gentle receptive music for stimulation and comfort is indicated when the child is unable to actively or physically participate. Songs selected by the music therapist may offer reassurance to deal with anxiety by offering familiar experiences. Songs used are familiar to the child and may be associated with earlier pleasant situations (Ghetti, 2009).

Children who are sedated may be unable to move physically or respond vocally, so receptive music therapy allows the child to rest and listen, the familiar music helping him to feel less anxious while also being stimulated in a gentle way. The music therapist will determine if the child can tolerate stimulation by checking with medical staff, as stimulation may need to be kept simple if the child is sedated. The music therapist reduces any other stimulation in the room, as in other examples above. Sometimes the music therapist will use small objects for visual stimulation and guitar for accompaniment if space in the environment permits.

What to observe. Very sick children fatigue quickly; therefore, the music therapist will observe signs that they are not coping well with the stimulation. If the child is being monitored, signs that the music therapist will observe include unreasonable sustained increase in heart rate (an initial increase in heart rate is acceptable as they alert to the stimulus), drop in oxygen saturation, or increase in blood pressure, indicating the body is not coping well with the new stimulus.

Alternatively, the music therapist will observe whether the child's breathing and heart rate settle and oxygen saturation increases, and he appears calmer and less anxious, less withdrawn and more engaged. This may include the child remaining alert and looking with interest at any objects used (for example, his eyes follow the movement of the object).

Procedures. The music therapist will talk quietly to the child at first, alerting him to the presence of another person in the room. She will introduce any visual objects and begin singing quietly, altering tempo, volume, and pitch as needed to engage the child further, or to calm and settle further if required. Depending on the level of sedation of the child, the music therapist will not ask the child questions, or require any verbal or physical response, but will continue to talk and sing to the child in a calm and moderate voice.

Charlie, four years old, had undergone an HSCT and was suffering from Graft vs. Host Disease. He had become very unwell, experiencing pain and discomfort. He was mildly sedated and required an oxygen mask. He had not been able to participate in anything or verbally communicate for some time, and, shutting his eyes for most of the time, had withdrawn from his environment. The music therapist had just purchased some new magnet animals and brought them in to show Charlie. She placed them on a magnet board and held the board close to his face so that he could see them. She sang "Five Little Ducks," moving the ducks over the board, with one "disappearing" with each verse. Charlie's eyes remained open for the entire song, as he watched with interest, his breathing settled, and he attempted a smile. His parents and nurse reported that this was the most interest he had shown in anything for some days, and the first time he had smiled in weeks.

If the child is sedated, only familiar music should be played, and it should be kept to only one or two songs with simple accompaniment due to the effects of sedation. Unfamiliar music requires more cognitive brain activity to attend to the new stimulus and may also induce a negative emotional response, and a child under sedation will have reduced cognitive capacity and ability to regulate emotions. Familiar music, on the other hand, may be readily identified with little cognitive effort and is more likely to activate a broad, rather than specific, response in the brain and a positive emotional response (Särkämö & Soto, 2012).

Song Lyric Discussion

Overview. This is particularly indicated for adolescent patients, as adolescents generally relate to the lyrics of existing song material, and song listening is one of the most popular activities amongst adolescents (O'Callaghan et al., 2012). Playing a favorite song and inviting adolescents to reflect on the lyrical content of the song can lead to discussion about feelings about their diagnosis, hospitalization, and treatment (Kennelly, 2001). The level of song lyric discussion can be structured by adjusting from basic to insight-oriented, according to the needs of the adolescent (Grocke & Wigram, 2007).

What to observe. The music therapist listens carefully to the responses of the adolescent, using them as cues to the level of discussion that is appropriate for him in the moment (Grocke & Wigram, 2007).

Procedures. The music therapist prepares the session by having a selection of recorded music and lyrics available for the young person to browse (for example, on an MP3 player, with songs categorized by artist, and also according to issues and emotions). The music therapist suggests that the adolescent look through the music and see if there are any songs that are relevant for him right now (McFerran, 2010). The adolescent may also be given the option of choosing a song from his own collection. The music is played and listened to together, after which the music therapist asks questions based on the level of discussion chosen for the session. A basic-level question might focus on the band, singer, and what the adolescent liked about the music (Grocke & Wigram, 2007). A more insight-oriented level of question might focus on the meaning of the lyrics and how he feels about the song (Grocke & Wigram, 2007). The music therapist continues asking questions related to what the adolescent has offered in his reply, seeking further descriptions and leading to deeper understandings (McFerran, 2010).

GUIDELINES FOR IMPROVISATIONAL MUSIC THERAPY

The use of improvisational music therapy can be planned as a segment of a music therapy session, or could be spontaneously offered. As with other techniques with children with cancer, the music therapist will observe how the child presents on any given day or moment, and will use whatever technique meets the child's need at that time. Improvisation can emerge as a session progresses, and the music therapist will be open to the reactions of the child and adapt accordingly.

Dramatic Play Free-Flowing Improvisation

Overview. As children naturally use play to explore and make sense of their world, working through play can be a nonthreatening way of dealing with difficult issues and expressing emotions associated with them (Sweeney, 2003). When a child explores his situation through musical play, the instruments he uses and the music that he creates form transitional objects (Winnicott, 1971) through which communication of unconscious material occurs (Sweeney, 2003). These transitional objects may represent people and situations related to the child or can be used to express a sense of self in relation to others through a kind of play where the musical instruments "come to life." Children will make sense of their experiences with their available resources and, even when not communicating, can think or worry about their situation (Aasgaard & Edwards, 1999).

This intervention is indicated for children who are at an age where "pretend" play has emerged or is beginning to emerge or is a major part of their play. The child may feel restricted in his environment and may need to extend boundaries, explore feelings, and make sense of the world and what is happening to him. The child will feel safe in the therapeutic relationship and have a good rapport with the music therapist formed over time. The interactive use of improvisation encourages problem-solving because it is flexible rather than predictable. It also engages the child in expression that will bring pleasure and meet his emotional needs in the moment.

What to observe. The music therapist carefully observes whether the child appears engaged with the characters and is contributing ideas and suggestions about the actions of the characters. If emotions surface that are too intense for the child and the child shows signs of distress, the music therapist will move the activity to something with which the child feels more at ease and comfortable, such as singing a familiar song. The music therapist remains with the child until he returns to a settled and calm state.

Procedures. The music therapist ensures that the environment feels safe for the child, with few interruptions. The child may be bedbound, or sitting beside his bed, in an isolated environment, or in a single room. The child may be less willing to explore when other children or parents are present. Sometimes, if there is a parent in attendance, the music therapist may prepare and/or coach the parent to not intervene with encouragement of the child to "sing songs" rather than play out stories. A selection of instruments is visible and readily accessible. The music therapist sits near the child, guitar ready to accompany play. A child who is fatigued, with little energy, may not be willing, or have the energy, to engage in this kind of play.

Most often, the child will instigate the play and initiate the characters, but sometimes the play may be encouraged by the music therapist making an initial suggestion—"Let's play a game with the instruments" or "Let's make a story about the maraca"—and may start by improvising a question about the instrument characters, for example, singing "What is the maraca doing today?" or "Where is the maraca going today?" or "Who is the maraca going to play with," etc. The music therapist provides a "vamp"-style accompaniment, repeating until the child provides the next line. She may echo the line the child provides, improvising with it as the child plays (Ghetti & Walker, 2009), and then, if needed, sing a prompting line such as "What happens next?," vamping again until the child replies. This continues until there is a conclusion to the story. The music therapist might need to cue the child to bring closure to the story by asking the child how he wants it to end (Ghetti & Walker, 2009). Much of the session consists of improvising by elaborating and collaborating on the child's dramatic play (Rubin-Bosco, 2002).

Lisa, a five-year-old girl hospitalized for a bone marrow transplant, had been isolated for six weeks. She was becoming increasingly frustrated with the lengthy separation from family and friends and limited experiences available to her. Lisa had previously enjoyed the re-creative music experiences that were part of the regular weekly group music therapy sessions. However, she was beginning to show signs of becoming bored with the same choices and options and initiated an exploration of different ways of playing instruments. Lisa started to attribute characters to some of the instruments: She turned the small timpani drum upside down, saying that it was the "prison"; the maraca was the "guard"; the animal castanet, which she put inside the drum, was the "prisoner," who, she stated, was trapped. The monkey bells were coming to save the prisoner (castanet), but were stopped by the guard (maraca). The music therapist accompanied this dramatic play with improvised guitar chords, and a repeated sung motif question throughout—"What happens next?"—with which Lisa took the play further, for the music therapist to then reflect back through improvised song. Lisa was able to express her sense of being isolated and trapped through her play and was affirmed by the reflections of the music therapist.

Adaptations. A nonverbal child will not easily engage with this activity, but the music therapist might encourage a nonverbal child to play with the characters and reflect the child's play through improvised song, watching for signs that the reflections are not overly interpretative, as, if the interpretations are incorrect, the child will show signs of disengagement by looking away and discontinuing to play. However, if interpretations are correct, the child will remain engaged.

Instrumental Improvisation

Overview. Instrumental improvisation is indicated for children for whom nonverbal expression appears to be their preferred method of communication, children from non–English speaking backgrounds, children with little verbal communication, and/or children who show an interest in playing instruments. It is also indicated for children with mucositus, for whom speaking or vocalizing is uncomfortable, and is also suitable for children who need to have an outlet for their emotions related to cancer diagnosis and cancer treatment but who may not be able to express these via words. It can also be used to stimulate playful interactions between child and family. Often the families are so worried that they may need some help in initiating playful interactions with their child. Goals include to express emotions nonverbally through engaging in instrumental improvisation, to engage with family and/or music therapist nonverbally through improvising on instruments simultaneously, to experience control over the environment through selecting instruments to play and leading the "start/stop" game, to experience mastery of instruments, and to feel connected with others. Children experience creative freedom as they determine the tempo, dynamics, rhythmic structure, and form of their musical creations (Robb, 2003).

This activity is not suitable for children who are too physically weak to play instruments or who are tired, lethargic, or severely unwell. The child needs to be physically feeling well enough to actively play an instrument and have adequate energy levels to sustain playing instruments for at least a few minutes.

What to observe. The music therapist will observe whether the child is becoming "bored" or tired of being the leader. This may be indicated by a lessening of energy in playing or a stopping of playing. The child may become distracted and less focused on playing and may look around the room or to other instruments. The child may begin to play destructively (e.g., banging on the drums in an aggressive manner) to the point that he may hurt himself or others in the room.

Procedures. The music therapist will have a variety of instruments available for selection, but will limit choices. For example, a nonverbal child can be shown instruments and asked to choose and take an instrument, rather than asked an open-ended question to which he is required to answer verbally. If there are family members present, they too can be offered a choice of instruments to play. The music therapist will choose her instrument based on the child's choice so that she can provide appropriate accompaniment. The music therapist will allow the child to lead by freely playing on his instrument and will follow by providing matching accompaniment, usually with structural elements such as rhythm and melodic contour (Robb, 2003). When the child is showing signs of tiring as the leader, the music therapist will suggest a change of instruments or a change in leader, allowing the activity to be extended and offering the child further challenges.

The music therapist directs the involvement of any family members who are present, to prevent them from inadvertently "taking over" the improvisation. This might be done by setting up the parameters of the session and/or discussing the process with the family members before the session begins, and if necessary guiding the involvement of the family members during the session.

Thomas was a six-year-old boy in the consolidation *phase of his treatment for ALL and during this hospital admission was isolated due to* febrile neutropenia. *Thomas was previously very quiet and shy during both individual and group sessions during inpatient admissions and in outpatients. It was very rare for him to respond verbally, and most times his mother, father, or siblings would respond on his behalf when he was asked a question. He would indicate his preferences by pointing and using one-word responses. Thomas needed to gain some mastery and control over his environment, to have choices and gain confidence to engage and interact with others in this environment.*

In this session, his grandmother was present. At the beginning of the session, the music therapist showed Thomas two instruments—a small guitar and bongo drums—and invited him to choose one. He pointed to the small guitar. The grandmother was also offered a choice of two instruments and chose the small keyboard. The music therapist chose the guitar with the intention of providing a melodic and structured accompaniment.

Thomas began playing and was joined by music therapist and grandmother. Without verbalizing instructions, the music therapist followed Thomas's lead, playing when Thomas played, stopping when he stopped. Thomas became the "leader" and music therapist and grandmother followed. The music therapist played the guitar by strumming the guitar in a I, IV, V chordal progression, matching the loud dynamic and the fast rhythms of Thomas playing on the guitar. The music therapist stopped as soon as Thomas stopped playing and picked up where the chord progression had left when he recommenced playing. The music therapist shifted to a more Spanish style, playing root chord A on the guitar and sliding it up a fret to give it a freer, more improvised accompaniment. Instruments were swapped a number of times, and each had turns at being the leader. Thomas smiled with delight when he noticed that the music therapist and his grandmother were following his lead. He found great joy in trying to "trick" the music therapist and his grandmother by stopping at different times (e.g., after long periods of playing or really short periods). Thomas initiated changing instruments by pointing at his grandmother's keyboard, so they both swapped and the musical improvisation game started again. The session continued, with lots of changes of instruments as additional instruments were introduced.

When Thomas appeared to be tiring of this, and in order to engage him further, to encourage greater activity, and to challenge him more, the music therapist suggested that the grandmother lead and Thomas and the music therapist follow. Thomas smiled at this suggestion and pointed to Grandma to acknowledge that she was to lead. When it seemed that Thomas had had enough of the "musical improvisation game" (noted by Thomas appearing to look around the room and playing the instruments with less intent), the music therapist arranged a mini drum "kit" for Thomas to play (i.e., bongo drum, small djembe, lollypop drum [held by Grandma in the air], and tambourine [held by the music therapist]). Thomas improvised on this drum "kit" for some time with mallets. The music therapist moved the tambourine as a target so that Thomas had to keep looking and reaching to different locations to play it. Grandma followed and repeated this with the lollypop drum. To provide a structure within which Thomas could feel supported to continue his playing for an extended period, the music therapist improvised vocally and melodically using the words "Thomas is a fine musician and loves to play the drums." Thomas laughed and smiled as he played his drum kit.

By the end of the session, Thomas was talking to the music therapist and asked his grandmother to show the music therapist her camera, which had photos of his new sandpit at home. The music therapist felt that the improvisation activity gave Thomas control over his environment and the confidence and rapport with the music therapist to initiate talking with the music therapist, which he had not done in previous sessions (Annette Baron, personal communication, May, 2012).

Adaptations. If the child is showing signs of uncertainty as to what and/or how to play, or seems unwilling to explore and play freely, the music therapist can provide a more structured improvisation by making suggestions to direct the activity. This may be done using colors or imagery, for example, "Let's make the sound of the beach" or "Let's make the sound of thunder," etc. The music therapist might get things started with a rhythmic ground and encourage the child's participation. Alternatively, the music therapist may use a structured improvisation exercise such as ABA, where A is a structured, familiar song that the music therapist plays while the child plays along on their instrument, and then B is the improvised section, followed by a return to A (Ghetti & Walker, 2009). The child experiences the structure but also the freedom of expression in the B section. This could build coping skills and resilience by testing out a new experience and then returning to the security of something familiar.

Song Improvisation

Overview. Song improvisation can be a powerful way for children to become aware of and express thoughts and feelings. Children can tell their stories and explore issues that may otherwise feel overwhelming or frightening. The musical structure and the context of the song make it safer for children to experience feelings that may not have been in their consciousness (Bruscia, 1987; Turry & Turry, 1999). Song improvisation can offer an avenue for processing a child's experience directly or metaphorically. This can happen either in the moment or over time within the context of an ongoing process. The inclusion of the element of lyrics adds a level of expression that is concrete (Turry, 1999).

What to observe. The music therapist will observe the level of engagement and verbal involvement of the child. If the child is quiet and not forthcoming with active verbal interaction, the therapist changes the activity to meet the needs of the child, perhaps to something less verbal. Conversely, if the child is "chatty" and easy to engage verbally, song improvisation is indicated.

Procedures. Spontaneous song can evolve naturally from the child's active participation in music interaction (Ghetti & Walker, 2009) or from conversation with the therapist. For example, after a conversation with the child about his soft toy, the therapist may encourage the child to make up a song about the toy. Children may sing their songs on their own in order to express the identified feelings and take ownership of their feelings. At times, the therapist sings with the child, especially after the child has sung alone in order to reinforce the ego and provide grounding (Turry, 1999). At other times, the music therapist supports and validates the child's contribution by echoing back the child's verbalizations or themes (Ghetti & Walker, 2009).

GUIDELINES FOR RE-CREATIVE MUSIC THERAPY

Re-creative music therapy may be used as part of a session, or for the whole session, depending on the needs of the child in the moment. Re-creative music most often consists of songs or pieces of music that are familiar to the child; sometimes new songs or pieces of music are also used.

Group Music-Making for Normalization

Overview. Participation in group music-making sessions in the cancer unit is indicated particularly for newly diagnosed patients and their families. This helps with their initial coming to terms with the diagnosis by observing others participating in a normal and positive way (Ghetti & Walker,

2009). For "regular" patients who have previously been admitted to the unit, the familiar experience is something to which they look forward. The session format is familiar and, as they know what to expect, they can feel confident in participating (Robb, 2003). For children who spend a lot of time in bed, it can be motivation to get out of bed for a short time and to be physically involved in an experience outside of their room. For children who are missing friends, siblings, and other social experiences, it is an opportunity to socialize with others. Choices offered in this environment encourage autonomy and engagement (Robb, 2003).

What to observe. The music therapist will note varying levels of physical capabilities and energy. For example, there may be children with a lot of energy—healthy, able siblings—and conversely, unwell children who are fatigued. Most children who are inpatients are likely to be attached to an IV pole and therefore will be physically limited in movement activities.

Procedures. The music therapist sets up the space prior to children arriving. Depending on individual settings, the room is set up invitingly with chairs in a circle, with space for IV poles. Sometimes the music therapist might place a box of instruments in the middle of the circle for the children to initiate choices throughout the session; at other times, the music therapist might prefer to contain the experience by offering certain instruments at particular times throughout the session. The music therapist will make this choice based on the dynamics of the group at the time.

Prior to approaching children to invite them to attend the group, the music therapist will verify with nursing staff which children are allowed out of their room to attend the group and which are not. This individual invitation can be effective for newly diagnosed patients and their parents who may be unsure and nervous about attending. Children who need to remain isolated for medical reasons and cannot socialize with others (for example, HSCT patients) can unfortunately not participate in these social music therapy groups.

Regular music therapy groups in the cancer unit can be targeted at different age groups. For example, there may be a primary school age–focused group and an adolescent-focused group. A school-age group could include camp songs and other familiar songs. Adolescents can choose music which best suits their individual preferences and share those songs with others in the group. The music therapist needs to have a wide variety of contemporary songs in her repertoire for this type of group.

Music therapists use a regular greeting or familiar song to welcome children to the group and to mark the beginning of the group (Ghetti & Walker, 2009). The songs used in the group will be chosen based on what is developmentally appropriate for the ages of the children attending. For instance, for toddlers and preschoolers, animated play songs and nursery rhymes are used, often with small handheld rhythm instruments related to the songs. Children can play duck-shaped castanets during duck-themed songs, frog castanets during frog-themed songs, and monkey-shaped bells during monkey songs, etc. Props may also be used to accompany songs to engage children when the energy is waning and quieter, less noisy songs are warranted. For example, during "Eency Weency Spider," children can manipulate spiders made from egg cartons and pipe cleaners, and during "Old MacDonald Had a Farm," they can play with soft plastic toy animals.

Choices are offered throughout the session. For example, the music therapist may offer each child an opportunity to choose a song and/or an instrument to play. Toward the end of the session, quieter, slower songs might be sung, putting the instruments and props away, using hand actions instead to reduce the energy, allowing the children to leave feeling settled. For example, "Twinkle, Twinkle, Little Star" may be sung using hand actions. A closing song is usually sung, often a good-bye song, to indicate the end of the session. Many music therapists personalize the song to include children's names.

Lara was a three-year-old girl, newly diagnosed with ALL. Just two days after admission for her induction phase, the music therapist invited Lara and her mother to join the group music session which was offered to all children in the cancer unit once a week in the playroom. Lara's mother looked tired but indicated that Lara loved music and singing and they would come right along. Lara, however, was very tentative when she arrived, clinging to her mother and nervously looking around. The music therapist encouraged Lara and her mother to participate in the group whenever they liked, but if they chose to just observe that day, then that was fine, too. There were three other young children, all under five years of age, with their parents participating in the group that day, all of whom had attended the regular group many times previously and were in varying stages of their treatment. Two had lost their hair and had nasogastric tubes, and all three had IV poles. Lara and her mother observed these other children with apparent curiosity.

The session included songs that the children all knew, which immediately and readily engaged them and encouraged confident participation. A box of small percussion instruments was available for the children to access and to play if they chose to. As Lara appeared too shy to access the box on her own, her mother chose an instrument for her and helped her to play it. The music therapist also gave each child an opportunity to choose a song for the group to sing, to promote independence, and when it came to Lara's turn, she also chose a song that she knew, assisted by her mother. The other children readily participated as the format of the session was very familiar to them, and they confidently accessed the instruments and played self-assuredly and independently. The other parents in the group also participated, often singing and playing along themselves, assisting their child when needed, but otherwise relaxed and enjoyed observing their child's participation in a normal fun activity. As the group progressed, Lara appeared more comfortable and started to smile and interact more with her mother. She watched the other children participate, and copied their actions to one of the songs, which required frog castanets to "jump" into the pond (throwing the frogs into the box).

As the group came to an end and the good-bye song was sung, including each child's name, Lara observed as each child packed up their instrument and waved good-bye. When her name was sung, she waved good-bye as she shyly smiled at the group. After the session, one of the other mothers spoke to Lara's mother on the way out of the playroom, introducing herself and her child.

For Lara and her mother, this was the first time that they had had any social interaction with other cancer patients and their families. It was also the first time since diagnosis that they had participated in an activity that was familiar and "normal." They were able to observe the comfortable and relaxed way other children and their families interacted and had adapted to life in the hospital. This helped them with their acceptance of their situation and perhaps gave them some ways to manage their new situation.

Instrumental Instruction

Overview. Teaching a child to play an instrument can be beneficial for several reasons. There are potential cognitive deficits associated with long-term hospitalization and some cancer treatments; therefore, the challenge of learning an instrument is indicated for these children to encourage continuing cognitive development. For adolescents who are struggling with the lack of independence and autonomy, particularly in long-term hospital admissions, it provides opportunities for mastery, empowerment, self-expression, and control.

Preparation. The decision to learn to play an instrument will come as a request from the child, or the music therapist will offer it as an option if it is observed that the process of learning an instrument would be beneficial to the child. If possible, the music therapist will encourage them to choose the "terms" of the lessons—which instrument (if there is a choice, for example, such as guitar, keyboard, or ukulele), how often the lessons occur and when, and what would they like to learn. The music therapist prepares songs and/or pieces of music from which the child can choose that are simple enough to learn within a short time frame and not beyond the capabilities of the child for use in generating success.

What to observe. The music therapist first ensures that the young person is physically capable of playing the instrument and/or if there are any obstacles to him playing an instrument. For example, if the IV is in his hand, this would prevent him from playing freely. The music therapist will note the energy level and concentration capacity of the child. The child may only be able to concentrate for a few minutes in each session, especially if the effort of learning the instrument is challenging for the child. They may become frustrated if success at playing the instrument is not immediate, and they have little patience to persist.

Procedures. After setting up the "terms" of the lessons, the music therapist will provide lessons to the child as per these terms. The music therapist usually teaches or models small achievable tasks on the instrument, constantly encouraging and praising the child for any step achieved. Where possible, the musical instrument can be left in the child's room for him to practice with, if he chooses. This will depend on the instrument, for example, if it belongs to the patient or is available (or not) for loan. Also taken into consideration is the space available in the room to store the instrument when not in use, as some hospital rooms have limited space, and also whether the room is shared with other patients.

Jake, a 15-year-old with AML having an HSCT, was reported as becoming withdrawn and disengaged and subsequently referred to music therapy. The music therapist suggested that he borrow a guitar from the music therapy department and learn guitar while isolated in his room. He agreed to give it a go, a guitar was provided, and lessons commenced. Some days, Jake was too unwell to pick up the guitar, but his parents reported that whenever he felt well enough he would play, even if only for a few minutes. At each music therapy session, the music therapist would encourage Jake in the progress he was making, and challenge him with new material if requested. Jake seemed to be enjoying the discovery of playing the guitar and the opportunities for self-expression and self-regard it gave him. His levels of motivation, engagement, and communication were reported to increase. As his treatment was coming to an end and discharge was in sight, his parents bought him a guitar similar to the one he had been using while in hospital, so he could continue playing at home.

GUIDELINES FOR COMPOSITIONAL MUSIC THERAPY

Songwriting

Overview. Songwriting provides a flexible yet structured musical medium for the expression and communication of thoughts and feelings. It can provide insight about how the child is adjusting to the illness or coping with the treatment, and provide opportunities to acknowledge, support, and explore feelings regarding hospitalization (Kennelly, 2001). Songwriting is indicated for older children and adolescents who are alert and able to engage in a cognitive activity.

What to observe. The music therapist will note the energy levels and concentration capacity of the child, offering a simpler technique if the child shows signs of having low energy. For example, if the child is lying in bed and talking is requiring effort, the music therapist will provide simple songwriting choices. On the other hand, if the child is sitting up, alert, and chatting easily, then the music therapist will offer more leadership of the songwriting process to the child.

Procedures. There are a number of approaches to songwriting which have been outlined in the music therapy literature. Hadley (1996) outlines them according to the level of structure provided:

- The cloze technique, or fill-in-the-blanks: Some of the original words are deleted and the child is prompted to fill in the blanks with his own words. This type of songwriting provides the highest level of structure to the child.
- Song Parody, also called Song Augmentation (Edwards, 1998): Here, the child or adolescent substitutes his own lyrics for words to a pre-existing melody, or adds a new verse to an existing song. This provides not only an opportunity for expression, but also a unique sense of accomplishment (Ledger, 2001).
- The blues: The child's or adolescent's song is in the musical and lyrical form of the blues style, and may grow from musical storytelling or from verbal improvisation built on a blues accompaniment (Aasgaard, 2002).
- Original songs: The child or adolescent creates both the music and the lyrics. This process may evolve from song improvisation or may involve the reworking of music and lyrics until the child is satisfied with the final product. The role of the music therapist is to facilitate the adolescent's involvement in composing the song. This may involve the music therapist providing most of the musical material and helping the young person structure his ideas into lyrics (McFerran, 2010).

Maria was an eight-year-old girl who was experiencing an extended hospital admission due to complications following an HSCT. She had become withdrawn, communicating little with anyone, and appeared to sleep most of the day. Despite previously engaging in sessions with the music therapist, she was no longer indicating any interest or willingness to participate in music-making or listening when offered. The music therapist asked her what would she have if she could have anything she wanted, and she replied that she would like everyone to leave her alone so that she could go to sleep. The music therapist began to improvise a song based on those words, and there was a hint of a smile on Maria's face. The music therapist suggested that perhaps together Maria and the music therapist could write a song about wanting to go to sleep. Maria didn't respond at first, so the music therapist began to make up song lines that required Maria to fill in the missing word. For example, "I just want to go to sleep, I hate it when ... ." Maria began to make suggestions, offering further lines. After a while, two verses had been written, and Maria had remained engaged for the entire time. Subsequent sessions involved improving on the song and adding a verse about what Maria would really like and what she was looking forward to, which was to get out of the hospital and live a normal life. On Maria's request, the song was written up on a large piece of paper and displayed above her bed. Her mother reported that when the doctors came in to examine her or otherwise bother her, she pointed to the song, indicating to them how she felt.

Music Artifacts

Overview. Children and adolescents can create their own music artifacts, such as CD or video products, or record their musical creations, which may include their singing voices (Aasgaard, 2002; O'Callaghan & Aasgaard, 2012). These artifacts can assist in decreasing anxiety and increase positive coping while also becoming mementos for family members. The children are invited to record their singing and musical compositions, or make sound effects and play instruments, so that they can hear themselves in the performances (O'Callaghan & Aasgaard, 2012). CD creations involve the child creating original music using interactive computer-based music software (Barry et al., 2010) and can be used during treatment and/or procedures. Video production as described by Burns et al. (2009) includes music selection, lyric writing, discussion, and digitally recording the song. Also included in the creating of the video artifact is photo and artwork selection, video design using story boards, and discussion.

What to observe. As with songwriting, the music therapist notes the energy levels and concentration capacity of the child.

Procedures. To create a CD artifact, the music therapist demonstrates the program and supports the child in choosing and creating their preferred musical sounds (Barry et al., 2010). The child's original music creations are "remixed" by the music therapist after the session, extending and adjusting elements of the musical material such as structure, tempo, pitch, and instrumentation so that the length of the CD matches the approximate duration of his treatment and is still compatible with the child's original composition (Barry et al., 2010). The child is then given the option of using it during his treatment.

Burns et al. (2009) describe the process of creating a video artifact in the context of a research protocol for admission for a bone marrow transplant. The process in the course of regular music therapy services is similar. To create a video artifact, the music therapist first discusses this option with the child, and then explains the process. Over a number of sessions, the music therapist supports the child's efforts in creating a video. Typically, the more active participation aspects of this intervention, including songwriting (see previous section), discussion, and digitally recording the child's song, occur during a time in the child's hospital admission when they are not experiencing high levels of fatigue and physiological side effects (Burns et al., 2009). When the child is experiencing these side effects, the music therapist engages the child in the more passive aspects of creating a video artifact, including photo and artwork selection, video design, discussion, and encouraging the child in making independent choices and decisions (Robb, 2000).

WORKING WITH CAREGIVERS

Music therapists help or guide parents in using music supportively with their children. Many parents already use music to help their children through aversive cancer experiences and to remain connected with, and inspire, their children's "normalcy," aesthetic, and enjoyable experiences (O'Callaghan et al., 2011). Parents can provide recorded music, musical instruments, online music videos, and other resources, such as karaoke machines. This often helps their children through treatment and coping with symptoms and procedures, or can assist sleep.

Many hospitals follow a family-centered model of care to minimize psychological distress in sick children, and families are encouraged to spend as much time as possible with the hospitalized child. Thus, children who are with a parent at the time of a music therapy session have the option of having a session with or without parent(s) present. Equally important as the child's experience of pleasure is the need for the parent to witness their child having fun and being autonomous and to actively participate in music therapy sessions, thereby experiencing fun together with their child (O'Neill & Pavlicevic, 2003).

RESEARCH EVIDENCE

In pediatric oncology treatment contexts, quantitative and qualitative research provides evidence for music therapy's beneficial effects (Hilliard, 2006; Standley & Hanser, 1995). This section will provide a summary of the available evidence to date.

Many studies of music therapy in pediatric oncology refer to the use of interactive music, which may include a combination of receptive, re-creative, improvisational, and compositional methods without singling out any particular method for examination. Therefore, the studies below are organized according to the outcomes they addressed rather than by specific methods.

Anxiety and Pain Reduction

Barrera, Rykov, and Doyle (2002) report on the use of interactive and developmentally appropriate music-making with 65 children with cancer and their families. The music therapy sessions included one or more of the following activities: singing, songwriting, instrumental improvisation, and listening to prerecorded music of their choice. This study used a single group pretest-posttest design. The results indicate statistically significant yet minimal improvements ($p < .001$) in children's ratings of their feelings from pretest ($M = 2.55$, $SD = 0.61$) to posttest ($M = 2.76$, $SD = 0.35$). Parents' satisfaction scores were high, with 64% of the parents rating music therapy as very helpful in comforting their child, 58% stating that music therapy helped reduce their child's anxiety, and 48% stating that music therapy brought comfort and anxiety reduction to themselves.

A research study by Bufalini (2009) examined the impact of interactive music on anxiety in 39 pediatric oncology patients undergoing painful procedures. In this controlled clinical trial, children in the music therapy treatment group received interactive music therapy prior to and during conscious sedation, whereas children in the control group received standard care conscious sedation. The results demonstrated significantly less anxiety in the children in the music group ($M = 36.3$, $SD = 11.5$) than those in the control group ($M = 56.9$, $SD = 16.3$) ($p < .05$) and indicated that music therapy has a significant effect on the reduction of anticipatory anxiety and induction compliance on pediatric oncology patients undergoing procedures.

The effect of music-assisted relaxation on the fear and pain of six pediatric patients ages 6 to 15 years undergoing bone marrow aspirations (BMA) was evaluated in a study by Pfaff, Smith, and Gowan (1989). Music-assisted relaxation consisted of patient-preferred relaxation music provided by a music therapist. The study utilized a self-report scale to measure pain and fear and a behavioral observation scale to measure the children's distress. Patients were observed during a baseline BMA procedure (without music therapy intervention) and then received music-assisted relaxation during the second of two consecutive bone marrow aspirations. Analysis of the children's responses on the self-report measures suggested trends for reductions in anticipatory fear ($p \leq .06$), experienced fear ($p \leq .09$), and experienced pain ($p \leq 0.12$) during the music therapy sessions, but these were not statistically significant. This is not surprising given the small sample size. The hypothesis that music-assisted relaxation would result in a reduction in total observed behavioral distress was not supported ($p \geq .05$). However, a significant reduction in crying behavior was found during music-assisted relaxation ($p \leq .03$).

Daveson (2001) describes a session with a three-year-old girl newly diagnosed with leukemia who was referred to music therapy for anxiety reduction. The girl presented as withdrawn and anxious as indicated by a lack of eye contact, muscular tension, minimal verbal responses, and a reluctance to interact with any persons entering the room. During the session, the author used familiar song singing and opportunities for choice and control. The outcome was that the patient's level of anxiety appeared to reduce as indicated by an observable decrease in muscular tension, an increase in eye contact, and an increase in the frequency of spontaneous verbal responses.

Sahler et al. (2003) explored the feasibility of providing a combined music therapy and relaxation imagery intervention to patients in a bone marrow transplant (BMT) unit and examined the effects on the frequency and intensity of pain and nausea, the two most common side effects associated with transplantation. This case-controlled study used a nonrandomized convenience sample. The protocol intervention involved a 45-minute assisted relaxation and relaxation imagery session provided twice weekly by a music therapist. There were 23 participants in the treatment group and 19 in the control group. Subjects rated pain and nausea at the beginning and the end of each music therapy session on a 10 cm visual analog scale grounded at each end as least pain (or nausea) or worst pain (or nausea). Self-reported pain and nausea were significantly decreased after music/relaxation imagery intervention, compared to ratings before the intervention. Self-reported pain decreased from 7.7 (*SE* = 1.9) to 4.9 (*SE* = 1.3) (*p* < .004). Self-reported nausea decreased from 7.9 (*SE* = 1.8) to 5.0 (*SE* = 1.5) (*p* < .001). Limitations of the study included that the intervention was typically delayed until after transplantation, probably reducing its potency in modulating stress during one of the most vulnerable times in the transplantation process. The frequency of the intervention was lower than planned because of the misperception among staff that certain patients were "too sick" to participate.

Coping

A study by Robb (2000) examined a contextual support model of music therapy which is based on Skinner and Wellborn's (1994) motivational theory of coping. The theory maintains that children who remain engaged with their environment generally cope with stress in an active, flexible, and positive manner. This study examined three basic hypotheses of the theory: (a) that music interventions create supportive environments, (b) that music interventions increase children's active engagement, and (c) that relationships exist between supportive environments and engaging behavior. Ten pediatric oncology patients ages four to seven years who were restricted to an isolated environment participated in the study. Participants, serving as their own controls, experienced four different environmental conditions. The data revealed that therapeutic music interventions possess more environmental support elements than other activities and events experienced by children in an isolated hospital environment. Scores from the behavioral observation data support the assertion that music interventions increase children's active engagement with the environment. Other findings from the study indicate that positive behavioral effects of music interventions were not maintained in hospital experiences that followed the music session, and that environmental support elements were related to some positive behaviors, but these behaviors were not consistent across environments.

Based on the above study, a multisite randomized controlled trial was conducted to examine the effect of music therapy on the coping behavior of 83 oncology patients ages four to seven years (Robb et al., 2008). The purpose of this trial was to determine the efficacy of the Active Music Engagement (AME) intervention on three coping-related behaviors (i.e., positive facial affect, active engagement, and initiation). Participants were randomly assigned to one of three conditions: AME (N = 27), music listening (ML) (N = 28), or audio storybooks (ASB) (N = 28). Active music engagement involved age-appropriate, music-based activities to create a predictable environment that supports the actions of children. Children were given opportunities to choose materials, and the inherent flexibility of live music was used to support initiated actions of children. Interventions were guided by a music therapist who kept the child's decisions and actions central to the activity at hand. AME activities were subdivided into five categories: (a) greeting song, (b) instrument-playing to live music, (c) action songs, (d) illustrated songs in storybook form, and (e) closing song. After adjusting for baseline differences, results indicated that AME participants had a significantly higher frequency of coping-related behaviors compared with ML or ASB. Positive facial affect and active engagement were significantly higher during AME, compared with ML and ASB (*p* < .0001). Verbal and gestural initiation was significantly higher during AME than ASB (*p* < .05).

A two-part study by Robb and Ebberts (2003a, 2003b) examined the effect of a music therapy treatment protocol for young patients undergoing a bone marrow transplant. Part one of the study examined patient anxiety levels and depressive symptoms. Part two of the study investigated the lyrical content of patient-generated songs, providing insight into the coping strategies used by these patients and issues patients expressed. Six pediatric BMT patients ranging in age from 9 to 17 years were randomly assigned to the music condition and the no–music contact condition. Both conditions consisted of six one-hour sessions that occurred over a three-week period. The treatment protocol involved a combination of songwriting and music video production strategies. Participants in the control group met with an interventionist and played patient-selected board, card, and video games. Graphic analysis of scores from the Children Depression Inventory and The State Trait Anxiety Inventory for Children indicated a consistent downward trend in depression and anxiety levels for all participants. Content analysis of the song lyrics revealed expression of issues related to the following themes: hope, positive coping, appreciation, mental status, control, time, bewilderment, treatment, and diagnosis. Examination of positive coping strategies included in the children's song lyrics were independent coping (i.e., feelings of independence and self-control; confronting a situation) and family, peer, and professional support. Initial outcomes from this pilot study suggested that the proposed music-based intervention may help patients undergoing BMT identify and develop personal strengths that will enable them to cope positively with stress related to diagnosis and treatment.

Outcomes from the above study were used to inform a study by Burns, Robb, and Haase (2009) which explored the feasibility and preliminary efficacy of a therapeutic music video (TMV) intervention for adolescents and young adults (AYAs) undergoing stem-cell transplantation (SCT). The TMV was designed to diminish symptom distress and improve coping, derived meaning, resilience, and quality of life by supporting AYAs in exploring thoughts and feelings. Twelve participants were randomized to either the TMV intervention or an audio-book control group. Both groups received six one-hour sessions, delivered during the acute phase of SCT. Children in the intervention group participated in the TMV protocol with a music therapist, while those randomized to the low-dose control group listened to patient-selected audio books with a child life specialist. The results suggested positive trends in the TMV group for hope, spirituality, confidence/mastery, self-transcendence, high levels of participation and satisfaction, and improvement in symptom distress, self-efficacy and coping, and quality of life.

A mixed methods research study by Barry and colleagues (2010) investigating the effects of a music therapy CD (MTCD) creation intervention on pediatric oncology patients' distress and coping during their first radiation therapy treatment showed that ratings of distress were low. Eleven pediatric radiation therapy outpatients ages 6 to 13 years were randomly assigned to either the MTCD creation group, in which they could create a music CD prior to their initial treatment to listen to during radiation therapy, or to a standard care group. Data sources included pediatric interview, parent questionnaire, staff questionnaire, and the music therapist researcher's clinical reflexive journal. Ratings of distress during initial radiation therapy treatment were low for all children. The quantitative analysis suggested that distraction and cognitive restructuring were the most helpful and most frequently used coping strategies. In addition, results indicated that 67% of the children in the standard care group used social withdrawal as a coping strategy, compared to 0% of the children in the music therapy group. Analysis of the qualitative data indicated that MTCD creation was considered a fun, engaging, and developmentally appropriate intervention which offered a positive experience and aided use of effective coping strategies to meet the demands of initial radiation therapy treatment.

Expression/Communication

A study by O'Callaghan et al. (2011) examined pediatric cancer patients' and their parents' perspectives about music and music therapy's role in the children's lives using a constructivist research approach with grounded theory design. Twenty-six children up to 14 years old with cancer and 28 parents participated. Data included transcripts from semistructured research interviews and observations of children's music behaviors. The results indicated that children's adverse cancer experiences are often alleviated by music usages. Four main themes were identified: (a) children's cancer experiences can be helped by their own music; (b) children's cancer experiences can be helped by musical interactions within their families, social networks, and electronic (including online) connections; (c) children's cancer experiences can be helped by hospital music therapy and creative programs, which can also vicariously support their families; and (d) parents are grateful for music therapy and related care, and recommend more supportive musical and sound hospital environments.

Summary and Conclusions

Children's cancers are rare and differ from adults, and have a higher rate of cure than for adults. The main types of childhood cancer include leukemia, lymphoma, solid tumors, and brain tumors. Cancer treatments depend on the type and severity of cancer and the child's age. Forms of treatment include chemotherapy, radiotherapy, and/or surgery and typically take place in a center or hospital that specializes in treating childhood cancers. Treatment can suppress the immune system, leaving children at risk of contracting infections, and at times this may mean the child needs to be isolated; however, at different times they can manage normal routines. Treatments also carry the risk of both short-term and long-term side effects.

A diagnosis of cancer usually heralds the start of a long and uncertain journey with many stages—diagnosis; period of treatment, which could be short and intense or long and complex; end of treatment; and long-term follow-up stage. The experience of the journey varies for each individual child and their family, and is dependent on a wide variety of variables. Initially the child and family are confronted with a multitude of stresses, not the least of which includes coming to terms with the ramifications of diagnosis and treatment. This varies widely based on age.

Initially, the needs of this population include the reduction of anxiety and adjustment to diagnosis and hospital environment. For children hospitalized for lengthy periods, the psychosocial impact will be great. There is a need for interventions that diminish the negative effects of hospitalization and that provide supportive environments that encourage coping. Creative and age-appropriate opportunities are required to help maintain and/or attain developmental milestones. Some children will require rehabilitation. Normal experiences help families manage the roller-coaster ups and downs of the cancer journey.

Music therapy with this population needs to be flexible and take into account the child's current condition, energy, and needs, which vary across the course of treatment. Music therapy sessions may involve the application of multiple techniques as appropriate to the needs of the child in that session. Specific techniques can be planned for an entire session or as a segment of a session, or spontaneously offered within the session. Music therapists use receptive music therapy, improvisational music therapy, re-creative music therapy, and compositional music therapy.

There are only a handful of research studies on music therapy with pediatric oncology patients. These studies typically refer to the use of interactive music, which may include a combination of receptive, re-creative, improvisational, and compositional methods without singling out any particular method for examination. Several case studies have been published that support the use of music therapy with this population, but more research is needed to build and support evidence-based practice in this area of work.

Glossary

The following definitions are adapted from Murphy, K. (Ed.). (2011). *Family handbook for children with cancer,* 2nd ed. The Children's Oncology Group.

Audiogram: An audiogram measures hearing by testing how well a child can hear sounds of different pitches and different degrees of loudness.

Biopsy: the removal of a small piece of tissue from the body to test for cancer cells.

Blood count: a laboratory study to evaluate the number of white blood cells, red blood cells, and platelets in the blood.

Blood cultures: If the child has signs of infection, the blood may be tested to see if bacteria, viruses, or fungi are present. This helps the health care team know how to best treat the infection.

Bone marrow aspiration and biopsy: a procedure in which a needle is placed into the cavity of the bone, usually the hip bone, to remove a small amount of bone marrow for examination under the microscope.

Bone scan: an imaging method that provides important information about the bones, including the location of cancer that may have spread to the bones. A low-dose radioactive substance is injected into a vein, and pictures are taken to see where the radioactivity collects, pointing to an abnormality.

Central venous line: a method of giving intravenous fluids, blood products, and medicines by surgically inserting a catheter into a large vein (usually in the neck) that passes into other large blood vessels. There are many different types of central line catheters that may have multiple ports or lumens. Multiple ports allow more than one IV solution to be given simultaneously. Blood can also be withdrawn from this type of catheter.

CT scan: a series of detailed pictures of areas inside the body taken from different angles. The pictures are created by a computer linked to an X-ray machine; also called a CAT scan, computed tomography scan, and computerized axial tomography.

Echocardiogram (echo): a test of the strength and function of the heart. The test is done using an ultrasound machine. A clear jelly is placed on the child's chest. The technician will move a small round probe (transducer) around on the chest. This probe sends sound waves to the heart, and the returning sound waves create a picture of the heart.

Electrocardiogram (ECG or EKG): a method of evaluating heart rhythms and muscle functions by the measure of the heart's electrical impulses.

Febrile: fever; raised body temperature.

Gallium scan: a test that uses a radioactive material called gallium to look for swelling (inflammation), infection, or cancer in the body.

Glomerular filtration rate: a test used to check how well the kidneys are working. Specifically, it estimates how much blood passes through the tiny filters in the kidneys, called glomeruli, each minute.

Graft vs. Host Disease (GVH or GVHD): the condition that results when the immune cells of a transplant (usually of hematopoietic stem cells) from a donor attack the tissues of the person receiving the transplant.

Insuflon® catheter: This is a small soft tube placed into the fatty tissue (subcutaneous tissue) of the body. Some children need to receive repeated shots of medicine into their subcutaneous tissue. Instead of having to get several pokes into the skin, this small soft tube can be placed into the fatty tissue of the body. Then, the injections that would normally be given through the skin can be placed into this tube instead.

Intrathecal: describes the fluid-filled space between the thin layers of tissue that covers the brain and spinal cord. Medicine can be injected into the fluid, or a sample of the fluid can be removed for testing. Chemotherapy given intrathecally can kill cancer cells throughout the brain and spinal cord.

Intravenous (IV): the administration of a drug or fluid directly into the vein.

Lumbar puncture: a procedure in which a thin needle is placed in the spinal cord to withdraw a small amount of spinal fluid or to give medicine into the central nervous system through the spinal fluid. Also called a spinal tap.

Magnetic Resonance Imaging (MRI): a method of taking pictures of the inside of the body. Instead of using X-rays, MRI uses a powerful magnet and transmits radio waves through the body; the images appear on a computer screen as well as on film. As with X-rays, the procedure is physically painless, but some people may find it psychologically uncomfortable to be inside the MRI machine.

Mucositus: Oral mucositus is an inflammation or an ulceration of the mucous membranes of the surface of the inside of the mouth (e.g., the lips, tongue, and palate).

Nasogastic insertion: By inserting a nasogastric tube, access is gained to the stomach and its contents. This enables drainage of gastric contents, decompression of the stomach, or obtaining a specimen of the gastric contents.

Neutropenia: less than the normal number of neutrophils (infection-controlling white blood cells) in the circulating blood.

PET scan (positron emission tomography scan): PET scans look for tumor activity in the body. They can also show infections or inflammations. A PET scan is done by injecting a small amount of radioactive isotrope or tracer into a vein. The tracer travels to places in the body where there is tumor activity. After the tracer is injected, the child needs to lie very still on the scanner table while pictures are being taken. Sometimes there are special dietary instructions to follow, and there may be additional instructions if sedation is required.

Remission: complete or partial disappearance of the signs and symptoms of cancer in response to treatment; the period during which a disease is under control. A remission may not be a cure.

Ultrasound: an imaging method in which high-frequency sound waves are used to outline a part of the body. The procedure can be done to any part of the body—the presence, progression or regression of a tumor or infection can be monitored in this way. Also called ultrasonography.

X-rays: one form of radiation that can be used at low levels to produce an image of the body on film or at high levels to destroy cancer cells.

References

Aasgaard, T. (2000). 'A suspiciously cheerful lady.' A study of a song's life in the pediatric oncology ward, and beyond. *British Journal of Music Therapy, 14*(2), 70–82.

Aasgaard, T. (2002). Song creations by children with cancer: Process and meaning. Unpublished doctoral dissertation. Aalborg University, Denmark.

Aasgaard, T., & Edwards, M. (2012). Children expressing themselves. In A. Goldman, R. Hain, & S. Liben (Eds.), *Oxford textbook of palliative care for children* (pp. 100–107). Oxford: OUP.

Abad, V. (2003). A time of turmoil: Music therapy interventions for adolescents in a pediatric oncology ward. *Australian Journal of Music Therapy, 14,* 20–37.

Baggott, C. R., Kelly, K. P., Fochtman, D., & Foley, G. V. (2011). *Nursing care of children & adolescents with cancer* (4th ed.). Philadelphia: W. B. Saunders.

Barnes, C., Downie, P., Chalkiadis, G., Camilleri, S., Monagle, P., & Waters, K. (2002). Sedation practices for Australian and New Zealand pediatric oncology patient. *Journal of Paediatric Child Health, 38,* 170–172.

Barrera, M., Rykov, M., & Doyle, S. (2002). The effects of interactive music therapy on hospitalized children with cancer: A pilot study. *Psycho-Oncology, 11*(5), 379–388.

Barry, P., O'Callaghan, C., Wheeler, G., & Grocke, D. (2010). Music therapy CD creation for initial pediatric radiation therapy: A mixed methods analysis. *Journal of Music Therapy, 47*(3), 233–263.

Blount, R. L., Piira, T., Cohen, L. L., & Cheng, P. S. (2006). Pediatric procedural pain. *Behavior Modification, 30,* 24–49.

Boldt, S. (1996). The effects of music therapy on motivation, psychological well-being, physical comfort and exercise endurance of bone marrow transplant patients. *Journal of Music Therapy, 33*(3), 164–188.

Brodsky, W. (1989). Music therapy as an intervention for children with cancer in isolation rooms. *Music Therapy, 8*(1), 17–34.

Bruscia, K. E. (1987). Improvisational models of music therapy. Springfield, IL: Charles C. Thomas.

Bufalini, A. (2009). Role of interactive music in oncological pediatric patients undergoing painful procedures. *Minerva Pediatrica, 61*(4), 379–389.

Burns, D. S., Robb, S. L., & Haase, J. E. (2009). Exploring the feasibility of a therapeutic music video intervention in adolescents and young adults during stem-cell transplantation. *Cancer Nursing, 32*(5), E8.

Daveson, B. (2001). Music therapy and childhood cancer: Goals, methods, patient choice and control during diagnosis, intensive treatment, transplant and palliative care. *Music Therapy Perspectives, 19,* 114–120.

Davis, W., Gfeller, K., & Thaut, M. (2008). *An introduction to music therapy: Theory and practice* (3rd ed.). Silver Spring, MD: American Music Therapy Association.

DeGraves, S., & Aranda, S. (2008). Living with hope and fear the uncertainty of childhood cancer after relapse. *Cancer Nursing, 31*(4), 292.

Douglass, E. T. (2006). The development of a music therapy assessment tool for hospitalized children. *Music Therapy Perspectives, 24*(2), 73–80.

Dun, B. (1999). Creativity and communication: Aspects of music therapy in a children's hospital. In D. Aldridge (Ed.), *Music therapy in palliative care: New voices.* Philadelphia, PA: Jessica Kingsley.

Dun, B. (2001). Journeying with Olivia: Bricolage as a framework for understanding music therapy in paediatric oncology. *Voices: A World Forum for Music Therapy, 7,* 1.

Dun, B. (2011). All in Good Time: A music therapist's reflection of providing a music therapy program in a pediatric cancer center over 20 years. *Music and Medicine, 3*(1), 15–19.

Ghetti, C., & Walker, J. (2009). Hematology, oncology, and bone marrow transplant. In D. Hanson-Abromeit & C. Colwell (Eds.), *Medical music therapy for pediatrics in hospital settings* (pp. 147–194). Silver Spring, MD: American Music Therapy Association.

Grocke, D. E., & Wigram, T. (2007). *Receptive methods in music therapy. Techniques and clinical applications for music therapy clinicians, educators and students.* Philadelphia, PA: Jessica Kingsley.

Hadley, S. (1996). A rationale for the use of songs with children undergoing bone marrow transplantation. *Australian Journal of Music Therapy, 7,* 16–27.

Hedstrom, M., Haglund, K., Skolin, I., & von Essen, L. (2003). Distressing events for children and adolescents with cancer: Child, parent, and nurse perceptions. *Journal of Pediatric Oncology Nursing, 20,* 120–132.

Hilliard, R. E. (2006). Music therapy in pediatric oncology: A review of the literature. *Journal of the Society of Integrative Oncology, 4*(2), 75–78.

Hirst, S. (2009). *Developing a best practice and sustainable service model for future bone marrow transplant services.* RCH Children's Cancer Centre Bone marrow transplant service. Future service model. Melbourne: Royal Children's Hospital.

Hirst, S. (2009). *Strengthening services for children with cancer and their families from a culturally and linguistically diverse (CALD) background.* Summary report. Pediatric Integrated Cancer Services. Melbourne: Royal Children's Hospital.

Hockenberry, M. J. (1988). Relaxation techniques in children with cancer: The nurse's role. *Journal of the Association of Pediatric Oncology Nursing, 5*(1, 2), 7–11.

Jacob, E., Hesselgrave, J., Sambuco, G., & Hockenberry, M. (2007). Variations in pain, sleep, and activity during hospitalization in children with cancer. *Journal of Pediatric Oncology Nursing, 24,* 208–219.

Kazak, A., Rourke, M., Alderfer, M., Pai, A., Reilly, A., & Meadows, A. (2007). Evidence-based assessment, intervention and psychosocial care in pediatric oncology: A blueprint for comprehensive services across treatment. *Journal of Pediatric Psychology, 32*(9), 1099–1110.

Kennelly, J. (1999). Don't give up providing music therapy to an adolescent boy in the bone marrow transplant unit. In R. Pratt & D. Erdonmez Grocke (Eds.), *Music Medicine 3. Music medicine and music therapy: Expanding horizons* (pp. 228–235). Melbourne: University of Melbourne.

Kennelly, J. (2001). Music therapy in the bone marrow transplant unit: Providing emotional support during adolescence. *Music Therapy Perspectives, 19*(2), 104–108.

Kupst, M. (1992). Long-term family coping with acute lymphoblastic leukemia in childhood. In A. M. La Greca, L. J. Siegel, J. L. Wallander, & C. E. Walker (Eds.), Stress and coping in child health. New York: Guilford.

Lane, D. (1996). Music therapy interventions with pediatric oncology patients. In M. A. Froehlich (Ed.), *Music therapy with hospitalized children: A creative arts child life approach* (pp. 109–116). Cherry Hill, NJ: Jeffrey Books.

Ledger, A. (2001). Song parody for adolescents with cancer. *Australian Journal of Music Therapy, 12,* 21–28.

McFerran, K., & Wigram, T. (2010). *Adolescents, music and music therapy: Methods and techniques for clinicians, educators and students.* Philadelphia, PA: Jessica Kingsley.

Munet-Vilaro, F. (2004). Delivery of culturally competent care to children with cancer and their families—The Latino experience. *Journal of Pediatric Oncology Nursing, 2,* 155–159.

Murphy, K. (Ed.). (2011). *Family handbook for children with cancer* (2nd ed.). The Children's Oncology Group.

Nguyen, T., Nilsson, S., Hellström, A., & Bengtson, A. (2010). Music therapy to reduce pain and anxiety in children with cancer undergoing lumbar puncture: A randomized clinical trial. *Journal of Pediatric Oncology Nursing, 27*(3), 146–155.

O'Callaghan, C., Baron, A., Barry, P., & Dun, B. (2011). Music's relevance for pediatric cancer patients: A constructivist and mosaic research approach. *Supportive Care in Cancer, 19*(6), 779–788.

O'Callaghan, C, Sexton, M., & Wheeler, G. (2007). Music therapy as a nonpharmacological anxiolytic for pediatric radiation therapy patients. *Australasian Radiology, 51,* 159–162.

O'Callaghan, C., Barry, P., & Thompson, K. (2012). Music's relevance for adolescents and young adults with cancer: A constructivist research approach. *Supportive Care in Cancer,* 1–11.

O'Neill, N., & Pavlicevic, M. (2003). What am I doing here?: Exploring a role for music therapy with children undergoing bone marrow transplantation at Great Ormond Street Hospital, London. *British Journal of Music Therapy, 17*(1), 8–16.

Pfaff, V. K., Smith, K. E., & Gowan, D. (1989). The effects of music-assisted relaxation on the distress of pediatric cancer patients undergoing bone marrow aspirations. *Children's Health Care, 18*(4), 232–236.

Phipps, S., Peasant, C., Barrera, M., Alderfer, M., Huang, Q., & Vannatta, K. (2012). Resilience in children undergoing stem cell transplantation: Results of a complementary intervention trial. *Pediatrics,* 129, e762–e770.

Robb, S. L. (2000). The effect of therapeutic music interventions on the behavior of hospitalized children in isolation: Developing a contextual support model of music therapy. *Journal of Music Therapy, 37,* 118–146.

Robb, S. L. (2003). Designing music therapy interventions for hospitalized children and adolescents using a contextual support model of music therapy. *Music Therapy Perspectives, 21,* 27–39.

Robb, S. L., Clair, A. A., Watanabe, M., Monohan, P. O., Azzouz, F., & Stouffer, J. W., et al. (2008). Randomized controlled trial of the active music engagement (AME) intervention on children with cancer. *Psycho-Oncology, 1*(7), 699–708.

Robb, S. L., & Ebberts, A. G. (2003a). Songwriting and digital video production interventions for pediatric patients undergoing bone marrow transplantation, part I: An analysis of depression and anxiety levels according to phase of treatment. *Journal of Pediatric Oncology Nursing, 20*(1), 2–15.

Robb, S. L., & Ebberts, A. (2003b). Songwriting and digital video production interventions for pediatric patients undergoing bone marrow transplantation, part II: An analysis of patient-generated songs and patient perceptions regarding intervention efficacy. *Journal of Pediatric Oncology Nursing, 20*(1), 16–25.

Rubin-Bosco, J. (2002). Resolution vs. re-enactment: A story song approach to working with trauma. In J. Loewy & A. Hara (Eds.), *Caring for the caregiver: The use of music and music therapy in grief and trauma* (pp. 118–127). Silver Spring, MD: American Music Therapy Association.

Sahler, O. J., Hunter, B. C., & Liesveld, J. L. (2003). The effect of using music therapy with relaxation imagery in the management of patients undergoing bone marrow transplantation: A pilot feasibility study. *Alternative Therapies in Health and Medicine, 9*(6), 70–74.

Särkämö, T., & Soto, D. (2012). Music listening after stroke: Beneficial effects and potential neural mechanisms. *Annals of the New York Academy of Sciences, 1252,* 266–281.

Snyder Cowan, D. (1997). Managing sickle cell pain with music therapy. In J. Loewy (Ed.), Music therapy and pediatric pain (pp. 115–123). Cherry Hill, NJ: Jeffrey Books.

Standley, J. M. (1996). Music research in medical/dental treatment: An update of a prior meta-analysis. In C. Furman (Ed.), *Effectiveness of music therapy procedures: Documentation of research and clinical practice* (2nd ed., pp. 1–60). Silver Spring, MD: National Association for Music Therapy.

Standley, J. M., & Hanser, S. B. (1995). Music therapy research and applications in pediatric oncology treatment. *Journal of Pediatric Oncology Nursing, 12*(1), 3–8.

Stewart, J. (2003). "Getting used to it": Children finding the ordinary and routine in the uncertain context of cancer. *Qualitative Health Research, 13*(3), 394–407.

Sweeney, C. (2003). "Couldn't put Humpty together again": Symbolic play with a terminally ill child. In S. Hadley (Ed.), *Psychodynamic music therapy: Case studies.* Gilsum, NH: Barcelona Publishers.

Taylor, L., Reeves, C., McCart, M., Bushardt, R., Jensen, S., Elkin, T., Borntrager, C., Brown, R., Simpson, K., & Boll, T. (2007). A preliminary investigation of cognitive late effects and the impact of disease versus treatment among pediatric brain tumor patients. *Children's Health Care, 36*(4), 373–384.

Thibodeaux, A., & Deatrick, J. (2007). Cultural influence on family management of children with cancer. *Journal of Pediatric Oncology Nursing, 24,* 227–233.

Turry, A. (1999). A song of life: Improvised songs with children with cancer and serious blood disorders. In T. Wigram, & J. De Backer (Eds.), *Clinical applications of music therapy in developmental disability, pediatrics and neurology* (pp. 13–31). Philadelphia, PA: Jessica Kingsley.

Turry, A., & Turry, A. E. (1999). Creative song improvisations with children and adults with cancer. In C. Dileo (Ed.), *Music therapy and medicine: Theoretical and clinical applications* (pp. 167–178). Silver Spring, MD: The American Music Therapy Association, Inc.

Winnicott, D. W. (1971). *Playing and reality.* London: Tavistock.

Chapter 9

Palliative and End-of-Life Care for Children

Kathryn Lindenfelser

*"I'd like to sing about the angels that came last night
to tell me I don't have to go through this anymore,"
said eight-year-old Maria.* (Lindenfelser, 2011)

Providing music therapy for children or adolescents diagnosed with a life-limiting condition and their families can be a way of altering the perception of the situation, enhancing communication and expression (Amadoru & McFerran, 2007; Lindenfelser, Grocke, & McFerran, 2008), improving the child's physical state, and fostering positive experiences (Lindenfelser, Hense, & McFerran, 2012). In many instances, music therapy also brings hope to what may be a horrifying experience for a family facing the possible death of a child because it provides a new avenue for meaningful communication, addressing pain, nurturing relationships, and creating a legacy. Because of the uncertainty related to the prognosis of many pediatric conditions that are life-limiting, children and families are searching for ways to keep hope alive and to continue living in the midst of letting go. We continue to learn more about the impact that music therapy has at this crucial time in a family's life.

Music therapy has been integrated in North America as a service for adults receiving palliative or end-of-life care for several decades (Munro & Mount, 1978). It is in more recent years, however, that palliative care has been provided to children and their families (Behrman & Field, 2003). Evidence is growing to demonstrate that music therapy is a valued service within the continuum of care for children and families in this setting (Knapp, Madden, Wang, Curtis, Sloyer, & Shenkman, 2009; Lindenfelser et al., 2008, 2012). As the needs of children and families become better defined and understood within this context, it becomes clearer how to provide music therapy.

This chapter includes clinical examples from my own clinical practice with infants, children, and teens receiving palliative and end-of-life care in the hospital, hospice, or home environment and their families. As a clinician and researcher, I find that the growing research in this setting supports the experiences I have witnessed of music therapy inspiring a child who has not spoken or responded for months to begin to smile and vocalize. The studies that are mainly qualitative are bringing validity to the inclusion of music therapy in this setting. Because children may be near the end-of-life for so many different reasons and with a wide array of conditions, there are no limits to how a child or family may engage in music therapy at this time in life.

DIAGNOSTIC INFORMATION

Pediatric Palliative Care

Pediatric palliative care refers to the philosophy of caring for or comforting a child living with a progressive, life-threatening or life-limiting illness as well as his family by providing physical, emotional, spiritual, and psychosocial comfort (Knapp & Contro, 2009; World Health Organization, 2012). "Palliative" means to care or to comfort as opposed to cure, as well as to enhance quality of life in the midst of a life-limiting condition (American Academy of Pediatrics, 2000). It aims to maintain and improve quality of life, not just in the dying stages, but in the weeks, months, and years before death (Gilmer, 2002; World Health Organization, 2012). Palliative care for children and young people is an active and total approach to care. It consists of managing pain and symptoms, offering emotional and spiritual support, providing respite (restful) care, and supporting the family through bereavement.

End-of-Life or Hospice Care

In our culture, we use the term "hospice" care when it has been determined by a medical doctor that a person has six months or less to live and when the patient or family feels ready to forgo any additional curative treatments that will prolong life. Often families that care for a child who has a life-limiting condition are hesitant to transition to hospice care and choose to continue receiving treatment of some sort through the end-of-life. The care provided to a child at the end-of-life and his family may look similar to a child receiving palliative care in that holistic care is being provided. The difference often relates to how the care is being billed and covered by the child's insurance provider or Medicaid, which is a benefit provided by the state for families who are eligible. Ultimately, the goal of end-of-life and hospice care is similar to palliative care, ensuring that the child and family are receiving pain and symptom management, emotional and spiritual support, and support following the death of a child through bereavement. The difference is that a child on palliative care is often receiving some type of treatment and a child who is on "hospice" is no longer receiving treatments other than those to maintain comfort addressing the symptoms that are arising.

Life-Limiting Conditions

Children die from a variety of causes. If a diagnosis is made and it is believed by the medical team that the condition will shorten the child's life so that the child will most likely not live until adulthood, the condition is considered to be life-limiting. Life-limiting conditions are those for which long-term survival is a challenge; there is no reasonable hope of a cure and a young person is likely to die prior to adulthood (Liben, Papadatou, & Wolfe, 2008). It may be difficult, however, to predict when or in what manner the death may occur.

Life-limiting conditions cover a wide spectrum of conditions, including neurologic, muscular, metabolic, cardiac, renal, immunologic, oncologic, gastrointestinal, and chromosomal, of which four broad groups may be identified (Armstrong-Dailey & Zarbock, 2010; Goldman, 1998; Hynson & Sawyer, 2001):

> 1) Life-threatening conditions for which curative treatment may be feasible but can fail (i.e., cancer, irreversible organ failure of heart, liver, kidney).

2) Conditions where premature death is inevitable but where there may be long periods of intense treatment aimed at prolonging life and allowing participation in normal activities (i.e., *cystic fibrosis*, malignancies, HIV/AIDS).

3) Progressive conditions without curative treatment options, where treatment is exclusively palliative and may commonly extend over many years (i.e., neurodegenerative, metabolic diseases such as *Batten's disease, mucopolysaccharidoses, Muscular Dystrophy, Spinal Muscular Atrophy*).

4) Irreversible but nonprogressive conditions causing severe disability leading to susceptibility to health complications and the likelihood of premature death (i.e., severe cerebral palsy, multiple disabilities such as following brain or spinal cord injuries).

Each year in the United States, approximately 500,000 children cope with a life-limiting illness (Huang, Shenkman, Madden, Vadaparampil, Quinn, & Knapp, 2010). Of these 500,000 children, approximately 50,000 die. More than half of these deaths are within the first year of the child's life, while an additional 8% of the remaining deaths are from prolonged illnesses (Hinds, Schum, Baker, & Wolfe, 2005).

Adult Palliative Care vs. Pediatric Palliative Care

It is important to consider the differences between adult palliative care and pediatric palliative care. These differences lend reason to why clinical training and provision of services differ as well. Caring for a child requires a different set of skills than that for the care of an adult. Some of the reasons why the model for adult palliative and end-of-life care differs from the model of care for children are as follows (Children's Hospice International, 2010; Friebert, 2009):

- Childhood diseases are often treated as aggressively as possible, with the overall goal of extending the life of the child as much as possible at any cost.
- Parents identify the point of diagnosis as the most devastating time of emotional/spiritual adjustment, and often desire to do everything possible to extend the child's life.
- Families often experience undue stress due to strained finances, yet are in need of physical and emotional relief and respite from the challenges of daily cares for their child.
- The expertise and skills involved with children (developmental issues/needs, medication dosages, etc.) are not inherent in the skill base of staff who care predominantly for an elderly population.
- Reimbursement, not best clinical practice nor what is often in the best interest of the child, drives choices made available to children/parents/guardians. Access to reimbursement for pediatric palliative and end-of-life care is changing in the United States. The provision of reimbursement for services differs between pediatric and adult populations.

These reasons correlate with the sometimes unmet needs in pediatric palliative care such as the need for financial assistance, more in-depth psychosocial/emotional support for families, including siblings, respite care, and prolonged bereavement (Friebert, 2009; Knapp, Madden, Curtis, Sloyer, & Shenkman, 2010). Support for children and families continues to be developed as unique needs are identified as well as tools to adequately measure and improve quality of life (Huanet al., 2010).

The conditions and symptoms vary greatly from child to child within the context of pediatric palliative and hospice care. Sometimes the prognosis of a given condition is unknown because of the rarity of many pediatric life-limiting conditions. When providing music therapy within this context, it is important to meet the needs of each individual child and family. New and unfamiliar symptoms often arise and there are often unique considerations. Ultimately, inviting and finding ways to involve and support the family is central to pediatric palliative and end-of-life care.

NEEDS AND RESOURCES

Focus on Family-Centered Care

The family is at the core of the interdisciplinary team caring for a child who is receiving palliative or end-of-life care (Knapp & Contro, 2009). To know that a child may die is considered one of the most devastating experiences (Hinds et al., 2005; Kubler-Ross, 1983). The stress of such a diagnosis jolts a family with uncertainty, unexpected challenges, and changes in routines and wishes (Knapp & Contro, 2009). While the stress may lessen over time as a family establishes a new norm, fear, sadness, and worry often remain. Thus there are unique challenges presented to health care providers in order to best support families (Gilmer, 2002).

Families' lives may be enhanced when services are integrated early on during the course of a child's diagnosis (Gilmer, 2002). Pediatric palliative care, therefore, aims to involve the child and family in the decision-making process and to evaluate together the best approach to care and treatment (Goldfarb, Devine, Yingling, Hill, Moss, Ogburn, & Roberts, 2010). The advantages of providing support to the whole family are great if and when available (Hynso & Sawyer, 2001; Knapp et al., 2010). In order to meet a family's needs, it is important to understand the family dynamics and cultural background in order to provide effective communication and support (Gilmer, 2002).

Loss of Control

With the diagnosis of a condition that may be life-limiting, life changes dramatically for a family. Families often experience a loss of control on many levels (Burgess, 1994). This loss of control may be related to the family's value and belief system (Bartell & Kissane, 2005). For example, a family's spiritual belief may be questioned or challenged. Beliefs that were firm and clear to a family one day may no longer provide the same comfort. A family may also struggle with significant and often unpredictable changes in their child over the course of the illness, including the child's loss of physical abilities. Furthermore, many changes take place within family dynamics as well as within relationships with others, as the child and family may not be able to participate in the same ways they had been in their community. Finally, there is the loss of a potential future that the family had envisioned with the child (Burgess, 1994). It is important, therefore, for the health care team to facilitate opportunities for families to maintain a sense of control. In order to lessen the experience of loss that the child feels himself, it is important to encourage the child to participate as much as possible in daily activities, to attend school, and to engage with friends and family. By acknowledging the child and family's desires and needs, the experience of loss of control may be reduced.

Communication

Communicating openly about the child's situation and diagnosis assists in reducing the experience of loss of control and allows children and families to cope and be involved through the dramatic changes of illness and death. Adequate communication also helps to reduce feelings of isolation, anger, and anxiety that children may feel in regard to their condition (Faulkner, 2001). Children typically have questions and concerns about dying, and it is important for children to be validated and acknowledged in their quest for information (Doka, 1995). Certainly it is important to consider the child's developmental stage, emotional response and temperament, and wishes when determining the timing and content to be shared about the child's prognosis and reality of potential death (Behrman & Field, 2003). Children have their own sense of what is happening and are aware of nonverbal cues from caregivers and family members, and may become angry and isolated when truth is not shared. Ultimately, it is easiest for children and families to adjust and cope when their questions are answered as honestly and compassionately as possible (Kubler-Ross, 1983).

Leaving Legacies

Providing opportunities for children to leave a legacy may be empowering at the end of life (Behrman & Field, 2003). Music therapists have the unique ability to assist with this, as it is through the creation of videos, songs, journals, and pictures that children and families are able to create memories together that continue the child's legacy. Such projects provide an outlet for expression and intimacy at the end of life (Behrman & Field, 2003). Additionally, it is through nonverbal communication during the creation of art, music, and play that death can be explored (Faulkner, 2001). As children and families create legacies together, the child may feel empowered in regard to his own death and feel reassurance that he is loved and cared for, that his pain will be managed, and that family and friends will be present (Faulkner, 2001). In interviewing bereaved parents about their experiences of music therapy when their child was terminally ill, many parents shared legacy projects such as songs written for or by the child who was dying and stated that these serve as a significant component of remembrance (Lindenfelser et al., 2008). These ways of keeping the child's memory alive help parents to maintain their connection to their child (Woodgate, 2006) and continue to bond to their child (Klass, Nickman, & Silverman, 1996).

Multicultural Considerations

The cultural identity of the family impacts the interplay of dialogue and decision-making related to care and treatment options for a child with a life-limiting condition. Honoring and respecting cultural beliefs, rituals, and traditions helps to establish a trusting relationship. The following are some areas to consider and to investigate when working with families in the pediatric palliative and end-of-life care setting.

Religious beliefs. Depending on the religious background of the family, the conversation related to the child having a condition that is life-limiting may be more challenging to have. In the Muslim faith, for example, death is not spoken of until it happens. The provision of palliative care is still possible as palliative care is the affirmation of life (Gilmer, 2002), yet the discussion with the family may center on the possibilities for treatment rather than the emotional and spiritual support provided considering that the child's life span may be short. Families are often willing to share what their religious beliefs are and how they prefer to receive support based on their beliefs. It is important to note, however, that immigrant families from countries where they may have been prosecuted for their religious beliefs may be cautious in sharing their beliefs even with clinical staff. It is important to assure families that their beliefs are respected and that they will not be judged or treated any differently.

Religious beliefs are identified in intake forms when a child is first admitted to receive palliative or end-of-life services. A chaplain or spiritual care provider is typically involved with the interdisciplinary team and available to provide support so that religious or spiritual beliefs and values are honored. A Catholic family, for example, may wish to have their priest provide spiritual care, so the chaplain may contact the family's priest to provide support and to administer specific sacraments related to the Catholic faith. It is important not to confuse religious affiliation and belief in a deity with spirituality. Families who do not have a specific religious affiliation or who identify with atheism or agnostic beliefs may find as much comfort in receiving spiritual support as families with strong religious beliefs. Many families may question why such a situation has come upon them or why God would allow for such suffering. These questions are often shared and discussed with a spiritual care provider or chaplain. While the chaplain may not have specific answers, the opportunity to ask such questions can be helpful.

Acknowledging questions related to finding meaning and feeling helpless within the context of religious beliefs is vital. As Gilmer (2002) states, "one task of the palliative care providers is to learn to live with the dualism of meaning and meaninglessness and to listen with well-trained ears to the spiritual anguish of families without using religious platitudes in an effort to comfort them" (p. 211). In music therapy, we can be present to the uncertainty and simultaneous search for meaning and hope.

Gender roles. The voice and perspective of each family member, regardless of age or gender, is honored within a family-centered approach. Within some cultures, however, the male or female gender may be more dominant. It may be that discussion and decisions take place within the family but are communicated back to the clinical team by one family member who represents the voice for the whole family. The music therapist should be respectful of these roles even if it conflicts with their own personal values or cultural norms.

Language. When a family's first language is a language other than that of the clinical team, it is imperative to involve an interpreter. Ensuring that information around the child's condition and the family's needs are understood requires that language is not a barrier. The first step in any relationship, including one that is centered on the care of a child and family, is to ensure that information and communication is accessible. This is essential in building a trusting relationship among all involved.

While music is considered a universal language and can often speak through language barriers, it is always important to invite an interpreter to the music therapy sessions for families who do not speak English fluently. This is important to ensure that key emotions or needs expressed are understood correctly. There are times when the child speaks fluent English, yet other family members do not. It is not appropriate in these cases to rely on the child as the interpreter. This puts unnecessary responsibility and pressure on the child. Depending on the setting, most palliative care programs have access to companies that provide interpretation both over the phone and during visits.

Considering multicultural needs and desires honors the uniqueness of each family and celebrates their identity. The aspects of multiculturalism described above provide opportunities for clinicians to consider how they can provide the best care possible while honoring the family's history, culture, and beliefs. The period leading up to the death of a child provides opportunities for families to identify and rely on their strengths. Spiritual beliefs, for example, are often strengthened and assist a family in finding a level of acceptance and renewed hope. Music therapists have the opportunity to provide music interventions that heighten families' awareness of their strengths.

REFERRAL AND ASSESSMENT PROCEDURES

Music therapy sessions with a child who has a life-limiting condition and his family may take place at a number of locations including the hospital, home, children's residential hospice facility, or the school. Typically, children receiving palliative or end-of-life care will only attend school when they are feeling physically up to it, though this may differ from child to child depending on the importance of maintaining a "normal" routine. Each setting requires the music therapist to correspond with a number of individuals, including other family members, clinicians, or teachers.

Because the conditions of children with life-limiting conditions can change in a moment, it is essential to respond very quickly to a referral. Daveson and Kennelly (2000) and McFerran and Hogan (2005) point out the necessity of collaborating with other clinicians and responding to referrals in a timely manner in order to develop and implement effective music therapy services.

The assessment and referral process may look different depending on the setting where the music therapy sessions will take place. For example, the music therapist may need to consider whether or not other family members will be present, what session times will best meet the needs of the child and family, the timing of medical treatments, and working around school routines.

Hospital

In the hospital environment, there is often a clear process for receiving a music therapy referral, typically from another clinician such as a nurse, child family life specialist, doctor, or social worker. Following receipt of the referral, which documents why the referring clinician believes that music therapy will be beneficial for the child/family, the music therapist will complete an assessment. Some hospitals have a predetermined assessment form for each discipline, while others will expect the music therapist to create an assessment form. Information for the assessment may be gathered from the child's medical chart, from talking with the clinicians who are currently caring for the child in the hospital, and from family members present upon introduction of the service. The timing of a session in the hospital usually depends on other treatments that are being provided and is worked into a semistructured routine agreed upon by the interdisciplinary team.

Home Care

The child who is receiving palliative or end-of-life care in the home may or may not be receiving this from a home care agency connected with the pediatric hospital where the child receives inpatient care. The presence of such connection will determine the amount of information already available to the music therapist. In either case, a new referral is typically needed in order to make a music therapy visit in the home. A referral will most likely be made in writing and received via email since clinicians providing home care are in the field rather than working out of one facility. This is usually followed up with a phone call confirming receipt and answering any questions the music therapist may have prior to visiting the child and family in their home. Home care visits require consideration for the appropriate timing of the session. For example, the parents or guardians may work, yet may wish to be home during the time of the visit. Sometimes families may wish for siblings to be included. In addition, the music therapist needs to consider the child's daily routine at home. It is important that the assessment capture this information to assist with future scheduling.

School

A music therapy referral in the school setting may be received from the child's teacher, nurse, social worker, paraprofessional, or parent. The timing of a music therapy session at school is typically integrated into the overall schedule of the school day and may or may not be the ideal time for providing music therapy for the child. This requires the music therapist to respond creatively to the needs of the child and to integrate music therapy goals as appropriate. Often, music therapy goals for a child with a life-limiting condition in the school setting are quite different compared to the other settings. For example, for a child with an Individualized Education Plan (IEP), the music therapy goals will likely relate to IEP goals that focus on academic skills, activities of daily living, or communication skills. In contrast, music therapy goals in other settings typically relate more to the emotional, spiritual, or physical needs of the child and family.

Residential Pediatric Palliative Respite/Hospice Home

There are a growing number of homes in the United States where children with life-limiting conditions may stay with their family for a short stay, called a "respite stay," to have a break from the 24/7 care routine or where they may be cared for as a family while the child is in the dying process. Typically, each child will automatically be referred for music therapy upon their admission whether it be for a short respite visit or for end-of-life care. Information for the assessment may be drawn from the clinicians and care providers who admitted the child and/or documentation from previous respite stays, as well as from the family. In the case where a child is actively dying in the hospice home, the music therapist will most likely offer music and assess the needs in the moment. For a child who visits the home for respite stays periodically, it is important to reassess because the child's needs and abilities may change drastically between each visit as their disease or diagnosis progresses.

Considering the Child and Family

It is important that the music therapy assessment of a child who has a life-limiting condition also involve assessment of the family's coping and family dynamics. For example, sometimes the child or young adult acquires the emotional state of a parent or sibling, whether that involves feeling at peace, panicked, depressed, or afraid. On the other hand, children have a way of holding on to their own emotional or spiritual state and impact that of other family members. For example, it is not uncommon to hear family members say "I am so angry and sad, but can see that he is peaceful and that brings me peace" or "She is so strong and that makes me feel strong." Because a child's emotional state can impact that of other family members and vice versa, it is imperative to have a clear understanding of each family member's emotions in order to enhance the music therapy experience. The assessment of physical and cognitive needs typically centers on the child's needs, yet it is important to consider family members' needs in these areas as well. Due to the stress involved in caring for a child who has a life-limiting condition, it is common for parents and other family members to be dealing with their own physical or cognitive issues. For example, family members may be dealing with headaches, migraines, constipation, or even more serious issues that arise because of stress. When family members have difficulty articulating their wants or needs, integrating music without too much verbal dialogue in the assessment may be helpful as the assessment will continue to occur throughout the music.

Assessment of Emotional State

Children who are receiving palliative or end-of-life care, as well as their family members, may experience a wide array of emotions ranging from anger, frustration, fear, and anxiety to joy, peace, and calm. Some families may openly express their emotions, while others may not be readily able to share how they are feeling. The family's emotional expressivity typically impacts the child's willingness to express emotions himself. When assessing a child's emotional state, it is important to understand that disease symptoms may affect the child's ability to adequately communicate his emotional state. Therefore, it is essential not only to ask about emotions and to sing about them, but also to observe a child's facial affect for expression of fear, sadness, anger, or distress. This is especially important for children who are unable to verbally express themselves. This may be due to their developmental level, increase in medications, or impact of the disease progression on cognitive functioning, resulting in a different way of expressing and processing emotions.

Anxiety and fear. With many life-limiting conditions, there is a lot of uncertainty around the prognosis and the course the disease may take. For this reason, it can be difficult for a child and family to grasp what may be happening in the coming days, weeks, months, or years. This reality can evoke feelings of anxiety and fear. Fagen (1982) describes the fear that may be associated with hallucinations that may arise from large dosages of pain medications. Images described by children may be explored more willingly through music, and in turn the meaning of these images may bring comfort for both the child and the family. Children may also be more willing to explore through music any anxiety or fears they may have related to impending death. However, often the anxiety and fear are most felt by family members. For example, in providing music therapy for an infant with *Trisomy* who periodically stopped breathing, the parents and older brother stated how anxious they felt from moment to moment, always anticipating the baby's last breath. Music can help to transform anxiety and fear into comfort and even hope.

Depression. Children who were active and engaged in many activities until the symptoms of their illness began to take over may experience isolation, anger, and depression. Depression is often observed in children whose lives drastically change due to their diagnosis. Referrals are often made to music therapists to address depression because of the opportunities for self-expression through songwriting or song analysis. Hilliard (2003) describes a session with a young girl who was referred for music therapy due to depression. The music therapy sessions resulted in "exploration, discussion, and acknowledgement of the patient's positive attributes and abilities" (p. 36). Signs of depression should be reported to the interdisciplinary team so that the child can receive comprehensive treatment.

Anger. Anger can often easily be detected in a child or parents' posture, vocal tone, or behavior. Anger is easy to identify when it is expressed through outward behaviors such as hitting, swinging, or loud, vocal outbursts. However, sometimes a child or family member may internalize the anger and let it build up over time. Music therapy interventions can provide the opportunity for anger to be expressed safely. This is important, as it is difficult to address other emotions until the anger is able to be expressed.

Assessment of Physical State

Depending on the child's diagnosis, the child may have a variety of physical needs. It cannot be assumed that because a child has dealt with a life-limiting diagnosis for any amount of time they are either comfortable or in pain. A child's comfort impacts the child and family's quality of life and it is imperative to assess it at all times.

Pain. The ability of a child with a life-limiting condition to respond to questions related to pain or comfort can vary greatly. Some children will be able to verbally identify and state their level of comfort or pain. In these cases, the use of pain scales outlined in Chapter 2 is appropriate. However, many children with life-limiting conditions may have limited cognitive or verbal skills, so it may be difficult to know how the child is feeling physically. If the child is not verbal, due to having a *tracheotomy,* yet has highly attuned cognitive skills, using a graphic rating scale where the child is able to point may be appropriate. For children who are not able to communicate their level of pain, it is important to follow the pain assessment scale identified as best to use by the family and health care team. This will most likely be a passive observation scale that the clinician uses to rate how it appears the child is feeling. This often involves careful observations of the child's facial affect, posture, vocal sounds, and eye gaze. Because the experience or observation of pain is subjective, it is important to take each response seriously and to immediately report to other clinical team members if a child continues to experience pain during or following a music therapy visit.

Physical function. In most instances, a child's ability to function physically declines over time due to the child's diagnosis. The reality of declining physical abilities can be frustrating for a child who was physically capable prior to the disease. A decrease in a child's mobility often results in increased swelling or *edema* due to a decrease in circulation. Increased edema, in turn, can make it difficult for organs to function properly and may impact other physiological processes necessary for life. If a child experiences pain upon movement, his interest or motivation toward mobility may greatly decrease.

It is important to assess and evaluate any changes in the child's physical function, including all aspects of mobility. During music therapy, a child who is otherwise not moving independently may be inspired to make independent movements. Children may extend themselves physically in order to engage actively in making music, but may be quite exhausted at the end of the music therapy session. Because of music's motivational power, it is not uncommon for the music therapist and other interdisciplinary team members to notice extreme differences in physical functioning. For example:

A four-year-old girl with a terminal brain tumor was quite lethargic the last month of her life. It was difficult to arouse her to engage in any way, and the nurse and social worker reported that this little girl was no longer moving her arms or legs and slept during most of the day. However, during music therapy the little girl exerted herself and would swing her legs and arms to play the drum, stay awake for a half-hour session, and giggle throughout music therapy.

As a child nears the end-of-life, he may become tired easier and faster and may be more lethargic and even unresponsive. The smallest amounts of interaction and engagement can bring great joy and special memories for the child and family.

Shortness of breath. Shortness of breath can be symptomatic of pain, a slowing respiratory response due to decrease in circulation, or anxiety. When a child is near the end of life, breathing patterns change. It is important to notice the child's breathing pattern at the start of a music therapy session. If breathing appears to be labored or heavy, almost like panting, it is important to inform the nurse or medical doctor, as this may indicate a change in the child's condition. If the child is unable to indicate whether or not his shortness of breath or heavy breathing is due to pain, the family may be able to help evaluate whether this represents a change from the child's usual breathing pattern. In any case, music therapy can assist in regulating a child's breathing by entraining the breath to live music.

Assessment of Spiritual State

It is important to assess a child and family's spiritual well-being. Sometimes families' spiritual or religious beliefs provide great comfort for what they are experiencing, and other times families feel great anger toward once-held beliefs (Davies, 2002). As in all areas of care, it is important to be aware of our countertransferences or our own emotions in relation to those we are witnessing so that we do not mix our feelings and spiritual beliefs with the child's or family's. As discussed earlier in the chapter, it is important to understand a family's religious beliefs and values so that information is communicated adequately. Sometimes it can be difficult to know just how to assess a family's spirituality until music is chosen and shared in a session and dialogue begins. For example:

During musical improvisation and songwriting with a four-year-old child whose one-year old brother was receiving palliative care services due to a rare genetic condition, the four-year-old sang, "I'll be so sad when you die and I hope that you go to heaven." His mother cried and said she didn't realize the four-year-old had an understanding or beliefs around what was happening to his brother, as this was not something they had previously talked about.

Assessment of Cognitive State

Assessing a child's cognitive state involves understanding the child's developmental level and his level of alertness. A child's cognition can be impacted by medications or narcotics and may differ from visit to visit. The child's parents or caregivers are a good resource for assessment of this area of functioning. If the child is able to verbally communicate and functions at a developmental level appropriate for his age, it is appropriate to ask the child some questions related to his day or who came to visit him recently. Slurring in a child's speech can indicate changing cognition. A varying level of alertness may provide information related to the child's cognitive functioning as well. If a child is typically awake and alert and able to speak and interact, but is now lethargic, has slurred speech, and is unable to make eye contact, this may indicate a change in the child's cognitive state.

INTRODUCTION TO MUSIC THERAPY METHODS

Information gathered from the referral and assessment will inform the appropriate music therapy methods to be used (See Appendix A). A music therapist may encounter quite radical changes from session to session in a child's level of functioning and energy, especially if the duration between sessions is more than a few days. Prior to each session, it is important to review previously documented notes from other clinicians' visits and to inquire with the child's parent or caregiver to get a sense of the child's status on the day of the session.

Because of these rapid shifts in functioning and well-being, an assessment is conducted at each visit and provides information that will direct how the music therapy session progresses. For example, the child may have just received pain medication, which causes him to feel tired and not interested in completing the song he has been working on in previous sessions. In this case, it is important to be prepared with receptive music therapy interventions. Or, a child who is typically quiet and restful may have a burst of energy and be eager to engage in improvisation. In this case, having melodic and rhythmic instruments ready to meet the child's needs in the moment is vital.

Preparation. Before starting a music therapy session, it is important to begin each session by adequately preparing the space. This may include asking if the lighting in the room is comfortable for the child or family members and making any necessary changes such as opening or closing a curtain. The therapist should also check for any sources of sound that may be disruptive or distractive during the session. This may include turning of the television or radio or closing a door. Creating a space that is conducive to a child or family engaging in meaningful dialogue or feeling comfortable drumming and expressing anger or agitation or simply being able to fall asleep during the music is important.

Another important aspect in preparing for a session is ensuring that infection control procedures are followed. Each setting has its own infection control policies, so it is important to find out what these are prior to entering a space. The music therapist should wash her own hands either prior to entering or just upon entering the space where the session will take place. Also, the equipment and instruments need to be appropriately sanitized. This may involve wiping each instrument or tool with an antibacterial wipe. In the hospital setting, some children are considered to be in isolation due to their compromised immune system. This may require that a gown and gloves are worn during the session. This can make playing the guitar challenging, but still possible. Be sure to follow the procedures indicated.

What to observe. In determining which music therapy intervention would be most appropriate to use, it is important to observe at the beginning and throughout the music therapy session if the child is comfortable or in pain. Grimacing, tight facial muscles, or fists or cries, as well as the child's breathing pattern, should be noted. These observations will direct the intervention and may indicate a need to shift the musical elements so that the experience heightens the comfort of the child and/or family. It is also important to observe emotional expressions, whether they be tears and crying or smiles and giggles. Typically, if other family members are engaged in the session, each person may have a different emotional response as discussed earlier. In these cases, it is important to validate either vocally or through music that it is okay to feel and express emotions. One mother, when offered music therapy, stated that while she knew it would be beneficial for her son, it would make her emotionally vulnerable (Lindenfelser, Grocke, & McFerran, 2008). It is important to respect the willingness of children and families to express emotions, and while music therapy may be a joyful experience for one family, it may evoke emotions that feel uncomfortable to be expressed for others.

OVERVIEW OF MUSIC THERAPY METHODS AND PROCEDURES

An overview of music therapy methods and procedures included in this chapter are listed below. They are not listed in any particular order in terms of priority or frequency of use.

Receptive Music Therapy

- Live Music Listening: the use of live preferred familiar song or improvised music to build a therapeutic relationship, find meaning in the midst of a challenging situation, and validate and acknowledge feelings, values, and beliefs.
- Recorded Music Listening: listening to prerecorded music to increase the opportunity to make choices, express individuality, and increase comfort.
- Song Analysis: listening to a song and reflecting on the lyrics and elements of the music to assist the child and family in telling their story or assist in their search for meaning.
- Music-Guided Imagery for Relaxation: the use of music-guided imagery to enhance relaxation, self-awareness or to decrease pain and anxiety.

Improvisational Music Therapy

- Instrumental Improvisation: Instrumental improvisation allows children to express or communicate their feelings and thoughts in a novel way, and it helps to remind parents that their child is first and foremost a child, rather than focusing on their child as being sick and dying.
- Vocal Improvisation: improvising music with the voice to improve self-expression and providing opportunities for choice and control.
- Storytelling and Symbolic Play: This intervention uses stories and symbolic play through music and instruments to facilitate communication and expression of emotions, thoughts, and worries.

Re-creative Music Therapy

- Song Singing: singing familiar songs to normalize the experience and to validate children's interests and identity.

Compositional Music Therapy

- Songwriting: Songs written for, by, or with a child can help facilitate communication of the child's experiences and feelings and are often a treasured and tangible part for the family as they forever remember their child and find support from the songs through bereavement.

GUIDELINES FOR RECEPTIVE MUSIC THERAPY

Receptive music therapy methods involve the patient listening to music without active participation in the music-making. For one patient, the music therapist may be accompanying herself while singing the patient's favorite song and for another, the music therapist may be providing soft music on the guitar or piano while providing verbal cues for relaxation and imagery. Receptive music therapy methods are almost always utilized during music therapy sessions with a child or teen receiving palliative or end-of-life care. Soft instrumental accompaniment can hold the space for a grieving family or be the impetus to a deeper conversation within the family. Sometimes, simply playing a familiar, preferred song that a child or family has requested may bring comfort and remind them and bring validation of who they are, their interests and beliefs. It furthermore provides a "normal" experience for which they may be longing. Families have reported that listening to music helps take their mind off the horrendous reality they are facing and is comforting (Lindenfelser et al., 2008). At other times, integrating cues for imagery and relaxation over a soft instrumental accompaniment can assist in addressing and relieving pain, anxiety, and fear and experiencing transcendence with the situation at hand.

Live Music Listening

Overview. Live music listening may include the music therapist playing a preferred familiar song or improvising on an instrument. Selecting songs that are meaningful to a child or young adult can provide the means to strengthen trust, build a therapeutic relationship, find meaning in the midst of a challenging situation, and validate and acknowledge feelings, values, and beliefs (Grocke, 2007). Actively engaging family members in selecting songs for the child can be empowering, as this creates an opportunity for choice and control (Sheridan & McFerran, 2005). Depending on the child's diagnosis, he may or may not be able to select a song of choice. In this case, the child's family may be able to recommend the child's music preference.

Preparation. It is important to know the genre or type of music the child and family enjoy. If live music is being provided, the music therapist should plan to bring an accompanying instrument and know the music and songs by memory or plan to bring the music necessary to play the preferred songs live.

During a music therapy visit with a family who had three young daughters of whom the youngest had been diagnosed with a rare genetic disease, the family members were asked to select songs that they thought the child would enjoy. This helped them to feel like they were "helping" their sister as they noticed her relaxing, cooing, and closing her eyes. Another example was a teen nearing the end of his battle with brain cancer who selected the song "Drift Away" by the Doobie Brothers. His father felt that his son asking the music therapist to play this song was a way of him communicating that he was beginning to "drift away."

Hilliard (2003) also shares examples of how song listening supports families while their child is in the dying process. Songs can tell one's story, help to be present in the moment, bring comfort and peace, or give clarity around the situation and feelings at hand without needing to go into deep dialogue. The songs that were shared during and at the end of a child's life are remembered and often felt as a strong, continuing bond after the child has died (Lindenfelser et al., 2008).

Procedures. When providing live music for a child or family, the therapist needs to have clear goals in mind. Once the goals are established, particular songs and accompaniment styles may be selected to meet those goals. Sometimes live music played on the guitar or piano is provided without the inclusion of lyrics. The various elements of the music can assist in either further relaxation or increased engagement and stimulation. Aasgaard (2001) describes playing the pentatonic scale as his client Peter was dying. No words needed to be spoken as the tones filled the room and supported Peter's mother as she held her son at the end of his life. Indeed, providing live music can create a revered space. Depending on the type and style of music provided, the opposite can also occur.

When providing live music through improvisation on an accompanying instrument, the music therapist should carefully choose the appropriate chordal structure to best support a child and family. Families have stated how the vibrations of the music shift the energy of the home or room where the child is being cared for. It makes them feel comforted as the music matches their emotional and spiritual state and often takes them to a new place of understanding and peace. It is not uncommon for music to set the stage for deeper therapeutic work by impacting the milieu or environment (Aasgaard, 1999).

Providing live music for a child and family is quite different from a music performance. While technique and skill are vital to creating a therapeutic experience, it is not important to play overly complicated chords or melodies or virtuoso as you would onstage. The focus of the music provided is always on what will best meet the goals of the child and family. Simple accompaniment and sometimes slower tempi with moments of silence are often integrated. By observing and assessing the child and family throughout the music, indications will be given as to the appropriate tempo and feel of the music. For example, if the goal of the music is to increase relaxation, it may be important to slow the tempo over time and to observe the body language and breathing patterns of the child. As the child takes deeper and slower breaths, the tempo of the music can continue to decrease. Family members often smile as they witness their child relaxing, and this in turn often helps the family to relax as well. The opposite is true if a child's energy begins to increase, and therefore a more upbeat tempo may ensue.

Depending on the child's state, there is often time between the songs for simple reflection and feedback. When emotions are expressed during the music, such as tears or smiles, this indicates an opportunity to inquire about the emotions unveiled due to the music. It may be appropriate to state "I noticed that this song brought tears to your eyes" and to allow time for more to be shared if the child or family member is comfortable. A child or family member may nod or go into great detail as to the meaning of the song and emotions experienced without any further questions. There may be situations, however, depending on how comfortable the child or family feels, where asking more questions is indicated. For example, some children and family members may not feel comfortable verbally expressing emotions unless they feel invited to do so. In such instances, it may be appropriate to ask, "Would you tell me more about your tears during the music?" Or, it may be important to validate such emotions by saying, "It is okay to have tears, and music often brings up emotions that we were not aware of. Is there anything that you would like to talk about that came to mind during the music?" It is okay to hold quiet space as a child or family member determines what they will share and to listen both compassionately and actively by nodding or reflecting what is shared. It can be very therapeutic for emotions to be expressed during music, and it is important to feel comfortable welcoming this expression.

Determining when to stop playing and providing music depends on the state of the child and family. It may take just a few minutes of live music matching the child's state to allow the child to deeply relax and perhaps even fall asleep, or it may take providing live music for an extensive amount of time before the goal of the music is reached. A session may begin with providing familiar songs to the child or family, and they may want to listen and hear the words to their favorite songs before settling in to relax. As a child begins taking deeper breaths and appears to have more relaxed posture during the music, it may indicate an opportunity to invite the child to continue to gently relax as you provide live, gentle improvisation and invite the child to rest or close his eyes. If the child has fallen asleep, the tempo can continue to decrease, with more moments of silence in between gentle arpeggios until the music has ended. It is important to depart the room quietly if it is wished that the child remain asleep. If it is anticipated that the child may wake up wondering when or where the music therapist went, it may be appropriate to leave a note upon departure. On the other hand, when more upbeat, live music is provided and continues throughout a session, it may become clear that the session is coming to a close when a child or family member mentions how the music was for them or if they express appreciation, as this can indicate they are finished with the session. Or, the music therapist may openly say, "How was it to listen to the music today? We will finish with this last song." If a child remains awake, alert, and engaged and the session is coming to a close, it is important to indicate this prior to the last song so that it does not feel like the music ends abruptly.

Recorded Music Listening

Overview. The simplest and most basic way of introducing music as a therapeutic tool within pediatric palliative and end-of-life care may be through suggesting listening to preferred recorded music. Selecting preferred, recorded music to be played provides an opportunity for the child or family to make choices and express their individuality and may increase their comfort and help to manage discomfort and pain. Recorded music may be played during a music therapy session and involve reflection, or the access to recorded music may be coordinated by the music therapist so that the child or family can listen to their preferred music at varying times of the day, not just during music therapy sessions. There are many tasks and decisions that families are making each day related to their child's care, and sometimes remembering to incorporate preferred, recorded music goes overlooked but can make a difference in how the child and family feel.

Procedures. Prior to the initial music therapy visit, a music therapist may have a phone conversation with a family and suggest playing recorded music as a way of providing comfort, assisting with restlessness and decreasing pain. For example:

Upon suggesting playing recorded music to a family, the mother of the child said, "Of course, I didn't even think of that, but we all love music and should have it on more often." The family quickly found that selecting recorded songs was a task that other siblings could help with, and in turn they felt they were helping their sister.

When recorded music is provided during a music therapy session, the music therapist then deepens the child's and family's awareness of the potential benefits of listening to recorded music. If families are already using recorded music to create a comforting environment for their child, it can be advantageous toward gently establishing a therapeutic relationship if the music therapist listens to the selected songs with the child and/or family. As McFerran (2010) writes, asking "What kinds of music do you like?" (p. 87) can be a great way to engage children in selecting recorded music that they may be willing or interested to share. While perhaps obvious, it also helps to establish a therapeutic relationship as interest is shown in the child's preferences. A child's ability to respond to such questions depends on their diagnosis or condition. If their ability to communicate is compromised, siblings or parents may be invited to make suggestions or recommendations.

When listening to prerecorded songs, the child and family may have equipment necessary to play songs they enjoy and want to hear, and other times it is important for the music therapist to provide this equipment and have access to a variety of recorded songs that can be played over speakers. Listening to preferred songs can lead to discussions about specific aspects of the song(s) that the child likes and may become a song analysis intervention. It is important for the music therapist to take note of this so that future live performances of these songs can capture this if possible.

Additionally, adding other sensory experiences while listening to recorded music can provide opportunities for validating and supporting the child (Grocke, 2007). Having a variety of textures available such as a feather, streamers, soft blankets, bubbles, or silky cloth may invite the child to relax further or engage physically by making vocalizations, stretching limbs, or taking deeper breaths. Providing gentle touch such as holding a child's hand or gently rubbing their back, hands, or feet during the recorded music may also be comforting. When providing tactile stimulation, it is important to first evaluate whether the child has any tactile defenses so that the experience does not cause distress. Whether the recorded music is selected by the child, family, or music therapist, it is important to assess if the music is assisting in meeting the needs of the child, whether that be to help relax, decrease pain or agitation, or stimulate engagement while gentle touch or tactile experiences are provided.

Song Analysis

Overview. Song analysis may be used to reflect on a song that is shared either live or recorded. The song lyrics may help the child and family tell their story or search for meaning. Grocke (2007) suggests that song analysis may provide the child and family opportunities to enjoy preferred music, project and express difficult emotions, encourage insight, and understand how they are feeling about the situation. *One mother of a young child who was near the end of life selected "What a Wonderful World" by Louis Armstrong. She described the beauty and challenges her baby brought for her. While she knew he would not live much longer and that she could not imagine life without him, she stated that he made her world more beautiful and bright, and she felt she would hold on to that reality following his death.* Comforting words, familiar melodies, and tempo all contribute to the meaning a song has for a child or family.

Procedures. Song analysis begins by inquiring with the child or family what song is meaningful to them or, as stated above, by asking what music or songs a child or family enjoys. If the intervention is preplanned, it may be appropriate to bring a copy of the lyrics for the child or family to follow. Once it has been determined which song will be played either live or recorded, it may be appropriate to invite the child and/or family members to take in whatever may be meaningful for them about the song. It is important that the music therapist allows for some silence following the song. Following listening to a live or prerecorded version of the song, questions may be asked such as "How was that for you to hear?" or "What is it about that song that is meaningful to you?' The child or family member may already be having an emotional response, so it is important to first acknowledge the emotion that arose during the song and build further discussions and/or subsequent interventions onto that initial reaction.

Grocke (2007) shares various levels of questions that deepen a song analysis experience. For example, a first-level question, as described by Grocke (2007), may include simply asking, "What do you like about this song?" A second-level question may be to invite the child or family member to share more deeply by asking, "Are there particular lyrics that stand out as being meaningful to you?" (p. 166). Or, "does the song remind you of anyone or anything in your life?" (pp. 166–167). A third-level question goes even deeper by asking, "Is there something about the song that relates to your life at the moment?" (p. 167).

Songs can bring up memories and emotions. As emotions are expressed, it is important to invite the child or family member to share more if they feel comfortable and to know that it is common for songs to bring up emotions. For example:

When discussing music therapy experiences a bereaved mom had with her deceased infant son, she stated *"at first [when offered music therapy] I was not sure I wanted music therapy because I knew that it would make me vulnerable emotionally." She continued by saying that she sang particular lullabies to her son, and that while she knew her son would love to hear the music and familiar songs played by the music therapist, it would make her aware of how horrendously sad she felt and she was trying to "hold it together."*

We can sometimes think of songs and the music we share as always bringing a positive experience, and it is important to remember how vulnerable or sometimes threatening music can be when it brings emotions that one may not wish to feel at that time. Providing adequate support when the depth of emotion is experienced during music is vital, and that is our job as music therapists. We have a powerful tool with music, and we must be prepared to support a child or family member.

Emotions discussed or shed in relation to songs may not otherwise be expressed. For example:

A *young woman found the song "Wonder" by Natalie Merchant to tell her story. She felt that everyone was looking her over as if she was not a person, and as the song says, "they had no explanation." Following the song, she acknowledged her impending death and found comfort in the words "She'll find her way," as she trusted she would, though she felt alone on the journey.*

Following further discussion around the lyrics and other elements of the song and depending on the emotional response of the child or family members, it may be appropriate to transition to another intervention so that the session finishes with a gentle experience. Song analysis can be quite emotional and sometimes exhausting to someone who has short bouts of energy with which to focus on such an intervention. Following the song analysis intervention with the client who enjoyed the song "Wonder" by Natalie Merchant, we would often close the session with a music listening or music-guided relaxation intervention.

Music-Guided Imagery for Relaxation

Overview. There are a number of different styles of guided imagery. The type of guided imagery and music suggested for purposes of use within pediatric palliative care incorporates techniques for providing vocal cues for relaxation and imagery. Using imagery with children and teens can be quite effective, and the way that it is utilized depends on the child's developmental, cognitive, and verbal abilities. This intervention may be useful when the child's goals relate to increasing relaxation and self-awareness or decreasing pain and anxiety. It may not be indicated, however, for children with declining cognitive functioning, as it may be confusing or cause more anxiety. That being said, there have been times when this author has used this intervention with children with end-stage brain cancer. While their cognitive functioning was declining, these particular children found comfort accessing imagery as they talked about being at the ocean, for example, so such imagery was incorporated.

Preparation. It is important to determine whether live or recorded music will be used during the experience. Having the appropriate equipment or instruments is important. Live music is preferred for this intervention in most instances, as it provides the opportunity for the music therapist to adjust the tempo and dynamics when the child or family member becomes more relaxed.

Procedures. This intervention may be the conclusion to a music therapy session that involved another intervention or may be the sole intervention used during a session. In either case, to begin a music-guided imagery experience, the child or family members are invited to find a comfortable position either lying down or sitting in a comfortable chair. As stated in the introduction to this section, adjusting the lighting and environmental sounds certainly applies here. Once the child or family member appears comfortable, begin by informing them that this is a time for them to relax and engage in experiencing imagery. Welcome them to close or leave open their eyes and that they are welcome to adjust themselves for better comfort at any time. Especially when in the hospital environment, it is important to state that the sounds outside and within their room can fade away from their awareness and that if any alarming sounds occur, to know that they are being attended to by someone else. You may invite the child or family member to take a few gentle breaths as they settle into a relaxed position prior to the music beginning.

For some children or family members, it may be necessary to offer a relaxation induction before starting the music. A relaxation induction is the verbal instruction given to allow someone to move into a more relaxed place, which helps prior to inviting imagery. It allows the mind to quiet.

As the child or family member becomes more relaxed, it may be appropriate to suggest an image. An image such as a flower, house, or special place to the child may be used and may provide a sense of control by managing pain or stress and allowing mental "escape" to a place that may be less stressful (Grocke, 2007). Sometimes just asking the child or other family members to imagine a color that is comforting can be an easy way to begin. It is important to first ask either the child or other family members if in fact the image that will be used is of comfort. Most often, it is best to invite a comforting image from the child or family member and to welcome deeper descriptions of that image or experience. If a child is verbal and descriptions of images are accessible, the music therapist may deepen the experience by asking more about what is seen, felt, and heard. Children are often quite capable of quickly accessing imagery that can provide information about how they are processing their experience, sometimes without even closing their eyes. For a child who is in pain, using imagery may be effective in redirecting the child's focus and allowing the pain to be transformed.

Once the child or family member is in a comfortable position, the accompaniment begins, which may include soft picking of a repetitive chord structure on the guitar or arpeggios and simple melody on the piano or keyboard. The music therapist may begin to speak with a soft vocal tone to offer relaxation instructions. The following relaxation instructions are appropriate for most children:

"As you hear the sounds of the music, allow yourself to take a gentle, comforting breath. Notice the warmth of your breath as it softens the muscles of your body. Continue to breathe in and out and notice how this calms your body and your mind." For some children, it is important that the therapist maintains a vocal presence throughout by continuing cues for relaxation such as "Allow your breath to gently relax as you listen to the music," as some children may become anxious when they no longer hear the therapist's voice. It is important, however, that these continuing instructions remain general enough that the imagery a child may be having is not disrupted. After inviting gentle breaths, it may then be appropriate to invite the simple imagery of a color by saying, *"As you are breathing gently, notice a comforting color that joins your breath. If it feels comfortable, invite this color to enter your body, bringing more comfort to each part of your body."*

It may be appropriate to ask "What color are you noticing?" and to then repeat this color if/when the child states the color they are noticing. For example, if the color is yellow, you may say: *"Notice the yellow color slowly and gently entering your body with your breath and bringing comfort and peace. If the color changes, allow it to do so. There may even be more than one color that helps to comfort your body. Allow your breath and this color to move gently from your head down into your shoulders, bringing comfort and peace [or another positive quality] into your shoulders and down your arms into your hands and fingers. As you continue to breathe gently, allow your breath and color down into your chest and tummy, bringing comfort and helping your body to feel peaceful. As you breathe gently, notice your breath and color moving down your spine and into your hips and legs, allowing comfort and peace to reach all the way down into your feet and toes. If there is any part of your body that feels uncomfortable, bring your breath and the color to that part of your body so that it feels comfort and peace. Continue to allow your breath to be gentle as you welcome your imagination to take you to a beautiful place where you like to be.*

This concludes the relaxation induction and is a bridge to inviting an imagery experience. Inviting open-ended questions about this place or feeling is important so that the child can determine how much he wants to engage in the imagery. Asking nondirective questions may feel less threatening if the child appears to have the energy to do so. This may not always be the case, and then it may be appropriate to ask the child at the start of the session or to confirm with a family member that a particular image is appropriate to integrate. At this point, you would then invite that particular image preselected by the child by saying, for example, *"Begin to notice yourself at the river and find a restful place to sit on the edge of the river. You can take in the gentle breeze and feel it on your face as you sit by the side of the river. Begin to smell the fresh air and smell of the trees and flowers nearby. If you would like, you can touch them and feel them on your hands."*

If open-ended questions are appropriate, you would then continue from the relaxation induction and into the imagery experience by saying, *"What do you notice about this beautiful place? Is there anything that stands out to you or anything you are drawn to? Feel free to move closer, to feel your body moving in a way that feels comfortable. Notice the colors around this place. Is there anyone with you here? Is there anything you would like to say or any messages that you are hearing? Take that in and feel free to interact as much or little as you would like.*

The questions help to open up opportunities for imagery, but do not necessarily each need to be answered. The child or family member may appear restful and relaxed throughout or may choose to answer the questions. Leave space between the questions and continue the soft arpeggios. It takes practice to continue a steady accompanying pattern with vocal cues. Take the time necessary to practice speaking over your playing and adjusting your tempo, chordal structure, and vocal tone as each takes time to refine.

Once you feel that the child has engaged for an appropriate amount of time in the imagery, you may say, *"Take a few more moments to explore anything else that you would like while you are here. Notice how beautiful this place is. You are always welcome to return to this place if you would like [continue music with no vocal cues for a moment]. It is now time to begin to slowly return from this place. Begin to notice your breath again and notice how calm your body feels. Keep that feeling as you slowly begin to feel your body again. When you are ready, feel your fingers and your toes and gently move them. Begin to hear the sounds of this space again and notice the light coming in. When you are ready, you may open your eyes [slowly create more rhythm to ground the child or family member back in this space]. As the music comes to an end, you can continue to feel calm and peace. As your eyes open, feel free to gently stretch if you would like or continue to rest.*

If a child has fallen asleep during the intervention and is in a safe environment such that there are others around when the child awakens, it is okay to quietly leave the session upon ending the music. If the child is gently awake following the relaxation and imagery experience, it is important to ask how that was for them and to allow the child or family member to express their experiences. Finding a comforting place, even if in the imagination, can bring comfort and peace, especially considering that this place is within them, when it can otherwise feel that life is quite chaotic and challenging. As the child or family shares more about their experience in a more alert space, they are often able to integrate it and keep the images with them when times are challenging, or they can be reminded to "return to the river in their imagination" when they want to be away from a challenging situation or to feel more calm.

An 11-year-old boy was in the hospital receiving end-of-life care. His home was many hours away, and when asked where he would like to "be" in his imagination, he said "on the river by my home." He had been experiencing excruciating abdominal pain and rated his pain at a 7 on a scale from 1 to 10. Pain medication had already been administered prior to the start of the session. The boy followed cues for deeper breathing and engaged in an imagery experience as accompanying music was provided on the guitar with the suggested image of being by the river. The boy fell asleep, and the grimace from experiencing abdominal pain was wiped from his face.

It is important to note that this particular intervention is distinctly different from the Bonny Method of Guided Imagery and Music (BMGIM). The BMGIM requires additional training and utilizes prearranged, recorded classical music. Open-ended questions are also asked by the therapist, and a dialogue ensues throughout the music as the client's experience deepens both due to the music and to the interventions used by the therapist. The BMGIM is often not indicated within this context, as children in this setting do not often have the energy to engage in the depths of this method. The description of this intervention is drawn from my training in the BMGIM, though it is not necessary to have this training to facilitate an effective music-guided imagery for relaxation session.

GUIDELINES FOR IMPROVISATIONAL MUSIC THERAPY

Vocal or instrumental improvisation can provide a means for releasing tension, anger, and pain within pediatric palliative and end-of-life care. It can also provide an avenue for expressing emotions that may not otherwise be acknowledged.

Instrumental Improvisation

Overview. Playing instruments is accessible to anyone regardless of skills or abilities. Instrumental improvisation allows children or young people to explore different sounds and ways to express or communicate their feelings and thoughts. It can help to remind parents that their child is first and foremost a child, rather than focusing on their child as being sick and dying (Lindenfelser et al., 2008). There are many times when parents express pure joy as they witness their child's ability to muster up enough energy and skill to wiggle their toes or fingers to play the chimes or feel the texture of the drumhead, both simplified forms of instrumental improvisation.

Preparation. It is important to determine which instruments will be offered during the improvisation and to be sure that they are all in working order and cleaned prior to use. Ensuring that the child has a variety of rhythmic instruments to choose from provides the means for a successful experience in improvising. Improvisations can become quite loud, so another aspect to consider in preparing for the session is to ensure that the sound level will not be disruptive if and when in a hospital environment. If a child is sleeping next door, it may be best to consider a different time for the improvisation or to consider moving to a general playroom on the floor if it is safe for the child to move to a different space.

Procedures. Instruments can look intimidating to children who have not been around instruments before. So, it may be helpful to begin by sharing one instrument at time so that the child does not feel overwhelmed. Introducing each instrument by name and then demonstrating how an instrument is played and the variety of ways to play it may help the child begin to feel more comfortable and confident in his ability to play the instrument on his own. After each instrument has been introduced, the child may indicate an interest or preference by reaching toward the preferred instrument or grabbing it independently. If the child is still hesitant, he may enjoy watching another family member play an instrument that he selected for that person to play. Once comfort and interest have been established for the child and other family members, instrumental improvisation can take many forms.

A child who is angry and having trouble finding appropriate ways to express feelings such as anger can use playing instruments to be a means of release. For example, *a six-year-old boy diagnosed with end-stage leukemia was swearing and hitting his mother and brothers. In addition to dealing with a life-threatening diagnosis, his parents were in the midst of a divorce. Other interdisciplinary team members warned one another of this child's physical outbursts. A soft, familiar song selected by the child's mother was being played as the child woke up from his nap. Rather than waking and expressing immediate anger and pain, as was usually the case, the child said "I know that song, it's 'Baby Beluga'" and joined in singing. Shortly after, the child asked about the drum. Shyly, his brothers gathered in the room, tentatively, as their brother was typically quite belligerent. Within moments, each of the brothers had their own drum and they were taking turns playing as loudly as possible. After letting out their energy on the drum, they began to synchronize their rhythm and added words and melody about things they enjoyed and missed being able to do together due to their brother's condition. The instruments provided a safe means to release anger and tension, and the interventions moved from providing familiar, live singing to instrumental improvisation to vocal improvisation and storytelling through music.*

Integrating instruments in a session even as a child is actively dying can validate and connect the child's previous experiences during music therapy and may bring comfort for a family. *While he was in the Pediatric Intensive Care Unit, music therapy was provided for a two-year-old boy who had just been extubated and was near the end-of-life. Music therapy was provided for the little boy as well as for his family, who was at his bedside as he took his last breaths. I took out the green frog castanet that the little boy had loved to play and set it under his tiny, lifeless hands. Even though the little boy was no longer able to play the castanet on his own, it validated his enjoyment of life previously and reminded his family of the times they experienced joy together. After the little boy's death, his mother stated that it meant so much to her that his interests and preferences were still honored even though he was unable to express them.* Sometimes the instrument or song played or improvised is a link to the healthy and happier days and times, and this becomes a strong part of what is remembered (Lindenfelser et al., 2008).

As stated above, once comfort with the instruments is established, each person involved in the session may select their preferred instrument, or an opportunity for additional choice and control may be provided if the child determines which instrument each person plays. The music therapist may consider using the drum or another instrument to keep a steady beat to begin the improvisation if that is indicated, or the child may be invited to "play how he feels" and there may be very little rhythmic grounding. The improvisation may then continue with everyone playing their instrument to match how the child is feeling. The tempo, of course may vary greatly, and if the tempo and dynamic has grown quite loud, the music therapist may direct a "stop" and "start again" motion using the sound of the instrument stopping and starting or by using vocal cues. This cue may then be directed by the child if the child is interested in having some control with the improvisation. Asking the child to play as quietly and then as loudly as he is able to can help a child to feel the varying ways of expressing himself through music.

If there was very little rhythmic grounding during the majority of the improvisation, it may be important to finish with a final improvisation that has a steady rhythm, depending on the mood of those involved. If the energy of the room feels unsettled following an unstructured improvisation, it may be indicated to continue with a final improvisation that has a steady rhythm. The child may determine what this rhythm is, and it may be important for the music therapist to quickly engage in this steady rhythm so that others will follow.

Improvisation allows for a child to express himself, as well as any others involved in the improvisation. It is important to keep the focus of the improvisation on the child's needs primarily, while simultaneously observing the participation of others involved. If a child is cautiously engaging, it is important to honor that. Parents, however, sometimes want to overly encourage their child to engage at a level that they wish. If this is not comfortable for the child, it is important to acknowledge that and invite the parents to follow the child's cues with the improvisation. Giving the child as much control and opportunities for decision-making as possible will allow for trust to build and emotions to be expressed through music that maybe would not otherwise be expressed.

Vocal Improvisation

Overview. The primary goals for vocal improvisation involve improving self-expression and providing opportunities for choice and control. In this setting, depending on the child's developmental abilities, vocal improvisation could be as simple as singing or humming vowel tones such as "oo" or "ahh" or as complex as creating and adding words and lyrics to simple or pre-existing melodies.

Procedures. Vocal improvisation may take place a cappella or with the support of an underlying rhythm or chordal structure provided on an accompanying or rhythmic instrument by the music therapist.

Children who do not otherwise make vocalizations may be inspired to freely create vocal sounds. These sounds may be imitated or initiated by the child and then imitated by the music therapist. Such interactive vocalizations validate the child's interest in communicating. While they may appear very simple, the sounds made by a child with a rare chromosomal disorder or genetic condition, who does not otherwise verbalize or vocalize, are quite profound. This can be very moving for family members who do not otherwise hear their child's voice, and it can empower family members to realize new ways that their child can communicate. To begin, the music therapist may sing a simple melody on "oo" or "ahhh" and then wait for the child to respond. If the child does not respond, the music therapist may sing again, repeating the same simple melody and then waiting for the child to respond as if inviting a dialogue. *During music therapy, a little boy with a complex medical condition who typically did not communicate verbally other than to cry began toning or vocalizing soft vowel sounds. His family and other staff imitated the sounds he was making, to which the little boy smiled and vocalized again.*

For children able to create their own words within a vocal improvisation, the music therapist may begin by creating an accompaniment and chordal structure and then melodically singing "my favorite thing to do is ..." and allowing the child to melodically add his "favorite thing to do." This may continue with a number of questions and answers from the child. The questions may start with the child's likes and dislikes and move to feelings and deeper emotions. *The six-year-old sibling of a little boy with a rare genetic condition engaged in vocal improvisation, answering questions through melody. I sang "I love my little brother and I wish that we could ...." The sibling continued by singing a whole list of things he wished he could do with his brother, like "I wish I could play soccer" ['jump on the trampoline," "hold him," etc.]. I continued by singing "I'm so glad that I can ...," and the brother sang "I can sing to him and read to him and dance for him." This validated his feelings and helped his mother to see how much he was feeling that she didn't realize. For another family that also had a baby with a rare genetic condition, the older siblings sang about the things they "wished for their brother." One brother sang, "I wish that he wouldn't die, I want to be able to play with him."*

Storytelling and Symbolic Play

Overview. Telling stories and engaging in symbolic play can be an effective way to express what may otherwise be challenging for a child or sibling to communicate. Storytelling and symbolic play invite the child or young person to creatively describe something of meaning to them and, in music therapy, it also involves the use of instruments and music to aid in the story being shared. Instruments often begin to represent a feeling or experience.

Preparations. In addition to having rhythmic and accompanying instruments available, it may be appropriate to have puppets or other small, washable toys that the child may use as a tool for telling their story.

Procedures. Typically, music therapy interventions such as song listening or singing or guided imagery may precede the child's willingness to engage in storytelling or symbolic play. These previous interventions may inspire the child to begin creatively describing his own experiences or story. This intervention may be used for something as simple as asking the child which instrument he most relates to and why. It may be more complex as the child builds an identity for different instruments or props and continues by mimicking feelings that instruments or props may feel that relate to the child's experiences. Children may project their needs on instruments or toys that become part of a music therapy session. They may willingly share how a toy or instrument is feeling or what they might be going through as a way of playfully expressing their own experience. Sweeney (2003) reports on the use of an instrument as a transitional object used in play and demonstrating a little boy Matthew's understanding of his own impending death. Using imagination and fantasy (Roberts, 2004), sometimes nursery rhymes [in the case of Matthew, relating to Humpty Dumpty (Sweeney, 2003)] can facilitate expression of the child's experiences. The symbolism drawn from play and storytelling with music can be an effective means of understanding the child's inner awareness of their situation.

GUIDELINES FOR RE-CREATIVE MUSIC THERAPY

Song Singing

Overview. The means of engaging children in singing songs occurs all over the world and is a normalizing experience for children who have a life-limiting condition. Parents who participate in music therapy sessions with their child who is receiving palliative care services have stated that it makes them feel normal because parents of a child who is healthy and typically developing often bring their child to music and singing groups. Children are often uninhibited when it comes to singing and creating music. Singing familiar songs or teaching new songs validates children as children or may validate the identity and interests of a teenager.

Procedures. If a child's preferred music has not yet been identified, it is important to begin by asking the child or young person about the songs they particularly enjoy or the artists whose music they most often listen to. This intervention is quite similar to providing live music; however, it often involves the child creating the music and/or singing himself. Sometimes the song itself is playful and shared or chosen purely for enjoyment because the song is familiar and comforting for the child. At other times, songs may be used because of the content, which may highlight themes such as hope, sadness, or love. The way in which songs are sung depends on the state of the child. Sometimes a song that was otherwise shared quite rhythmically and vigorously when a child was feeling well, strong, and engaged may be shared at a slower tempo to match the child's energy level as he becomes weaker. Accompaniment may be provided for the song by the music therapist, and the child may engage in playing a rhythmic instrument while singing the lyrics. This intervention can begin to merge with compositional music therapy if the child would like to adapt the lyrics. The music therapist may ask the child if there are other words or feelings they would like to incorporate in place of the words that exist in the song.

GUIDELINES FOR COMPOSITIONAL MUSIC THERAPY

Children and family members often have many things to say or express during this end-of-life period that can be difficult through words and made easier through music. Songwriting can be a powerful way for children and family members to express what otherwise may not be shared.

Songwriting

Overview. Songs may be written for, by, or with a child or teen receiving palliative care and involve creating a rhythm and melody that shares something important about a child's or family's life and experiences. These songs are often a treasured and tangible part of remembering the child into bereavement (Lindenfelser et al., 2008). Hilliard (2003) wrote about a young girl who wrote a song not only to express her feelings about death, but also as a gift to her friend as she saw how sad her impending death made her best friend. Aasgaard (2003) writes about the creation of music as an act of love, as his patient also wrote a song to give away and as a legacy of her life. Sometimes songs are an expression of the child's wishes rather than an expression of the way things actually are for them. Aasgaard (2001) shares how his client Brian accesses feelings of normalcy by writing a song. When the child is unable to write his own song, it can be empowering for family members to write a song for the child.

Preparation. Songwriting can sometimes happen spontaneously, so it is important to have the means to capture a child's or family's words that they want put to song. Bringing paper and writing materials or a computer or recording device to each session allows for these moments to be captured. Because songwriting may be somewhat spontaneous and the opportunity to continue the process is not always available because of a child's changing or declining condition, it is important to have equipment ready to record the experience if that is a wish of the child or family. In this setting, a music therapist may sometimes complete the song for a child or family member and present it to the family after the death of a child if the intervention took place near the end of the child's life.

Procedures. The process involved in songwriting depends on the child or family's interest. Songwriting may be presented as an option at each session and declined for many weeks until it suddenly is the wish of the child or family to write a song to express what they want expressed. Parents who have engaged in this process have stated that it feels like it is a meaningful gift they are giving to their child as well as to themselves. It can be difficult to put words to the horrendous experience of losing a child, so starting by singing about what the child brings to their life, how they love their child, and what they wish for their child may be an effective way to begin. *A song written by parents of an infant with Trisomy 18 started by writing together outside of the music therapy sessions how they loved their daughter. They were journaling each day about their daughter and decided that it would be meaningful to turn the wishes they were journaling into a song. Together we brainstormed whether they wanted the song to be more of a ballad, lullaby, or folk song. From there, they were able to select the tempo when given a number of options, as well as the chordal structure.* Children and families may not be able to easily select exactly how they want a song to sound until they are given some options that help them to define and decide just how they want their song to be shared.

The process of writing a song may look different when it is written by the child. Often this happens more fluidly and in the moment, with the child or music therapist creating a sustaining rhythm on an accompanying instrument and adding words or lyrics in the moment. The music therapist may ask the child about his feelings or what he wishes for, and this turns into a song. At other times, it may involve a thoughtful structure to the words that the patient wants to share. Some children want to write a more serious song that they are intentionally leaving behind, or they may want to be playful and sing about things that make them giggle.

Songwriting provided a powerful means to communicate the wishes of a little girl who is quoted at the start of this chapter. The medical team had suggested that music therapy may not be appropriate on this particular day with this little girl, as she was quite aggressive, hitting and biting, and it was feared that she might throw instruments and hurt someone. I offered to try, as our previous music therapy sessions had been quite effective in allowing the little girl opportunities to engage in expressing her emotions through drumming and symbolic play with the music as well as for an opportunity for bonding with her younger sister, who spent many days in the hospital by her side. As I walked in the room on this particular day, the little girl shouted, "I'd like to sing about the angels that came last night to tell me I don't have to go through this anymore." She pointed to the corners of the room where she saw the angels and continued that no one was listening to her. Her song was shared with her mom and medical providers, who heard that she did not want another round of chemotherapy and that she was going to be okay.

This example beautifully demonstrates how songwriting can be a powerful tool for children who want their voice to be heard.

WORKING WITH CAREGIVERS

As stated previously, the care of the family or those caring for the child who is receiving palliative or end-of-life care is just as important as the care of the child with the life-limiting condition. From the assessment and treatment to evaluation, each aspect of the provision of music therapy may involve the family or other caregivers. Flower (2008) writes that parents bear significant witness to the spirit and uniqueness of their child's life, no matter what their child's skills, disability, or life span may be. In addition to the emotional support that can be provided when parents or caregivers engage in a session, there may also be logistical reasons why it is important to involve caregivers. For example, some children may need their airway to be suctioned periodically or may need to be repositioned every several minutes or hours, and parents or medically trained caregivers would be necessary to perform these tasks to ensure that the child is comfortable throughout the session. Most importantly, the music is reaching and affecting the state of the child as well as that of the family or caregivers, so knowing what the needs are of the child's caregivers is also important. Family members know the child and his needs best and desire for his needs to be met at all times, yet family members also have their own needs. Including family members in a session or offering for them to have some free time when the session is in the family's home and they are the primary caregiver can be a relief as well. There may be times when the child is unresponsive and the focus of the music therapy session is really for the comfort, ease, and support of the family. Supporting parents and siblings who care for a child receiving palliative or end-of-life care is essential to the overall health and wellness of the family and the overarching quality of life for the family (Lindenfelser, 2005).

RESEARCH EVIDENCE

Evidence supporting music therapy within pediatric palliative and end-of-life care is sparse, yet growing. There is a recent growth in qualitative evidence supporting the value that parents and caregivers witness and experience when music therapy is provided to their child receiving palliative or end-of-life care (Amadoru & McFerran, 2007; Knapp et al., 2009; Lindenfelser et al., 2008; Lindenfelser et al., 2012).

This evidence suggests that families who receive music therapy services while their child is receiving palliative or end-of-life care experience an improved quality of life (Lindenfelser et al., 2008, 2012) and improved satisfaction in the services that they receive overall (Knapp et al., 2009). Data from surveys and follow-up interviews with families asking about their overall satisfaction and quality of care found that those who received music therapy with their child responded more positively overall (Knapp et al., 2009). A study by Lindenfelser, Grocke, and McFerran (2008) investigated bereaved parents' experiences of music therapy when their child was terminally ill. Interviews were conducted with bereaved parents and then analyzed using a phenomenological approach. The first theme illustrated that music therapy is "valued as a means of altering the child's and family's perception of their situation in the midst of adversity" (Lindenfelser et al., 2008, p. 330). Additional themes suggest that music therapy is a significant component of remembrance, is a multifaceted experience, and enhances communication and expression; most families wished for more music therapy. Lindenfelser, McFerran, and Hense (2012) then investigated the quality of life of parents and the experiences witnessed during music therapy sessions with children receiving palliative care in the home setting through a multisite, mixed-method design. A PedsQL Family Impact Module revealed that there was little change in the parents' emotional, physical, and social functioning levels, which is to be expected in this context. For example, following the completion of the survey, one mother commented that the survey did not capture how much she and her daughter enjoyed music therapy. However, through a phenomenological analysis of in-depth interviews with these same parents who participated in the sessions with their child, it was found that music therapy (a) draws on the healthy aspects of the child and helps the child to continue to thrive, (b) is fun and contributes to a soothing experience, (c) enhances communication and is an outlet for expressing a variety of emotions, and (d) allows the therapeutic benefit to extend beyond the needs of the child as well as the session, such that it is a means to continuing the bond following the death of a child. Positive responses to music therapy were also noted in a phenomenological analysis of interviews with caregivers and clinical staff at a homelike facility where children with life-limiting conditions receive music therapy during their short stays for respite care or end-of-life (Amadoru & McFerran, 2007). Themes such as that music therapy transcends the ordinary as children's positive reactions "are beyond the expectations people have of them" (p. 125) and that music therapy brings happiness and a better quality of life by soothing a child who is distressed or restless and allows for the freedom to be loud and creative also demonstrate the value of music therapy in this setting (Amadoru & McFerran, 2007).

Additionally, there is anecdotal evidence demonstrating the important role of music therapy within pediatric palliative and end-of-life care to address and reduce anxiety and fear (Fagen, 1982; Ibberson, 1996; Sweeney, 2003), to decrease pain through imagery and symbolic play (Sweeney, 2003), to bring comfort and support (Froehlich, 1996; Hilliard, 2003), to increase opportunities for communication and validate interactions within the family (Aasgaard, 2003; Amadoru & McFerran, 2007; Daveson & Kennelly, 2000; Hilliard, 2003; Pavlicevic, 2005), and to provide opportunities for choice and control (Ibberson, 1996; Sheridan & McFerran, 2004).

There are, however, currently no randomized controlled trials conducted to demonstrate the effectiveness of any given music therapy method or modality on particular symptoms that children or teens who receive palliative or end-of-life care may be experiencing. One reason may be that it can be unethical and oftentimes unfeasible to expect children or teens to contribute to data collection as they are in the dying process (Lindenfelser et al., 2012). Also, it is challenging to quantify the effectiveness of music therapy in this setting, when there are many changing variables considering the child's declining state. Additionally, there is such a wide range of symptoms related to the wide variety of life-limiting conditions that a child or teen who is receiving palliative or end-of-life care may have that it is very difficult to look at the specific needs of a large population. Bradt and Dileo (2009) report in a Cochrane Review of music therapy in end-of-life care that the challenge

> in conducting research with those in end-of-life care is the conflict between the requirement of providing an intervention that is sufficiently standardized so as to be adequately evaluated versus the imperative to tailor the intervention to the particular needs of each participant. This conflict is of utmost concern for

persons who are dying because of the urgency of providing appropriate and meaningful treatment while the patients are still alive as well as the lack of predictability regarding when death may occur. To address this issue, studies should utilize a standardized treatment that will also allow for flexibility in the music therapy methods used to address the needs of each patient ... the importance of qualitative research and non-RCT research to gain a better understanding of the qualitative aspects of the experiences of patients and their loved ones, as well as to identify factors that may contribute to or limit the effectiveness of music therapy interventions. (p. 14)

As palliative and end-of-life services become more available to children and teens as health care policies regarding reimbursement for services begin to change (American Academy of Pediatrics, 2000), it is essential that future studies begin to target the effectiveness of music therapy within a session. Tools such as quality of life indicators and comfort and pain measurements continue to be developed and improved so that the quality of life of a child and family can be evaluated more adequately (Huang et al., 2010). The music therapy research that we are able to draw on in this setting does highlight the value and improved support felt by families, which demonstrates what a vital resource music therapy is for children and teens receiving palliative and end-of-life care, as well as for their families.

SUMMARY AND CONCLUSION

Whether it is sharing receptive music therapy methods such as listening to a favorite song together or discussing the meaning of the lyrics to create a song that expresses the challenges and joys faced by children or teens receiving palliative or end-of-life care and by their siblings or parents, music therapy is a means to altering the perception of the horrendous reality that these families face as it brings joy, relief, and happiness. Relieving distress or pain using music adds another level, as this experience may be long held in the memory of the excruciating days leading up to a child's death. If there is a way to bring any amount of comfort or relief, if even so that the family remembers are able to access or provide something that was life-giving and comforting at such a dire time, this is of great value. Music can be enjoyed regardless of physical or developmental limitations and reaches through cultural barriers that may limit other services provided to children and families in this setting. It validates the life, values, and beliefs of all involved and open to experiencing the music. As such, music therapy is an essential component of pediatric palliative and end-of-life care.

GLOSSARY

The following definitions are based on the *Taber's Cyclopedic Medical Dictionary* (1997).

Batten Disease. A hereditary disturbance of metabolism that results in blindness and mental retardation.
Cystic Fibrosis. A single-gene defect manifestation in multiple body systems such as chronic obstructive pulmonary disease, pancreatic exocrine deficiency, urogenital dysfunction, and abnormally high electrolyte concentration in the sweat. Cystic Fibrosis usually begins in infancy and is the major cause of severe chronic lung disease in children.
Edema. A local or generalized condition in which the body tissues contain an excessive amount of tissue fluid.

Mucopolysaccharidoses. A group of inherited disorders characterized by a deficiency of enzymes that are essential for the degradation of the mucopolysaccharides heparin sulfate, dermatan sulfate, and keratin sulfate. This deficiency may cause a number of symptoms including retina degeneration, skeletal dysplasia, cardiac lesions, deafness, and retardation.

Muscular Dystrophy. A hereditary disease usually beginning in childhood in which muscular ability is lost.

Spinal Muscular Atrophy. A hereditary disease usually beginning in childhood in which muscular ability is lost. At first there is muscular pseudohypertrophy, followed by atrophy.

Tracheotomy. The operation of incising the skin over the trachea and making a surgical wound in the trachea to permit an airway during tracheal obstruction. This technique is used to provide an airway in emergency situations and to replace the airway provided by an endotracheal tube that has been in place for more than several weeks.

Trisomy 13 or Trisomy 18. In genetics, having three homologous chromosomes per cell instead of two; both cause severe congenital deformation and mental retardation. Children with Trisomy 13 or Trisomy 18 do not usually survive beyond the first year of life.

REFERENCES

Aasgaard, T. (1999). Music therapy as milieu in the hospice and paediatric oncology ward. In D. Aldridge (Ed.), *Music therapy in palliative care: New voices* (pp. 29–42). Philadelphia, PA: Jessica Kingsley Publishers.

Aasgard, T. (2001). An ecology of love: Aspects of music therapy in the pediatric oncology environment. *Journal of Palliative Care, 17*(3), 177–181.

Aasgaard, T. (2003, August 1). Musical acts of love in the care of severely ill and dying children and their families. Retrieved from http://www.musictherapyworld.de/modules/archive/papers/show_abstract.php?id=51

Amadoru, S., & McFerran, K. (2007). The role of music therapy in children's hospices. *European Journal of Palliative Care, 14*(3), 124–127.

American Academy of Pediatrics, Committee on Bioethics & Committee on Hospital Care. (2000). Palliative Care for Children. *Pediatrics, 106*(2), 351–357.

Armstrong-Dailey, A., & Zarbock, S. (2009). *Hospice care for children.* New York: Oxford University Press.

Bartell, A. S., & Kissane, D. W. (2005). Issues in pediatric palliative care: Understanding families. *Journal of Palliative Care, 21*(93), 165–172.

Behrman, R. E., & Field, M. J. (2003). *When children die: Improving palliative and end-of-life care for children and their families.* Washington, DC: The National Academies Press.

Bradt, J., & Dileo, C. (2010). Music therapy for end-of-life care. *Cochrane Database of Systematic Reviews.* 2010, Issue 1. Art. no.: CD007169. DOI: 10.1002/14651858.CD007169.pub2.

Burgess, D. (1994). Denial and terminal illness. *The American Journal of Hospice and Palliative Care, 11*(2), 46–48.

Children's Hospice International. (2010, September 10). Retrieved from http://www.chionline.org/

Curran, E. (2001). *Guided imagery for healing children and teens: Wellness through visualization.* Hillsboro, OR: Beyond Words Publishing.

Daveson, B., & Kennelly, J. (2000). Music therapy in palliative care for hospitalized children and adolescents. *Journal of Palliative Care, 16*(1), 35–38.

Davies, B., Brenner, P., Orloff, S., Sumner, L., & Worden, W. (2002). Addressing spirituality in pediatric hospice and palliative care. *Journal of Palliative Care, 18*(1), 59–67.

Doka, K. J. (1995). Talking to children about illness. In K. J. Doka (Ed.), *Children mourning, mourning children* (pp. 31–39). Washington, DC: Hospice Foundation of America.

Fagen, T. S. (1982). Music therapy in the treatment of anxiety and fear in terminal pediatric patients. *Music Therapy, 2*(1), 13–23.

Faulkner, K. (2001). Children's understanding of death. In A. Armstrong-Dailey & S. Zarbock (Eds.), *Hospice care for children* (2nd ed., pp. 9–22). New York: Oxford University Press, Inc.

Flower, C. (2008). Living with dying: Reflections on family music therapy with children near the end of life. In A. Oldfield & C. Flower (Eds.), *Music therapy with children and their families* (pp. 177–190). Philadelphia, PA Jessica Kingsley.

Friebert, S. (2009, December 8). National Hospice Palliative Care Organization Facts & Figures: Pediatric Palliative and Hospice Care in America. Retrieved from http://www.nhpco.org/files/public/quality/Pediatric-Facts-Figures.pdf

Froehlich, M. (1996). Music therapy with the terminally ill child. In M. Froehlich (Ed.), *Music therapy with hospitalized children: A creative arts approach* (pp. 209–217). Cherry Hill, NJ: Jeffrey Books.

Gilmer, M. (2002). Pediatric palliative care: A family-centered model for critical care. *Critical Care Nursing Clinics of North America, 14,* 207–214.

Goldfarb, F. D., Devine, K., Yingling, J. T., Hill, A., Moss, J., Ogburn, E. S., & Roberts, R. J. (2010). Partnering with professionals: Family-centered care from the parent perspective. *Journal of Family Social Work, 13,* 91–99.

Goldman, A. (1998). ABC of palliative care: Special problems of children. *British Medical Journal, 316,* 49–52.

Grocke, E., & Wigram, T. (2007). *Receptive methods in music therapy: Techniques and clinical applications for music therapy clinicians, educators and students.* Philadelphia, PA: Jessica Kingsley.

Hilliard, R. E. (2003). Music therapy in pediatric palliative care: Complementing the interdisciplinary approach. *Journal of Palliative Care, 19*(2), 127–132.

Hinds, P. S., Schum, L., Baker, J. N., & Wolfe, J. (2005). Key factors affecting dying children and their families. *Journal of Palliative Medicine, 8*(1), 70–78.

Huang, I., Shenkman, E. A., Madden, V. L., Vadaparampil, S., Quinn, G., & Knapp, C. A. (2010). Measuring quality of life in pediatric palliative care: Challenges and potential solutions. *Palliative Medicine, 24*(2), 175–182.

Hynson, J., & Sawyer, S. (2001). Paediatric palliative care: Distinctive needs and emerging issues. *Journal of Paediatric Child Health, 37,* 323–325.

Ibberson, C. (1996). A natural end: One story about Catherine. *British Journal of Music Therapy, 10*(1), 24–31.

Klass, D., Nickman, L. L., & Silverman, P. R. (1996). *Continuing bonds: New understandings of grief.* Bristol, PA: Taylor and Francis Publishers.

Knapp, C. A., & Contro, N. (2009). Family support services in pediatric palliative care. *American Journal of Hospice and Palliative Medicine, 26*(6), 476–482.

Knapp, C., Madden, V., Wang, H., Curtis, C., Sloyer, P., & Shenkman, E. (2009). Music therapy in an integrated pediatric palliative care program. *The American Journal of Hospice & Palliative Care, 26*(6), 449–455.

Kubler-Ross, E. (1983). *On children and death: How children and their parents can and do cope with death.* New York: Touchstone of Simon and Schuster, Inc.

Liben, S., Papadatou, D., & Wolfe, J. (2008). Paediatric palliative care: Challenges and emerging ideas. *The Lancet, 371,* 852–864.

Lindenfelser, K. J. (2011). Music therapy at end of life: Bringing comfort to patients and families. *Minnesota Health Care News, 9*(11), 26–27.

Lindenfelser, K. J., Grocke, D., & McFerran, K. (2008). Bereaved parents' experiences of music therapy with their terminally ill child. *Journal of Music Therapy, 45*(3), 330–348.

Lindenfelser, K. J., Hense, C., & McFerran, K. (2012). Music therapy in pediatric palliative care: Family-centered care to enhance quality of life. *American Journal of Hospice and Palliative Medicine, 29*(3), 219–226.

McFerran, K. (2010). *Adolescents, music and music therapy: Methods and techniques for clinicians, educators and students.* Philadelphia, PA: Jessica Kingsley.

McFerran, K., & Hogan, B. (2005). The overture: Initiating discussion on the role of music therapy in paediatric palliative care. *Progress in Palliative Care, 13*(1), 7–9.

Munro, S., & Mount, B. (1978). Music therapy in palliative care. *Canadian Medical Association Journal, 119*(9), 1029–1034.

Pavlicevic, M. (Ed.). (2005). *Music therapy in children's hospices: Jessie's fund in action.* Philadelphia, PA: Jessica Kingsley.

Roberts, R., & Sparling, P. (2006, February 2). Creative care for children at home: A palliative music therapy initiative. *The Healthline.* Retrieved from http://www.thehealthline.ca/palliative_care/index.asp?pid=61(a

Sheridan, J., & McFerran, K. (2004). Exploring the value of opportunities for choice and control in music therapy within a paediatric hospice setting. *Australian Journal of Music Therapy, 15,* 18–32.

Sweeney, C. (2003). "Couldn't put Humpty together again": Symbolic play with a terminally ill child. In S. Hadley (Ed.), *Psychodynamic music therapy: Case studies* (pp.23–35). Gilsum, NH: Barcelona Publishers.

Thomas, C. L. (Ed.). (1997). *Taber's Cyclopedic Medical Dictionary* (18th ed.). Philadelphia: F. A. Davis Company.

Woodgate, R. L. (2006). Living in a world without closure: Reality for parents who have experienced the death of a child. *Journal of Palliative Care, 22*(2), 75–82.

World Health Organization. (2012). WHO Definition of Palliative Care. Retrieved April 3, 2012, from http://www.who.int/cancer/palliative/definition/en/

APPENDIX A

ASSESSMENT FORM—MUSIC THERAPY IN PEDIATRIC PALLIATIVE AND END-OF-LIFE CARE

Patient Name:

Parents/Guardians:

Address:

Phone:

Date of birth/Age:

Referred by: _____ Date: _____

Reason for Referral: □ Quality of Life □ Coping Patient □ Coping Family □ Anxiety □ Agitation

□ Actively Dying □ Dyspnea □ Pain related to:_____

Primary Diagnosis:_____

Physical Limitations: _____

Limits to Communication:_____

Religion:_____ Cultural/Ethnic Background:_____

Music Background

□ Vocal □ Plays Instrument □ Movement/Dance □ Music Listening

Preferred Music:_____

Favorite Musicians:_____

Favorite Songs:_____

Observed Responses to Music Therapy Interventions:

□ Heightened affect/mood □ Increased Verbalizations/Vocalizations □ Increased Alertness

□ Reported/Observed Increase Comfort □ Increased Energy □ Closed Eyes □ Fell Asleep

□ Slower/Deeper Breathing □ Expressed Emotions (as evidenced by):

□ Tears □ Smiles □ Laughter

Participation: □ Singing □ Instrument Playing □ Movement □ Music/Song Choice

Music Therapy Goals

□ Patient or Family will exhibit increased comfort/relaxation

□ Pt./Family will exhibit increased coping ability, esteem, well-being

□ Pt./Family will exhibit decreased anxiety

□ Pt. will exhibit decreased shortness of breath

□ Pt. will exhibit/report decreased pain/discomfort

□ Pt./Family will express loss and grief

□ Pt./Family will verbalize spiritual or cultural needs/support

□ Pt./Family will plan music for memorial/funeral

□ Pt./Family will respond to music therapy interventions by: Engaging in music, incl. expression

Interventions—Plan of Care

□ Provide music for relaxation/comfort

□ Provide music for decreased pain/agitation/anxiety/discomfort

□ Encourage emotional expression and response

□ Provide music and guided imagery

□ Assist Pt./Family in songwriting or song analysis

□ Encourage Pt./Family participation in improvisation/rhythmic play

□ Provide music to validate and support Pt./Family spiritual beliefs

□ Provide music to validate Pt./Family's cultural heritage

Clinician's Signature/Title:	Time In:	Time Out:	Date:

Chapter 10

Brain Injuries and Rehabilitation in Children

Jeanette Kennelly

INTRODUCTION

Music therapy practice in pediatric rehabilitation is slowly expanding in relation to research evidence and descriptive practice reports. In the past 30 years, music therapy researchers and clinicians who specialize in this particular field have published results of studies and descriptions of casework which inform clinical practice (Gilbertson, 2009). This chapter begins by providing the reader with guidance and information about the diagnosis, needs, and resources of the child with an acquired brain injury, considerations for working with caregivers, and referral and assessment procedures. The second part of this chapter focuses specifically on music therapy guidelines used with this population and the music therapy competencies required to conduct these methods safely and effectively. The chapter concludes with multicultural considerations which are important when working with this population and a description of the current research evidence to support pediatric music therapy rehabilitation practice. This chapter is based on the clinical and research practice and publications by this author and other music therapists. It is hoped that it will provide the reader with practical information and guidelines regarding this specialized form of therapy. Working with these children, their families and rehabilitation staff have been both professionally and personally rewarding experiences for the author. This chapter is dedicated to all who have contributed to these experiences.[i]

DIAGNOSTIC INFORMATION

Children and adolescents may acquire neurological damage through traumatic brain injury (TBI), cerebral vascular accident (CVA), or brain injuries acquired from other causes. Injuries received as a result of limited oxygen flow to the brain (hypoxia) can also result in an acquired brain injury (ABI). An ABI refers to any injury to the brain that occurs after birth (Australian Institute of Health and Welfare, 2007). A TBI refers to injury caused as a result of trauma to the head such as a blow or wound (Anderson, 2004). The main causes of TBI in young children include motor vehicle accidents (MVA), blows to the head, and falls. A CVA occurs when blood flow to the brain is interrupted due to a hemorrhage, tumor, or stroke, and as a result the brain ceases to function properly. Young children may also acquire trauma to the brain as a result of a hypoxic brain injury, where, for example, in a near-drowning incident, the brain has received little or no oxygen supply.

Traumatic brain injury remains a leading cause of death and disability among children and young adolescents in the United States (NCIPC, 2002–2006). This includes an estimated average of 473,000 emergency department visits, 35,000 hospitalisations, and 2,000 deaths recorded annually for children up to 14 years old. Children 4 years old and younger have the highest rate of TBI-related emergency department visits, followed by older adolescents from 15 to 19 years old (NCIPC, 2002–2006).

Due to the high incidence of TBI with children and adolescents as compared with other causes of brain injury which require rehabilitation, the scope of this chapter will predominantly focus on TBI.

It is imperative that the music therapist practicing in the field of neurorehabilitation be knowledgeable regarding the pathophysiological aspects of ABI and implications for music therapy practice. While it is beyond the scope of this chapter to include specific detail regarding each of these aspects, a broad knowledge of the brain and its areas of functioning are mandatory for every music therapist practicing with this population.

The human brain is structured into three main areas: the cerebrum, the cerebellum, and the brainstem. The cerebrum consists of two hemispheres (left and right), which are divided into four lobes: the frontal, parietal, occipital, and parietal (Figure 1). Each of these lobes is responsible for different types of human functioning. The inner layer of the cerebrum is referred to as white matter, while the outer layer is known as the gray matter or cerebral cortex (Watson, Kirkcaldie, & Paxinos, 2010).

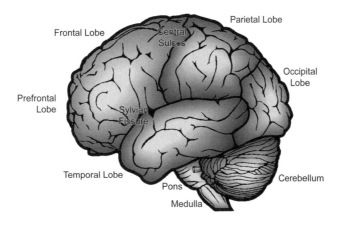

Figure 1. The Brain

The general functional areas of the frontal lobe include the primary motor cortex and the premotor and supplementary motor areas, which involve the initiation of voluntary movements; the Broca's area, which concerns written and spoken language; and the prefrontal cortex, which is associated with personality and insight (Nolte, 2009). The parietal lobe processes tactile stimuli and proprioceptive information or the ability to perceive oneself in space, and is responsible for awareness of spatial dimensions; it furthermore is important to the understanding of language. The occipital lobe is mainly associated with visual functioning, while the temporal lobe involves the processing of learning and memory, complex processing of visual information, hearing, and language comprehension (Nolte, 2009).

The cerebellum can be found at the base of the brain near the brainstem and is important for posture and motor coordination. The brainstem is located underneath the cerebrum and connects with the spinal cord. It is involved in many important functions, such as the communication of signals between the brain and the spinal cord, sleep regulation, breathing, and heart rate (Watson et al., 2010). Injury to any of these areas creates a particular type of impairment and causes a degree of dysfunction depending on the level of injury received (Blosser & De Pompei, 2003). Referenced texts in the fields of neuroanatomy will assist music therapists to further their knowledge of these dysfunctions. Music therapy articles and textbooks focused on music therapy for neurorehabilitation are also useful for further consultation. As two renowned and accomplished neurorehabilitation music therapy clinicians and researchers, Baker and Tamplin (2006) have produced a comprehensive text which extends the content of this chapter regarding diagnoses, needs, and strengths of this population. This textbook is highly recommended for any music therapist working in neurorehabilitation.

It is important early in this chapter to define the different stages of care and the different phases of neurorehabilitation. For the purpose of this chapter, descriptions provided by Anderson, Northam, Hendy, and Wrennall (2001) will be used to define the different phases of rehabilitation:

1) Acute phase (early rehabilitation): The acute phase is defined as one of "survival," as the child with a more severe TBI remains unconscious and requires constant medical care.
2) Subacute phase (intensive rehabilitation): As the child emerges from coma and presents with posttraumatic amnesia (PTA), he enters a period of "recovery/adjustment" where the period of intensive rehabilitation begins.
3) Chronic phase: The final phase is defined as one of acceptance and adjustment as the child is supported with his reintegration into the community.

The guidelines presented in this chapter focus on supporting the patient in the subacute phase of pediatric rehabilitation (Anderson et al., 2001). The music therapist is to select music therapy interventions carefully after consideration of the presented guidelines and recommendations, the research evidence, and, most importantly, the needs of each child as he moves through the trajectory of rehabilitation recovery. The terms "child" and "children" will be used throughout the chapter to represent children as well as adolescents.

The music therapist working with this population may encounter common terminology in relation to impairments following an ABI. An example of these terms is given below and grouped according to the nature of the impairment (Anderson, 2004; Anderson et al., 2001):

1) Cognitive and Behavioral:
   - *Perseverative*—continuous repetition of a response or action which presents as inappropriate and out of context
   - *Lability*—sudden change in mood and behavior
   - *Disinhibition*—reduced ability to manage behaviors and impulsive responses
2) Physical:
   - *Hemiparesis*—loss of skills or weakness to one side of the body
   - *Contracture*—tightening of the skin, skin tissue, muscles, tendons, ligaments, and joint areas
   - *Dyspraxia*—motor learning impairment when signals from the brain to different parts of the body are interrupted or damaged
3) Communicative:
   - *Aphasia*—the inability to use language such as word recall or the inability to read and write
   - *Expressive Aphasia*—the loss of the ability to produce language (spoken or written)
   - *Receptive Aphasia*—people with receptive aphasia can speak with normal grammar, syntax, rate, intonation, and stress, but they are unable to understand language in its written or spoken form
   - *Dysarthria*—motor speech disorder which results in impaired articulation

- *Apraxia*—impaired ability to perform different types of movement (Nolte, 2009)

Changes in the child's personality may also occur following a TBI. These include demonstrations of physical aggression, irritability, and immature behaviors (Feeney & Ylvisaker, 2003). Family members observing these behavioral changes often experience difficulty in adjusting to the development of a new and different child postinjury. The impacts of a TBI therefore have diverse implications for both child and family members.

NEEDS AND RESOURCES

Management of the needs of children with TBI is complex and presents diagnostic and therapeutic challenges to the rehabilitation team (Kochanek, Belle, & Bayir, 2010). When children sustain a TBI, their needs are distinguished from that of adults. Regardless of their age at the time of injury, children's developmental skills are still being acquired. Neurological trauma sustained during a period of growth and development places physiological and psychological stress on the acquisition of these skills (Kennelly, 2006).

As children are placed in an environment of daily rehabilitation treatment (usually a rehabilitation unit), they are faced with the challenge of learning and relearning skills; this, in turn, places stressful demands on their physiological and psychological well-being. Although these children may initially appear overwhelmed by the rehabilitation environment and its intensive therapy program, they often present amazing inner strength and resilience. This author's extensive clinical experience with this population has indicated that many of these children often possess an inner drive to return to their premorbid self, regardless of their developmental age. This positive self-drive and their participation and endurance of repetitive daily tasks and routines are to be admired. In addition, incredible support is often provided by their family network. It is important that music therapists remember and acknowledge these strengths and qualities as they engage in pediatric neurorehabilitation programs. It is also important to remember that children (together with their family) possess diverse characteristics and strengths and, when faced with the trauma of a brain injury, may respond in ways that potentially hinder their rehabilitation progress. For example, a child's self-drive may compromise treatment goals, particularly if he is unable to comprehend that a return to his premorbid state of functioning is not possible. It is imperative that the music therapist consider the broad range of strengths and needs in children and their families.

Brain Development

The development of the central nervous system (CNS) and brain maturation hold particular significance for the child diagnosed with a TBI. Growth spurts of the CNS, which typically take place between seven and nine years of age and 16 and 19 years, may be disrupted by injury and may alter or cease the course of development (Anderson et al., 2001). Research regarding brain maturation has debated the hierarchical progression vs. the continuing development of the brain. Prior to the 1970s, it was assumed that the earlier in age a child received an injury, the better the outcome would be (Kolb & Gibb, 2010). However, current research no longer supports this idea. Instead, evidence suggests a differential recovery from injury dependent upon age of injury (Anderson, Spencer-Smith, Leventer, Coleman, Anderson, Williams, Greenham, & Jacobs, 2009; Hessen, Nestvold, & Anderson, 2007). Anderson and colleagues found that injury received prior to the age of two leads to greater cognitive dysfunction, compared to injuries received at an older age. It is imperative that the music therapist working in rehabilitation be knowledgeable of this type of evidence and the implications of this research on clinical practice (Kennelly, 2006). Recommended reading to support practice includes topics of cerebral development and biomechanics of traumatic brain injury in pediatrics (Anderson & Yeates, 2010; Blosser & De Pompei, 2003).

Considerations for Recovery in Pediatric Rehabilitation

It is important for the music therapist not to treat their pediatric patient like a "little adult" (Blosser & De Pompei, 2003, p. 32). While adult rehabilitation models of practice may still be useful to adopt when working in pediatrics, a different way of practice is required when working with children. "Because children are a 'work in progress,' brain injury has the potential not only to rob a child of knowledge and skills already acquired ... but also to jeopardize the child's ability to master new skills" (Ylvisaker, Chorazy, Feeney, & Russell, 1999, p. 356). Consideration of a child's premorbid skill development and acquisition is vital during treatment planning. The child and adolescent experience many periods of rapid developmental change and constantly move in and out of these stages as they mature physically, emotionally, cognitively, and spiritually (Kennelly, 2006). The child with a TBI may experience an interruption to skills acquisition and be required to learn new skills without previous knowledge or experience of that skill.

Three areas of attention must be considered when working with these children: (a) long-term effects of the trauma; (b) delayed onset of deficits where, due to the child's age and time of injury, the full impact of their deficits may not be known or evident; and (c) age variability (Blosser & De Pompei, 2003). It is important that the music therapist be knowledgeable regarding the critical periods of brain development in relation to developmental stages (e.g., major changes are noted in the parietal, occipital, and temporal regions for children ages one to six years) (Blosser & De Pompei, 2003).

Needs Addressed in Pediatric Music Therapy Rehabilitation

The needs of children in rehabilitation, regardless their type or level, are complex and impacted by the phase of their current treatment (Kennelly & Brien-Elliott, 2001). Whether for the semiconscious child who presents as irritable (Kennelly & Edwards, 1997) or the child who struggles to speak clearly (Kennelly, Hamilton, & Cross, 2001), music therapy has a role to play in meeting these individualized needs. Adopting the phases of rehabilitation according to Anderson and colleagues (2001), the following needs of the child and adolescent are presented:

1) *Acute phase (early rehabilitation):* Depending on the severity of injury, the child's main need during this phase is survival. The goal of the medical, nursing, and therapy team is to medically stabilize the child. It is imperative during this stage that the music therapist consults with the team regarding the purpose and appropriateness of music therapy interventions. Depending on the protocol adopted by each team, music therapy may not be indicated during this stage. As the child's immediate needs concern medical stability, music therapy may be used to provide physical and emotional support. Depending on the child's level of consciousness, his need to remain calm and relaxed in order to increase recovery rate is of primary concern when adopting any potential music therapy interventions. The child's family may also require emotional support during this time. It may be appropriate to conduct sessions at bedside with the family members present in order to provide opportunities for meaningful interaction.

2) *Subacute phase (intensive rehabilitation):* During this phase, the child's needs are broadly categorized into two areas, namely functional and psychosocial. Functional needs include needs in (a) physical areas, such as improved tolerance for sitting and motivation for activities of daily living in order to regain gross and fine motor skills; improved gait, balance, and posture; pain management; and muscle relaxation; (b) cognitive and behavioral domains, such as improved orientation and arousal, self-control, ability to follow directions, attention, learning, and conversational skills; and (c) communicative areas, such as improved rate and articulation of speech, intonation, and respiratory control. Psychosocial needs encompass emotional support and adjustment following the injury. Typical psychosocial needs include anxiety and fear concerning hospitalization and treatment, isolation from family and home, and issues of grief and loss (Baker & Tamplin, 2006).

3) *Chronic phase:* The child's needs in this final phase may include functional and psychosocial areas as previously described; however, the focus in these domains may differ as the preparation for discharge to home or another rehabilitation setting is made. Functional needs may include reintegration into the home and school environment (e.g., the ability for the school-age child to mobilize independently around the school environment and communicate effectively with teachers and peers). Psychosocial needs may also focus on this reintegration period as the child returns to his home and school environment in a potentially different emotional state that his premorbid self. Ongoing rehabilitation may be required through outpatient services. This will place different demands on the family as they juggle life outside the hospital setting with a continuing therapy program.

While the focus of this chapter is the child requiring neurorehabilitation, there are other chapters in this volume which may assist the reader in the planning and delivering of clinical practice with this population (Chapter 2 by Bradt on pain management; Chapter 8 by Dun on children with cancer; and Chapter 12 by Townsend on medically fragile children). Guidelines in the area of pain management will be useful for working with the patient in rehabilitation as the therapist addresses the area of high muscle tension and associated pain. Children who are diagnosed with brain or spinal cord tumors may also require rehabilitation. Reading Dun's chapter will assist the pediatric rehabilitation music therapist in understanding these patients' diagnoses and associated needs. Readers are encouraged to access the chapter by Townsend for content regarding patients in a minimally conscious or persistent vegetative state. Trauma, burns, postinfective complications, and malignancy may result in amputation and limb deficiency and require patients to receive rehabilitation. Other chapters in the volume relating to these client groups may also assist the clinician's knowledge and practice when working in pediatric rehabilitation.

WORKING WITH CAREGIVERS

As described by Lehr (1996), "acquired brain injury sustained by children and adolescents is very much a family affair" (p. 53). In caring for the needs of the child, the role of the family and significant carers must be considered. The child may require emotional support during all phases of rehabilitation treatment and, depending on his age at time of injury, will often look for this support from their primary carers (Blosser & De Pompei, 2003; Kennelly, 2006).

As the child with an ABI faces different issues through each rehabilitation phase, his family also moves and adjusts within these phases accordingly (Anderson et al., 2001). During the acute phase, parents and siblings are concerned with the survival of the child and often feel helpless or responsible for the injury. The family members may become physically separated by location due to the needs of the child. This separation may create financial pressures. As the child enters the subacute phase, other issues concerning adjustment to the changes in the child, managing the rehabilitation needs of the child with the rest of the family's requirements, as well as ongoing financial and employment concerns, continue to place stress on the family. The final chronic phase places the family in a space of continued support for their child. Sourcing educational and housing options and managing behavioral and physical problems are just a few of their concerns (Anderson et al., 2001). In order for the physical, cognitive, and emotional needs of the child to be successfully addressed and managed, multiple support mechanisms are required in pediatric rehabilitation for both child and family.

Music therapy programs can be used to address the needs of the child and his family members. It is important that the therapist be specific with the goals addressed in each program in order to ensure that appropriate needs are being met (e.g., if the focus of the session is the child, and family members are present, program goals should be centred on the child's needs). It is possible that during the use of music therapy, some of the family members' concerns or anxieties can become inadvertently addressed. Parents may be able to engage in the session with their child and assist the therapist in providing a supportive space for the child to musically express himself. Older siblings may provide leadership and guidance to a child who feels frightened and insecure. Appendix A presents issues faced by children and their family members during the different rehabilitation phases and the music therapy role/interventions that can address their required needs (Kennelly, 2006, pp. 229–231).

Referral and Assessment

Music therapy practice models can be used to guide the pediatric rehabilitation music therapist in the development of referral criteria and assessment protocols and delivery of quality therapy programs. As the child presents with various needs throughout their rehabilitation, the therapist may need to consider different models of approach for each recovery stage. This author recommends the use of a meta-model in neurorehabilitation, developed by Daveson (2008), to assist the planning and evaluation of music therapy programs and associated interventions. The three approaches presented in this meta-model, namely restorative, compensatory, and psycho-social-emotional, provide a flexible framework which guides the therapist in delivering "patient-centred and patient-led care" (Daveson, 2008, p.74).

The child with a TBI may initially present as unconscious and be admitted to the pediatric intensive care unit (PICU). During this acute phase, the goals of the music therapy interventions will depend on the child's level of injury and prognosis. While some authors define this phase as acute or early rehabilitation care, it is important for the rehabilitation music therapist to consult their department's guidelines regarding procedures and appropriate timing for assessment. It is possible that the PICU music therapist (as opposed to the rehabilitation music therapist) may begin a program with this child. If so, it is important that the rehabilitation music therapist remain in consultation with the PICU music therapist regarding the child's progress and responses to therapy in order to ensure continuity in care should a handover be required. The reader can consult Chapter 5 by Ghetti on music therapy interventions in the PICU.

There are some cases where the child is only referred to the rehabilitation team when his medical condition is regarded as stable and he presents with PTA. Similar considerations for therapy program planning must be made for children diagnosed with a brain or spinal cord tumor. At the time of admission to the oncology unit, they may receive music therapy interventions from the oncology music therapist; however, because of damage caused by the tumor, they may also require a period of rehabilitation. Music therapy department guidelines and a rehabilitation unit's admission criteria may require the patient to be no longer receiving active chemotherapy or radiation treatment in order to receive rehabilitation. This requirement may stem from concerns regarding side effects from cancer treatments and any possible contraindications which may result if both forms of treatment are engaged in simultaneously.

Referral Procedures

Each rehabilitation unit maintains their own set of referral procedures. It is important for the music therapist to consult these guidelines when establishing processes in relation to music therapy referrals. Guidelines for the acceptance of referrals can assist in determining the quality and quantity of the music therapy clinical caseload. This is particularly important for the new therapist working with this population, e.g., working with a large number of patients who have PTA can be emotionally draining for the therapist and time restrictions may also prevent the acceptance of all such referrals. Prioritization criteria for caseload management maintained by each rehabilitation unit may assist the music therapist in this area. A separate document outlining referral guidelines may include a brief description of how music therapy can address various rehabilitation needs following an ABI, as outlined earlier in this chapter.

In order to ensure an efficient referral process, it is important that the referral document be concise, informative, and user-friendly. The document should include the name of the child; the date, the name, and professional details (e.g., medical, nursing, physical therapy) of the person responsible for the referral; reason(s) for referral; and space for a brief description of the child's personal and medical history. To simplify the referral process, reasons for referral may be prelisted on the form, organized by categories of needs. For example,

Behavioral/Cognitive Domains:
- Improve orientation
- Decrease agitation

Emotional Domains:
- Provide opportunities for self-expression
- Promote adjustment to illness and/or injury

Communication Domains:
- Increase rate of speech
- Improve clarity of speech

The referral form should also allow for options of self-referral (by the child) and referral from family members (Edwards & Kennelly, 1999; Kennelly & Brien-Elliott, 2002, 2001).

Another form useful for consideration when working in pediatric rehabilitation is a fact sheet for hospital staff and families These publications may assist those unfamiliar with music therapy by providing an understanding of the definition and role of music therapy/music therapist, reasons for referral, and the goals of music therapy programs (AMTA, 2011). Separate fact sheets can be provided for staff and families, as the publication for staff may require a more formal approach in relation to definition, role of music therapy, and evidence to support interventions.

Assessment

Assessment of the child with an ABI involves a wide range of tests and tools; however, not all are available for use by music therapists. Different tests require specific training for administration and interpretation, while others may only be administered by particular members of the medical, nursing, or therapy team. Each tool serves a different purpose in the examination of a child's medical, physical, behavioral, cognitive, communicative, emotional, and social status. While it is beyond the scope of this chapter to provide detailed information for each tool, it is imperative that the music therapist working with this population be knowledgeable regarding the purpose and results of each assessment and the ways it may inform their own music therapy assessments. The music therapist should also consult their rehabilitation unit on the type of preferred tools used by each health discipline. For example, measurements of recovery from coma can include the Glasgow Coma Scale (GCS) (Teasdale & Jennett, 1974), the Ranchos Los Amigos Scale of Cognitive Functioning (Hagen, Malkmus, Durham, & Stenderup, 1979), and the Children's Orientation and Amnesia Test (COAT) (Erwing-Cobbs, Levin, Fletcher, Miner, & Eisenberg, 1990) to evaluate posttraumatic amnesia (Blosser & De Pompei, 2003). Following an ABI, a child's level of consciousness can be determined by their GCS score, indicated by a number between 3 and 15, with higher scores representing greater awareness. The total score is based on the patient's motor and verbal responses and eye opening. As the GCS was originally designed for use with adults, a modified version of the GCS, the Paediatric Glasgow Coma Scale, is used with infants and young children under two years of age (James, 1986). The COAT is structured into three sections: general orientation (such as their own name and age), temporal orientation (such as the current day of the week or year), and memory (such as recalling the name of the tester). Scores are provided for each section and range from 5 to 15 points per question, with higher scores representing a higher level of orientation. The Ranchos Los Amigos Scale measures states of consciousness according to eight levels, from the first level demonstrating no response to purposeful and appropriate responses at level 8. The reader is encouraged to access the texts by Baker and Tamplin (2006) and Blosser and DePompei (2003) to extend their understanding of common assessment tools such as the GCS and the COAT.

A number of measures for assessing TBI outcomes in children have been published in the United States (NCIPC, 2002–2006). These include quality of life assessments such as the Child Health & Illness Profile (CHIP); behavioral and cognitive assessments; functional assessments such as the Functional Independence Measure for Children (WeeFIM); educational, vocation, and recreation assessments; and assessments of family functioning, depression, and posttraumatic stress disorder (NCIPC, 2002–2006). The WeeFIM is a common functional assessment tool which can be administered by a variety of trained and credentialed health care staff (AROC, 2012). Eighteen items of daily activities including motor and cognitive domains are scored according to the rates of dependence and independence. The score ranges from 1 to 7 for each item, with higher scores representing increased independence. This tool may be useful for music therapists to support their own assessments and assist individual and joint therapy goal planning.

The development of a tool to musically assess levels of consciousness in children with ABI provides some guidance toward the selection and appropriateness of music therapy methods (Whitehead, 1998). The "Music Therapy Assessment Continuum" consists of 15 categories across five levels of consciousness, ranging from no response to initiating a musical response with and without the music therapist. The tool was developed based on the researcher's clinical experience and a review of music therapy and non–music therapy assessment tools in rehabilitation. The researcher provides a clinical vignette of a nine-year-old girl who received an anoxic brain injury, which demonstrates practice applications for this assessment tool. Examples of the recording of musical and nonmusical responses are useful for music therapists in considering the role of assessment. However, this instrument has not yet been standardized and therefore may be limited in its use as an assessment instrument.

Music therapy assessment tools in pediatric rehabilitation may incorporate the Pediatric Inpatient Music Therapy Assessment Form (PIMTAF) developed by Douglass (2006). While the form does not specifically address the needs of a child recovering from an ABI, the tool contains relevant assessment criteria which may apply to this population. The form is structured according to areas related to a patient's background, referral and physiological information, physical/motor and cognitive skills, social and emotional behavior, communication skills, and musical behaviors. Questions dealing with the patient's musical background, their favorite music, and special interests are also addressed. The final section contains information regarding the recommended treatment modality, goal areas to be addressed, music therapy interventions to be used, and a summary or plan for treatment (Douglass, 2006).

Another useful assessment tool, though not specifically designed for the pediatric population, is the Individual Music Therapy Assessment Profile (IMTAP) form developed by Baxter, Berghofer, MacEwan, Nelson, Peters, and Roberts (2007). This tool provides opportunities for detailed information to be recorded on diverse rehabilitation needs, including gross motor, fine motor, oral motor, sensory perception, communication, cognition, emotional responses, social skills, and musical skills. As a criterion-based assessment tool that is not standardized by age or age range, the IMTAP presents as a comprehensive and detailed tool useful for the pediatric rehabilitation setting.

The music therapist may need to consult family members for information regarding a child's music preferences, including any history detailing the child's experiences and exposure to music. This typically occurs when the child is unable to provide this information due to the extent of his injury. Contact with the child's school teachers may also provide useful information regarding music preferences and experiences, including important peer friendships prior to his injury (Kennelly, 2006).

INTRODUCTION TO MUSIC THERAPY METHODS

The music therapist working in pediatric neurorehabilitation is challenged with a wide array of developmental factors and age ranges that impact a child's recovery from a brain injury. Children in the first 12 months of life respond differently to hospitalization and their injury as compared with a five-year-old, 12-year-old or adolescent (Robb, 2003). Their understanding and ability to cope with potentially stressful experiences must be considered by the therapist when assessing, planning, and evaluating client-related goals (Edwards & Kennelly, 2011). The music therapist should observe physical, cognitive, social, and emotional responses of the child prior to, during, and after interventions.

Each guideline in this chapter must be considered according to the premorbid and current assessment of the patient's developmental status, whether in the physical, cognitive, social, or emotional domain. The reader is encouraged to access literature on the topic of milestone attainment in childhood development, including models and frameworks adopted in pediatric music therapy practice (Edwards & Kennelly, 2011; Robb, 2003). General pediatric music therapy literature (non–rehabilitation-specific) will also be useful in supporting the therapist's understanding and knowledge of this area (Edwards, 2005; Edwards & Kennelly, 2011; Kennelly, 2000; Robb, 2003).

Throughout the guidelines in this chapter, contraindications have been included as a point of importance in guiding the selection of therapy techniques. Besides these specific contraindications, it is recommended that the music therapist, prior to assessment, be aware of the etiology of the patient's injury and have a working knowledge of the regions of the brain and their associated functions. This will allow the music therapist to have an understanding, prior to the actual assessment, of potential deficits or impairments resulting from damage to specific brain regions in the child and implications for the neural processing of music. It is also imperative that the music therapist carefully consider the selection and use of methods in order to reduce potential overstimulation for the child, particularly when the child is diagnosed with PTA. Presented guidelines include recommended length of session or intervention times in order to minimize levels of fatigue and overstimulation. As the child recovering from an ABI requires time to process auditory information, sufficient time must be given by the music therapist to observe any response to the music therapy methods employed. It is important that the music therapist remain patient and flexible in her use of these methods and provide sufficient time for the child to respond accordingly before any change to the method is made.

Competencies of the Pediatric Rehabilitation Music Therapist

As described in the introduction to this chapter, in order to practice competently and effectively, it is important for the pediatric rehabilitation music therapist to be knowledgeable and demonstrate an understanding of a variety of areas which can impact the selection of music therapy methods with this population. These include child and family developmental factors, neuroanatomy, stages of recovery, implications for therapy interventions within each recovery stage, and assessment and evaluation procedures adopted by the multidisciplinary team (Baker & Tamplin, 2006; Kennelly, 2006).

Specialist training in Neurologic Music Therapy (NMT) is available and is based on a model whereby specific techniques have been designed and scientifically researched to produce efficacy (Thaut, 1999). These techniques target the areas of sensorimotor, speech and language, and cognitive rehabilitation. This training provides the music therapist with a set of specialized skills which may be adapted when addressing the various needs of a child recovering from an ABI. Collaboration and communication with other neurorehabilitation music therapists can also extend practice skills and knowledge for the developing therapist. Further information regarding these training programs and supportive networks is located in the Appendix under Resources.

When considering clinical practice guidelines, it is important for the pediatric rehabilitation music therapist to be familiar and competent in a range of musical styles and genres. As the age range of patients will vary considerably from newborn infants to adolescents, so too will their preferences and musical tastes for repertoire. The use of live vs. recorded music must be carefully considered as the music therapist examines her abilities to replicate musical material which may be complex in structure and timbre. Adolescent song material requires a broad range of practice expertise, including competency in a number of instruments such as electronic keyboards and acoustic/electric guitars (Kennelly, 2006).

Digital recording equipment such as iPods, MP3 devices, and the use of iPad applications may prove helpful when considering the use of music technology in clinical practice. The use of iTunes provides greater opportunities for song listening and offering song choices. Computer software programs for song composition and song recording include the Super Dooper Music Looper, Acid Pro 6, Sound Forge, and GarageBand. Other useful music technology resources have been listed toward the end of this chapter. It is important that the music therapist plan for the use of these resources and consider any contraindications for the inclusion of music technology (Whitehead-Pleaux, Clark, & Spall, 2011).

Literature in Pediatric Rehabilitation Music Therapy

While the research evidence for various music therapy methods is presented toward the end of this chapter, it is important to recognize and value the impact of all types of literature which support and describe clinical practice. As described by Gilberston (2009), "systematic analyses and meta-analyses [of controlled clinical trials] will not be able to capture the clinical diversity described in the complete spectrum of types of publications on music therapy with children with traumatic brain injury" (p. 135). Gilbertson developed a reference standard bibliography of literature pertaining to pediatric ABI as a useful way of searching for and establishing a broader scope of available music therapy literature. A table describing the various music therapy techniques adopted in each report or study provides a different way of viewing and understanding clinical practice (Gilberston, 2009). It is recommended that this literature be sourced as an additional support to the practice of pediatric rehabilitation methods.

Music therapy research which focuses on the techniques adopted within music therapy methods and procedures provides us with a different way of understanding clinical practice. A study by Edwards and Kennelly (2004) used modified grounded theory to identify categories of non–music therapy techniques used by a music therapist while working with three children. Its findings revealed that additional techniques such as cuing, synchrony, and orientation were integrated and enmeshed with the traditional use of music therapy interventions. This research suggests that music therapists working in pediatric rehabilitation need to consider a variety of techniques, both musical and nonmusical, when practicing and interacting with children and their families.

Finally, music therapists have described their clinical practice in pediatric rehabilitation to address cognitive/behavioral needs (Magee, Baker, Daveson, Hitchen, Kennelly, Leung, & Tamplin, 2011), psychosocial needs (Baker, Kennelly, & Tamplin, 2005a; Bower & Shoemark, 2012; Robb, 1996), communication and interaction (Bower & Shoemark, 2009; Gilbertson, 1999; Kennelly, Hamilton, & Cross, 2001; Leung, 2008), and a combined range of needs including physical functioning (Hurt-Thaut & Johnson, 2003; Kennelly & Brien-Elliott, 2001; Rosenfeld & Dun, 1999). The aim of this chapter is not to provide a comprehensive discussion of the pediatric music therapy rehabilitation literature but rather to formulate practice guidelines based on the existing literature as well as this author's extensive clinical experience. It is therefore recommended that the reader further consult these articles in view of the presented clinical guidelines.

OVERVIEW OF MUSIC THERAPY METHODS AND PROCEDURES

An overview of music therapy methods and procedures included in this chapter is listed below. The methods and procedures are not presented in a specific order.

Receptive Music Therapy

- Music Listening for Orientation and Arousal: use of live and recorded music to increase orientation and arousal in a child who emerges from a coma.
- Structured Music Experiences to Promote Physical Functioning: use of music listening as a structured and predictable focus point during targeted work on range, flexibility, and strength of movement.
- Songs as Reinforcer and Cue for Self-Control: Songs are utilized as an effective reinforcer of desired behavior as well as a cue or prompt for following directions.
- Music-assisted Pain Management: use of music listening to support children in their reported experiences of pain and assist them to achieve a more relaxed state.
- Music-assisted Relaxation: use of music listening to offer much needed periods of relaxation during the intensive treatment schedule typical for ABI rehabilitation.
- Music Listening for Emotional Support: use of music listening to offer support and validation as the child with ABI deals with a range of emotional challenges.

Improvisational Music Therapy

- Instrumental Improvisation for Emotional Support: use of instrumental improvisations with various levels of structure to enhance exploration and expression of emotions related to the challenges of having an ABI.
- Instrumental Improvisation to Promote Physical Functioning: use of instrumental improvisation to provide individualized cues and prompts for directed movement.
- Instrumental Improvisation to Reduce Perseverations: use of instrumental improvisation to reduce verbal and behavioral perseverations

- Improvisational Music Therapy to Promote Direction-Following: Improvised music is used to prompt and cue the child to listen attentively and engage in musical conversations which encourage imitation and turn-taking.

Re-creative Music Therapy

- Modified Melodic Intonation Therapy: use of short phrases based on simple melodic and harmonic structures to enhance functional verbal communication.
- Singing to Improve Articulation and Rate of Speech: use of songs to improve articulation and increase the rate of speech in children with ABI by stimulating areas of the brain which do not respond effectively to these routine of drills in spoken form.
- Singing to Improve Intonation: use of singing songs, scale exercises, and vocal interval matching to expand the child's vocal range and improve intonation.
- Re-creative Music Therapy to Improve Respiratory Control: Song singing is used to improve breath control and increase speech phrasing with children recovering from an ABI.
- Rhythmic Auditory Stimulation (RAS): Neurologic Music Therapy technique using song singing to improve gait rehabilitation.

Compositional Music Therapy

- Songwriting to Promote Learning: writing of songs with lyrics that provide structure and sequential order for physical or cognitive tasks, aid memory and conversational skills through the use of musical prompts and cues, and promote learning.
- Songwriting to Provide Emotional Support: writing songs to provide opportunities for self-expression in regard to different dimensions of the rehabilitation experience for children experiencing difficulties adjusting to their injuries, disabilities, and period of hospitalization; difficulties interacting with family and staff; and feelings of anger and anxiety.

GUIDELINES FOR RECEPTIVE MUSIC THERAPY

The use of receptive music therapy interventions requires a noise reduced environment in order to maximize the benefits of this method. Sessions may take place at the child's bedside, in a treatment room on the hospital ward, or in the rehabilitation unit. Prior knowledge of the child's rehabilitation routine or daily therapy timetable is important for scheduling an optimal time for these interventions. Consultation with medical, nursing, or rehabilitation therapy staff may be necessary in ensuring minimal disturbances and distractions from other interventions (medical and nonmedical). Prior assessment of the child's musical preferences is required to determine and prepare repertoire appropriate for the individual child. The music therapist should observe physical and emotional responses of the child prior to, during, and after interventions.

Music Listening for Orientation and Arousal

Overview. As children emerge from an unconsciousness state, they may experience a period of confusion and agitation which is described as PTA. This phase refers to a period of time following an ABI or when the child emerges from coma where memory and sense of orientation is impaired (Anderson, 2004). Music therapy may be used alone or additionally with other allied health therapies (such as occupational therapy) in order to increase a child's state of orientation and arousal. The state of arousal can be determined by positive changes in awareness (such as smiles and positive affect) and the ability to engage comfortably with presented stimuli, e.g., remaining settled and calm. Signs of overstimulation may present as irritability, agitation, grimacing, and increased fatigue (Baker & Tamplin, 2006). However, these observations require careful and consistent monitoring and testing in order to determine overstimulation (Baker & Tamplin, 2006). Research literature supports the use of music therapy with adults (Baker, 2001) and children in PTA (Bower, 2010). Receptive techniques described in this guideline are based on this evidence. As the research by Baker also incorporated the use of recorded music, this guideline will also contain references and recommendations for this form of music. Working with a child in PTA requires careful observation of fatigue levels and the potential ability for music to overstimulate and increase agitation. Duration of the session should be 10 to 15 minutes and include the use of familiar and preferred music which is structured simply and predictable. The therapist should also monitor use of combined vocal/instrumental music, as this presentation of material may overstimulate the child. Considerations of using only voice or only an accompanying instrument such as the guitar are also suggested.

Preparation. The child in PTA is usually located in a private setting away from other patients so as to minimize agitation levels and maintain a quiet environment. The music therapist must ensure that other staff and family members are aware of the goals of this music therapy intervention in order to maximize the potential benefits. The therapist may be required to plan ahead for the use of this method, particularly if the child is already engaged in a full-time rehabilitation program.

What to observe. Prior to the session, the child may present as disoriented, which may include varying levels of agitation and confusion. Assessment of the child's PTA state for that day may have already taken place; therefore, it is imperative that the music therapist be aware of these results before commencing therapy. Questions adapted from pediatric PTA scales (Erwing-Cobbs et al., 1990) may assist in orientating the child according to the following areas: identifying the music therapist by name and face, past therapy sessions, and songs used within these sessions. The music therapist should plan and consult for this type of assessment with the rehabilitation team in order to avoid overstimulation and overtiring the child with additional forms of questioning.

Procedures. This guideline is based on research by Baker (2001) with adult patients in PTA. The music therapist introduces herself to the child using a calm, supportive tone and explains in simple terms the purpose of the session. All musical repertoire used should be familiar and preferred by the patient, not overstimulating in terms of tempo or rhythmic structure and contain positive lyrics. When the first song is played or sung a capella for the child, whether the complete song or only a verse and/or chorus, the child is asked to relax and listen to the music. The therapist may also decide to sing a capella only with the first song (or the chorus and then introduce an accompanying instrument) in order to monitor the child's responses to the musical stimuli and avoid overstimulation. The accompanying style should be soft in dynamics, slow in tempo, and simple in rhythm, such as a compound time. During the music, the therapist observes the child's responses. Following the music, the therapist may present questions to the child about the music, depending on their PTA state. For example, if the child appears disoriented at the start of the session, the therapist may choose to ask only one question after the music, such as "Do you like that song?," before proceeding to ask the child if he recalled hearing that song from before. The number of songs/instrumental compositions used in any session will vary according to the child's fatigue levels. The suggested initial length for each session is 10 to 15 minutes, using three pieces of music with the same selection of repertoire for each session to promote orientation (Baker & Tamplin, 2006). At the end of the session, final observations are made in relation to the child's physical, communicative, and emotional responses. Posttraumatic amnesia testing by a health care staff member may occur again at this time. This receptive guideline may also be useful in addressing other areas of need for children in PTA, including relaxation and decreasing agitation and distress (Baker, 2001; Baker & Tamplin, 2006; Magee et al., 2011).

Recorded music may be used in place of live music for orientation and arousal (Baker, 2001). Considerations of recordings using only voice or an instrument require review from the music therapist in relation to appropriate musical elements such as tempo, volume and texture, and style. Particular consideration must be given to the type of audio equipment used in the environment (by the child, their carers, or staff). Use of earphones and free-field music require close monitoring as each child may respond differently to their use. In addition, volume levels and duration of listening time need to be evaluated to avoid fatigue and a decrease in arousal. It is important for the music therapist to provide detailed guidelines to staff and family members for the use of music listening for orientation and arousal, particularly when the therapist is unable to be present during the implementation. A list of recommended guidelines can be placed at the child's bedside or placed in his clinical chart for reference. The music therapist should furthermore provide education regarding these guidelines to both carers and staff. Instructions for this guideline may include changing from one music track to another if the child appeared overstimulated; increasing or decreasing volume levels; or terminating the use of the recording. It is recommended that time be allowed in between musical material for the child to process the stimuli, rest, and prepare for the next listening activity. This should be considered for the use of live music as well. As the child is unable to regulate the use of the recording, it is imperative that a responsible carer or staff member (if the music therapist is not present) attend to the use of the recording equipment and monitor the child's responses to the music at all times. The music therapist needs to emphasize to the carers and staff the importance of never leaving the child alone while the music is playing.

While acknowledging the use of recorded music to increase orientation and arousal levels, the author recommends that where possible, the music therapist be present during implementation of music listening to address this need and that live music be used instead. Research suggests that music results in improvements in orientation and agitation with the adult in PTA, regardless of the type of music (live or recorded) (Baker, 2001). However, the presence of a music therapist provides greater flexibility to more easily address the changing needs of a child (i.e., the ability for a therapist to subtly change and adapt the music's tempo, dynamics, and timbre in response to the child's reactions as opposed to the use of recorded music). Still, it is important to note that the music therapist may not be able to provide daily therapy face-to-face and the use of recorded music to address this area of support has its benefits. It is the role of the therapist to provide clear and structured guidelines and educate those caring for the child in their use of recorded music.

Depending on the level of PTA, it is possible that the child may attempt to sing spontaneously with the music therapist or demonstrate purposeful or unintentional movements in response to the music. The child may also attempt to move toward the music therapist and her instrument with an intention of engaging in instrumental play. According to Baker and Tamplin (2006) and Bower (2010), these responses may be acknowledged by the therapist at the time; however, the therapist needs to be aware that engaging the child in music-making during the PTA stage may impact negatively on the session goals because of potential overstimulation. At the same time, it is possible that engaging in song singing may assist the child's orientation and arousal state (Bower, 2010). Careful observations of the child's responses are needed before deciding to change from receptive to re-creative methods.

Structured Music Experiences to Promote Physical Functioning

Overview. Music listening is often used in rehabilitation to promote physical functioning (i.e., increase, improve, assist, or encourage fine or gross motor movements). The rationale for using music in this area is based on evidence which supports the link between rhythmic auditory stimulation (RAS) and improved physical movement in rehabilitation (Hurt, Rice, & McIntosh, 1998; Thaut, 2005; Thaut et al., 1996). These links between the auditory and motor components in the brain can be influenced by rhythm, helping to control movement (Thaut, 2005). Listening to music provides a child with a structured and predictable focus point during targeted work on range, flexibility, and strength of movement (Kennelly & Brien-Elliott, 2001). Children with ABI are faced with many challenges in the rehabilitation of their physical skills. For example, many patients who need to relearn to transition from sitting to standing (and vice versa) often face difficulties with weight bearing, balance, and posture and require assistance to perform this type of movement safely and effectively. In addition, this movement may evoke intense fear in the child. This example will be used below to explain how music listening can assist with this learning process. It is recommended that the reader consult Baker and Tamplin (2006) for detailed instruction concerning the use of music therapy interventions for rehabilitation of many other physical impairments (e.g., addressing wrist movement; grasp and release).

Referrals focused on improving physical functioning are usually received from the rehabilitation physiotherapist and/or occupational therapist. The child may feel unmotivated to participate in therapy sessions and reluctant to perform gross or fine motor movements because of pain or fear associated with the movement. The music therapist works collaboratively with these therapists in providing appropriate music which offers structure, stimulation, and motivation for different forms of exercise (Kennelly & Brien-Elliott, 2001).

Preparation. The music therapist places herself and her accompanying instrument in an appropriate space near the child and any other therapy staff present. This may include standing, sitting, kneeling near the child, and being flexible in moving to various positions if required to do so. The use of the acoustic guitar is useful in this type of session, as the therapist is able to move freely around the room while maintaining eye contact with the child.

What to observe. While the goal of the session focuses on physical functioning, it is imperative that the therapist observe a range of responses from the child, including their vocal/verbal responses. These observations may communicate the emotional aspect of the physical task at hand and assist the therapist in monitoring their use of this intervention. As the child engages in the physical activity, the music therapist observes any changes in their functioning, however minimal, and adjusts the musical parameters such as tempo and accompaniment style accordingly. Therefore, it is important that the therapist maintain communication with other therapy staff present as they work toward a common session goal.

Procedures. As stated above, the procedural steps provided here are for music therapy assistance with movement from sitting to standing position, or vice versa. These procedures will vary according to the specific tasks and the child's developmental age. For example, the tasks could range from assisting a child to reach for the guitar while in prone/supine positions to promote trunk extension to preparing a child for standing and weight bearing or transferring from wheelchair to his hospital bed. The range of target areas in promoting physical functioning is endless and unable to be covered comprehensively in this chapter. Therefore, only a few examples will be provided here. Songs should be used with lyrics that give instructions specific to the task. When assisting a child to transition from sitting to standing or vice versa, the music therapist should attempt to explain to the child the purpose of the song and ask the child to listen to the lyrics carefully. Again, the instructions provided by the song lyrics will depend on the age of the child and his ability to follow directions. For the younger child, parents may be asked to assist the child with these cues. Using verbal and physical cues from any other therapists present and the musical cues of the song, the child listens to the lyrics and music and is encouraged to perform the instructed movement. A short instrumental introduction of four bars before the song can prepare the child for the required movement. The child's favorite songs or song parodies may be used to focus, prompt, or cue the child for the selected task, extend his physical ability, and maintain concentration. The music should be structured simply with the use of repeated melodic/rhythmic motifs in even phrases to provide a predictable holding environment. Fatigue and concentration levels of the child should be closely monitored during the session. An example of a standing and sitting song is provided below, where the child is preparing to transition from sitting to standing and vice versa (Kennelly, 2006, p. 232).

Steven's "Standing" Song.[ii] This song was created with assistance from Steven's physiotherapist and occupational therapist to assist him with the steps necessary for preparation to stand. The melody used was *Twinkle, Twinkle, Little Star*.

<blockquote>

My legs are apart, my feet are straight
My trunk is in the middle
Arms straight by my side
Looking straight ahead
Now I'm ready for standing
Look at me, I'm standing

</blockquote>

Steven's "Sitting" Song.[iii]Another song was also written for Steven to assist him with balance/trunk control in a sitting position. The music was *Take It Easy* by the Eagles, one of Steven's favorite songs.

<blockquote>

Verse:
Now my feet are back and my feet are flat and my trunk is in the middle
Looking straight ahead, hands on my lap, my fingers out and loose

Chorus:
It's my sitting song, this is my sitting song
My body is straight and tall and I'm ready to play
It's my sitting song, this is my sitting song
My hands on my lap, my fingers out and loose

</blockquote>

When conducting joint therapy sessions, it is imperative that the goals are discussed among the team members prior to the session in order to maximize the benefits of the music intervention and enhance the understanding of the music therapy goals by non–music therapy staff. During this intervention, it is possible that the child may begin to sing with or desire to play an instrument with the therapist. The music therapist must decide if this response requires a shift in methods (e.g., shift to improvisational music therapy) and, importantly, if this change will enhance or detract from the goal of the session.

Recorded music may also be used to meet the goals of physical functioning. It is imperative that if the music therapist has not prepared these audio recordings herself (i.e., recorded her own singing or playing of music or recorded original versions of the song), all music material be presented to the music therapist for assessment prior to its use with the child. The use of recorded music which is unfamiliar or not preferred by the child may prove unsuccessful in meeting the goals of this session. Guidelines for the use of music listening should be given to rehabilitation staff. A staff member or carer can be given the responsibility of monitoring the use of the recording equipment (i.e., stopping and starting the music, increasing or decreasing the volume according to the child's responses and directions from therapy staff). Recorded music used in past sessions and prepared by the music therapist may be played to the child.

Songs as Reinforcer and Cue for Self-Control

Overview. A child may be referred by a variety of rehabilitation therapists to address the need for improved self-control. Cognitive dysfunctions in relation to memory, learning, and attention are common for many children following an ABI (Anderson, 2004). Depending on the locality and degree of injury, the child may experience difficulty in managing their behaviors, which prevents their ability to listen and follow directions from therapy staff. The ability for the child to communicate effectively with all therapy staff is vital to the progress of rehabilitation goals and impacts each area of impairment. Songs can also function as an effective reinforcer of desired behaviors as well as a cue or prompt for following directions. This intervention can be used in individual music therapy and group music therapy as well as cotreatment sessions. The volume of the music should be closely monitored, particularly when using material that is engaging and energetic in tempo, rhythm, and timbre. Music has the potential to overstimulate a child recovering from an ABI, and selection of suitable tempi, meters, rhythms, timbres, and volumes must be considered.

Preparation. Prior consultation and planning with other therapy staff working on this goal is required in order to maintain consistency and clarity across all therapy programs.

What to observe. During the session, the music therapist observes the verbal and nonverbal responses of the child (e.g., evaluating the number of times an appropriate/inappropriate response is made). Observations will include the maintenance of eye contact; level of engagement; ability to turn-take (if involved in a group session); ability to follow directions; maintenance of seated position; and concentration during the music listening.

Procedures. Sessions focused on self-control involve supporting the child to maintain focus and a settled stance (usually sitting). This can be accomplished in a variety of ways. First, music can function as a positive reinforcer for the desired behavior. Preferred and known songs are presented to the child, who is encouraged to select material, one piece of music at a time, for listening. Song material may include compositions written by the child and therapist. The child is instructed to sit and listen to the music without interruption (such as inappropriate or irrelevant comments which do not relate to the musical material). The music therapist may decide to play only a chorus or a verse at a time, depending on the attention span of the child. During the music, the music therapist maintains eye contact with the child and monitors his responses. If the child remains settled and does not call out, the second song is introduced and the procedure is repeated.

Second, songs can be used as a cue or prompt for following directions. For the younger child, this intervention can be welcomed as a game where the therapist sings prompts such as "stop, look, and listen" and provides musical and verbal cues to support the intended use of this song. The instructions or cues provided in the song can focus on self-control or can be aimed at helping the child follow directions related to specific physical skills a child needs to learn (e.g., "lift your right arm way up high, lift your left arm, too" when a child is relearning how to dress and undress himself). Song material can be used to assist daily living activities and prompt the child to prepare and action the correct sequencing of each step (Baker & Tamplin, 2006).

Finally, songs can be used in group work to encourage turn-taking (Baker & Tamplin, 2006). Each group member may be asked to bring in song material to share and be required to listen attentively when other children present their songs. It is possible that the children begin to sing along during this intervention, which may enhance concentration and improve their ability for self-control. Should this occur, a shift to the use of a re-creative method may be indicated.

Music-assisted Pain Management

Overview. Different levels of brain impairment following an ABI may impact a child's perception, experience, and communication of pain. This can make adequate pain management challenging. An increase in muscle tone which includes a perceived painful response is common with this population (Baker & Tamplin, 2006). Children face the additional difficulty of being unable to clearly articulate the locality and severity of this pain if their ability to communicate is impaired. Music listening can be used to support children in their reported experiences of pain and assist them to achieve a more relaxed state. Consideration of the child's phase of rehabilitation is important. For example, for those who are in PTA, the use of this intervention may be inappropriate as the child may be unable to clearly communicate his experience of pain.

Preparation. Pain perception is a complex phenomenon. In order to provide effective pain management interventions, the music therapist should have a thorough understanding of the multidimensional nature of pain perception and the various factors that can enhance the child's management of his pain. Parameters concerning volume, tempo, and overall style of music must be considered carefully to avoid the possibility of increasing the child's reported pain perception and risk overstimulation. Some popular music which consists of fast tempi and complex textures and rhythms may not be suitable for children who seem to want to withdraw from stimulation because of the pain. For other children, complex music may be effective in focusing the child away from the pain. The reader is encouraged to read Chapter 2 in this volume for further guidelines on this topic.

What to observe. Continuous assessment of the impact of the music throughout the session is required by the therapist in order to determine its effectiveness or possible contraindication. Musical material should be used for short durations (approximately 10 minutes) in order to minimize fatigue and overstimulation.

Procedures. The music therapist begins by slowly and quietly playing the music with the aim of engaging the child and focusing their attention. Depending on the age of the child, his level of brain impairment, and perceived pain, different musical parameters can be emphasized in order to gain his focus. For example, the child with increased muscle tone can often scream or yell loudly, and his breathing becomes short and rapid. The therapist must carefully consider what musical elements should become most salient to calm and settle the child. The therapist may decide to first match the rhythm and tempo of the child's rapid breathing with a simple chord progression and, using the entrainment principle, may gradually slow down the live music and replace the rapid rhythms with melodic contours. Alternatively, the therapist may first want to match the strength of the child's screaming with some loud chords on the piano and then introduce more musical structure by adding a simple rhythmic pattern with a distinct melody line. Where possible, the child is encouraged to select favorite repertoire for the therapist to perform. Some children enjoy listening to lullaby-type vocal improvisations with soft instrumental accompaniment, as such music is able to communicate care and love for the child. If appropriate, family members present during the session may be involved in the singing and/or selection of the songs and can support the child. The music therapist must carefully monitor the responses of the family members to the child and ensure that the child's needs are supported effectively and not compromised.

Music for pain management can be used in individual music therapy or combined therapy sessions (e.g., a physiotherapist or occupational therapist who may also be responsible for pain management). If the sessions are multidisciplinary, the music therapist should plan for the use of this intervention in collaboration with other staff to ensure a consistent and clear approach toward the child's pain management. In planning the intervention, the music therapist must also consider the type and anticipated intensity of the pain. For example, pain perceived during joint therapy sessions to improve physical functioning may require a different approach than that to pain perceived during a dressing change procedure.

Similar procedural steps can be adopted for the use of re-creative music therapy and pain management. It is possible that during the use of receptive techniques, the child will spontaneously sing. As the goal of this session remains the same, the music therapist must consider the implications of the child's engagement and any possible contraindications. Depending on the nature of the pain management scenario, the child may be required to sit or lie still (e.g., during injections) and not engage in singing or instrumental play to avoid interference with the procedure.

Music-assisted Relaxation

Overview. As the child continues with the recovery and daily grind of their rehabilitation program, his tolerance for ongoing therapy with repetitive instructions of tasks and routines can become overwhelming. While attempts are made to schedule periods of relaxation and "time out," children can often appear frustrated and encounter difficulty understanding the need for such intensive treatment (Kennelly, 2006). Therefore, opportunities for relaxation may be required at various points during recovery. As the term "relaxation" can refer to a number of physical and emotional needs (e.g., muscle relaxation; anxiety management) (Baker & Tamplin, 2006), the guidelines provided here focus on the emotional needs of the patient. Contraindications as discussed for pain management must also be considered within this method.

Preparation. As this intervention is focused on providing opportunities for relaxation in relation to emotional support, individual sessions are recommended. It is imperative that the session be conducted in a quiet and private space in order to optimize the child's relaxed state. This may be scheduled as the child's final session of the day if the goal is to assist the child to fall asleep. Otherwise, the session may be planned just before a meal break to ensure a sense of "work-free space"—a perception of music therapy as a fun and enjoyable time which is void of work and routine (Kennelly, 2006).

What to observe. If the child demonstrates a lack of relaxation response, such as increased agitation or restlessness, the intervention should be stopped and where appropriate modified according to either the child's response and/or observed responses from the music therapist, other staff, and/or carers. For example, for the child who presents as frustrated or aggressive, the intervention may require the music therapist to present the music in either a strong, "attention-grabbing" way, where the child can be distracted from their position of frustration, or in an opposite way, using music to gently focus the child using soft dynamics and a slow tempo. Positive changes in the child's physical or emotional responses may indicate that the intervention is effective. It is recommended that musical material be used for short durations (i.e., total session duration of approximately 10 minutes) in order to minimize fatigue levels and reduce overstimulation. The use of a behavior assessment scale to assess agitation before and after the session may be useful (Corrigan, 1989).

Procedures. The procedural steps for music-assisted relaxation are similar to those for music-assisted pain management. The music therapist uses preferred and known music to support the child. The music therapist adapts this method according to the presented needs of the child. For example, a child who initially presents as restless may require music which engages him visually and aurally before moving to music with more sedative qualities. For the younger child, the therapist can use active facial expressions to engage and interact with the child in order to establish an empathic connection. Using the song "Twinkle, Twinkle," the therapist can sing unaccompanied and use hand actions and associated facial expressions to support the child emotionally. Visually and aurally engaging with a known song can promote a sense of safety and support (Kennelly & Brien-Elliott, 2001). During this singing, the child's restless state may change and the child become more settled and focused on the therapist. Music using arpeggiated accompaniments sung or played at a slow tempo, matching the patient's heart or respiratory rate (if attempting to fall asleep), can be used at this time. Vocal timbre may mirror the accompanying style, and provide a sense of support and engagement (Magee et al., 2011). The session may only use between one and three songs and conclude with the child falling asleep or appearing relaxed and settled.

Music Listening for Emotional Support

Overview. As the child moves through different phases of recovery from an ABI, their emotional needs also change depending on a number of factors, including his rate of recovery, his coping mechanisms, and levels of family and community support (Anderson et al., 2001). Children and adolescents experience a range of emotional challenges, including grief and loss, isolation from family and their community, difficulties with their self-expression and adjustment to hospital life (Kennelly, 2006; Kennelly & Brien-Elliott, 2001). The following guidelines may be used as a general intervention to provide emotional support following a TBI. Music listening for emotional support (as opposed to improvisation or composition interventions) is recommended for children in the acute rehabilitation phase or the initial stage of the therapeutic relationship, as their medical status may dictate their ability to participate in the session. The music therapist must make an informed clinical decision as to the use and appropriateness of this method with children in PTA, as their disoriented state may not always clearly indicate a need for this type of intervention.

Preparation. Depending on the child's emotional state and required needs, this intervention may be more suitably conducted in a private setting (in a separate room away from other patients on the ward or rehabilitation unit). It may also be necessary to schedule this session in the child's daily rehabilitation routine in order to secure an optimal time free from sessions focused on functional activity.

What to observe. It is important when working within the area of psychosocial support that the therapist carefully monitor the child's responses in the music therapy session and allow adequate time for a trust relationship to develop. Children might be withdrawn and distrustful of medical staff. Flexibility and patience on the part of the music therapist will communicate care and support to the child and will allow for rapport to develop.

Procedures. When a child feels angry, scared, frustrated, or sad, he can respond in many different ways. The music therapist must empathically listen to the child, be mindful of the stage of the therapeutic relationship, and keep the allotted session time in mind when deciding on the session content and sequence of interventions. If rapport and trust have not yet been established, the music therapist may begin by singing familiar songs with lyrics that communicate care and support. Care should be taken not to use songs that evoke reflection or discussion of intense emotions at the early stage of the therapeutic relationship, although this author acknowledges that elicitation of specific emotions is often beyond the control of the music therapist or may be unrelated to the music selected. Whenever possible, choice of music is provided in order to create a sense of familiarity and control (Kennelly & Brien-Elliott, 2001). Some children may indicate their choice verbally or gesturally, while others may remain withdrawn or even ask the therapist to leave. Responses to music listening may range from no response, initiating eye contact with the therapist, smiling and acknowledging the significance of the music, and singing with the therapist (which then transitions to the use of re-creative methods). Other positive changes in the child's responses include an increase in vocal and verbal communication with the therapist (often dependent on the developmental age of the child) and changes in the child's affect. If the child demonstrates little change in his emotional state, the music therapist should consider gently changing her approach in relation to the way the musical material is presented and her interaction with the child. Considerations may involve pausing at the end of phrases to observe the child or ask the child how he may be feeling and varying the parameters such as tempo, style, and timbre in order to engage the child in a different manner. It is possible that the child may refuse to engage with the music and/or the therapist and instead ask for the session to end. The therapist may choose to continue discussions with the child about his emotional state (without music) and then offer to visit the child at another time. Alternatively, the therapist may choose to refocus the session with any family members present and engage in song listening with them. It is possible that the child, after viewing the interaction of these family members in music therapy, may then actively choose (or unconsciously choose) to receive music therapy. It is important for the therapist to monitor the child's reaction to re-focusing on another family member to ensure that the child does not view such a shift as being misunderstood or neglected by the therapist.

Even when the therapist does not shift her focus to the family members, whenever family members are present in the room, the music therapist must be clear with her intentions and purpose in relation to their involvement. This is to ensure that the child remains the primary client in the session. The use of music listening for emotional support can certainly be impacted by the responses of others present who are responding emotionally to the music provided. While at times these responses may enhance the emotional state of the child, they may also create experiences which remove the child as the central focus of support. A holding experience may be provided for all present; however, the primary goal remains providing emotional support to the child.

The guidelines provided here are similar when using re-creative methods for emotional support such as singing songs or active music-making with the child. It is advised that the therapist be prepared to move from receptive methods to re-creative music therapy methods within a session. Therefore, when providing sessions in patient rooms, the music therapist should bring age-appropriate instruments to the session. These instruments can be stored on a cart in the hallway until transition to active music-making is indicated. Actively singing songs and instrument playing is often indicated when enhanced communication between the child and significant others is desired.

Finally, music listening as well as actively singing songs can also be used in group settings. When formulating goals for group sessions, it is important that the music therapist consider the individual needs of each child together with the needs of the group. Careful consideration of selected song material preferred by all children must be taken in order to meet goals and display respect and sensitivity to group needs.

GUIDELINES FOR IMPROVISATIONAL MUSIC THERAPY

When using improvisational music therapy interventions, the therapist should ensure that age-appropriate instruments are provided and that adaptations have been made (or are able to be made during the session if the physical therapist or occupational therapist is also present). In order to minimize interruptions from the child during the session, ensure that the environment does not contain any objects or distractions which may shift the client's focus (e.g., television or other audio/visual equipment).

Instrumental Improvisation for Emotional Support

Overview. The need for emotional support in children with ABI usually changes throughout the course of their recovery. As the therapeutic relationship develops and trust and rapport have been established, children may feel more confident and secure in their use of improvisation to express feelings and emotions. The use of this intervention usually takes place in the subacute phase of rehabilitation.

However, it is important to note that some children are readily able and even eager to engage in improvisational music-making at an earlier stage in their recovery.

Preparation. The music therapist should ensure that a variety of age-appropriate instruments are provided to facilitate opportunities for engagement.

What to observe. Musical and nonmusical responses of the child in relation to the improvisation should be observed. If improvising alone, the following areas can be considered: choice of instrument(s); creative use/exploration of instrument(s); creative use of musical elements (e.g., rhythm, melody, scale, form); and interaction with others while playing. The music therapist may use this information to describe the abilities of the child in relation to self-expression within a musical context and compare these responses to those observed outside the music therapy environment. If improvising with the therapist or with others, the following areas (musical and nonmusical) could be observed: the level of participation with others; the level of communication with others; ability to turn-take; role in the improvisation (e.g., leader vs. follower); and so on. Here too, interactive responses during music therapy can be compared to such responses in other environments.

Procedures. The deliverance of this intervention is influenced by the developmental age of the child and their level of current communication. Instruments may be first presented with an invitation to engage musically with the therapist. For example, for the young preverbal child who appears withdrawn, the instruments may be placed near him and the therapist awaits a response or sings an initial known song to establish rapport; for a four-year-old child who is distressed, a choice of two instruments may be given, accompanied with suggestions for story-making; and for the older child, a conversation on the topic of instrument playing (exploring prior experiences and interests) may lead to the use of different instruments. The older child or adolescent who is able to communicate his feelings of anger may use improvisation as a way to further ventilate these feelings. Those unable to do so may require additional support from the therapist in the form of verbal discussion to elicit expression of these feelings or use of receptive techniques to provide emotional support. The therapist is required to be flexible in the way she presents music improvisation opportunities to the child, given the range of developmental age, readiness to engage in music-making, and physical abilities and limitations.

Improvisations with younger children can often appear free in their form and structure. The therapist may be guided by the child's spontaneous playing and singing and provide a simple and repetitive chordal framework for this music (I, IV, V, and I). As the child improvises, the therapist provides a supportive accompaniment which at times involves the child playing alone. Improvisations with older children or adolescents may focus on a particular theme, idea, or story. Such improvisations are called referential improvisations (Bruscia, 1987). A traditional 12-bar blues framework can be offered to children who require more musical support to create their improvisations. The therapist may discuss these ideas with the child prior to the improvisation or allow the music to develop without prior planning. Improvisations can be recorded (with the child's or his carer's permission) where appropriate and used for discussion during later sessions. This material may be useful for evaluation purposes such as improvements in self-expression.

An example of this was Peter, a 13-year-old boy engaged in instrumental improvisation for emotional support. The music therapist (who participated in the improvisation) observed Peter's responses according to his musically expressed motifs. His ability to engage musically with the therapist using mirroring and matching techniques demonstrated a nonmusical form of interaction as opposed to a verbal discussion of his feelings.

Music improvisation focused on providing emotional support can also be used in group work, especially with adolescents. Discussion of feelings and emotions in relation to their injury and rehabilitation can be facilitated by music-making with their peers. As hospitalization for a brain injury and subsequent rehabilitation can be lengthy, these teenagers are often isolated from their classmates and other peers in their home life. Therefore, building supportive relationships among teens in the hospital becomes an important psychosocial part of the teen's recovery.

Instrumental Improvisation to Promote Physical Functioning

Overview. As indicated in "Receptive Music Therapy to Promote Physical Functioning," goals related in this area can be targeted through a medium which provides cues and prompts for directed movement, including the motivation to complete these tasks successfully. Improvisational music therapy allows for cues and directions to be modified according to the child's in-the-moment physical needs and abilities. This is important, as the child may exhibit an unexpected leap in physical ability within a given session or, conversely, experience a set-back because of increased pain or discomfort. As the range of gross and fine motor skills (including coordination) of all age ranges cannot be covered in this chapter, the following guidelines are given as an example of improvisational music therapy to promote bilateral lower limb movement. Again, the music therapist working with this population should consult the Baker & Tamplin (2006) textbook, as it addresses many different interventions to target a wide range of physical skills. A list of music technology resources which can be used to target functional movement are provided at the end of the chapter.

Preparation. The therapist should ensure that age-appropriate instruments are provided and that adaptations to the instruments have been made (or are able to be made during the session if the physical therapist or occupational therapist is also present). Modifications may include built-up handles on mallets or portable platforms for keyboards which provide increased flexibility for the therapist and promote range of movement for the child. In the case of this clinical example, a drum kit modified to incorporate a kick pedal on both left and right sides is used to promote bilateral movement.

What to observe. The music therapist observes the physical and musical responses of the child during the improvisation, being careful to adapt or modify the music as required. If the child sings during the improvisation, the therapist should structure his musical responses according to the goals of the session. For example, if the improvisation is focused on improving range of movement and the child sings about moving his right foot to kick the drum, the therapist should incorporate these lyrics in the improvisation. Conversely, if the therapist is singing about prompts for alternating between left and right foot movements, she needs to observe the child's responses and either praise the child for his correct movement or cue the child again for the appropriate response.

Procedures. This guideline is based on Thaut's (2005) Therapeutic Instrumental Music Performance (TIMP), where the playing of musical instruments is used to target and improve functional movement. Key elements of the use of improvisation in this guideline are rhythm, phrasing, tempo, use of lyrics, and dynamics. However, unlike TIMP, where the music is directed by the therapist particularly in relation to tempo and rhythm, this method is guided by the responses of the child. The aim is to initially meet and support the child at his current level of functioning through improvisation and provide ongoing support throughout the use of this method. The therapist begins by either inviting the child to begin the improvisation using his left and right foot and supporting his rhythm and beat or by providing a rhythmic framework to encourage his participation. The therapist continues to provide a supportive rhythmic base (e.g., four crotchet beat with emphasis on first and third beat and sings about using "left on 1 and 3" and "right on 2 and 4") while monitoring the child's movements and rhythmic responses. If the child encounters difficulties initiating or maintaining this movement, the therapist may focus on one side only (e.g., left foot kick and improvises music according to the child's response). Tonal and melodic frameworks should be simply structured to aid and focus the child's movements. If the child successfully completes this movement, the improvisation may be extended and the child encouraged to increase the number of repeated kicks between left and right feet. This can be achieved by increasing the tempo, altering the rhythm or phrasing, and so on. This can be further supported by the use of the therapist's improvised lyrics targeting the desired change in movement. The music therapist can use improvised rhyming, chanting, or rapping to motivate and maintain the child's interest. An example of using a chant in a slow-paced 4/4 could be:

> *Hey there, Timothy*
> *I can see you move your feet.*
> *Left and right side, watch them move*
> *Now let's try to change your groove*
> *Listen to the rhythm, listen to your feet*
> *Listen to the pattern change, 1, 2, 3!*

The use of singing and instrumental playing or either technique in isolation may be dependent on a number of factors, including the child's ability or interest in using his voice and the particular goal of the session. Simple, repetitive melodies (or chants) with predictable phrasing provide a stable baseline and also contain enough "musical space" for the necessary changes to promote the attainment of physical functioning goals. It is important that the therapist monitor the fatigue levels of the child during these sessions, as multiple concurrent uses of physical and cognitive domains of the brain can tire and overstimulate.

Similar guidelines may be applied to the use of re-creative music therapy to promote physical functioning. Further description of methods used in adult rehabilitation (which can be generally used to inform pediatric practice), such as rhythmic auditory stimulation (RAS), patterned sensory enhancement (PSE), and TIMP may be found in Baker and Tamplin (2006) and Thaut (2005). A description of RAS as a method in pediatric rehabilitation is included later in this chapter.

Instrumental Improvisation to Decrease Perseveration

Overview. A common impairment in communicative functioning for children recovering from an ABI is their continuous repetition of a response or action which presents as inappropriate and out of context (Baker & Tamplin, 2006). Perseveration often occurs in conversations, e.g., when a child repeats a phrase such as "I like it" as a response to any given question, which may not always indicate that he does "like it." The child's perseverative tendency may limit his ability to interact appropriately with others and provide limited ways of expressing his thoughts and feelings. The goal of this intervention is to decrease perseverative response or actions during improvised music.

What to observe. During the improvisation, the child may demonstrate repeated musical patterns, such as rhythmic or melodic phrases which he is unable to explore or change in any way. The music therapist should observe the following elements: the duration of time the child is able to engage in improvisation without perseverative behaviors (musical and/or verbal); the ability for the child to engage musically through his use of rhythm, melody, and the selection of instrumentation with minimal display of perseveration; and the amount and type of cues (visual, verbal, physical, and musical) required from the music therapist to change his style of musical interaction (Baker & Tamplin, 2006). The therapist needs to monitor the fatigue levels of the child during the session and begin with session lengths between 10 and 15 minutes (Baker & Tamplin, 2006).

Procedures. When a child exhibits perseverative behavior during a session, the music therapist invites the child to improvise with his choice of instrument. As the music begins, the therapist provides an accompaniment that replicates the repetitive and perseverative structure of the child's verbalizations or behaviors and prompts the child to experiment creatively with his selected instrument(s). For example, an eight-year-old boy may verbally and musically perseverate during a session by repeating words or phrases such as "go away" and may be imitating the rhythmic structure of this word or phrase on the drum. The therapist begins by first matching this perseveration and then gradually introduces a different word or phrase (both musically and verbally), such as "listen to the bongo," which possesses a different rhythmic structure than "go away." If the child does not respond well to this change, the therapist may choose to focus on using the rhythm alone (without the verbal utterance), so as to provide a simpler instruction, and then gradually introduce the complete phrase. This phrase may be used as a chant or presented in more melodic form, depending on the child's initial type of perseverative response.

If the aim is to decrease perseveration of musical elements while playing the bongo, such as inability or refusal to engage in bilateral playing, similar procedures can be used to target a change in this area. Singing or chanting different words or phrases which focus on "left" and "right" may cue the child to creatively explore the dimensions of this instrument.

This intervention may also be used to promote attention behaviors. Improvising on an instrument such as the bongo, which promotes bilateral playing, can encourage a child to maintain and extend his focus. Joint improvisations with the therapist, using the bongo alone or with the voice, involve an interactive process which demands various types of attention. For further description of methods to promote focused, sustained, selective and alternating attention, please refer to Baker and Tamplin (2006).

Improvisational Music Therapy to Promote Direction-Following

Overview. In this intervention, improvised music is used to prompt and cue the child to listen attentively and engage in musical conversations which encourage imitation and turn-taking. It is important that the music therapist considers the child's ability to imitate rhythmic or melodic motifs so that the appropriate standard of musical material can be introduced. Complex motifs accompanied with complicated directions may confuse the child and also overstimulate him.

What to observe. The music therapist evaluates the number of times the child successfully completes the set tasks, taking note when errors are made and the number and type of cues required to complete the task (Baker & Tamplin, 2006).

Procedures. Depending on the child's age, it may be necessary to discuss the aims of this session with carers in order to address this goal. For younger children, the intervention may be presented as a "listening game" where the reward includes a free choice of song/instrumental play at the end of the session. In order to play the game, the child needs to listen carefully and do as the music therapist says, as in a "Simon Says" game. For example, using a simple and repetitive rhythm or melody, the therapist sings a song about listening and incorporates lyrics which present tasks such as "beat the drum like this" and then plays a 4 crotchet beat and waits for the child's response. If the pattern is repeated successfully, the therapist moves to a new instruction within the improvisation which is more rhythmically complicated. It is important to gradually introduce new directions and fall back on the previous direction if the new task is too difficult. If the child is unable to follow the first direction, the therapist repeats the rhythm or melody using the same instruction. Depending on the child's ability and range of response, it is useful to invite the child to take the role as "leader" and provide patterns for the therapist to imitate. This facilitates a sense of control and mastery, which is important for children at this developmental stage. Vocal improvisations may also be used, or a combination of instrumental and vocal. Young children enjoy using their voice when playing games. The music therapist can experiment with changes in timbre, tonality, and dynamics accompanied by different facial expressions to encourage the child's participation and focus. These musical patterns can be accompanied by gross motor movements, which can further motivate the child—for example, pretending to be an elephant or a lion in a jungle, marching around the room with a drum and improvising call-and-response patterns (for the older child above eight years), or more simple imitations (for the younger child of ages two to six years).

GUIDELINES FOR RE-CREATIVE MUSIC THERAPY

In order to optimize outcomes in re-creative music-making, sessions should be conducted in a quiet room free from distractions. Sessions may be conducted by the music therapist alone or in conjunction with other professional therapists. It is important that prior planning take place with joint therapy sessions in order to ensure clarity regarding treatment goals.

Modified Melodic Intonation Therapy

Overview. The impact of an ABI on speech and language domains of the brain can affect many areas of daily living (Blosser & De Pompei, 2003). Communicating with staff, family, and friends is a function which is integral to coping with these daily activities and to relationships formed with these significant others. For the young child who sustains a brain injury, the process of acquiring verbal skills has been disrupted, and development of speech and language milestones becomes a priority for all therapy programs (Blosser & De Pompei, 2003). In addition to receiving speech therapy, children may be referred to music therapy to address their speech and language impairments (Kennelly et al., 2001; Leung, 2008). The rationale for using music in this area is based on evidence which supports the structural similarities between speech and music (Patterson, Uppenkamp Johnsrude, & Griffiths, 2002). The elements of pitch, rhythm, and timbre are shared in music-making and speech production, which further supports the rationale for music therapy methods in this area of rehabilitation (Baker & Tamplin, 2006). Modified Melodic Intonation Therapy (MMIT) is used to enhance functional verbal communication (Baker, 2000; Baker & Tamplin, 2006).

What to observe. The music therapist monitors the child's attempts to sing/speak functional phrases with and without the therapist and outside the therapy session. The music therapist monitors the child's responses in relation to using preferred song material as a form of singing exercise. Adolescents may find this form of drill challenging as their preferred song material is changed into an activity which demands a new focus.

Procedures. This technique was developed by Baker (2000) for adult patients with aphasia, but can also be used with the pediatric and adolescent population. Guidelines for melodic intonation therapy (MIT) prepared by the Music Therapy Department at the Royal Children's Hospital (Children's Health Services, Brisbane, Australia) provide a stepwise introduction to the use of this method (RCH, 2011). This hospital guideline includes three treatment protocols: two for MIT and one for MMIT (developed by Baker, 2000). The guidelines presented below will focus on the MMIT protocol.

In MMIT, the child is first engaged in singing familiar songs to encourage and promote his ability to sing. Once the child is comfortable singing with the music therapist, the therapist introduces a small number of functional phrases. These phrases are based on simple melodic and harmonic structures but are musically different to each other so as not to confuse the child. It is important that the melodic range for the phrases be limited to the interval of an octave (preferably a fifth or sixth for children) and the rhythm match the inherent rhythmic structure of the words in the phrase. In addition to carefully composing the musical structure of the phrases, the therapist needs to attend to the placement of target words. Target words should be placed at the end of the phrase. For example, "I would like four calamari rings" or "I would like to buy a Coke" where "calamari rings" and "Coke" are the target words.

As the music therapist plays and sings these phrases several times, the child is invited to listen and eventually join in singing with the therapist. Gradually, as the child gains confidence with singing this phrase, the therapist withdraws her participation and the child is encouraged to sing the phrases without the therapist's assistance. As confidence and skill in this area increases, the child is asked questions which prompt the functional phrase as a response, e.g., the therapist may ask the child "What would you like to buy?," and the child can respond accordingly using normal conversation speech. This type of practice can be reinforced by the child's carers and other therapy staff when the music therapist is not present, particularly in the non-therapy setting, which is the aim of this technique. Some children may respond more successfully to phrases which focus on rhythm rather than melody, and the same procedural steps can apply (without reference to the use of melody) (Baker & Tamplin, 2006).

Baker and Tamplin recommend that familiar melodies should not be used as the content for these functional phrases so as to avoid confusion and potential error for the patient. The author of this chapter acknowledges this recommendation; however, in her past clinical experience, she has adopted the use of familiar melodies in MMIT and noted that some children were able to respond positively to the adaptation of this technique. It is important to consider the applicability of using both familiar and unfamiliar music and to base this selection on the perceived benefits and preferences of the child.

Singing to Improve Articulation and Rate of Speech

Overview. One area of communication impairment as a result of an ABI is a slower rate of speech, which may be further complicated by poor articulation (Blosser & De Pompei, 2003). Because of damage to the cerebellum, children can possess difficulties with lip closure to effectively reproduce words beginning or ending with letters such as /p/, /b/ or /d/ or facilitate particular tongue movements for words beginning and ending with letters such as /s/ or /th/. Song singing can be used effectively to improve articulation and increase the rate of speech for children with ABI (Bower & Shoemark, 2009; Kennelly et al., 2001). Music can motivate and encourage children to engage in speech exercises (both traditional and in song form) and also stimulate areas of the brain (i.e., the limbic system) which may not respond effectively to these routine of drills in spoken form (Bower & Shoemark, 2009).

What to observe. The music therapist should monitor the child's level of fatigue and engagement during the session, as overuse of this method may impact on his ability to participate effectively. The therapist monitors the child's responses according to rate of speech, number of intelligible words using the target sound, and number of times the target phoneme is used (Baker & Tamplin, 2006). It is important to monitor the use of tempo throughout this method in modeling an appropriate singing rate. Prior assessment of a child's functional speech by the speech pathologist will assist to inform the number and type of words required. The number of target sounds may begin with one per set of lyrics and gradually increase as the child improves.

Procedures. The following steps are based on communication interventions described by Baker and Tamplin (2006) and Thaut's (2005) Rhythmic Speech Cuing. The music therapist selects preferred songs of the child which incorporate the required target word and/or phoneme. For example, the nursery rhyme "Baa, Baa, Black Sheep" incorporates the /b/ sound for three words and the /p/ for one word and can be used to encourage lip closure. The steady tempo can also be used to reinforce speech rate, especially when a child is speaking slowly. The use of percussion instruments such as drums played by the therapist or the child if appropriate can support the increased or decreased rate of speech required. Songs which place the target word at the end of each line of lyrics are usually the easiest to first achieve. The difficulty of sound pattern articulation in singing ranges from placement at the end of a sentence to the more challenging placement of a sound in multiple places within each phrase (Baker & Tamplin, 2006). The advantage of using singing to enhance articulation and improve rate of speech is that both goals can be addressed simultaneously due to the use of temporal cues in music (Baker & Tamplin, 2006). Depending on the age of the child, the focus of these target words/phonemes may be made explicit or just simply overemphasised (as with the younger child) to encourage and motivate their participation. This method can also be used with older children or adolescents. Songs such as "Don't Worry, Be Happy" can be used to target the /b/ and /ooo/ sounds effectively.

Songs that promote movement such as clapping or swaying side to side may interfere with the achievement of this speech goal, as they have the potential to distract and overstimulate. However, these spontaneous movements, if controlled to some degree by the child or the music therapist (and speech pathologist if present), can assist speech rate. The therapists can ask the child to refrain from using movements during the song and suggest that opportunities to move to the song will come later in the session.

An illustration of this was 12-year-old Mary, who enjoyed spontaneously moving to songs by the Spice Girls. Despite the assistance of the speech pathologist, who attempted to restrain Mary's hands, she proceeded to move the rest of her body while engaged in song singing. Each time she made a movement, she slowed her rate of speech and at times stopped singing. In order to improve Mary's responses, the music therapist decided to introduce a game and asked Mary to sit on her hands (while in the wheelchair) for the entire song. If Mary managed to do this successfully, the song was sung again and Mary was permitted to move accordingly. This strategy appeared effective, as Mary was able to restrain herself rather than rely on an adult to do this for her. She was then able to focus solely on her singing and not be distracted by her spontaneous movements.

Compositional music therapy may also be used to address this area of need. New song material may be created either with therapist and client or therapist alone to target the required words and phonemes. Song material can be recorded, and the child is encouraged to practice these target sounds or sing along with the song.

Singing to Improve Intonation

Overview. Another area of communication impairment following an ABI is poor intonation. Children can experience difficulty in maintaining an appropriate pitch range, which, in turn, may make the speech difficult to understand by others (Baker & Tamplin, 2006). The tone of their speech is often low in pitch and monotonous. They are unable to freely vary the pitch of their speech and, as a result, often sound "robotic." Singing songs or engaging in scale exercises may assist the child in expanding his vocal range (Kennelly et al., 2001). Songs with simple variations in the melody line can motivate the child to try to match the intervals used in the song, resulting in improved intonation.

While the preference is to use the child's known song material, some repertoire may be inappropriate for use if the melodic range is too broad and difficult for the child to reproduce effectively (e.g., adolescent song material). However, it may be possible for the therapist to use sections of these songs, such as the chorus only, to reinforce the goals of the session.

What to observe. The music therapist monitors the child's responses to pitch range exercises, i.e., lowest and highest note achieved in each session. The child's ability to sing in tune with and without the music therapist's involvement should also be observed.

Procedures. A combination of pitch exercises and the singing of preferred songs may be used to address this area of need. This method is based on descriptions of communication interventions by Baker and Tamplin (2006) and Thaut's use of Vocal Intonation Therapy (2005). The therapist begins by using warm-up vocal exercises to increase vocal range (e.g., scale patterns or arpeggiated patterns) and then gradually moves on to repetitions of melodic contours using known song material. These exercises may be conducted with or without musical accompaniment (piano or guitar), depending on the needs of the child and his level of speech impairment. Some children respond effectively to the use of an accompanying instrument, as it provides an additional musical support aside from the therapist's singing voice. However, others, particularly younger children, may be distracted by the use of an instrument, and gestural hand movements may be used to visually cue the child to increase or decrease the pitch level. Following these exercises, the therapist can begin to use phrases from a preferred song. She begins with phrases that shift between two notes (ascending or descending, depending on the song's melodic line). The child practices these two note intervals repeatedly until an improvement is observed. When ready, the child is invited to sing the complete line of lyrics (where these intervals originated), and the therapist observes his ability to sing the various pitches and intervals.

Other variations of this method include exercises to improve dynamic modulations, increase sound prolongation, and reduce hypernasality. Vocal exercises that promote various oral motor skills such as tongue placement to increase or decrease hypernasality may be incorporated in sessions. Scale passages using "la, lay, li, lo, loo" can encourage more open vocalizations. Breath work, which is described in the next section, may also address the issue of hypernasality. Other methods to improve intonation with adult rehabilitation patients may be adapted for the pediatric population, and the reader is encouraged to access texts by Baker and Tamplin (2006) and Thaut (2005) for further reading.

Re-creative Music Therapy to Improve Respiratory Control

Overview. The ability of a child with an ABI to breathe effectively has implications for many activities of daily living. Engaging in physical rehabilitation such as learning to walk and relearning speech skills requires sufficient and effective breath support and control. Children recovering from an ABI often present with breathing difficulties. They can appear short of breath, which is particularly noticed in their slower rate of speech or their inability to deliver well-phrased and coordinated sentences (Anderson, 2004). Song singing can be used effectively to improve breath control and increase speech phrasing with children recovering from an ABI (Kennelly et al., 2001; Leung, 2008). Familiar song repertoire and accompanying vocal exercises can motivate the child to engage in an activity which is enjoyable and fun.

What to observe. The therapist monitors the posture of the child during song singing or different exercises, his ability to sustain a single note or type of phoneme, the quality of the tone produced, and the duration of each note. The music therapist needs to carefully monitor the use of this method so as not to fatigue or increase respiratory difficulties for the child. Overstimulation of the child should also be considered during the use of this method.

Procedures. The therapist begins by engaging the child in a variety of breathing exercises which focus on use of the diaphragm and the chest. This method is based on descriptions of communication interventions by Baker and Tamplin (2006) and Thaut's (2005) oral motor and respiratory exercises (OMREX). Depending on the age of the child, this activity may need to be incorporated into a game between the child and the therapist. For example, using the song "The Wheels on the Bus," sounds and activities on the bus can be used to promote extended breaths—"the children on the bus go ha-ha-ha," where the focus is a short but controlled exhalation, or "the siren on the truck goes 'wheeeeeeeeeee,'" encouraging a prolonged exhalation which modulates in pitch. The exercises may be practiced independently of the song first and then slowly incorporated within the song. This is to ensure that the child learns to correctly focus on the necessary breath support required for the particular phrase (as a separate form of learning) before singing the song in its traditional form.

The music therapist examines the phrasing of each preferred song in order to establish its appropriateness for this activity. Due to complex phrasing, some adolescent song material may not be suitable for this method. However, it is possible that short excerpts of this style of song may be used (such as a chorus only) to target this therapy goal.

A variety of exercises focusing on volume and pitch control, together with different phonemes such as vowel sounds, can also be used to improve respiratory control (Baker & Tamplin, 2006). The reader is encouraged to access this text for further description of these methods.

Rhythmic Auditory Stimulation (RAS) for Gait Rehabilitation (Thaut, 1999)

Overview. Specialist training in Neurologic Music Therapy equips the therapist with a wide range of skills and techniques which address functional rehabilitation (Thaut, 1999, 2005). One of these techniques, RAS, aims to improve gait rehabilitation. Children recovering from an ABI often experience difficulties in learning to walk again due to injury of the motor cortex. These difficulties include impaired coordination, hemiplegia, and sequencing of movement (Anderson, 2004). Although RAS has not been researched in children with an ABI, evidence supports its use within adult rehabilitation. Pediatric music therapists who have completed this specialist training may find this technique useful in addressing this functional area of need.

Gait improvement through RAS is based on a rhythmic entrainment effect where rhythm, as an external auditory cue, is used to synchronize movement (Thaut, 2005). Therefore, RAS can be used as an entrainment stimulus where rhythm is used to cue movement as it occurs in the session or as a facilitated stimulus where clients can practice using RAS and eventually achieve improved gait without this technique (Thaut, 2005). Adapting RAS for the pediatric ABI population requires several considerations in order for the technique to be applied appropriately and successfully. Aside from the degree of brain impairment, age and premorbid physical and cognitive development must also be considered. The use of RAS requires the patient to concentrate on the rhythmic cues for an extended period of time; therefore, the proposed session length times for adults of 30 to 60 minutes (Baker & Tamplin, 2006) may be inappropriate to use with children under the age of 6 or with older children recovering from severe brain injuries.

What to observe. The music therapist observes the child's ability to modify his gait patterns according to the presence and absence of the RAS. It is important that consultation take place with the physical therapist in order to evaluate the child's gait pattern and potential risk for falls. This may take place prior to music therapy or during joint therapy sessions. This consultation will also assist the music therapist in program planning and determine the need for the physical therapist's presence during the use of RAS. The child's fatigue and concentration levels should also be monitored throughout the use of this technique.

Procedures. RAS for gait training consists of six steps: assessment, resonant frequency entrainment/pregait exercises, frequency modulation, advanced adaptive gait, fading, and reassessment (Thaut, 1999). The music therapist begins by assessing the child's cadence (steps per minute), velocity (meters or feet per minute), and stride length. The RAS frequency is matched to gait cadence and is gradually increased or decreased to promote improvement. Toward the end of the session, RAS is faded and the child is encouraged to maintain the new cadence without RAS assistance. The cadence of movement is reassessed and overall gait pattern re-evaluated (Thaut, 1999). The music therapist uses familiar music with a guitar or drum accompaniment, and the RAS frequency is always matched to a metronome beat. If an accompanying instrument is used, it is important that an additional therapist such as the physical therapist be physically located nearby in order to closely monitor the child for potential falls. Hand clapping by the therapist can also be used during song singing as a noninstrumental form of accompaniment. If the child is having significant difficulties concentrating on the music, the metronome alone can be used to maintain the required beat. The child may choose or find it easier to concentrate on the music alone than sing with the therapist. It is important that the music therapist strictly attends to this beat in order to maintain a consistent frequency. Language impairment such as receptive aphasia may also prevent a child from concentrating on song singing during RAS. The combination of music and language may distract and confuse the child; therefore, a rhythmic pulse such as drumbeat can be used instead. The therapist listens to the metronome beat via the use of headphones in order to maintain a steady beat and minimize distraction for the child.

While the duration of RAS for adults with ABI is recommended to be between 30 and 60 minutes (depending on fatigue and endurance) (Baker & Tamplin, 2006), children may experience difficulty concentrating and maintaining their physical functioning for this period of time. It may be more appropriate to use this technique several times a day for short periods of time, e.g., 5 to 10 minutes at a time or multiple times during a session with other physical rehabilitation activities used in between. This may improve the child's concentration and reduce the potential for fatigue. RAS can also be used to slow gait patterns in children whose walking is unsteady or unusually fast, to practice walking up and down stairs, and to manage different types of surfaces (Thaut, 2005). Recordings of music used during sessions may be given to the child for use outside of the music therapy session. These recordings need to be updated regularly to reflect the child's progress.

GUIDELINES FOR COMPOSITIONAL MUSIC THERAPY

Songwriting to Promote Learning

Overview. Throughout the rehabilitation process, the child is faced with relearning or learning new ways of coping with the activities of daily living (Anderson, 2004). Prior to receiving the injury, a school-age child generally knows how to wash and dress himself and demonstrates independence in completing different tasks, such as reciting the alphabet or writing his name. The impact of an ABI may affect the child's ability to recall prior learning, including the sequencing of steps involved to complete a task such as showering or brushing his teeth. Songwriting can be used to provide structure and sequential order for these steps, aid memory through the use of musical prompts and cues, and promote learning (Baker & Tamplin, 2006). The example provided below focuses on the goal of learning and recalling information related to a set task such as showering, dressing, or making a cake. Depending on the child's level of injury and ability to concentrate, the songwriting process can be introduced in stages, e.g., focusing on one verse at a time while monitoring fatigue levels.

Preparation. The therapist should familiarize herself with the preferred music style of the child or adolescent in preparation for a songwriting session. In addition, the therapist may consider using songwriting software such as GarageBand or Super Dooper Music Looper and also bring equipment to record the song. Descriptions of this software and other suitable programs are provided at the end of this chapter.

What to observe. The music therapist observes the child's ability to sing the song with and without assistance. The child's ability to sing the lyrics and recall procedural steps (in correct order) for completing the task should also be recorded. The child's involvement in the songwriting process, such as his ability to create the lyrics and music, should also be observed.

Procedures. This method is based on Thaut's Musical Mnemonics Training (2005) and Baker and Tamplin's songs as mnemonic strategies (2006). The process described may take place over a number of sessions, as sufficient time must be allowed for the child to think about the steps, select the music, and learn to sing the song. The music therapist introduces the concept and purpose of songwriting to the child. The therapists (if an occupational therapist is involved) begin by asking the child the types of steps involved in making a cake. The child may at times require prompts or visual aids such as pictures illustrating the activity in order to recall the correct information. If the child is able to recall the steps but in the incorrect order, the therapists should continue with recording this information and can return to the task of reordering once all steps have been identified. Once this is achieved, the music therapist can examine the information for suitability in composition form, e.g., using four lines for a verse or looking for rhyming words at the end of each line, and assign the text to verse and chorus formatting. Depending on the child's level of cognition and developmental age, he may also be invited to assist the therapist during this stage.

The music can be freely composed by the child or the therapist can use fill-in-the-blank original song composition or song parody (Baker, Kennelly, & Tamplin, 2005a). Assistance can be provided by the music therapist as required. The verse outlining the first steps of the activity is usually composed first. The therapist sings the first line and invites the child to sing with her (always checking with the child if his song has been interpreted correctly by the therapist). This can be achieved by asking the child to express his opinion in relation to the therapist's musical representation of the song. This can assist the child in feeling empowered through the songwriting process. These first lyrics are repeated until the child can sing the verse alone and recall the procedural steps correctly. The song must contain a clear, simple and predictable melodic, rhythmic, and harmonic structure. Yet, the music must be appealing to the child so that it will be successful in promoting further motivation. The complete first verse is finished before moving on either to a second verse with further steps or the chorus. The chorus often describes the completion of the activity, such as the following:

Look at Sarah she has baked a cake, baked a cake baked a cake
Look at Sarah she has baked a cake, can't wait to try a piece!

The song can be recorded and used by the child to practice outside of the therapy session, such as in the home environment if the child is an outpatient. Family members may be incorporated in this session to encourage the child in his song singing, particularly outside the music therapy context. This intervention is also appropriate for group sessions where each member can be asked to sing/identify the next step/line of lyrics. Other goals which may incorporate similar guidelines include areas of organizational skills, problem-solving, and disorientation. Here the similar principles of planning, conducting the tasks, investigating the solution, and self-evaluation can be broken down into small steps and incorporated using this songwriting technique (Baker & Tamplin, 2006).

Songwriting for Psychosocial Support

Overview. As previously described in receptive and improvisational music therapy for emotional support, music can be used to provide opportunities for self-expression in regard to different dimensions of the rehabilitation experience. The child's ability to communicate effectively with family, friends, and hospital staff is paramount to a successful rehabilitation experience (Blosser & De Pompei, 2003). Whether conducting conversations with staff about daily therapy programs or engaging in social dialogue with their family and peers, his need to communicate clearly and effectively is important. When this ability is impaired, the results may impact functional aspects of daily living and the child's confidence, self-esteem, and emotional well-being. Compositional music therapy can be used to promote skills in conversation (Baker & Tamplin, 2006). This intervention may be more appropriate to use with older children and adolescents, particularly those preparing to return to the school environment.

Writing songs can also be a supportive medium for children experiencing difficulties adjusting to their injuries, disabilities, and period of hospitalization, and feelings of anger and anxiety. This intervention can be used effectively with children from different cultural backgrounds, as the process provides opportunities to incorporate their own language to portray important feelings, emotions, and messages. Working with the non–English-speaking child and the use of songwriting require a different level of flexibility and readiness from the therapist. Support required to work with a non–English-speaking family may include the use of interpreters to meet his needs. The use of this intervention usually takes place in the subacute and chronic phases of rehabilitation.

What to observe. The use of this guideline must be considered alongside the child's ability to engage in "insight-oriented therapy" (Baker & Tamplin, 2006, p. 199). Fatigue levels of the child should also be monitored, as engaging in songwriting may increase emotional responses and impact the cognitive ability required to create the material. Depending on the child's developmental age, his level of injury, and his ability to concentrate, this songwriting task can be introduced in short sections while monitoring fatigue and interest levels. The music therapist monitors the child's ability to provide suitable and relevant material for the song, his ability to self-evaluate his progress, and his degree of perseveration during the activity. Further detail regarding the evaluation of this method in adult rehabilitation can be found in Baker and Tamplin (2006, p. 182). The authors provide a table of target skills areas for evaluation, such as degree of perseveration or ability to order ideas into groups, which can be modified for the pediatric population.

Procedures. The nine-stage framework adopted by Baker, Kennelly, and Tamplin (2005a) and Baker (2005) is a useful model for this intervention. The model involves a series of stages which move both the child and therapist through the songwriting journey. The purpose of this songwriting intervention is explained to the child according to the goal of the session, i.e., if the goal is to promote good conversation skills, the therapist can begin by stressing the importance of these skills in the child's everyday contact within the community and the way songs (as opposed to pure verbal interaction) can be used to communicate his intentions and feelings.

The therapist and child begin with a discussion of the topic (stage 1) and explore different ideas which interest the child. These discussions can range from topics concerning the hospital or rehabilitation experience to his family and friends, or, for the younger child, can relate to his favorite toy or a family pet. A topic is selected (stage 2), and related ideas are explored together (stage 3). Depending on the age of the child, this exploration can take in different ways ranging from song singing and imaginary play involving toys or books to exploring diary or journal entries with adolescents. The main concepts related to the selected topic are developed by the child (or with assistance from the therapist) (stage 4) and developed into a chorus. A discussion on the extension of these ideas (stage 5) then takes place, which helps form the verses of the song (stage 6). Here the child is presented with any ideas gathered during stage 3 which were not included in the chorus but can be considered for the song's verses. The child, with or without the therapist's assistance, may set aside ideas or points which he feels do not need to be included in the song (stage 7). An outline of the main topics of the song is prepared by the therapist and child (stage 8), and the song lyrics are finally written (stage 9).

Other less traditional songwriting formats may also be used, such as free-form (with no particular chorus). After the song is composed, it is practiced during subsequent sessions and the child is encouraged to sing it independently. This experience can provide a feeling of empowerment and enhance the child's self-expression. The song may be recorded and given to the child prior to/on discharge from the rehabilitation unit. This composition can be used to facilitate conversation skills between (a) the child and family members (e.g., the song may contain messages about the child's hopes for his return home, including activities he wants to engage in) or (b) the child and his friends (e.g., the song may contain messages about the child's desire to re-engage with social activities and reminders to friends about changes in the child's physical and emotional state). The song can be used as a prompt for these conversational skills and also reminds the child of his contribution to the song (i.e., his ability to tell others what is important to him as described by the song's content). Moving through each stage of the songwriting process is dependent on the developmental age of the child. Younger children may not be able to identify extended topics and ideas, and the structure or outline of material may be presented more simply and concisely. Music therapy techniques used to facilitate this intervention include fill-in-the-blank, song parody, or original lyrics (Baker & Tamplin, 2006). An example of a song parody technique used to support a young girl as she prepared for discharge is included below (Kennelly, 2006, p. 232). Other techniques adopted by Baker and Tamplin (2006) include song collage or the use of multiple selections of different song lyrics to create a composition and the use of rhyme, which can be adapted for the pediatric population.

The following song was written to the tune of the Spice Girls' song called "Stop" and compiled with lyrics by a young patient as she prepared to leave hospital and return home.

Tracey's "Going Home" Song[iv]

Stop right there, I need a dog
And I'm getting it for Christmas it's before my birthday
Hey you, I'm going to Dreamworld
And there I'm going on the Tower of Terror
Du du du du, du du du du, du du du du I can't wait to walk again
Ba ba ba ba, ba ba ba ba, ba ba ba ba dog's are great!!
Sally, Bill, Dad, Mum and I we are all going to Dreamworld
Just Dreamworld it is the best, just the best place in Australia
I'm looking forward to Christmas then I'll get my dog
Just got to get that fence finished
So when I get my dog it can run around

Family members can also be involved in the songwriting process. However, it is imperative that the child's needs are of primary focus during the sessions. Some family members, while initially intending to support their child, may inadvertently "take over" the songwriting process and either place their own needs ahead of their child's or instruct their child to write the song in a particular style so as to produce an acceptable piece of work. It is important that the music therapist explain the purpose and goals of the session and acknowledge any concerns or difficulties the family members may be experiencing in relation to the child. The following song parody was written by the music therapist and family members of a child who received multiple head injuries. The song was based on an Australian country and western song by Slim Dusty, "The Pub With No Beer," and the lyrics include anecdotes from members of Bobby's family. While the child was recovering in ICU and emerging from coma, the song was used to provide emotional support and facilitate appropriate interaction among family members as they attempted to communicate with the child (Kennelly, 2006, p. 231).

Bobby's "Hello" Song[v]

Oh it's great to be here with Bobby today
He's lying in bed hearing all that I say
And I know he loves music and singing as well
So listen very closely 'cause I've got lots to tell
You love old Slim Dusty, his songs are true blue
There's the Pub with no Beer and lots of others too
There's "Slim, Live at Wagga," you know this the best
Having a beer with Duncan will beat all the rest

And then there's another group different to Slim
They're a favorite of Bobby's, Why don't you ask him
Kiss that's their name and it's Dad's favorite too
They even spit blood when they're singing a tune
Now Bobby loves drawing and playing football
Any toys full of batteries, big, large or small
He loves pulling things apart so Grandma tells me
"I'm gonna be a mechanic, just wait and see"
He loves playing dress-up with Sue and Grandma
He dressed as the bridegroom, the best looking by far
He's got magic fingers and Grandma has said
He can make you feel better just by touching your head
So let those magic fingers cast their spell
And see if they can make Bobby well
This song's nearly over, it's time to go
I'll come and see you again to sing more songs that you know

MULTICULTURAL CONSIDERATIONS

The issue of the cultural identity of the child and his family is important to consider throughout each phase of rehabilitation (Ponsford, Sloan, & Snow, 1995). A phenomenological study in the United States by Roscigno and Swanson (2011) of parents of children diagnosed with a severe TBI found that cultural barriers impacted upon understandings of their child's injury and progress. Parents commented on the importance of being understood and listened to with respect to their cultural differences and reported clashes between themselves and hospital staff when this did not occur. This took place when hospital staff provided medical information about their child's recovery and presumed parents understood details regarding diagnosis and prognosis. Another example of difficulties encountered by parents focused on the perceived inability for staff to "humanely engage" with families and being unaware of the cultural dimensions of the family's experiences of trauma. Findings from this study recommended that ongoing research was required in understanding how culture-based beliefs and attitudes impacted a family's responses to their child's TBI.

Culture may also influence the way an ABI is understood as a form of disability (Uomoto, 2005). A qualitative study with adult patients with TBI from Italian, Lebanese, and Vietnamese backgrounds (Simpson, Mohr, and Redman, 2000) indicated that understandings of rehabilitation varied widely across the different cultural groups and that shame and stigma were associated with brain injury in patients from all backgrounds. The music therapist may be able to address these areas of concern for the child or his family through the use of improvisational music therapy where music can support and validate the expression of feelings. Compositional interventions may also be used to support or promote awareness of feelings and thoughts regarding cultural perceptions of brain injury.

A family's cultural background and their beliefs and value systems must be considered when planning and delivering therapy programs. Each of these areas may impact on the assessment (including the use of appropriate measurement tools), planning, and delivering of treatment and evaluation of goals. Assessment of the psychosocial background and emotional state of the child and family may require adaptations of current tools, particularly when cultural factors prevent the exploration of such material. During assessment, the music therapist gathers information regarding the child's cultural background which may impact not only on their musical preferences and experiences of music, but also on the ways in which music is perceived and valued by the family. Indigenous families may hold different opinions and views on the role of music, and therefore a one-dimensional view of this role cannot be held by the therapist when planning programs.

Research Evidence

Research evidence in the practice of rehabilitation music therapy has mainly focused on the adult population. Systematic reviews of the effects of music therapy in adults with ABI (Bradt, Magee, Dileo, Wheeler, & McGilloway, 2010) or specifically the effects of music in the treatment of neurological language and speech disorders for adults (Hurkmans, de Bruij, Boonstra, Jonkers, Bastiaanse, Arendzen, & Reindeers-Messelink, 2012) are useful in providing efficacy information for music therapy practice in this clinical area. However, despite this evidence, limited research has been conducted to date within the pediatric ABI population. As previously described in this chapter, working clinically with a child or adolescent with these injuries requires specific knowledge and expertise and, therefore, demands a strong, evidence-based practice framework to support clinical practice.

A review of the research literature on the use of music therapy within pediatric rehabilitation revealed a mixed methods study using an intrinsic single case study design (Bower, 2010); a case study design using therapeutic narrative analysis (Gilbertson, 2005); and a modified content analysis of song lyrics (Baker, Kennelly, & Tamplin, 2005b, 2005c). Each of these studies is reviewed below. No randomized controlled trials, cohort studies, crossover design, case-control studies, or cross-sectional surveys were found in the current literature.

A mixed methods study by Bower (2010) explored the use of music therapy with a 10-year-old girl recovering from a severe TBI. The study incorporated a quantitative repeated measures design and qualitative, intrinsic single case study. The study investigated the effects of music therapy on agitation levels during PTA and explored the child's and therapist's responses during sessions using a tri-tiered analysis of videotaped data. The music therapist's responses during the music therapy interventions were analyzed according to the child's behaviors. Data was collected during the first 10 days of the PTA period; the music therapy intervention used was live singing of familiar songs (with and without guitar accompaniment). This intervention was presented to the child using receptive and re-creative music therapy methods. Quantitative data analysis revealed inconclusive results regarding the effect of music therapy on agitation levels during and after therapy. Factors influencing these results included poor inter-reviewer agreement in relation to the rating of agitation levels, the appropriateness of the tool to measure these levels, and time constraints (Bower, 2010). Findings from the qualitative analysis produced four behavioral categories for the child, described as adjectives: neutral, acceptance, recruitment, and rejection. Neutral behaviors were described as no response to the music, while acceptance, recruitment, and rejection behaviors indicated a response to the music therapy interventions. Acceptance behaviors included a calm, relaxed state where neutral behaviors were reduced or paused for some time. Recruitment behaviors included a physical change in the child's body such as a tensing of the muscles followed by a vocalization. The final category of rejection behaviors included responses which indicated increased agitation and potential overstimulation. Further analysis revealed that the music therapist responded to the child's behaviors in four different ways. Holding responses were described as providing a structured musical support for the child during the observation of the child's neutral behaviors. Affirming responses were used in relation to the child's acceptance behaviors in order to maintain a more relaxed state, while enticing responses from the therapist encouraged responses (or recruitment behaviors) from the child. The final category of therapist responses was described as "containing," where levels of music stimulation were changed in order to reduce rejection behaviors. Whether to promote a more relaxed state or provide opportunity for engagement in the sessions, the findings revealed that receptive and re-creative interventions may be used to support, encourage, or change a child's behaviors during PTA. The researcher acknowledges the limitations of this single case, although stressing the importance and significance of such in-depth analysis in order to reveal new insight and knowledge regarding the behaviors of a child with a TBI.

Gilbertson (2005) used therapeutic narrative analysis to examine clinical changes during improvised music therapy with clients in early neurorehabilitation (Gilbertson, 2005). In this case study design, Gilbertson examined audio and video recordings of clinical music therapy with three clients who had a severe TBI, two of whom were children (Neil, age nine, and Bert, age 14). Moving through a series of five phases, the researcher qualitatively analyzed 12 episodes of purposively selected clinical material in order to discover meanings and understandings of clinical change in therapeutic practice. The music therapy method used in this study was the Nordoff-Robbins creative music therapy approach, which involves in-depth analysis of improvisations; accordingly, musical material transcribed from clinical sessions was included in the analysis. Music therapy improvisation methods provided opportunities for meaningful connection by engaging in a relationship which supported and extended each client's ability to communicate. Different types of relationships created through improvised music therapy (e.g., between the client, the therapist, and the music) may enable clients to feel empowered and encouraged as they re-engage with themselves and their new life following a TBI. Similar to Bower's, this study was "an inquiry into processes" (p. 232) and did not suggest the effectiveness of one method over another. Moreover, findings from both studies demonstrate a link between responses of children with a severe ABI to the musical events and interventions used by music therapists. This is important to consider when planning therapy programs, as children receiving rehabilitation, particularly in the acute and subacute phases, are surrounded by a variety of different stimuli which may not promote appropriate responses.

A retrospective analysis of 82 songs written by clients with a TBI identified general themes (Baker, Kennelly, & Tamplin, 2005b) and differences within these themes across the life span (Baker, Kennelly, & Tamplin, 2005c). Thirteen of the 82 songs were written by a nonadult group: children (n=3), early adolescents (n=3) and mid-adolescents (n=7). A variety of songwriting approaches were used by the researchers in each clinical setting; however, the differences in their approaches could not be controlled for in this study. These included word substitution, adding new words to known songs, and creating original song material. A modified content analysis approach was used to analyze the lyrics. Prior to analysis, researchers constructed categories within themes which were informed by past music therapy research findings, themes within the literature on adjustment to disability, and the researchers' clinical experience. These included self-reflections, messages, memories, reflections upon significant others, expression of adversity, concern for the future, imagery, and spirituality.

The theme of self-reflection in song lyrics was most common across the life span, with the early adolescent group rating as the highest in this category. The majority of self-reflections in this category focused on "what makes me happy." The mid-adolescent group recorded the highest incidence of "messages" as a theme in song lyrics as they searched for new ways to communicate their feelings and newfound identities. The inclusion of "memories" in songs was frequently found in children and early/mid-adolescence as they spoke of relationships with significant others; however, minimal explanation was provided by the authors for this finding. The remaining themes recorded lower incidence for these age groups in comparison to older clients. Findings from this research highlight the need to consider age-related and developmental factors when adapting compositional music therapy methods with this population.

A search for research evidence focusing specifically on re-creative music therapy in pediatric ABI revealed no published studies.

SUMMARY AND CONCLUSIONS

In order to work effectively with children with ABI, music therapists need to have knowledge of the impact of brain injuries on the child's cognitive and physical development as well as their psychosocial well-being. This chapter provided basic information related to brain anatomy and rehabilitation stages. However, therapists wishing to work with this population will need to deepen their knowledge of cerebral development and the biomechanics of traumatic brain injury. It is recommended that the music therapists practicing in the clinical area of pediatric rehabilitation, regardless their level of experience in the field, consult a wide variety of literature in order to extend their knowledge and clinical expertise. Opportunities for training and education in music therapy and non–music therapy-related disciplines relating to rehabilitation will also assist the developing practitioner. A variety of music therapy interventions using receptive, improvisation, re-creative, and compositional methods can support the child who is recovering from an ABI. These methods are designed to meet the child's physical, psychosocial, cognitive, behavioral, or communicative needs throughout each rehabilitation phase. In addition, the pediatric rehabilitation music therapist needs to be aware of the implications of working with caregivers, as their involvement in clinical music therapy sessions may determine the selection and use of therapy interventions. Similarly, multicultural considerations should be taken into account throughout each phase of recovery. A summary of research evidence in pediatric music therapy rehabilitation was presented to support the use of specific therapy interventions.

As previously described in this chapter, the child or adolescent with an ABI should not be treated as a "little adult" (Blosser & De Pompei, 2003, p. 32). Music therapy practice with this pediatric population requires carefully designed and implemented approaches which are appropriate to each developmental age level. While techniques and methods outlined with adult populations are useful, the need for continuing research with children and adolescents recovering from an ABI is needed in order to develop techniques grounded in evidence-based practice. In addition to this research, it is important for clinicians in their everyday practice to continue reporting their use of different and evolving music therapy interventions so that other therapists may learn and become aware of the wide variety of methods available in the international arena. "Lack of existence [of research] should not be confused with lack of evidence, and in the current situation of a wide diversity of clinical interventions, clinicians are encouraged to join researchers or become researchers themselves, to provide evidence of their daily clinical practice" (Gilbertson, 2009, p. 137).

REFERENCES

AMTA. (2011). *Bedside music—Music therapy in hospitals. Making Music Being Well Fact Sheet.* Victoria, Australia: Australian Music Therapy Association.

Anderson, V. (2004). Pediatric head injury. In M. Rizzo & P. Eslinger (Eds.), *Principles and practice of behavioral neurology and neuropsychology* (pp. 863–879). Philadelphia: W. B. Saunders.

Anderson, V., Northam, E., Hendy, J., & Wrennall, J. (2001). *Developmental neuropsychology: A clinical approach.* Hove, East Sussex: Psychology Press.

Anderson, V., Spencer-Smith, M., Leventer, R., Coleman, L., Anderson, P., Williams, J., Greenham, M., & Jacobs, R. (2009). Childhood brain insult: Can age at insult help us predict outcome? *Brain, 132*(1), 45–56. DOI: 10.1093/brain/awn293.

Anderson, V., & Yeates, K. (Eds.). (2010). *Pediatric traumatic brain injury—New frontiers in clinical and translational research.* Cambridge: Cambridge University Press.

AROC. (2012). Australasian Rehabilitation Outcomes Centre. Retrieved from http://ahsri.uow.edu.au/aroc/training/index.html

Australian Institute of Health and Welfare. (2007). *Disability in Australia: Acquired brain injury.* Bulletin 55, (December). Retrieved from http://www.aihw.gov.au/WorkArea/DownloadAsset.aspx?id=6442453666

Baker, F. (2000). Modifying melodic intonation therapy programs for adults with severe non-fluent aphasia. *Music Therapy Perspectives, 2*(2), 107–111.

Baker, F. (2001). Rationale for the effects of familiar music on agitation and orientation levels of people experiencing posttraumatic amnesia. *Nordic Journal of Music Therapy, 10*(1), 32–41. DOI: 10.1080/08098130109478011.

Baker, F. (2005). Working with impairments in pragmatics through songwriting following traumatic brain injury. In F. Baker & T. Wigram (Eds.), *Song writing methods, techniques and clinical applications for music therapy clinicians, educators and students* (pp. 134–153). Philadelphia, PA: Jessica Kingsley Publishers.

Baker, F., Kennelly, J., & Tamplin, J. (2005a). Song writing to explore identity change and sense of self/self-concept following traumatic brain injury. In F. Baker & T. Wigram (Eds.), *Song writing methods, techniques and clinical applications for music therapy clinicians, educators and students* (pp. 116–133). Philadelphia, PA: Jessica Kingsley Publishers.

Baker, F., Kennelly, J., & Tamplin, J. (2005b). Adjusting to change through song: Themes in songs written by clients with TBI. *Brain Impairment, 6*(3), 205–211.

Baker, F., Kennelly, J., & Tamplin, J. (2005c). Themes in songs written by clients with traumatic brain injury: Differences across the lifespan. *Australian Journal of Music Therapy, 16,* 25–42.

Baker, F., & Tamplin, J. (2006). *Music therapy methods in neurorehabilitation—A clinician's manual.* Philadelphia, PA: Jessica Kingsley.

Baxter, H., Berghofer, J., MacEwan, L., Nelson, J., Peters, K., & Roberts, P. (2007). *The individualized music therapy assessment profile: IMTAP.* Philadelphia, PA: Jessica Kingsley.

Blosser, J., & De Pompei, R. (2003*). Pediatric traumatic brain injury.* New York: Delmar Learning.

Bower, J. (2010). *Music therapy for a 10-year-old child experiencing agitation during posttraumatic amnesia: An intrinsic mixed methods study.* Master's thesis. Retrieved from http://repository.unimelb.edu.au/10187/8949

Bower, J., & Shoemark, H. (2012). Music therapy for the pediatric patient experiencing agitation during posttraumatic amnesia: Constructing a foundation from theory. *Music and Medicine, 4*(3), 146–152. DOI: 10.1177/1943862112442227.

Bower, J., & Shoemark, H. (2009). Music therapy to promote interpersonal interactions in early pediatric neurorehabilitation. *The Australian Journal of Music Therapy, 20,* 59–75.

Bradt, J., Magee, W., Dileo, C., Wheeler, B., & McGilloway, E. (2010). Music therapy for acquired brain injury. *Cochrane Database of Systematic Reviews.* Retrieved from http://onlinelibrary.wiley.com/doi/10.1002/14651858.CD006787.pub2/abstract

Bruscia, K. (1987). *Improvisational models of music therapy.* Springfield, IL: C. C. Thomas.

Corrigan, J. (1989). Development of a scale for assessment of agitation following TBI. *Journal of Clinical and Experimental Neuropsychology, 11*(2), 261–277.

Daveson, B. A. (2008). A description of a music therapy meta-model in neuro-disability and neuro-rehabilitation for use with children, adolescents and adults. *Australian Journal of Music Therapy, 19,* 70–85.

Douglass, E. (2006). The development of a music therapy assessment tool for hospitalized children. *Music Therapy Perspectives, 24*(2), 73–79.

Edwards, J. (2005). A reflection on the music therapist's role in developing a program in a children's hospital. *Music Therapy Perspectives, 23*(1), 36–44.

Edwards, J., & Kennelly, J. (1999). *Clinician's manual—Music Therapy for children in hospital.* Brisbane: University of Queensland Printery.

Edwards, J., & Kennelly, J. (2004). Music therapy in paediatric rehabilitation: The application of modified grounded theory to identify techniques used by a music therapist. *Nordic Journal of Music Therapy, 13*(2), 112–126. DOI: 10.1080/08098130409478106.

Edwards, J., & Kennelly, J. (2011). Music therapy for children in hospital care: A stress & coping framework for practice. In A. Meadows (Ed.), *Developments in music therapy practice: Case study perspectives* (pp. 150–165). Gilsum, NH: Barcelona Publishers.

Erwing-Cobbs, L., Levin, H., Fletcher, J., Miner, M., & Eisenberg, H. (1990). The child's orientation and amnesia test: relationship to severity of acute head injury and to recovery of memory. *Neurosurgery, 27,* 683–691.

Feeney, T., & Ylvisaker, M (2003). Context-sensitive behavioral supports for young children with TBI. *Journal of Head Trauma Rehabilitation, 18*(1), 33–51.

Gilberston, S. (1999). Music therapy in neurosurgical rehabilitation. In T. Wigram & J. De Backer (Eds.), *Clinical application of music therapy in development disability, paediatrics and neurology* (pp. 224–245). Philadelphia, PA: Jessica Kingsley Publishers.

Gilbertson, S. (2005). *Music therapy in early neurosurgical rehabilitation with people who have experienced traumatic brain injury.* Unpublished doctoral thesis. University Witten /Herdecke, Witten.

Gilbertson, S. (2009). A reference standard bibliography: Music therapy with children who have experienced traumatic brain injury. *Music and Medicine, 1*(2), 129–139. DOI: 10.1177/1943862109348967.

Hagen, C., Malkmus, D., Durham, P., & Stenderup, K. (1979). *Levels of cognitive functioning.* Downey, CA: Ranchos Los Amigos Hospital Inc.

Hessen, E., Nestvold, K., & Anderson, V. (2007). Neuropsychological function 23 years after mild traumatic brain injury: A comparison of outcome after paediatric and adult head injuries. *Brain Injury, 21*(9), 963–979.

Hurkmans, J., De Bruijn, M., Boonstra, A., Jonkers, R., Bastiaanse, R., Arendzen, H., & Reinders-Messelink, H. (2012). Music in the treatment of neurological language and speech disorders: A systematic review. *Aphasiology, 26*(1), 1–19. DOI: 10.1080/02687038.2011.602514.

Hurt, C., Rice, R., McIntosh, G., & Thaut, M. (1998). Rhythmic auditory stimulation in gait training for patients with traumatic brain injury. *Journal of Music Therapy, 35*(4), 228–241.

Hurt-Thaut, C., & Johnson, S. (2003). Neurologic music therapy with children: Scientific foundations and clinical application. In S. L. Robb (Ed.), *Music therapy in pediatric healthcare: Research and evidence-based practice* (pp. 81–100). Silver Spring, MD: AMTA, Inc.

James, H. (1986). Neurologic evaluation and support in the child with an acute brain insult. *Pediatric Annals, 15*(1), 16–22.

Kennelly, J. (2000). The specialist role of the music therapist in developmental programs for hospitalized children. *Journal of Paediatric Health Care, 14*(2), 56–59.

Kennelly, J. (2006). Music therapy in paediatric rehabilitation. In F. Baker & J. Tamplin (Eds.), *Music therapy methods in neurorehabilitation* (pp. 219–233). Philadelphia, PA: Jessica Kingsley..

Kennelly, J., & Brien-Elliot, K. (2001). The role of music therapy in paediatric rehabilitation. *Paediatric Rehabilitation, 4*(3), 137–143.

Kennelly, J., & Brien-Elliott, K. (2002). Music therapy for children in hospital. *Educating Young Children—Learning & Teaching in the Early Childhood Years, 8*(3), 37–40.

Kennelly, J., & Edwards, J. (1997). Providing music therapy to the unconscious child in the paediatric intensive care unit. *The Australian Journal of Music Therapy, 8,* 18–29.

Kennelly, J., Hamilton, L., & Cross, J. (2001). The interface of music therapy and speech pathology in the rehabilitation of children with acquired brain injury. *The Australian Journal of Music Therapy, 12,* 13–20.

Kochanek, P., Bell, M., & Bayir, H. (2010). Quo vadis. Carpe Diem: Challenges and opportunities in pediatric traumatic brain injury. *Developmental Neuroscience, 32,* 335–342. DOI: 10.1159/000323016.

Kolb, B., & Gibb, R. (2010). Integrating multidisciplinary research for translation from the laboratory to the clinic. In V. Anderson & K. Yeates (Eds.), *Pediatric traumatic brain injury* (pp. 207–224). Cambridge: Cambridge University Press.

Lehr, E. (1996). Parallel processes—stages of recovery and stages of family accommodation to ABI. In G. Singer, A. Glang, & J. Williams (Eds.), *Children with acquired brain injury: educating and supporting families.* Baltimore: Paul H. Brookes Publishing Company.

Leung, M. (2008). A collaboration between music therapy and speech pathology in a paediatric rehabilitation setting. *Voices: A World Forum for Music Therapy, 8*(3). Retrieved from https://normt.uib.no/index.php/voices/article/view/417/341

Magee, W. L., Baker, F., Daveson, B., Hitchen, H., Kennelly, J., Leung, M. & Tamplin, J. (2011). Music therapy method with children, adolescents, and adults with severe neurobehavioral disorders due to brain injury. *Music Therapy Perspectives, 29*(1), 5–13.

NCIPC. (2002–2006). *Traumatic brain injury in the United States: Assessing outcomes in children.* Atlanta, GA: National Center for Injury Prevention and Control. Retrieved from http://www.cdc.gov/traumaticbraininjury/assessing_outcomes_in_children.html#1

Nolte, J. (2009). *The human brain: An introduction to its functional anatomy.* Philadelphia: Mosby Elsevier.

Patterson, R., Uppenkamp, S., Johnsrude, I., & Griffiths, T. (2002). The processing of temporal pitch and melody information in auditory cortex. *Neuron, 36,* 767–776.

Ponsford, J., Sloan, S., & Snow, P. (1995). *Traumatic brain injury: Rehabilitation for every day adaptive living.* London: Lawrence Erlbaum.

RCH. (2011). *Guidelines for melodic intonation therapy.* Music Therapy Department, Royal Children's Hospital, Children's Health Services. Brisbane, Australia: Queensland Health.

Robb, S. (1996). Techniques in song writing: Restoring emotional and physical well-being in adolescents who have been traumatically injured. *Music Therapy Perspectives, 14*(1), 30–37.

Robb, S. (2003). Designing music therapy interventions for hospitalized children and adolescents using a contextual support model of music therapy. *Music Therapy Perspectives, 21*(1), 27–40.

Roscigno, C., & Swanson, K. (2011). Parents' experiences following children's moderate to severe traumatic brain injury: A clash of cultures. *Qualitative Health Research, 21*(10), 1413–1426. DOI: 10.1177/104973231141088.

Rosenfeld, J., & Dun, B. (1999). Music therapy in children with severe traumatic brain injury. In R. R. Pratt & D. E. Grocke (Eds.), *MusicMedicine 3: MusicMedicine and music therapy: Expanding horizons* (pp. 35–46). Victoria: University of Melbourne.

Simpson, G., Mohr, R., & Redman, A., (2000). Cultural variations in the understanding of traumatic brain injury and brain injury rehabilitation. *Brain Injury, 14*(2), 125–140.

Teasdale, G., & Jennett, B. (1974). Assessment of coma and impaired consciousness: a practical scale. *Lancet, 2,* 81–84.

Thaut, M. (1999). *Training manual for neurologic music therapy.* Colorado State University: Center for Biomedical Research in Music.

Thaut, M. (2005). *Rhythm, music and the brain—Scientific foundations and clinical applications.* New York: Routledge, Taylor and Francis Group.

Thaut, M., McIntosh, G., Rice, R., Miller, R., Rathbun, J., & Brault, J. (1996). Rhythmic auditory stimulation in gait training for Parkinson's disease patients. *Movement Disorders, 11*, 193–200.

Uomoto, J. (2005). Multicultural perspectives. In W. High, A. Sander, M. Struchen, & K. Hart (Eds.), *Rehabilitation for Traumatic Brain Injury* (pp. 247–267). Oxford: Oxford University Press.

Watson, C., Kirkcaldie, M., & Paxinos, G. (2010). *The brain: An introduction to functional neuroanatomy*. London: Elsevier, Inc.

Whitehead, D. (1998). *Awareness through the musical consciousness: A music therapy awareness continuum for children with severe brain injury. A tool to musically assess level of consciousness and to establish a treatment protocol*. Master's thesis. Retrieved from Theses Canada (26013118).

Whitehead-Pleaux, A., Clark, S., & Spall, L. (2011). Indications and counterindications for electronic music technologies in a pediatric medical setting. *Music and Medicine, 3*(3), 154–162. DOI: 10.1177/1943862111409241.

Ylvisaker, M., Chorazy, A., Feeney, T., & Russell, M. (1999). Traumatic brain injury in children and adolescents: assessment and rehabilitation. In M. Rosenthal, J. Kreutzer, E. Griffith, & B. Pentland (Eds.), *Rehabilitation of the adult and child with traumatic brain injury* (pp. 356–392). Philadelphia: F. A. Davis Company.

RESOURCES

Music Technology and Functional Rehabilitation

1) Adaptive Use Musical Instrument (AUMI) : Free and downloadable software for Mac and PC which allows a client to create musical sounds using the movement of a body part such as the head or hand. For further information, see http://www.musictherapywa.org/info/wp-content/uploads/2012/05/AUMIHandout.pdf (D. Knott, personal communication, May 8, 2012)

2) Alesis AirSynth: Useful for recovering function in upper limbs and arousal stimulation (D. Knott, personal communication, May 8, 2012)

3) Nintendo DS10's Kaos pad: Useful for stimulating movement and engagement in improvisation (D. Knott, personal communication, May 8, 2012)

Song Composition and Recording

1) Super Dooper Music Looper—easy-to-use music creation software, using precomposed loops of different instruments, sounds and styles.

2) Acid Pro—composition software which is useful for recording, mixing, and editing music.

3) Sound Forge—software which is useful for audio editing and mastering of music

4) GarageBand—music software that is similar to "Super Dooper Music Looper" in its use of precomposed loops, but has more complexity and variation in how it can be used (including recording live instruments into it). This is a useful and more suitable tool for engaging with adolescents.

Neurologic Music Therapy Training

http://www.colostate.edu/depts/CBRM

Neurologic Music Therapy Network Groups

https://www.jiscmail.ac.uk/cgi-bin/webadmin?A0=MTNEUROLOGYNETWORK
https://groups.google.com/d/forum/neurologic-music-therapists

APPENDIX A

CONSIDERATIONS WHEN WORKING WITH PEDIATRIC PATIENTS AND THEIR FAMILIES
(LEHR, 1996, ADAPTED BY KENNELLY, 2006).[vi]

The issues faced by a child and their family members during the different rehabilitation phases and the music therapy role/interventions that can address their required needs are presented:

Initial Injury Impact and Coma (Child)
- o   Family - Shock, grief, crisis, disruption of family routines and sense of loss of control over their lives
- o   Role of Music Therapy - Use music therapy to provide emotional support and assist grief process. Provide sense of control over hospital environment and daily routines
- o   Music Therapy Intervention - Invite family members to interact during music therapy sessions by singing, selecting their child's song material, and/or music-assisted discussion/reminiscence

Beginning response to commands (Child)
- o   Family - Resurgence of hope; continued disruption of family life; failure
- o   Role of Music Therapy - As described in *Initial Injury Impact and Coma*. Use music therapy sessions to provide encouragement to family members and give permission to 'take a break' and attend to their own needs
- o   Music Therapy Intervention - Continue to involve family during music therapy sessions through singing and/or contributing to improvised songs/song parody (e.g. prompt family members to ask questions in song form to encourage responses from the child (Endnote 5)

Agitation (Child)
- o   Family - Fear of regression and painful experiences. Continued disruption of family life
- o   Role of Music Therapy - Use familiar music to assist orientation and agitation levels through singing of familiar songs (Baker, 2002). This music may also assist family members emotionally during this difficult time
- o   Music Therapy Intervention - As described in *Initial Injury Impact and Coma* and *Beginning response to commands*. Invite family to use prepared song material at times outside therapy music therapy sessions to assist orientation and agitation

Early cognitive recovery (Child)
- o   Family - Initial fears of confusion resolve to recognition that their child and other family members, are expected to go through the motions of typical activities despite the state of the injured child
- o   Role of Music Therapy - Use song parody to address activities of daily living and promote and extend the child's functional skills
- o   Music Therapy Intervention - Involve family in the creation of musical material (Endnote 2 and 3). Also encourage the use of this material outside of music therapy sessions

Continued cognitive recovery (Child)
- o   Family - Re-establishment of family routines with adjustment for recovering child. Consideration of sibling reactions. Need for assistance with planning and management (hospital and home environments)
- o   Role of Music Therapy - Use music therapy with siblings (individual or group work) to work through grief responses to their sister or brother's injury
- o   Music Therapy Intervention - Songwriting/song parody to reflect changes within the family structure or preparations for going home (Endnote 4)

Socio-emotional recovery (Child)
- o Family - Emotional and behavioral concerns. Social rejection and isolation. Coping with child's reaction to injury. Emerging awareness of the extent and impact of child's limitations and changes on the child's and family's functioning
- o Role of Music Therapy - Provide emotional support and opportunity for self-expression through songs, for example Delta Goodrem's song *Out Of The Blue* or Anastasia's *Left Outside Alone*
- o Music Therapy Intervention - Use songwriting, song singing and improvisation techniques to provide this support

Developmental reinterpretation and readjustment to injury effects (Child)
- o Family - Beginning of long-term planning. Alteration of pre-injury plans both for family members and the injured child
- o Role of Music Therapy - Provide emotional support in terms of unresolved grief and loss issues through music therapy activities
- o Music Therapy Intervention - Use songwriting/song singing techniques. Involve family members where appropriate

ENDNOTES

---

[i] I would like to thank the children and families who I have worked with over the years that have inspired and helped shape the content of this chapter. In particular, I would like to acknowledge the rehabilitation music therapists from the Pediatric Health Reference Group in Australia, especially Helen Carrington from the Royal Children's Hospital, Brisbane (Children's Health Queensland Hospital and Health Service) for their assistance and input into the writing of these practice guidelines. Thank you also to other international music therapists working in this field who responded to my requests for assistance.

[ii]*Steven's "Standing" Song* reprinted by permission of Jessica Kingsley Publishers. Taken from J. Kennelly. (2006). Music Therapy in Paediatric Rehabilitation. In F. Baker & J. Tamplin (Eds.), *Music Therapy Methods in Neurorehabilitation* (p. 232). Philadelphia, PA: Jessica Kingsley.

[iii]*Steven's "Sitting" Song* reprinted by permission of Jessica Kingsley Publishers. Taken from J. Kennelly. (2006). Music Therapy in Paediatric Rehabilitation. In F. Baker & J. Tamplin (Eds.), *Music Therapy Methods in Neurorehabilitation* (p. 232). Philadelphia, PA: Jessica Kingsley.

[iv]*Tracey's "Going Home" Song* reprinted by permission of Jessica Kingsley Publishers. Taken from J. Kennelly. (2006). Music Therapy in Paediatric Rehabilitation. In F. Baker & J. Tamplin (Eds.), *Music Therapy Methods in Neurorehabilitation*. Philadelphia, PA: Jessica Kingsley.

[v]Kennelly, J. *"Bobby's Song"* reprinted by permission of Jessica Kingsley Publishers. Taken from J. Kennelly. (2006). Music Therapy in Paediatric Rehabilitation. In F. Baker & J. Tamplin (Eds.), *Music Therapy Methods in Neurorehabilitation*. Philadelphia, PA: Jessica Kingsley .

[vi] *Considerations when Working with Paediatric Patients and their Families* reprinted by permission of Jessica Kingsley Publishers. Taken from J. Kennelly (2006). Music Therapy in Paediatric Rehabilitation. In F. Baker & J. Tamplin (Eds.), *Music Therapy Methods in Neurorehabilitation*. Philadelphia, PA: Jessica Kingsley.

Chapter 10

Respiratory Care
For Children

Joanne Loewy

INTRODUCTION

Breathing: An Integrative Function

Inhaling and exhaling are physiological functions that represent both voluntary and involuntary mechanisms of the body and are necessary for survival. We are breathing all of the time, and in usual circumstances, we do not attend to our breath, nor do we need to closely monitor our pulmonary function. However, as breath's delivery of oxygen is critical to all aspects of physical vitality, our capacity to control and enhance breathing is an activity to which both clinicians and researchers are giving growing attention. The way we breathe may nurture critical aspects of general function.

Breathing has a direct impact on cardiac function. The way we breathe may also modulate our experience of anxiety and the way we handle it. The breath may influence how we think and feel, particularly at times of crisis, when we are prone to *cerebral hypoxia*.

As breathing is directly responsible for taking in and letting out, considerations of the environment and one's physical sensitivity to the atmosphere both materially and emotionally cannot be overlooked. This chapter will address pulmonary diseases and the roots of dysfunction, with particular attention to etiology and disease progression. To broaden the knowledge base of respiratory care, we will begin with a description of the most common respiratory diseases and proceed with a plethora of methods describing how music and music therapy may influence breathing function in both disease and wellness-prevention models. We will first begin with understanding the role of the lungs and pulmonary function and its relationship to the function of other organs in a holistic sense. The breath will be viewed as an integrative function, a timbre-metered element of flow that connects physical wellness to mental-spiritual function and vice versa. Aspects of rhythm, flow, intention, risk-taking, spontaneity, and control will become a central part of the methods discussed and will underline the way music therapy is prescribed.

Music therapy, provided as an integrated regimen that is recommended by doctors, nurses, and social workers, has strengthened the impact of traditional care in its capacity to influence one's ability to breathe in a direct way, as in singing or playing a wind instrument. Music therapy in respiratory care directly affects the breath and can advance inhalation and exhalation, particularly when attention is drawn to melodic theme and phrase sequencing. This chapter will enhance and advance the way we treat pulmonary challenges, providing alternatives to the standard model of care through the utilization of a music psychotherapy model.

Distinction between Music Medicine and Medical Music Psychotherapy

It is important to distinguish between the uses of music by non–music therapy medical personnel from the music that is used by trained music therapists. In music medicine, music is used to assist in medical treatment, and the music is used as the means of intervention or stimulus. The term was coined by Ralph Spintge (Pratt & Spintge, 1995; Spintge & Droh, 1987, 1993) and implies scientific evaluation of musical stimuli in medical settings through physiological, psychological, and medical research, as well as therapeutic applications to complement traditional medical treatment.

Medical music psychotherapy is related to music medicine but distinctly different. In medical music psychotherapy, we seek to integrate physical aspects of functioning with behavioral, cognitive, social, and spiritual orientations as presented in a music therapy context. Medical music psychotherapy in a medical setting involves treating the whole person—body, mind, and spirit. The approach warrants clinical interpretation and involves distinct parameters of physiological aspects of functioning that are contextualized within individualized and cultural-centered care.

DIAGNOSTIC INFORMATION

The Lungs

In usual circumstances, human beings have two lungs. The author has had the opportunity recently to work weekly in a clinic setting using music therapy with several patients of a wide range of ages (2–65 years old) who have functioned well with one lung, or a second lung transplanted. The lungs are the organs that are responsible for gas exchange. The process of breathing begins as oxygen comes into the mouth and nose and then passes through the trachea down toward the lungs, where blood is pumped in through the heart. The lungs are responsible for removing carbon dioxide from the blood. There is an exchange where oxygen comes in and carbon dioxide goes out. The lungs are our source of pulmonary function through inflow and outflow of air. The alveoli sacs within the lungs are receptors that monitor air's pressure and motion. The alveoli are sensitive and monitor blood pressure, speeding up the rate of breath if the pressure is low and slowing it down if it is high. The lungs work directly with the cardiovascular system.

The interchange between the lungs and the blood is known as pulmonary diffusion. Pulmonary diffusion is concerned with the exchange between gases and blood. In pulmonary evaluations, attention is paid to the measurement of the lung's capacity in transferring gases optimally (American Thoracic Society [ATS], 1995).

Pulmonary Diseases

Diseases of the lungs and airways are classified in a variety of ways. As this chapter is focused primarily on children (infants through teens), chronic obstructive pulmonary disease (COPD), the result of chronic *emphysema* or long-term *asthma* or lung disease, will not be presented. COPD has been studied in music therapy, and treatment recommendations related to the treatment of COPD with music therapy have been addressed (Azoulay & Raskin, 2008). The following section will define respiratory diseases beginning with premature infants and define the impact of disease progression, diagnoses, and secondary symptoms developmentally. This will be followed by definitions of common symptoms in breathing disorders and suggestions of how music therapy might seek to address such confounds.

Respiratory Distress Syndrome (RDS): Premature infants, whose lungs are not fully formed, may develop RDS. Most often, RDS occurs in infants born under 28 weeks. In 2005, 16,268 infants suffered from RDS, an incidence rate of 3.9 per 1,000 (Global Initiative for Asthma [GINA], 2010). Symptoms usually appear shortly after birth and become more severe as the infant grows. The infant's skin color, rhythm of breath, and depth and fluidity of breath are affected.

Respiratory Syncytial Virus (RSV): RSV is a major cause of respiratory illness in young children. It causes infection of the lungs and breathing passages and is highly contagious. As approximately 50% of children in the first year of life will be infected with RSV, and 30% to 70% of those will develop lower respiratory illnesses, these infants become an important population for Neonatal Intensive Care Unit (NICU) music therapists.

Asthma: Our body's capacity to breathe relies largely on our ability to inhale. As we inhale, we allow oxygen from the air to diffuse into the blood for use in respiration. Complications can arise in this distinct process and often do. The origin of repetitive struggles with breathing, which lead to chronic complications and a diagnosis of asthma, is argued among doctors and is not entirely understood as a disease (Osborne et al., 1992). Many argue that asthma is merely a host of symptoms without a distinct definition as a disease. This is surprising, as asthma has been a common disease among children and adults worldwide and for many years. Heredity, allergy, immune system, airway hyperresponsiveness, and environment are believed to be involved (Baroody & Naclerio, 2011).

Asthma symptoms can be triggered when the inhaling of allergy-causing substances (called allergens or triggers) causes a reaction in the airways. Whether allergens are the source or not, it is known that with asthma, nerve cells in the airways sense the presence of unwanted substances such as pollen, water, dust, fumes, or cigarette smoke. The respiratory centers then get signaled by these cells and contract the respiratory muscles, the result of which may present as a runny nose, itchy eyes, sneezing, or coughing. Symptoms, including aggressive sneezing and coughing, can affect the lungs and lead to inflammation. In an asthma exacerbation (the common term is "asthma attack"), the airway passage lining becomes swollen and air inhalation becomes obstructed (Bush & Saglani, 2010).

According to the World Health Organization, an estimated 235 million people suffer from asthma, and it is a public health problem for all countries and people of high and low economic social status, with over 80% of asthma deaths occurring in low- and lower-middle-income countries. This may be due to underdiagnosis and a lack of treatment (GINA, 2010).

Cystic Fibrosis: Cystic Fibrosis (CF) is an inherited disease that is not uncommon to children of northern European descent. It is a most serious disorder that causes severe lung damage and nutritional deficiencies. CF affects the cells that produce mucus, sweat, and digestive juices through secretions that block critical passages in the lungs and pancreas (Ratjen & Döring, 2003). Recommended CF airway clearance techniques have been developed, and it is useful to understand how music therapy might assist breathing, particularly with young patients who are diagnosed with CF (Griggs-Drane, in Azoulay and Loewy, 2008).

Pulmonary Hypertension: Hypertension that affects pulmonary function occurs in the blood vessels and is the result of increased blood pressure in the pulmonary artery, vein, or capillaries. This, in turn, affects the lung vasculature and might present as shortness of breath, dizziness, or fainting.

Pulmonary Fibrosis: a disease that involves scarring of the lung tissue. The damage can be caused by many different things, including airborne toxins in the workplace, certain lung diseases, and even some types of medical treatments.

Pulmonary Sarcoidosis: a disease less common in children than adults, involving the immune system cells that cluster and create lump *granulomas* in the lungs that often remain chronic. Many patients who develop sarcoidosis have a good prognosis; others make up a significant proportion that is prone to a more severe and prolonged disease course. It remains difficult to assess the predictors and outcomes of what precludes the severity of pulmonary sarcoidosis (Drent & Costabel, 2005).

Chronic Obstructive Pulmonary Disease: Chronic Obstructive Pulmonary Disease (COPD) is an adult lung disease characterized by chronic obstruction of lung airflow that interferes with normal breathing and is not fully reversible. It is the last stage of "chronic bronchitis" and "emphysema." This disease involves an obstruction on the exhalation.

Lung Function Evaluation and Treatment

It is important for music therapists to understand how the lungs function because the interventions prescribed in music therapy may directly and purposefully affect the airways. Therefore, comprehension of standard medical treatment will serve not only as a precautionary function, but also as a means by which integrative music medicine and music therapy interventions may or may not be indicated. The reason for referral is determined by the physician or nurse and documented, and ultimately should be well understood by all members of the team that are providing clinical care, including the parent and child/teen patient himself.

It is most common to test whether the lungs are functioning to their capacity through a Lung Function Test. There are several kinds of lung function tests that are usually employed and prescribed based on level of disease and diagnosis. Spirometry measures the volume of air and the ease or obstruction of air that is inhaled and exhaled. Lung volume measurement shows how much air stays within the lungs after a full exhale. Lung diffusion capacity measures how easily oxygen moves into the bloodstream from the lungs. Blood gas laboratories can determine how much oxygen is in the blood. A peak-flow meter may also be helpful in measuring lung volume, but it is prone to be more effort-dependent than spirometry, and therefore less accurate.

Standard treatments of care for children with respiratory diseases include but are not limited to *mechanical ventilation; continuous ventilation therapy,* or positive airway pressure; *surfactant therapy; bronchodilator therapy; aerosolized drug therapy; oxygen therapy; suctioning; tube care; postural drainage;* and percussion and vibration through *chest physiotherapy.*

There have been a host of studies seeking to substantiate the use of nonstandardized remedies in asthma care. There is research indicating that muscular relaxation may have the capacity to improve lung function of patients with asthma (Huntley, White, & Ernst, 2009). However, the evidence supporting any other relaxation therapies is scarce.

Studies involving breath training that would demonstrate changes in airways physiology, inflammation, or hyperresponsiveness have yet to be identified, although one trial did indicate that breath training resulted in improvements in asthma-specific health status and other patient-centered measures (such as anxiety) but not in asthma pathophysiology. The authors point out that although breathing exercises can assist patients whose quality of life is impaired by asthma, they are less than likely to reduce the need for anti-inflammatory treatments (Thomas et al., 2009).

NEEDS AND RESOURCES

The most common and perhaps obvious need of children facing respiratory challenges is the need to restore normal breathing so that they can have a well-regulated sense of control and mastery that will keep them functioning in their usual activities of daily living. Additional goals include but are not limited to self-awareness of breath control, which provides a means of regulation.

Practices and routine methods that can assist in motivating children to comply with their use of both conventional pharmacological regimens as well as nontraditional integrative strategies may well serve the child with respiratory challenges. Intervention offering preventative tools, particularly when children are healthy, may foster the strengthening and upkeep of positive lung health and avoidance of ER care which so often stems from avoidance of awareness and preventative strategies.

Inclusion of parents and significant others may serve as particularly beneficial for the infant, child, or teen who is prone to exercise-induced or stress-related exacerbations. A healthy diet, with nonfired foods, proper sleep, and avoidance of pollens and/or other allergens known to exacerbate asthma attacks can be monitored by parents and families of children with respiratory challenges.

REFERRAL AND ASSESSMENT PROCEDURES

It is understood by medical music therapists who are experienced hospitalists that functions of breath, rendered through clinical observation and through the knowledge of respiratory rate and oxygen saturation, reflect domains of the body that may be indicative of potential experiences of comfort or discomfort, anxiety or relief. In fact, particular aspects of breathing function are evaluated and included in a battery of assessments of other integral functions of the body that lead to diagnoses of a host of critical diseases. Although this chapter's focus is on how music and music therapy may influence children with respiratory challenges, the experiences provided in these pages may work in tandem with breath as an integral function and integrator within other symptoms and as part of the disease trajectory that may include a host of other illnesses.

Recommending prescriptive evidence-supported methods of music therapy particularly designed for children with respiratory disease requires a music therapy assessment. In an integrative music and medicine model, a music psychotherapy approach is integral to determine which assignment of interventions may ensue. This is particularly important in diseases in which breathing becomes obstructed because breath is intricately connected to emotion (Rietveld, van Beest, & Everaerd, 2005). Stress, in particular, can affect breathing and may lead to the child's perception and/or evidential lack of control in the breath process (Manusco, Peterson, & Charlson, 2000).

Referral Procedures

Appendix A presents a music therapy referral form for general pediatrics and Appendix B presents a referral for NICU infants. Both were developed at The Louis Armstrong Center for Music and Medicine at the Best Israel Medical Center, where both are currently being used. Referrals, both verbally and written, are documented and reviewed by staff within 24 hours.

Note that Appendix B includes specific check-offs denoted for referral parameters inclusive of breathing difficulties. Compromised breathing is an area notable to referring staff, and it is well understood that music therapists receiving verbal or written referrals for children who have respiratory illnesses will treat in two ways: physiologically and psychosocially. This is of general importance to each referring illness, as well as for diseases which are being ruled out. The check-off markers on the front of the form correspond with particular treatments which might ensue upon referral on the back of the form. In this way, this document serves as a "teaching" document for MDs and RNs who are newcomers to medical music therapy, particularly floating staff and/or new resident MDs.

Assessment

The assessment of psychotherapeutic function is included in the medical music psychotherapeutic approach. It is critical for the therapist to know the impact that the disease is having on the child's usual mode of function. For instance, how often does he experience shortness of breath and has it limited physical activity in the past? What other influences are at work in the child and family's lifeworld?

The lifeworld in the context of a child with a respiratory illness involves an explicit analysis of the child's physical environment. As the physiological process of breathing involves a direct taking in of the environmental atmosphere, the contact of children with potential allergens is important to be aware of. If the child's family has a new pet, or if there dust or mold in the house, the music therapist can note this by writing it in the assessment. It is best to err on the side of caution and not wear colognes or perfumes when working with children who have respiratory diseases.

A medical music psychotherapy assessment involves:

- Knowledge of each patient's unique mind-body connection (how the mind is affecting the body and how the body is affecting the mind).
- Identifying ways to support coping mechanisms that have been shown to enhance the immune system.
- Consideration of how to treat the rhythms, resonances, tones, and timbres of the body to promote harmonic balance.
- Assessing physical, emotional, cognitive, developmental, social, cultural, and spiritual needs of the person.
- Seeking ways to promote self-initiative, thereby enhancing one's sense of empowerment as a proactive force in his/her own healing.
(The Louis Armstrong Center for Music & Medicine, 2006)

Medical music psychotherapists consider specifically how former and current breathing challenges or asthma exacerbations have influenced the child's range of affect, willingness to invest in expression, or confinement of vocal production. A fear response might limit the child's sense of spontaneity and motivation. As therapists, we need to know the average level of everyday function for the child, which includes mood, activity level, and how the culture of his environment may affect treatment regimens. This is necessary in order to make an accurate determination of how significantly the disease process is or is not affecting the child's usual mode of functioning.

This author developed a music psychotherapy assessment that includes 13 Areas of Inquiry (Appendix C). This assessment defines critical areas of function revealed through musical behaviors and psychotherapeutic relationships developed both in and out of the music experience. The medical music psychotherapy assessment instruments included in the appendix indicate levels of baseline function and music preferences that may serve as a foundation for respiratory work that may ensue (Appendices D and E). Of note is the assessment of a child's choice of instrument and their preferred musical activity. The assessment also evaluates the voice. The Tour of the Room assessment approach (Loewy, 2000) includes demonstrating the musical instruments through a brief moment of sound and then encouraging the child during the assessment to express associations he has with those sounds. This should occur prior to choosing a particular instrument to play and/or prior to having any instrument played for any length of time by the therapist for the child. Another important element which ensues within the assessment is the child's revealing of a favorite song. The favorite song is usually an important road map into the child's psyche.

In respiratory illnesses, the voice is critical to assess, particularly because it is necessary to use the airways to speak and sing. As a child sings a favorite song, the therapist can assess the emotion and expression through analyses of phrasing and in particular the way in which the air is utilized to dynamically express potent lyrics. Medications such as steroids or inhalers may distort vocalization by affecting the vocal chords, resulting in a raspy, hoarse sound. The music therapist should be aware that such vocal discomfort may impair a child's expression.

Included within the Tour of the Room assessment (Loewy, 2000) is the display and therapist's sampling of instruments that have potential to target breathing projective qualities either directly or indirectly. The pan flute, recorder, melodica, horn reeds, and slide whistle require active breath participation in order to sound. The wind chimes, ocean drum, or synthesized wind or rain sounds might represent indirect air influence, in an unconscious process. In the selection of a wind instrument, a child might be revealing a direct or unconscious interest in exercising the airways, as the activation of producing a wind sound is contingent upon the use of lung exhalations. In playing a wind instrument, the breath can be used in a controllable manner. On the other hand, a wind instrument might emphasize the ability or inability to breathe, and horns or flutes might represent a potentially frustrating experience. Thinking about or listening to "blowing" could be representing an activity that is confining, especially if it is understood that the reason for hospitalization has to do with limited respiratory function. Instruments such as the accordion, shruti box, or harmonium require air and movement to be played and may be selected by children for this reason, as an indirect source of musical nourishment at a time when their own lungs are experiencing compromise.

INTRODUCTION TO MUSIC THERAPY METHODS

A review of early music therapy approaches in medicine reflects a plethora of studies seeking to validate the stimuli-response aspect of specific applications of music to influence specific behaviors. Behavioral models of music therapy utilize music as an activity for structuring responses and often include a "cue" that is determined to activate desired responses that are nonmusical.

As a medical orientation is scientific and seeks to define and predict the body's response to a treatment or agent, early studies in medical music therapy sought to quantify and standardize how a measurable music intervention might affect a particular aspect of function. Such studies typically involved the use of recorded music that could be replicated and easily quantified.

Behavioral approaches in medicine exist throughout the medical music therapy literature and in current times are at the forefront of some popular practices in nursing and in music therapy, such as Neurologic Music Therapy, where rhythmic gait training may be used to increase movement such as walking speed function, for instance. Another kind of behavioral music therapy approach involves the use of a Pacifier-Activated Lullaby (PAL) instrument whereby premature infants' non-nutritive sucking behaviors are sought to be reinforced through recorded music stimulation.

There are important behavioral aspects that can provide impetus and incentive for children with respiratory challenges. These include the selection and playing of instruments that utilize rhythm and breath. As cardiac function integrates with pulmonary activity, the utilization of rhythm may prompt regulation of breath. Additionally, using cued musical phrases to enhance breathing and exercise the lungs can strengthen and reinforce a child's control and willingness to breathe.

Little has been published on the use of music therapy for respiratory illness; therefore, most of the guidelines provided here are based on the research, symposia, and clinical work spanning the 20 years of inpatient and outpatient activity by music therapists who specialize in pulmonary function at The Louis Armstrong Center for Music & Medicine at Beth Israel Medical Center in New York City. Our asthma and COPD programs have moved patients through an integrated experience spanning from inpatient to outpatient adherence of music therapy practices. Continuity of care provides a unique forum that contributes to our hospital's approach in maximizing a "patient as doctor"–preventative strategy, post discharge. The clinical guidelines based on available music therapy publications relevant to respiratory practices in music therapy led to our institution of the AIP (Asthma Initiative Program) for children and teens and our AIR (Advances in Respiration) program for adults. More information on these programs is available at http://www.wnyc.org/articles/wnyc-news/2006/mar/11/music-is-medicine-for-kids-with-asthma and http://www.everydayhealth.com/opd/music-breathes-life-into-copd-patients-3061.aspx. The following guidelines provide an example of an asthma protocol which is meant to illustrate how a variety of methods may be implemented within asthma medical music psychotherapy sessions in order to provide an integrated experience.

Although the guidelines for describing particular approaches throughout this textbook are divided into parameters based on what a therapist provides and how a patient may respond, the Asthma Protocol as developed through research and clinical practice at The Louis Armstrong Center for Music & Medicine moves patients through an integrated experience. This means that a single music therapy experience ultimately includes receptive, improvisational, re-creative, and compositional elements within a single experience or activity. This should be taken into consideration by readers who are seeking to design a music therapy session for children and teens with respiratory challenges.

Most typically, the session will begin after the warm-up assessment music (Boxill, 1985; Loewy, 2000). With the body in a reclined position in the bed or settled on a reclined chair, or on a mat on the floor, we move into a tighten-and-release, cleansing breath experience followed by a music visualization activity wherein children are encouraged to imagine a favorite place. The children are moved into an imaginary experience as they breathe deeply into a relaxed or altered state and the therapist entrains the live music play to the child's breathing. Nolan (1998) writes about music having the capacity to both reflect and symbolize the entire spectrum of human experiences, "including those that are ineffable and those that contain seemingly illogical juxtapositions of opposites (for example, death and rebirth) within the same experiential time frame" (1998, p. 388). The music visualization experience may provide the means for random images associated with fear of death, or anxiety related to illness and wellness may be elicited. When brought back into awareness and as their attention is oriented back to the room, the children draw what was imaged. We then use re-created music, and learn a simple piece such as the Pachelbel "Canon" to show how the recorder is played, and we encourage the recorder to be used twice daily at home. This is followed by improvisational music-making wherein children are encouraged to create their own themes using the wind instruments (Harris & Rondina, 2009). The therapist frames their notes, meaning that a harmonic or bass contextual outline will provide a safe space wherein the patient feels free to play or fill in melodies or note sequences which are clinically improvised. After the therapist and child play spontaneously, the music can be recorded and the child may listen back to the music and the sounds of the recorder and process what the experience was like. The therapist may perhaps suggest creating an original title for the improvisation which provides further information metaphorically for how the creative process and music-making may have influenced breathing and lung function.

OVERVIEW OF MUSIC THERAPY METHODS AND PROCEDURES

Receptive Music Therapy

- Music-Guided Visualization as Integration: the use of music-guided visualization to relax and to enhance awareness and control of breath directly or through metaphoric imaging.
- Music-Assisted Relaxation and Sedation: the use of live music that moves from the original structure of a song, to triplet meter, to a wordless theme, to one note entrained to the patient's exhalation cycle to achieve sedation in the child.
- Musical Tighten-and-Release Informed by Breath Cleansing: the use of verbal directions with accompanying live music to encourage the child to tense and release particular group of muscles. This intervention is aimed at learning how to gain or restore control over a particular region that directly or indirectly is influenced by the breath.

- Remo Ocean Disc Breath Enhancement: This intervention, and its efficacy in inducing a relaxation response for infants, utilizes the Remo ocean disc to regulate the breathing of infants in the NICU with respiratory illnesses or distress.

Combined Use of Improvisational, Re-creative, and/or Compositional Music Therapy

- "No-Fail" Wind Play Interventions: the use of easy-to-play tunes with asthmatic children to deepen breathing.
- Interactive Music-Making with Children on Mechanical Ventilation: the creation of a musical dialogue with the child through their improvisatory breath response.
- Clinical Improvisation and Re-creative Music-Making for Active Lung Exercise: Singing and wind instrument play provides the means for a music-based way of working directly with the lungs.
- The AIP (Asthma Initiative Program) Protocol: This protocol, developed at The Louis Armstrong Center for Music & Medicine at Beth Israel Medical Center, uses wind playing to address actual control of the lungs and enhance adherence to maintaining wellness and prevention through monitoring of symptoms of the respiratory disease.

GUIDELINES FOR RECEPTIVE MUSIC THERAPY

When using receptive music therapy interventions for respiratory care, it may be easiest and most optimal to use a wind or string instrument in the therapy treatment. In playing a wind or string instrument, a theme is carried out with one breath or bow phrasing that is uncomplicated by harmony. The therapist can entrain the playing of a phrase to match and then deepen and relax (retard) the ease (length and flow) of the breath into a steady, predictable theme cycle. To motivate the breath in an effort to expand the lungs, we may consider moving the melody up in sequence. To relax and tone down the impact of the breath, we may consider moving the melody down in sequence. The music therapist in this circumstance is not thinking in "key" but rather in a melodic domain context. In the video listed here, one can observe the natural following of the music therapist whose simple single-lined flute playing is matching the breathing phrases of the patient (see www.pbs.org/wnet/musicinstinct/video/music-and-medicine/flute-therapy/74/). If a great deal of anxiety is present, the therapist might choose to play one note and perhaps implement a crescendo-diminuendo effect.

The music utilized in the session may be improvised or may come from the patient's request or perhaps the family's suggestion if the patient is on a ventilator or unable to speak. The assessment, including the therapist's use of transference and countertransference, will inform the music that will be implemented into the session. Transference within the music could occur when the patient asks or implies that the therapist should hold a musical idiom that the patient might desire to achieve himself. Countertransference would occur as the therapist contributes something musically that she feels might benefit the patient's desired effect. These terms are part of the clinical intuition within the developing musical interchange process.

Selection of music is a highly individualized choice but necessarily involves consideration of the patient's expressed desire, culture, and/or background. It may reference an image, feeling, or historical moment. In treating children with respiratory challenges, the metaphoric use of wind, water, and air in a nature context may serve as being quite therapeutic. Additionally, vocalizing entrained with the patient's meter of breath is an intimate way to provide a clinical context of support.

It is important that patients' vitals are within observable view. The music should stop if the heart rate (HR), respiratory rate (RR) or oxygen saturation level (O_2sats) move out of optimal range as specified in the nursing flow chart or determined through ongoing medical team consult. As music is related to an experience, the emotions elicited during listening might influence the patient's expression and the HR, RR, or O_2sats pulmonary function. Recorded music, particularly the preferred music of the child or his family, may be used by the child or family members during the hospital days, as may be their desire. Recorded music in the context of a music therapy session is not recommended, as the meter and thematic phrasing is fixed and therefore not part of the shifting vitals that medical music therapists can monitor and contextualize as part of the musical relationship. Recorded music does not lend opportunities to create an in-the-moment clinical musical relationship.

The timing of the music intervention is made in accordance with the child, depending on his individual needs and also with consideration to recommendations made by the medical team. For instance, if the child is having a treatment, such as a nebulizer treatment to ease breath, or a Chest Physical Therapy session to move sputum, it may be most optimal to have music therapy before, during, or after the treatment. This is part of the integrative teamwork that is an important aspect of session preparation for the care of any patient in the hospital who is under the jurisdiction of a nurse or doctor 24/7. With this kind of regular check-in, particularly in the planning of music therapy interventions, the recognition of music therapy as an "integrative" treatment in the hospital lifeworld becomes apparent. Furthermore, the timing of music interventions implies that music's effects are potent and can drive and influence the mind's intention directly and purposefully, changing the impact of the body's physiology (Loewy & Aldridge, 2009).

Referral (Appendices A and B), Assessment (Appendices D and E), and the treatment goals are planned based on the child's developmental, psychosocial, and medical presentations. Session plans are made after daily round attendance and in consultation with the team, and music therapy assessment with intervening sessions incorporating the above. Session experiences are based on the patient's projected length of stay, and closure should include activities for possible home use.

Music-Guided Visualization as Integration

Overview. Breathing is the primary means of connecting various aspects of functioning into what is perceived as a unified whole. Therefore, when a child is having an exacerbation, merely listening to a musical theme where breath is elongated can assist in one's incentive to breathe, orient, and integrate whatever part of the body one has explicated through gesture or words as having tension or constriction. Music is also helpful when children are encouraged to image their favorite place. Through the imagery, therapists can gain understanding of what inner resources (Bosco, 2002) the child may have access to. The child's imagery also provides information for how the traumatic effects of their obstructed breathing are affecting their anxiety level or ability to function.

In some cases, the child may not have easy access to the imagination of a "favorite place" or may not be able to close his eyes and sit still. In such cases, this kind of music experience may be contraindicated, particularly if it provokes anxiety.

What to observe. It is critical to observe the wake-and-sleep cycle of the patient receiving the music. Entrainment is a technique where the therapist observes and enters into the pulse and meter of the patient, in the moment. Effective entraining requires the therapist's moment-to-moment observation of the patient's breathing patterns so that the music is played in tempo with the pulmonary function expressed through breathing. It is implied that the music will be comforting or stimulating, but inquiry observably or verbally is a part of the feedback. As music is related to an experience, the emotions elicited during listening might influence the patient's expression and his HR, RR, or O_2sats. The observed and expressed emotion may have an impact on the course of therapy and should be not only observed, but also documented. The music therapist can be trained to use spirometry, which measures lung volume capacity and may be useful to implement as a best practice before and/or after a session to understand the impact of the music therapy.

Procedures. The therapist should first provide a physical "warm-up" for the patient's body awareness. Perhaps an ocean drum is used to create flow from the inhale to the exhale. The patient may be instructed to note any tightness or pain and to breathe to the particular place of tension and exhale for a long breath out. Another instrument for such a warm-up might be the piano or guitar. Movement from dissonance to consonance could induce a feeling of "settlement" or ease. Eventually, when each part of the body is relaxed, calm, and connected, the patient is asked to visualize a favorite place or a meaningful image.

Adaptations. Utilizing music visualization may be useful to implement in a group where members are encouraged to select an image, either a place or memory, or something they are hoping will occur. A safe special place or situation might serve as an anchor and ground their body as they focus on their breath. As the group of children pays attention to their breath, they can become attuned to their sensations within the body and the environment that surrounds them.

Music-Assisted Relaxation and Sedation

Overview. Deep breathing is a wonderful tool to use in order to treat respiratory function in a hands-on but indirect way. So often in respiratory illnesses, anxiety interferes with a child's ability to relax. Listening to music as a means of inducing a relaxation response (Bentson, 1973) or for the distinct purposes of sedation (Loewy, 2009) provides benefits integral to restoration and healing, both of which are critical to the relief of anxiety that may be associated with respiratory challenges.

A model of musical sedation was developed (Loewy, 2009) and may be useful in easing anxiety and feelings of being out of control that children might experience when they are having difficulty breathing. The author's model of sedation can take infants and children into a relaxed and/or sleep state. This can have a strong healthful impact particularly on patients who have had fear and sleepless nights due to anxiety that may be the result of the numerous interruptions that tend to be an invasive part of the pediatric hospital stay.

Preparation. When seeking to help children relax or sleep, the window shades can be pulled. A favorite stuffed animal or doll can be nestled in bed close to the child (infant through teen). Stuffed toys are prone to allergic experience, so nursing staff should be consulted. Knowledge of the sleep cycle or the scheduling of a test requiring sedation is useful to know.

What to observe. It is critical to observe the rapid eye movement (REM) sleep patterns of the patient as the breathing becomes settled. This generally ensues just prior to the child entering a deep sleep state. The length and level of sleep is useful to observe, and most hospitals have an instituted sleep/sedation scale.

Procedures. A method of music therapy sleep sedation has been researched and outlined step by step. In sleep sedation, music is played and implemented from full structure, to triplet meter, to a wordless theme. A "cadential effect" is instituted (Loewy, 2009), and then, finally, one note is entrained to the patient's exhalation cycle.

The music utilized in the sedation session starts in the format to which the child is accustomed and then slowly moves into a 3/4 or 6/8 holding meter before words and accompaniment (guitar) are removed; then the cadence is repeated over and over before the last note of the song and the syllable is entrained to the breath. The "ah" is repeated and entrained to the breath until the child enters a deep sleep state. The didgeridoo or shruti box with intervals or long breathed tones might provide optimal conditions for entrainment that enhance sleep state.

In relaxation and/or sleep sedation, the voice sung at the bedside may be the most effective musical intervention. It is particularly important to consider the general plan of respiratory care. The therapist can entrain through chant or on the "ah" vowel, which is the toned vowel affiliated with the heart and lung region (Rama et al., 1979). Other points of expressed pain or tension may also be accessed with correlated chakra body region vowels (Appendix F). Regulating the relaxation response (Bentson, 1975) in an effort to relax and elongate the impact of the breath, we may consider moving the melody down in sequence. The music therapist may use a glissando effect, elongating the words to lullabies of family- or patient-favored melodies. An example of this may be seen in the author's use of tonal vocal holding at www.nicumusictherapy.com.

At times, breathing difficulties can become so anxiety-provoking that the child may develop periods of apnea. Apnea is when breathing is suspended and the muscles involving respiration become compromised. Apnea can cause sleeplessness and may have a neurological or traumatic etiology. As apnea can cause a severe lack of oxygen in the blood, the Remo ocean disc may provide the perfect context for flow and can help to signal the mind and body to inhale and exhale continuously.

Musical Tighten-and-Release Informed by Breath Cleansing

Overview. Sound and music's capacity to enhance tension release is achievable through designed progressive muscle relaxation and visualization programs. This is not quite receptive, because the child is an active participant, but it is not improvisational, because the child is using the music in a directive and focused way. There are a host of clinical benefits in using "tighten-and-release"–oriented listening and movement activities in working with asthmatic children (Theodore & Peck, 2005). These include, but are not limited to, gaining a sense of control within the body, connecting aspects of function with desired feeling and form, and allowing for discharge of anger or repressed emotions.

What to observe. A release, by definition, is always surprising. It can be very small and subtle, or it can be not so small and not so subtle. One does not create a release. One lets go into a release. There are classic characteristics of releases that are consistent and reoccurring across cultures: Yawning, heat or cold in the body, quick repetitive rhythmic contractions in a part of the body, shaking, crying, laughing, and sweating all fall into a wide range of physical characteristics of a release (Sokolov, in Azoulay & Loewy, 2008). It is useful to observe the body and see if places where tension is stored or where pain occurs can become more relaxed using the tighten-and-release and then the cleansing breath focus.

Procedures. Prior to the playing of music, the child may be instructed on how to take a cleansing breath by inhaling slowly through the nose, "as if you are smelling your favorite food," and exhaling long and slowly through the mouth "as if you are a whistling wind." The exhale can be elongated to promote a relaxation response.

Through the isolation of a particular group of muscles whereby the child is directed to tense and then release, he learns how to gain or restore control over a particular region that directly or indirectly is influenced by the breath. Live music utilized to assist the child's relaxation response often starts with the use of dissonant or "tight"-sounding chords which beg to move into consonant chords or sonorities. This may be a suspended chord that is played as a tremolo and then crescendos into a consonant chord or a major 7th chord. The music implies "tension," which moves to "resolution" upon the cued breath and will of the child. The chord or sound of resolve may be followed by a long, pregnant pause, which allows for the experience of blood flow and ease, or rest. Using musical tension-and-release accentuates the verbal and physical cues used by the therapist.

Toning (Keyes, 1973) may be introduced to move the breath into areas where the child feels tension, areas that are "blocked." Tonal intervallic synthesis may provide vibratory support that may increase blood flow and ease of breath. Techniques that enhance release and flow through tonal intervallic synthesis are described in full in Loewy (2011). This technique involves the identification of obstructions or blockages and the careful use of vibratory vowel sounds with intervals of dissonance that move toward consonance, creating opportunities for flow and movement. Flow can occur within the bloodstream, in using toned extensions to bring oxygen into the veins, or flow might be used to connect one chakra to the next, as in head and nasal and throat passages to the chest or heart and lung synchrony. Tonal Intervallic Synthesis requires careful assessment, and medical consultation with the team is recommended.

Remo Ocean Disc Breath Enhancement (with or without Tonal Vocal Holding)

Overview. This intervention uses the Remo ocean disc to regulate the breathing of infants in the NICU with respiratory illnesses or distress. The Remo ocean disc is used to mimic the intrauterine sound environment. A study by this author indicates that the live womb sounds entrained with a baby's breath can induce and/or prolong a sleep state and can regulate HR (Loewy et al., 2013). Such breathing focus can often naturally expand into opportunities to vocalize, which can strengthen breath control and soothe the throat and vocal tract.

Preparation. In treating infants with RDS, an assessment is imperative for understanding the severity of the compromise so that interventions are informed and take into account the severity of the disease (see Chapter 3 for the Beth Israel Medical Center NICU Music Therapy Assessment). This assessment includes evaluation of the infant's vitals and his response to the Remo ocean disc and proprioceptive stimuli as well as breath and voice (Abrams et al., 2000; Loewy et al., 2013; Stewart, 2001). The therapist must also assess the infant's gestational age, medical status, and referral criteria prior to any toned voice sounds or ocean disc movement. This is achieved as the therapist attends multidisciplinary rounds and then, as a first step, simply observes the infant for 2–4 minutes prior to initiating any engagement in sound or vocalization.

In addition, the musicality of the caregivers and the timbre, range, and qualities of the parents' voices are important parameters to assess. Investigating the music preferences of the family, including Songs of Kin (Loewy et al., 2005), and the infant's potential exposure to music during pregnancy will indicate the infant's environment in the moment and will show parents that their sound environment and preferences will be a critical aspect of the care, including the music interventions that they will provide in tandem with the therapist.

A NICU baby with RDS who requires specialized NICU care must have medical consent, and infection control may be an issue. Hand-washing and the pinning of the therapist's hair so that it is up and away from the infant are a must.

What to observe. Careful attention to the premature infant or baby's vitals means that the entrained ocean disc womb sounds and the vocalizations should ideally stop after 3–5 minutes before starting again. In the silence, the therapist views the baby's vital signs to see the effect of the music and also observes the effects of the silence. Vitals are important to observe, and regulation is key.

Procedures. Music therapist Kristen Stewart (2009b) has considered the extensive variables that come together to inform treatment of the premature infant and young baby and which may be particularly effective when treating infants with RDS. She presents a sequential order of interventions from simplest to most musically complex. This approach of one intervention at a time is a standard rule in infant care that helps to avoid overstimulation.

To conduct breathing music therapy interventions that are inclusive of breath with the entrained ocean disc movement and voice use, Stewart arranges the breathing and voice interventions in order of complexity. Please see her chapter (Stewart, 2009b) for a complete discussion of these interventions and their role within the NICU treatment guidelines. The PATTERNS (Stewart, 2009a) approach includes respiration, vocalization, and children's folk songs, which would come in at the six months to one year marker.

The list of recommended progressive auditory input provided below begins with a simple sounding of air with the ocean disc that emphasizes the breath. This is followed by vocalise—a series of wordless vowel phrases through which infant-directed singing can organically develop between the infant and caregiver (Shoemark, 2006). Toning, or the singing of elongated vowels, is a "sonic massage that stimulates energy flow and releases tensions by targeting various parts of the body" (Bosco, in Stewart, 2008, p. 244). This can easily lead into tonal-vocal holding. Tonal-vocal holding is a technique (Loewy, 2004, 1995) inclusive of purposeful breathing and toning. The therapist purposefully uses the voice to match the tone and timbre of the infant's cry or coo. This matching is then developed into a two-tone holding pattern that provides "a long, steady blanket of vocal holding tones" (1995, p. 53) while remaining flexible to the infant. Integrating descending glissandi into the tonal pattern has been observed to facilitate release and stabilize infant respirations, while the use of ascending glissandi may help to create a gentle transition from sleep to quiet-alert states. The implementation of ascending or descending tonal patters may provide an enhancement for the breathing and respiratory function of babies.

The Song of Kin imbues the cultural heritage or traditions of the family. It signifies the most critical aspect of individualized, family-centered care. It may take the infant through transitions, sleep, beginnings, endings, and/or time of anxiety where comfort is warranted. Eventually, children's traditional folk songs can provide a mechanism for repetition of melody whereby the gradual development of word sequence and prosody may be reinforced. The repartee between parents and infants, which eventually develops through the participation of infant stimulation provided in the "Mommy/Daddy and me" type of group work, may serve as the foundation where families develop community through early socialization. This is well fostered through the singing of traditional children's music. These types of groups may include siblings of the infants who serve as role models within the music and whose singing voices will serve as exemplars throughout the baby's growing years.

Figure 1. Baseline Auditory Input from Environment (Stewart, in Azoulay & Loewy, 2009b)[1]

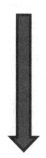

Audible Breath
Sounding
Vocalise
Infant-Directed Singing (Shoemark, 2006)
Toning (Keyes, 1973)
Tonal-Vocal Holding (Loewy, 1995)
Lullaby/Song of Kin (Loewy et al., 2005)
Traditional Children's Music

Isolettes, ventilators, pumps are all part of the auditory experience of the hospitalized infant or baby. A voiced "ah" tone may provide comfort, particularly during times of transition, which can be experienced as traumatic shifts in the lifeworld of a fragile baby.

Strengthening the parents' role in the provision of breathing support is a critical goal. As the compromised infant with RDS may experience breathlessness and periods of grunting, options inclusive of bonding, wherein parents' offerings of auditory breath sounds are entrained to the infant's meter of breath, can provide a supportive means of auditory stabilization, one that the vulnerable infant had been accustomed to in the womb. Live breath sounds can be encouraged by a parent, who should be instructed to hold the baby over the heart (Salk, 1973, Schwartz, 2000) while they exaggerate the breath sound made with a vocalized "sh-sh-sh" that is entrained to baby's breathing patterns. This is reminiscent of the "whoosh" of fluid through the placenta and can be used with an organized rhythmic pulse to enhance self-soothing behaviors (Loewy, 2013) and assist self-regulating and organized, fluid breathing (Abromeit, Shoemark, & Loewy, 2008).

GUIDELINES FOR COMBINED USE OF IMPROVISATIONAL,
RE-CREATIVE, AND/OR COMPOSITIONAL METHODS

When using combined improvisational, re-creative, and/or compositional music therapy interventions for respiratory care, it first and foremost must be clinically indicated that wind play is therapeutic. This may be most easily evaluated by the music therapist upon attending rounds and/or consulting with the attending physician, in particular the pulmonologist. In addition, the nurse will have significant updates on the patient's lung function, as will the medical chart. It often does serve optimal benefit to implement the use of a wind instrument into the therapy treatment plan.

Optimal guidelines for function are obtained through the referral and assessment procedures mentioned previously. In evaluating how to enhance lung function activity, the therapist can consider a host of structured and/or more free-flowing experiences that may or may not involve direct wind play.

Playing a wind instrument in and of itself will not necessarily serve as useful to a therapeutic relationship or physiological benefit if the child is not blowing correctly or if he is not invested. For young children, explaining this possible benefit to the lungs prior to the playful activity may have quite the opposite effect, inducing anxiety or turning him completely away from an opportune moment for "fun." In this way, the assessment is key; the music therapist needs to understand the child's interests, attractions, and sacred objects of everyday life, and then develop the activity to include areas of interest, which then might motivate a willingness to breathe and enable a process whereby the inhaling occurs more deeply and exhaling more fully.

The most critical and yet perhaps most understated guideline for implementing any music therapy "activity" is to make sure the experience presented will meet and greet the culture, interest, age, gender, and identified anxiety- and/or fear-related issues for the particular child being seen. This may be easily implemented through metaphoric play and therapeutic sensitivity and child-relating prowess.

Metaphoric play implies that the psychological issue and medical need will encompass a theme (issue and musical) that can be pursued by the option of "playing" a musical instrument. While the activity is presented and the child is invited in an appealing way, the child is enticed to "play" and in doing so has little or no awareness that such "play" is helpful to the breath or lungs. At a later time, such as in the closure-reflection period, perhaps, or later in the day, the therapist can revisit the memory of the experience and further explain how breath was addressed and well managed by the child through musical play. At that time, the "transfer" of the active music experience can be re-created by the child alone, or with the child and a sibling, or with the child and parent. The important concept in the revisit of the activity or in the explanation of "transfer" is that the child and/or significant other (sibling, parent, caregiver) can conceptualize how this may occur in other contexts at home or in school.

"No-Fail" Wind Play Interventions

Overview. The following interventions have proven useful in my clinical experiences with children who have asthma. Easy-to-play tunes where harmonizing can be enhanced as breathing deepens with elongated phrases provide asthmatic children with a way to productively use music successfully and playfully.

Procedures. Melodies such as the Pachelbel "Canon," "Hot Cross Buns," and "Merrily, We Roll Along," with five (or fewer) note steps that can be re-created with inclusion of other instrumental voicings, allow for opportunities for the child to lead and follow. This offers a sense of control of the breath. This experience is enhanced by the institution of accompanying sounds such as percussion and bass, which, blended with the wind structure, offer promising and sustained audible beauty for children of all ages.

In re-creating or improvising harmony voices or encouraging the child to do so, entraining with the played or blown phrases can suggest a slower tempo where exploration of feeling and physiologic response can occur through the observation of breath ease or tension. In this way, the play can be adapted, in the moment. The "No-Fail" wind play suggestions are:

1) Jazz-style "Take 4": Freely set melodic passages inspire improvisational melodies. The musical exploration stems from a tune that is familiar to the child. A musical style is easily formulated, particularly when it is based on the child's preference (rock, classical, country, light rock, show, etc.). This can be beneficial, as it fosters active play where the wind playing and assortment of notes within a I, V, I, harmonically supported riff can stimulate the child to fill in any combination or sequence of sounds within the four bars. Solos build self-esteem that can encourage ease of breath and provide the means for tension-and-release. Additionally, when the therapist is part of the play, the tempo of the "fours" can be slowed down to induce a relaxation response or sped up to enhance a more exertive lung exercise, encouraging diaphragmatic control, playfully.

2) Stop and Start or Lead and Follow: This intervention provides musical sounds in a group format, where the wind player leads four notes and the group has to answer in sung matched pitches. This can develop into a sung answer with words and then develop into an improvised song or reformat itself into a song that is well known and familiar.

3) Rap and Beat Boxing: This may work well, particularly for teens. Its clinical promise in working with patients who have asthma is that the focus is on the release of emotions, and this happens through the context of rhythm and movement. Teens can spontaneously rhyme and rap, using words and sounds to contextualize what is weighing heavy on their mind, body, and spirit and professing it in a raw and rugged, instinctual yet rhythmically organized format. Rap and beat boxing's releasing effects may clear the head and provide for better breathing because these experiences foster a sense of righteousness and control. This need is a most desired effect for teens.

4) Bird Song Improvisations: Winds often sound similar to birdcalls. Birds represent freedom, flight, and flow through their graceful flight through the breezy blue sky. A child's wind instrument may be representative of the character and expression of a bird that is flying high and flying freely for many miles to a desired place, set by the child. The therapist supports the musical voyage of melody with predictable and/or spontaneous unpredictable harmonies that are guided and informed by the tempo, rhythm, melodic patterns, and flow (or lack thereof) of the bird.

5) Story Song: Other effective interventions are presented for children through "Story Song" (Loewy & Stewart, 2003). Story Song is both re-creative and improvisational. Through the development of a plot distinctively and purposefully related to the interest of a child, the wind instrument can serve as an object or person or animal that needs to go somewhere or do something. Story Songs can be structured or freely created; the deftness of their use depends on the artistry of the therapist and the familiarity of the technique (Bosco, in Loewy & Frisch-Hara, 2002). The essence of the Story Song exists in its unique structure: a recitative, theme, countertheme or conflict, variations, resolution/recapitulation. Examples of Story Songs that might be useful for children with asthma could come from structured, already familiar (and loved) stories, such as "The Little Engine That Could." Perhaps the wind is assigned as the engine, and the conflict is that it breaks down. The child may select an instrument for the "break." The conflict may be improvised as whatever the child plays it out to be. Perhaps the train got stuck in mud (a big tom drum) or perhaps it slid off the track (out-of-control slide whistle play). The mechanism at work here is that the child creates the conflict and then has the opportunity to "muck around" with it in improvisational music play with the therapist.

The variations come into the Story Song play when the child is ready for them. The therapist works with the conflicts through the music. The conflict may be posed in a minor key. The variations come from re-creating solutions that the child introduces. Any and all options can be constructed. There is no wrong or right in the play, but there are significant themes musically, medically, and psychologically that may be signals of important information.

Sometimes the themes relate to issues in the child's lifeworld that the team had no idea about, but that had a direct effect on the symptoms of asthma.

I remember six-year-old Peter having an exacerbation, and the train broke down in his music again and again. It kept loading toys up to take to the neighborhood boys and girls, but as slow and evenly as he blew the recorder, the train could never make it up the hill. One time, his resolution was that the conductor needed more sleep, so we played and sang him a slow lullaby on "ah" (using our breath and the piano). By session 3, there was a baby girl doll on the tracks; it belonged to "Jessica," who was apparently this boy's next-door neighbor. Even though I thought it was strange that Jessica was an obstacle for the train (played as a spring drum), I also thought it was nice that this young boy was concerned about her. Yet, the variations of how to "save" her from the train never were quite complete.

When I later mentioned "Jessica" to his mother in the family lounge, she informed me that Peter was becoming very jealous about his peer neighbor and best friend Daniel's new baby sister. She mentioned a "monster" portrait of her that Peter had made in art. Apparently, Daniel was spending all his time with his family and new baby sister. This information was important to know, as it affected Peter's lifeworld, and there may have been repercussions on how his recent loneliness was impacting his breathing and anxiety-related symptoms. "Jessica" was clearly "in the way" of Peter's favorite playmate and threatened his fluidity. Knowing this informed the options I could suggest in the "variations"—the re-creative process that would ensue as options for Peter and wind-based characters in Story Song.

Story Songs with animals who can move swiftly though conflicts, perhaps through wind play, or people who make things or do things through selective rhythm or melodic phrasing can work to blend the fantasy-reality relationship between the imagined plot and the realized play. It is a mind-body relationship set into the child's construction of theme, conflict, variation, and resolution.

For older children and teens, Story Songs may be set to spirituals or the use of elements of nature, such as wind, air, light, water, sun, and moon. These may evoke improvisational play leading toward more mindful control of "flow," and, more distinctly, the identification of an obstacle that obstructs the mind and can certainly have a constricted impact upon the body, and in particular breathing. Live improvisation can be useful, again, through metaphoric play whereby the teen selects an image that has transformational qualities, such as a rose. The story may begin with the rose closed and quiet with the wind passing through it. Perhaps the pentatonic holds the beauty that is closed (perhaps a metaphor for the teen who feels shut down through the asthma or within the bumps of teenage-hood); maybe the wind is having less control but can still be representative of the potential for life energy through the teen's selection of the chimes. In playing the chimes, the teen may achieve some "sense" of feeling in control of the wind (though chime play).

There are often asthma exacerbations in teens. By offering an image such as a rose, or a root moving to tree, or a cocoon moving to butterfly, or a wave rolling into tide, the teen may choose and identify what the actual "block" or constriction is, and work through it improvisationally, with the therapist listening, musically mirroring, or holding/containing. The music used may be free-flowing or in the moment, or perhaps sophisticated thematic music might be brought in on a guitar, piano, viola, or wind. In the latter case, that theme can be rescored by the therapist and set up for the thematic conflict-resolution experience. Programmatic themes such as Elgar, Holst, Vivaldi, or Romantic Bach can work nicely for this.

The music utilized in the session may be improvised or may come from the patient's request or perhaps the family's suggestion, if they are invited to participate by the teen. For teenagers or even younger children, I invite the child to choose whom he would like to include in the session. Many times it can serve as useful and therapeutic to have the session with the child alone. This is because when parents fill in the blanks of therapeutic inquiries, the source of conflict is often lost. In music, and particularly within re-creative and improvisational music, the issues appear more pronounced because they are not defended or camouflaged with words, or colloquialisms. Instead, they are like aural Play-Doh™. Teen patients often can gain insight into the presented conflict and then can be coached on how to "shift" their constricting habits or tendencies in the moment by planning, imaging, creating alone, or co-creating with a friend or significant other.

Interactive Music-Making with Children on Mechanical Ventilation

Overview. Infants and children who require mechanical ventilation are unable to breathe on their own. Mechanical equipment delivers air to the lungs by creating positive pressure that will build intrathoracic pressure that expands the chest wall. The patients are treated in the NICU, Pediatric Intensive Care Unit (PICU), Surgical Intensive Care Unit(SICU), or respiratory Step-Down. While it may appear that these patients are unconscious or unable to respond to music, many are intricately connected to their sound environment, and improvisational music can mean the difference between feeling like an inanimate object or feeling like a human being. While tempting to place such patients under the Receptive Music Therapy category, the music improvisatory process becomes essential to their existence. Their breath response is improvisatory and may influence the activation of the equipment that is keeping them alive. Altering these patients' sound-making perception can provide a new context, and a host of musical dialogues may ensue. Hunter (2009) and his team write about implementing familiar melodies and songs in working with patients who are ventilated. Music therapists Wu and Ismail (2009) describe an approach where attention to a combination of the sounds of equipment and recognition of countertransference feelings might serve as the best orientation for informing improvisational music with patients who are minimally conscious. A child's awareness may be enhanced when developing music improvisations that are interactive with their machines.

Music therapist Brian Schreck (2012) created a soundscape with a patient nearing end of life, incorporating medical equipment sounds into a musical composition, which was helpful after the child died. The parents were able to grieve and reminisce, as the soundscape helped them to remember their child alive. In this way, the music served not only as a provision for awareness as he lived, but also as a remembrance for the family once this patient had died.

What to observe. Heart rate, respiratory rate, oxygen saturation, and ventilator and other equipment are critically important to these patients' survival and as such must be carefully observed from moment to moment. Nurses and doctors should be approached prior to and after each visit. The color of the child's skin may indicate effective or ineffective transfer of oxygen to the respiratory system, and the brow furrow may be indicative of stress or expressive reactions.

The music therapist must use descriptive language in the child's chart to record reactions and responses, particularly respiratory gurgles, arrests, and attempts to use the voice. In this work, particular with patients in very critical care, there is a risk of death, and the therapist must be prepared for any incident related to cardiac arrest or even death. The music must stop when a medical team member asks for it to be discontinued. This should happen without attitude or in-the-moment questions. The therapist stops the music and steps away from the patient in a moment's notice.

Procedures. Bradt (2009) wrote about the use of entrainment to alter breathing rate. Through the use of live music, the music's tempo is initially matched to the child's breathing rate and then continuously adapted to remain slightly below or above the patient's respiratory rate, resulting in effective manipulation of breathing patterns. When breathing is assisted by a machine, this may be easier to predict. However, the therapist must be familiar with the pitches, key, range, timbre, and rhythm of the machine.

Playing music or songs identified by significant friends and family might provide for a re-creative or receptive experience, depending on the advantage of either, which is evaluated by the therapist in the moment. The actual improvisational music set to the meter and key of the machine can provide the means for a symphony of sounds that can nurture the patient on temporary ventilation or at end-of-life support.

The voice might be preferable to other instruments, as it provides human contact. Hand-to-hand touch might also be warranted at this time. Inclusion of family members might provide for a supportive care environment where otherwise the family would feel hopeless and present as shut down and/or frustrated.

The implementation of musical idioms such as the blues, jazz, spiritual, pop, and country is generally improvised to enhance expression and enable synchronization of the music with the ventilator or other equipment. The source of inspiration for playing a particular musical idiom might stem from first playing a popular tune, brought in at the spur of the moment, after the warm-up has ensued. Eventually, depending on the mood and desire of the child (as advised, perhaps by family members) and the time of year (holiday), the weather (rain, sun, snow), and the child's report and experience of their breathing difficulties (or not), the therapist may move into a plethora of varying activities.

The music is characterized by moment-to-moment adaptations based on equipment and the sounds of the machines. When machine noise becomes loud and atonal, harmonic instruments may be implemented to create a holding consonant musical environment of support.

Whether using music improvisation, receptive music experiences, or compositional techniques, the procedure for how to conduct the session varies and is dependent upon the level of illness progression of the child. Interventions should be kept within a minimal time frame to prevent overstimulation and to ensure that the patient is able to have enough resting time.

Clinical Improvisation and Re-creative Music-Making for Active Lung Exercise

Overview. Singing and wind instrument play provide the means for a music-based way of working directly with the lungs. Encouraging children to participate in singing or wind playing can also be a health-inducing, meaningful way to suggest to children that their lungs are active, functional, and capable of making beautiful sounds. This is necessarily the opposite of what other health care practitioners may be relaying to children, because the frequent monitoring of lung function is suggestive to children of the fact that there is something wrong. Typically, instruments used to measure breathing produce a number, rather than a sound. In fact, the modern "spacers" have a toned note that is activated when a child inhales a medicine too quickly! This is actually a negative tone reinforcement and may not be the best instructional element for first-time users, particularly if they are not reading the directions. Children may conversely believe that as they inhale their medicine, they are seeking to activate the tone, rather than avoid it.

Preparation. Existing developmental or emotional issues defined by staff at rounds or by the parent/s, or revealed at assessment by the child directly, can be addressed through resourcing and accessing how the child's breathing is affected, as revealed through their playing (using the 13 Areas of Inquiry, Appendix C). The therapist can assess how freely or constricted the child's playing sounds. This is an intricately important part of the ongoing evaluation and is distinctly related to how the mind is affecting the body and vice versa.

Procedures. Different wind instruments provide a unique experience which will challenge the lungs as well as the coordination and technical aspects of play at a variety of levels. The slide whistle provides a no-fail experience of freedom. Notes are made freely by moving an effortless slide, requiring very little fine motor coordination and no adjustment of embouchure. The melodica requires the timing of breath with purposeful sequencing of the depressed key with the index and other fingers, which requires coordination of expiration of the lungs. Playing the melodica requires a good amount of air. The pan flute requires little exhalation volume, but one must form a specific embouchure for a note to be formed. The recorder requires coordination of air release and fine motor coordination of the fingers to cover the holes. The soprano recorder is the easiest recorder option for young children, as the holes are small and closely aligned, which prompts simplicity with pitch discovery and exploration. The alto recorder has larger holes and farther-spaced sound holes, yet the pitch can be less shrill; many children, particularly teens, may prefer the alto recorder as its sound timbre is deeper than that of the soprano recorder, even as it requires more concentrated agility and dexterity.

The AIP (Asthma Initiative Program) Protocol

Overview. The Asthma Initiative Program was developed at The Louis Armstrong Center for Music & Medicine at Beth Israel Medical Center. It was developed through research supported by the Recording Academy (the Grammy Foundation). It began as an inpatient method for children and teens hospitalized with severe asthma in the mid-1990s and eventually grew to be included in groups of children with asthma in the NYC public schools (Renner, 2006). Referrals to this program, both verbally and written, are currently documented and reviewed by staff in the Louis Armstrong Center for Music & Medicine (music therapist or intern) within 24 hours.

Preparation. Winds should be sterilized and labeled with masking tape and marker, indicating the child's name that is stored in a recorder case for reuse. The Beth Israel sterilizing procedure was approved by the hospital's Infectious Disease Committee and is available for readers (Appendix G).

Procedures. The AIP protocol includes the following:

1) Re-creative or Improvisational Wind Play: Each child in the AIP protocol receives a Yamaha recorder and learns the notes to the Pachelbel Canon. Group members are accompanied by the therapist on guitar or piano, playing one note with one breath and building up to an entire phrase in a single breath. More active children may use the slide whistle or harmonica to play random notes along with a therapist accompanied blues. Another kind of active play technique involves asking the children to imagine an animal and use the melodica to help it (walk, hop, run, skip, swim, or dance). The breath expresses the metaphor. The therapist frames and synchronizes the child's music on a matching melodica providing interesting harmonic accompaniments. For a child who is less active, or whose mood is quieter, blowing extended 'long tones' to achieve a lengthened exhale ,which activates the physiological relaxation response, may be warranted. Familiar or desired melodies can be introduced, and music of the child's culture with a variety of genres may be therapeutically significant affirming the diversity of peers and substantiating the inner-life culture of the group.

2) Breathing Entrainment: A central concept to the use of clinical wind improvisation that is paramount to the Armstrong approach is music entrainment. In therapeutic wind play, music

entrainment is the basis for a breathing relationship as the patient's tones are matched emotionally and physically though rhythmic and melodic/harmonic qualities of live music tones. These melodies may shift through synchrony and mutual transformation of phrasing and tone alignment as musical phrasing is co-created and sustained through the breath. The following description of music therapy's impact on breathing defines our core philosophy of wind playing and its effect on the mind and body.

Tension, fatigue, and fear tend to cause physical constriction and emotional contraction in the body and mind. Music, within its capacity to create flow and in its ability to enhance a feeling of space through the extension of open phrasing, can ease the fear and constraints of breathing. Wind playing provides a viable means whereby the breath can be consciously connected to intention. Entrainment, involving associated music played in tempo with the patient's blowing, can extend and increase the volume of breath and capacity to breathe, enhancing homeostasis (Loewy et al., 2009; The Louis Armstrong Center for Music & Medicine, 2009, para. 12).

Sputum may be triggered, and if coughing persists, rest periods should be encouraged. Children should be encouraged to play with their breath in a controlled but free way. Children who become overinvested or hyperactively involved may blow too loudly, and the instruments will buzz or create a high screeching noise. This should not be encouraged.

Music therapy experiences using the wind instruments should be conducted in a way that fosters creativity in children and a desire to play with increased interest. Increased wind play not only will address the actual control of the lungs, but also may enhance adherence toward maintaining wellness and prevention through monitoring of symptoms of the respiratory disease. Avoiding such self-monitoring runs the risk of sudden onset of respiratory exacerbation. Asthma is a chronic disease and a perfect example where adherence is not well maintained. This is why it is often called an "emergency room" illness.

It is helpful for children to keep journals of their experiences in playing winds at home. In this way, preventative care is encouraged, and the therapist will be able to see in outpatient treatment follow-up a written record of how the playing may be affecting the child's experience of breathing.

Each of these interventions requires the activity of verbal processing once the music has ended. The music psychotherapy approach warrants a check-in about what the child felt like when blowing the wind and the related difficulties of air or fluidity may address the emotional experience related to the content of the piece of music created, such as how the bird got lost or why was there no wind that day. The music experience with younger children in particular is symbolic; the animals or nature sounds or human roles played within the music may be seen as a metaphoric expression of the child's issues and thus may be intricately related to the physiological experience of being short on air or fully winded, or anywhere in between.

SUPPORT OF CAREGIVERS

As working with children who have respiratory challenges can bring about emotions of fear and anxiety in parents or caregivers, the assessment of whether to include caregivers in the music therapy sessions is one of critical importance. For infants, babies, and toddlers, inclusion of the parents is a must. In fact, parents can be educated and shown hands-on ways of using their bodies as integral instruments—such as the breath sounds a parent makes on "ah" as they are instructed to hold their infant over the heart (on the left side) with skin-to-skin contact as is recommended in kangaroo care. The "ah" sounds correlate with the heart-lung region (Appendix F) and can eventually replace the ocean disc as parents become comfortable using their sounds. They may be guided to assess and learn how to entrain with their infant's breath cycle.

This enhances bonding.

In the initial assessment of the child or teen, half of the session occurs with the caregiver, and the second half is with the therapist alone. In this way, the therapist can best determine whether or not the inclusion of the caregiver adds support or might evoke a feeling of "performance" stress in the child. Some children feel more comfortable to take musical risks or to stretch their imaginative musical playtime in their own space privately, without a parent present. In a medical music psychotherapy model, confidentiality is important. The story songs, clinical breath musical improvisations, or compositions made are considered as directly and intricately related to feelings, thoughts, and life circumstances of the child, or serve as indirect symbolic and metaphoric expressions of such. Either directly expressed or indirectly referenced, the experience may be intimate and should be treated as such, with confidentiality.

Outpatient Clinic or Within School Treatment Sessions

This chapter has not yet made mention of outpatient clinic or in-school treatment. The focus thus far has been on the acute care of children. In a global effort to build stronger prevention and adherence in the challenge of maintaining healthy respiratory function, medical centers and community practices are interested in developing better management of asthma through stronger methodological prevention practices with parents and children.

Since 2007, the AIP (Asthma Initiative Program) at The Louis Armstrong Center for Music & Medicine has expanded from hospitalized inpatient care to outpatient clinic, and is currently in the NYC public schools. This effort involved the development of personal and professional caregivers for children with asthma, guidance from the Department of Health (DOH), and support from a host of doctors at Beth Israel Medical Center, Long Island College Hospital, and principals in the NYC Board of Education within the schools. Our efficacy-based work is based on the protocol established through five-year research study conducted at Beth Israel.

The outcome of the study (in press) was the initiation and continuation of asthma music therapy groups in the public schools that are part of the weekly routine for children with asthma, a program which is part of their healthy routine for "well" school life. The groups have been offered in Harlem, Brooklyn, the Bronx, and Manhattan and have targeted children with mild, moderate, and severe asthma.

Collaborations with school nurses, principals, social workers, music teachers, and counselors, who all are considered professional caregivers, have been an intricate layer of the external and internal support for music therapy in the schools. The fact that the AIP is part of the students' school day implies that preventative care is integral to the avoidance of emergency room visits and hospitalizations. Working through music play and incentive building directly with the children themselves, using the above guidelines and providing take-home recorders from Yamaha and beautiful blank journals and symptom logs for journal writing with the children, reflects direct care and increases management at the patient level. This is a complement to their pharmacological regimen and may serve as reinforcement for medical treatments.

Activities that encourage an asthmatic child's capacity to organize and manage the asthma plan of care are instrumental to good health and asthma exacerbation prevention. This is due to the fact that asthma has an unpredictable nature. A plan that incorporates a daily diary is particularly useful and recommended by the National Heart, Lung, and Blood Institute (2007). Stress, in particular, can affect breathing and may lead to the child's perception and/or evidential lack of control in the breath process (Manusco, Peterson, & Charlson, 2000).

RESEARCH EVIDENCE

There is not yet promising evidence that supports effective inclusion of alternative or complementary therapies for children with asthma (Kealoha, 2009). Although pockets of studies including breathing, yoga, use of fish oil, and muscle relaxation therapy have shown inclinations of effectiveness, full reviews have not validated fully the use of any one alternative or complementary modality. There has been speculation that there is greater effectiveness than is reported or undertaken by researchers and that lack of reported evidence is due to the fact that parents do not share their CAM use with providers and providers fail to inquire about its use (Sidora-Arcoleo, 2008).

Music therapists are not excluded from the dearth of research activity investigating the impact of wind play in children with asthma. There is a single Cochrane Review in the literature that provides evidence that breathing exercises positively influence quality of life (Holloway & Ram, 2003). Playing a musical wind instrument provides a venue that is inherently child-friendly, and unlike ingested herbs or pharmacological agents, playing a wind instrument or singing involves breathing and has little, if any, associated risk. Addressing phrases in a musically explorative context provides an expressive means of honoring a child's intentionality that integrates their physiology with their thinking—and this elicits great potential for motivation. There is evidence that asthma exacerbation can be heightened by emotional upset. Lehrer, Isenberg, and Hochron (1993), through extensive literature review, showed that patients with asthma tend to experience high levels of negative emotion. According to their research, exacerbations can be associated with periods of high emotional influence. Panic disorders are not uncommon in children with asthma. Panic, other negative emotions, and a passive coping orientation may affect asthma by inducing hyperventilation and/or increased general autonomic liability, a specific pattern of autonomic arousal that may cause bronchoconstriction and/or detrimental effects on health care behaviors. Generalized panic is a risk factor for increased asthma (Lehrer, 1998).

In considering the aspect of panic and the role that anxiety may play in children who are asthmatic, it is necessary for the music therapist to understand normal ego function and its role in daily health maintenance. As children's ego formations are ever-developing, music-making as the result of breathing provides a no-fail means for them to learn how to control breathing in a way that is playful and noninvasive.

If we review details of the few studies undertaken with children and teens that have asthma, we find that engagement, recruitment, and retention are usually reported to be an interfering issue. A recent study (Eley, 2013; Eley et al., 2010) examined the effects of didgeridoo playing (for male participants) and singing (for female participants) on asthma management in 33 Aboriginal Australian children (mostly junior high–age and teenagers). These interventions were offered in an educational forum, with group lessons provided weekly for six months. Many people of this culture, according to the authors, believe that this instrument should not be touched by females—perhaps because of its weapon origin. The therapeutic value of wind playing showed significant rises in spirometry outcomes: Forced expiratory volume (FEV1) rose from 2.27 to 2.70 ($p < .01$), forced vital capacity (FVC) increased from 79.3±7.4% to 101.3±.3% ($p < .01$), and peak expiratory flow (PEF) improved from 67.7±5.5% to 81.2±5.5% ($p < .05$). The singing was less effective, but the PEF was still affected positively (from 70.8±7.7% to 98.4±4.9%). These results need to be interpreted with caution, given the small sample size and the fact that only 72% of 33 enrolled participants completed the entire treatment protocol.

Adherence, awareness, and compliance through the music activity and education were meaningful. The authors acknowledge that the timing of the lessons and enjoyment of the activity increased compliance. They reported that the expense of having a didgeridoo or an MP3 player is not realistic, but they also surmise that the quality of the instrument and equipment may have been a contributing factor or impetus for the breathing improvements. This is important for music therapists to take into account. This study was important because the impact of this project seemed to serve the needs of the underserved children in a culturally sensitive and diverse way.

In a UK "Bronchial Boogie" study, where school-age asthmatic children played wind instruments in a band several times a week and served as their own controls, it was found that two in three children with asthma who learned to use a wind instrument showed better inhaler technique and used rescue inhalers less often (Nursing Standard, 2004).

Early evidence, though not music therapy per se, showed that blowing a wind instrument can strengthen the muscles involved in breathing, especially the diaphragm (Bouhuys, 1964; Marks, 1974). These studies had interesting findings. As a baseline, Bouhuys (1964) found that professional wind players had greater lung vital capacity than non–wind player matches (N = 459). Although this study did not investigate people with lung disease such as asthma, this research has provided evidence that normal developing lungs can be influenced by wind playing. A decade later, Marks (1974) with a small sample size of 12children, found that constant practice with a wind instrument reduced the incidence of asthma, thereby sustaining strong pulmonary function. This study focused on children holding out long tones on winds; this seemed to improve their vital capacity, timed vital capacity, and total lung capacity and decreased residual volume and residual capacity, indicating breathing improvement.

In 1994, Lucia included 18 adolescents with asthma in a wind playing vs. control study for a 30-day period and found improvement in the teen players' "emotional response to asthma symptoms" (p.) as indicated by their responses to the standardized Selective Symptomology of Asthma Diary.

In a larger study (N = 106), Lehrer and colleagues (1994) compared progressive muscle relaxation to prerecorded music to no intervention. This was not a music therapy study but might be considered by some to qualify as a receptive activity. The music group produced greater decreases in peaks of tension than the progressive muscle relaxation, and greater compliance with relaxation practices.

There are gaping holes in the literature of studies including live music, which may provide greater benefits than music listening (Bailey, 1983), particularly in asthma, where evidence shows that moving air in a supported but relaxed fashion may improve breath capacity, mood, and quality of life.

In a Polish study, 96 male patients (18–23 years of age) were examined in two groups, one using traditional breathing exercises and the other using music therapy to enhance breathing. The study evaluated how singing could foster the control of breathing function. The study does not specify what kind of music was used. The goal of the treatment was to test the effects of rhythmic exercises on asthma by way of lung ventilation and psychological testing. Spirometry showed a positive value to their therapeutic method, indicating an improvement in the lungs through decreased resistance of the airways. The music group was reported to have decreased bronchial resistances, mood stabilization, increased sense of self, and reduced anxiety levels (Janiszewski, Kronenberger, Drozd, & Merkuriusz, 1996).

Finally, a music therapist (Wade, 2002) compared the effects of vocal exercising/singing with music-assisted relaxation on peak expiratory flow rates of nine children with asthma. In this study, there was an increase or maintenance of lung functioning shown through peak-flow metering after singing. However, peak flow is not the most effort independent gauge of symptomology available for such measurements. Spirometry may provide a more concise measurement and accurate reading because it is less effort-dependent than a peak-flow meter. Wade admits that results for the music-assisted relaxation group were not always consistent. It is notable, however, that she combines and integrates receptive, re-creative, and improvisational components of the music therapeutic process. The use of live music provides the therapy with in-the-moment shifts whereby the therapist may support the child to elongate their breathing, which can relax or stimulate breathing in an encouraging way.

SUMMARY AND CONCLUSIONS

While primary concerns and guidelines for music therapy interventions provided for infants, children, and teens with asthma have been defined, this chapter has meant to emphasize the critical components of breathing as an integrative function. It is important to recognize that the breath connects thinking to feeling, and expression to the voiding or release of tension. Music therapy experiences may encourage resilience through control of the body physiologically and intuitively as music enhances endurance and can provide meaningful opportunities for release. Breath is intricately connected to lung function, which operates in tandem with and as a result of motivation or lack thereof. Breathing not only is influenced by aspects of emotion as evaluated by a sensitive clinician, but also warrants careful assessment and perception through the child's own eyes. Daily functions, relationships, and self-perception all affect the way we breathe—whether within our experience of inspiration or of exhalation. The music activities presented in these pages are meant to be adapted to fit the issues and perspectives of the individual child with a respiratory disease. In infants, the caregiver's ability to use breath leading to the induction of tonal vocal holding inspired by their willingness to entrain their breath with their infant's is critical to respiration, vocalization, and bonding.

A child's awareness of music and air sounds and his ability to synchronize the breath through the therapist's use of creative receptive listening experiences may provide a basis for reflective music visualizations. Imaging or visualization is a way to resource (Bosco, 2002) and access, through fear, where breath may be limited. "Resourcing" is a trauma term that reflects how easy or difficult it may be for someone to access healthy anchors that exist conceptually within one's understanding of the body. Building resources within the music may offer an option for how the mind can expand and visualize options for new and refreshed air. This may be accessed through controlled and easeful music. Reflective drawings may reveal through unconscious fears or wishes, desires, and dreams that can then be played live, with fluid breath, supported harmonically or rhythmically by the therapist. Drawings can be shared with art therapists, who may provide insight into the child's confined and free expression that could be indicative of the child's experience of her body.

Whether improvising on a familiar piece of music through blowing sustained note phrases on a recorder or making harmonies with soulful improvised blues on the harmonica or melodica, music therapists are privy to the provisions of a host of clinical techniques and applications. From the Remo ocean disc for breath elongation, to the use of wind chimes in Story Song creations, to the train whistle cuing suggestive of direction and control of other played instruments, as in a wind ensemble at a school session, music therapy is a safe, nonconfrontational way to assist infants, children, and teens with breathing. The effects are far-reaching, and its efficacy will continue to grow as we honor the consistent use of winds in our sessions for children of all diagnoses and ages, but particularly children with breathing challenges. Music may provide important air cleansing sounds that can enhance and encourage relaxation. Entrained breath, body work through explorative wind play, and release opportunities lead to less fear and new assurances. Music therapy can be a way not only to inspire and deepen breath, but also to decrease the need for hospitalization as musical wind play increases compliance, regulation, and management, which collectively contribute to better self-care and fewer of the crises that are so common to the pediatric population.

GLOSSARY

The following definitions are adapted from online medical dictionaries (medlineplus.com and medical dictionary/the freedictionary.com) unless otherwise noted.

Aerosolized drug therapy: the delivery of a drug to the body via the airways by delivering it in an aerosolized form (Khilnani & Amit Banga, 2008).

Bronchodilator therapy: A bronchodilator is a substance that dilates the bronchi and bronchioles, decreasing resistance in the respiratory airway and increasing airflow to the lungs.

Cerebral hypoxia: Cerebral hypoxia refers to a condition in which there is decreased oxygen supply to the brain even though there is adequate blood flow. Drowning, strangling, choking, suffocation, cardiac arrest, head trauma, carbon monoxide poisoning, and complications of general anesthesia can create conditions that can lead to cerebral hypoxia.
(www.resoundinghealth.com/casebook/show/508)

Chest physiotherapy (CPT): a technique used to mobilize or loose secretions in the lungs and respiratory tract. Chest physiotherapy consists of external mechanical maneuvers, such as chest percussion, postural drainage, vibration, to augment mobilization and clearance of airway secretions, diaphragmatic breathing with pursed-lips, coughing and controlled coughing.
(http://currentnursing.com/reviews/chest_physiotherapy.html)

Continuous ventilation therapy or positive airway pressure: noninvasive respiratory support systems in the treatment of acute pulmonary edema used with patients as positive end-expiratory pressure. This process helps to keep the alveoli open upon inhalation and exhalation, thus increasing oxygenation and reducing the work of breathing.

Emphysema: an obstructive lung disease. The destruction of lung tissue around smaller sacs, called alveoli, makes these air sacs unable to hold their functional shape upon exhalation. Emphysema is most often caused by tobacco smoking and long-term exposure to air pollution.

Granulomas: any small nodular delimited aggregation of mononuclear inflammatory cells

Mechanical ventilation: a method to mechanically assist or replace spontaneous breathing. This may involve a machine called a ventilator or the breathing may be assisted by a physician, respiratory therapist or other suitable person compressing a bag or set of bellows. There are two main divisions of mechanical ventilation: invasive and noninvasive.

Nasal continuous positive airway pressure (nCPAP): a treatment that delivers slightly pressurized air during the breathing cycle. It is delivered via the nostrils and can assist in maintaining open airways.

Oxygen therapy: a noninvasive respiratory support system in the treatment of acute pulmonary edema.

Postural drainage: an important way to treat bronchiolitis (swelling and too much mucus in the airways of the lungs). It requires one to get into a position that drains fluid out of the lungs.
(www.nlm.nih.gov/medlineplus/ency/patientinstructions/000051.htm)

Respiratory Syncytial Virus (RSV): RSV causes infection of the lungs and breathing passages and is a common major cause of respiratory illness in young children. Infections often occur in epidemics that last from late fall through early spring. Respiratory illness caused by RSV—such as bronchiolitis or pneumonia—usually lasts about a week, but some cases may last several weeks.
(kidshealth.com)

Suctioning: Suctioning clears mucus from medical tubes with might threaten to block the airways. Suctioning of a tracheostomy tube is essential for proper breathing.
(www.hopkinsmedicine.org/tracheostomy/living/suctioning.html)

Surfactant therapy: Surfactant is a natural substance made of proteins and lipids (fats) normally produced in the lungs, which can be manufactured synthetically. It reduces the surface tension of the lungs which maximizes the surface area available for gas exchange. Without adequate surfactant, infants may be prone to breathing distress which results in limited oxygen and exhaustion. Manufactured surfactant is mixed with sterile water and is administered through a breathing tube (endotracheal tube) that is inserted in the baby's lungs.

Tube care: Tube care is the method of sterilizing tracheostomy tube so that it is kept clean and does not risk causing infection. (myclevelandclinic.org)

REFERENCES

Abromeit, D., Shoemark, H., & Loewy, J. (2008). Newborn intensive care unit (NICU). In D. Albromeit & C. Colwell (Eds.), *Medical music therapy for pediatrics in hospital settings* (pp. 15–70). Silver Spring, MD: American Music Therapy Association.

American Thoracic Society. (1995). Recommendations for a standard technique. *American Journal of Respiratory Critical Care Medicine, 152,* 2185–2198.

Bailey, L. (1983). The effects of live music versus tape-recorded music on hospitalized cancer patients. *Music Therapy, 3*(1), 17–28.

Baroody, F. M., & Naclerio, R. M. (2011). Nasal-ocular reflexes and their role in the management of allergic rhinoconjunctivitis with intranasal steroids. *World Allergy Organization Journal, 4*(1), S1–S5.

Benson, H. (1975). *The relaxation response.* New York: William Morrow & Company, Inc.

Bosco, F. (2002). Glossary. In J. V. Loewy & A. H. Frisch (Eds.), *Caring for the caregiver: The use of music and music therapy in grief and trauma (p. 174).* Silver Spring, MD: American Music Therapy Association.

Bouhuys, A. (1964). Lung volumes and breathing patterns in wind-instrument players. *Journal of Applied Physiology, 19, 967–975.*

Boxill, E. H. (1985). Music for the developmentally disabled. Rockville, MD: Aspen Systems.

Bradt, J. (2009). Music entrainment for breathing regulation. In R. Azoulay & J. V. Loewy (Eds.), *Music, the breath and health: Advances in integrative music therapy* (pp. 11–20). New York, NY: Satchnote Press.

Bush, A., & Saglani, S. (2010). Management of severe asthma in children. *The Lancet, 376*(9743), 814–825.

Drent, M., & Costabel, U. (2005). Sarcoidosis. (Monograph). *European Respiratory Society Monograph, 32,* 23–47. Retrieved from http://erm.ersjournals.com/content/ermsar/1.toc

Eley, R. (2013). The potential effects of the didgeridoo as an indigenous intervention for Australian Aborigines: A post analysis. *Music and Medicine.*(Advanced online publication) *DOI: 10.1177/1943862113476306.*

Eley, R., & Gorman, D. (2010). Didgeridoo playing and singing to support asthma management in aboriginal Australians. *The Journal of Rural Health, 26*(1), 100–104.

Global Initiative for Asthma. (2010). *Global strategy for asthma management and prevention.* Retrieved from http://www.ginasthma.org/pdf/GINA_Report_2010.pdf

Gregory, D. (2002). Four decades of music therapy behavioral research designs: A content analysis of Journal of Music Therapy articles. *Journal of Music Therapy, 39(1), 56–71.*

Griggs-Drane, E. (2009). The use of musical wind instruments with patients who have pulmonary diseases: Clinical recommendations for music therapists. In R. Azoulay & J. V. Loewy (Eds.), *Music, the breath and health: Advances in integrative music therapy* (pp. 103–116). New York, NY: Satchnote Press.

Harris, B., & Ronina, E. (2009). The asthma initiative program: Medical music psychotherapy with children and teens with asthma. In R. Azoulay & J. V. Loewy (Eds.), *Music, the breath and health: Advances in integrative music therapy* (pp. 135–150). New York, NY: Satchnote Press.

Holloway, E., & Ram, F. (2004). Breathing exercises for asthma. *Cochrane Database of Systematic Reviews, 2004*(1), CD001277.

Hulzebos, E. H. J. (2006). Preoperative intensive inspiratory muscle training to prevent postoperative pulmonary complications in high-risk patients undergoing CABG surgery: A randomized clinical trial. *The Journal of the American Medical Association, 296*(15), 1851–1857.

Huntley, A., White, A., & Ernst, E. (2002). Relaxation therapies for asthma: A systematic review. *Thorax, 57*(2), 127–131.

Janiszewski, M., Kronenberger, B., Drózd, P., & Merkuriusz, L. (1996). Muzykoterapii jako Formy ćwiczeń oddechowych wastmie oskrzelowej [Studies on the use of music therapy as a form of breathing exercise in bronchial asthma]. *Polski Merkuriusz Lekarski, 1*(1), 32–33.

Kealoha, M. (2009). What's new in alternative therapies for asthmatic children? *Journal of Community Health Nursing, 26*(4), 198–205.

Keyes, L. (1973). *Toning: The creative power of the voice.* Marina del Ray, CA: DeVorss.

Khilnani, C., & Amit Banga, A. (2008). Aerosol therapy. *The Indian Journal of Chest Diseases & Allied Sciences, 50*(3), 209–220.

Lehrer, P. M. (1998). Emotionally triggered asthma: A review of research literature and some hypotheses for self-regulation therapies. *Applied Psychophysiology and Biofeedback, 23*(1), 13–41.

Lehrer, P. M., Hochron, S., Mayne, T., Isenberg, S., Carlson, V., Lasoski, A. M., & Rausch, L. (1994). Relaxation and music therapies for asthma among patients prestabilized on asthma medication. *Journal of Behavioral Medicine, 17*, 1–24.

Lehrer P. M., Isenberg S., & Hochron, S. M. (1993). Asthma and emotions: A review. *Journal of Asthma, 30*, 5–21.

Loewy, J. V. (1995). The musical stages of speech: A developmental model of pre-verbal sound   making. *Music Therapy, 13*(1), 47–73.

Loewy, J. V. (1999). Music psychotherapy assessment in pediatric pain. In C. Dileo (Ed.), *Applications of music in medicine, vol. II: Theoretical and clinical perspectives.* Silver Spring, MD: AMTA.

Loewy, J. (2000). Music psychotherapy assessment. *Music Therapy Perspectives, 18*(1), 47–58.

Loewy, J. (2004). Integrating music, language, and the voice in music therapy. *Voices: A World Forum for Music Therapy, 4*(1). Retrieved from http://www.voices.no/mainissues/mi40004000140.html

Loewy, J. V. (2005). Sleep/sedation in children undergoing EEG testing: A comparison of chloral hydrate and music therapy. *Journal of PeriAnesthesia Nursing, 20*(5), 323–332.

Loewy, J. (2009). Musical sedation: Mechanisms of breathing entrainment. In R. Azoulay & J. V. Loewy (Eds.), *Music, the breath & health: Advances in integrative music therapy* (pp. 223–232). New York, NY: Satchnote Press.

Loewy, J. (2011). Tonal intervallic synthesis as integration in medical music therapy. In F. Baker & S. Uhlig (Eds.), *Voicework in music therapy: Research and practice* (pp. 253–266). Philadelphia, PA: Jessica Kingsley.

Loewy, J., & Aldridge, D. (2009). Prelude to music and medicine. *Music and Medicine, 1*(1), 5–8.

Loewy, J., Azoulay, R., Harris, B., & Rondina, E. (2009). Clinical improvisation with winds: Enhancing breath in music therapy. In R. Azoulay & J. V. Loewy (Eds.), *Music, the breath & health: Advances in integrative music therapy* (pp. 87–102). New York, NY: Satchnote Press.

Loewy, J., & Stewart, K. (2004). Music therapy to help traumatized children and caregivers. In N. Boyd Webb (Ed.), *Mass trauma and violence: Helping families and children cope* (pp. 191–215). New York, NY: Guilford Publications, Inc.

Loewy, J., Stewart, K., Dassler, A., Telsey, A., & Homel, P. (2013). The effects of music therapy on vital signs, feeding and sleep on premature infants. *Pediatrics.* Advance online publication. DOI: 10.1542/peds.2012-1367.

Lu, Y., Liu, M., Shi, S., Jiang, H., Yang, L., Liu, X.,...& Pan, F. (2010). Effects of stress in early life on immune functions in rats with asthma and the effects of music therapy. *The Journal of Asthma, 47*(5), 526–531.

Lucia, R. (1994). Effects of playing a musical wind instrument in asthmatic teenagers. *The Journal of Asthma, 31*(5), 375–385.

Manusco, C. A., Peterson, M. G., & Charlson, M. E. (2000). Effects of depressive symptoms on health-related quality of life in asthma patients. *Journal of General Internal Medicine, 15*(5), 301–310.

Marks, M. B. (1974). The Bela Schick Memorial Lecture. Musical wind instruments in rehabilitation of asthmatic children. *Annals of Allergy, 33*(6), 313–319.

Mondanaro, J. (2013). Music-based release strategies for acute and chronic pain: An individualized approach. In J. Mondanaro & G. Sara (Eds.), *Music and medicine: Integrative models in the treatment of pain* (pp. 133–148). New York, NY: Satchnote Press.

National Heart, Lung, and Blood Institute. (2007). *Guidelines for the diagnosis and management of asthma (EPR-3)*. Retrieved from http://www.nhlbi.nih.gov/guidelines/asthma/

Nolan, P. (1998). Countertransference in clinical songwriting. In K. Bruscia (Ed.), *The dynamics of music psychotherapy* (pp. 387–406). Gilsum, NH: Barcelona Publishers.

Nowobilski, R., Furgał, M., Czyz, P., De Barbaro, B., Polczyk, R., Bochenek, G., & Szczeklik, A. (2007). Psychopathology and personality factors modify perception of dyspnea in asthmatics. *Journal of Asthma, 44*(3), 203–207.

Osborne, M., Vollmer, W., & Buist, S. (1992). Diagnostic accuracy of asthma within a health maintenance organization. *Journal of Clinical Epidemiology, 45*(4), 403–411.

Philbin, M. K. (2000). The influence of auditory experience on the behavior of preterm   newborns. *Journal of Perinatology, 20*(8, part 2), S69–S76.

Pratt, R. R., & Spintge, R. (1995). *Music Medicine, vol. II*. St. Louis, MO: MMB.

Rama, S., Ballentine, R., & Hymes, A. (1979). *The science of the breath*. Honesdale, PA: Himalayan International Institute.

Raskin, J., & Azoulay, R. (2009). Music therapy and integrative pulmonary care. In R. Azoulay & J. V. Loewy (Eds.), *Music, the breath & health: Advances in integrative music therapy* (pp. 69–86). New York, NY: Satchnote Press.

Ratjen, F. & Döring, G. (2003). Cystic fibrosis. *Lancet, 361*, 681—689.

Renner, P. (2006, March 11). Music is medicine for kids with asthma. Retrieved from http://www.wnyc.org/articles/wnyc-news/2006/mar/11/music-is-medicine-for-kids-with-asthma/

Rietveld, S., van Beest, I., & Everaerd, W. (1999). Stress-induced breathlessness in asthma. *Psychological Medicine, 29*,1359–1366.

Rubin-Bosco, J. (2002). Resolution vs. re-enactment: A story song approach to working with trauma. In J. V. Loewy & A. F. Hara (Eds.), *Caring for the caregiver: The use of music and music therapy in grief and trauma* (pp. 118–127). Silver Spring, MD: ATMA.

Ryan-Wenger, N. A. (1996). Children, coping, and the stress of illness: A synthesis of the research. *Journal of the Society of Pediatric Nurses, 1*(3), 126–138.

Salk, L. (1973). The role of the heart in the relations between mother and infants. *Scientific American, 228*(5), 24–29.

Schreck, B. (2012, January). Innovative approaches to pain treatment panel. Paper presented at the Integrative Models in Pain Management Conference, Beth Israel Medical Center, New York, NY. Available at http://www.youtube.com/watch?v=lVE9wDvr52I

Schreck, B. (2013). A symphony of life: Harvesting emotions by preserving legacy and honoring pain. In J. Mondanaro & G. Sara (Eds.), *Music and medicine: Integrative models in the treatment of pain*(pp. 237–252). New York, NY: Satchnote Press.

Schwartz, F. (2000). Music and sound effect on perinatal brain development and the premature baby. In J. Loewy (Ed.), *Music therapy in the neonatal intensive care unit* (pp. 101–110). New York, NY: Satchnote Press.

Shoemark, H. (2006). Infant-directed singing as a vehicle for regulation rehearsal in the medically fragile full-term infant. *Australian Journal of Music Therapy, 17,* 54–63.

Sidora-Arcoleo, K., Yoos, L., Kitzman, H., McMullen, A., & Anson, E. (2008). Don't ask, don't tell: Parental disclosure of complementary and alternative medicine use among children with asthma. *Journal of Pediatric Healthcare, 22*(4), 221–229.

Sokolov, L. (2009). Opening to Breath: An examination of breath and process in embodied voicework. In R. Azoulay & J. V. Loewy (Eds.), *Music, the breath & health: Advances in integrative music therapy* (pp. 43–54). New York, NY: Satchnote Press.

Spintge, R., & Droh, R. (1987). Perioperatives Befinden mit anxiolytischer Musik und Rohypnol (Flunitrazepam) bei 1910 Spinalanaesthesien [Perioperative state with anxiolytic music and Rohypnol (Flunitrazepam) in 1919 cases with spinal anesthesia]. In R. Spintge & R. Droh (Eds.), *Musik in der Medizin—Music in Medicine* (pp. 175–178). Berlin: Springer.

Spintge, R., & Droh, R. (1993). *Music Medicine.* St. Louis, MO: MMB.

Stewart, K. (2009a). PATTERNS—A model for evaluating trauma in NICU music therapy: Part 2—Treatment parameters. *Music and Medicine, 1,* 123–128.

Stewart, K. (2009b). Dimensions of the voice: The use of voice and breath with infants and caregivers in the NICU. In R. Azoulay & J. V. Loewy (Eds.), *Music, the breath & health: Advances in integrative music therapy* (pp. 235–250). New York, NY: Satchnote Press.

The Louis Armstrong Center for Music & Medicine. (2008). *Music and health clinic.* Retrieved June 1, 2012, from http://www.wehealny.org/ services/bi_musictherapy/mhclinic.htm

Theodore, L., & Peck, H. (2005). Relaxation and guided imagery as an intervention for children with asthma: A replication. *Psychology in Schools, 42*(7), 707–720.

Thomas, M., McKinley, R. K., Mellor, S., Watkin, G., Holloway, E., Scullion, J.,...Pavord, I. (2009). Breathing exercises for asthma: A randomized controlled trial. *Thorax, 64*(1), 55–61.

Wade, L. M. (2002). A comparison of the effects of vocal exercises/singing versus music-assisted relaxation on peak expiratory flow rates of children with asthma. *Music Therapy Perspectives, 20,* 31–37.

Wu, L., & Ismail, A. (2009). The breath of innocents: Music therapy with children in states of severely impaired consciousness. In R. Azoulay & J. V. Loewy (Eds.), *Music, the breath & health: Advances in integrative music therapy* (pp. 199–212). New York, NY: Satchnote Press.

ENDNOTES

[1]Auditory Input from Environment reprinted by permission of Satchnote Press. Taken from K. Stewart (2009). Dimensions of the voice: The use of voice and breath with infants and caregivers in the NICU. In R. Azoulay & J. V. Loewy (Eds.), *Music, the breath & health: Advances in integrative music therapy* (p. 242). New York: Satchnote Press.

[2]13 Areas of Inquiry reprinted by permission of the American Music Therapy Association. Taken from J. Loewy (2000). Music Psychotherapy Assessment. *Music Therapy Perspectives, 18*(1), 47–58.

APPENDIX A – SIDE 1

REFERRAL FOR GENERAL PEDIATRICS

Beth Israel Medical Center
The Louis & Lucille Armstrong Department of Music Therapy

Name of PT: _____

Diagnosis: _____

Floor & Room: _____Primary Language of Patient:_____ English: ____ yes ____ no

Caretaker(s) Name: _____

Primary Language of Caretaker: _____ English: ___ yes ____ no

Relationship to patient:

_____ mother_____ father_____sibling_____foster parent_____ relative_____ friend

Reason (s) of Patient's Referral for Music Therapy (definitions on reverse side). Check areas that apply:

Anxiety/Fear:

    ( ) Separation Anxiety   ( ) Pre- or postoperative Anxiety ( ) General Anxiety

Pain/Stress:

    ( ) Breathing Difficulties   ( ) In need of tension release

Expressive Difficulties:

    ( ) Depression or Nonverbal ( ) Acting out or hyperactive

Coping:

    ( ) In Facing the Illness   ( ) Self Esteem   ( ) Communication/Socialization

In Loss of Consciousness:

    ( ) Increase awareness   ( ) Increase stimulation or use of imagery

Other
Specify:

_____

Comments:

_____

_____

Person Referring: _____ Ext: _____ Date:

_____

Please fax all referrals to 212-420-2726
Or call: John Mondanaro MA, LCAT, MT-BC, Clinical Director, 212-420-2722
Joanne Loewy DA, LCAT, MT-BC, Director, 212-420-3484

APPENDIX A: SIDE 2

MUSIC THERAPY REFERRAL CRITERIA

I. Anxiety/Fear: Music Therapy soothes, familiarizes, and/or activates:
  A. *Separation anxiety:* Chanting, musical holding and collaborative musical experiences create a feeling of safety in the hospital.
  B. *Pre-/Postoperative anxiety:* Making music relaxes and eases the mind and body of tension and fear stimulated by hospital procedures.
  C. *General anxiety:* Musical experiences help patients make sense of their fears through a nonthreatening medium.

II. Pain/Stress: Clinical improvisation provides an alternative, nonverbal means of release for a patient in discomfort:
  A. *Breathing & Vocalizing:* Life rhythms and tonal intervallic synthesis help a patient synchronize and deepen the breathing process. Toning stimulates the connection between the body breath and feeling states.
  B. *Tension release:* Opening channels of musical creativity stimulates the body's need to release tension

III. Expressivity
  A. *Depression, nonverbal/inactivity:* Structured and unstructured therapies help elicit feelings that may be "muted" or "blocked."
  B. *Acting out or hyperactivity:* The implicit structure of music therapy techniques such as African drumming song sensation, and instrumental composition offer patients a safe means of channeling their excessive amounts of energy

IV. Ego strength/Coping
  A. *Facing the illness:* The metaphoric use of music in song selection and composition offer patients a safe way into understanding and adjusting to their illness.
  B. *Self-esteem:* Performing and tape creating strengthen a patient's feeling of worth during this fragile time.
  C. *Communication/Socialization:* Community singing, drumming circles, and collaborative free improvisations foster communications between patients and within families

V. Loss of Consciousness/Coma/ICU
  A. *Awareness:* The use of familiar melodies help patients become oriented or tuned in to a state grounded, familiarized awareness.
  B. *Stimulation:* The use of music and guided imagery stimulates the healing process

APPENDIX B

MUSIC THERAPY NICU REFERRAL FORM

Beth Israel Medical Center

*Referrals may be made by the nurse practitioner, case manager, nurses, and residents but must have the consent of the attending physician and the parent/caretaker.

Age>32 weeks unless approved on a case-by-case basis by the Attending MD.

Questions/Concerns? Call Dr. Joanne Loewy 212-420-3484 or beeper 5208/917-537-1388

*Name*_____*Attending Contacted*_____

(name and beeper)

*Age-Gestational*_____ *Chronological*_____

*Family informed by:*_____

(name and beeper)

*Diagnosis*_____

Reason for Referral (Check all of the following that apply and write in any comments)

_____*Bonding (caretakers and infants that are in need of collaborative experiences).*

_____*Psychosocial Issues (ACS Hold, Intrauterine exposure to drugs/alcohol, Trauma, Stress, Violence, Family illness, Separation/divorce). Define:*

_____ *Respiratory difficulties*   _____ *Crying/Irritability*

_____ *Feeding/Sucking/Weight Gain*   _____ *Sedation/Sleep/Pain*
                                               _____ *Difficulty sleeping*
                                               _____ *Needs music for sedation during procedure*
                                               (date/time_____)

_____ *Self-regulation*

*Person referring*_____

(extension, beeper)

*Date*_____.

Please place this form in referral folder at nursing station

APPENDIX C

13 AREAS OF INQUIRY
(Loewy, 2000)[2]

13 Areas of Inquiry	*Qualitative Means*
Awareness of self and others & the moment	Musical, verbal, nonverbal reflection
Thematic Expression	Instrument, song choice, quality & style of singing and playing
Listening	Receptivity, ability to hear others
Performing	Speaking, playing, singing alone
Collaboration/Relationship	Willingness to interact in activity together, quality of expressing with others
Concentration	Ability to focus in and out of the music
Range of Affect	Qualities of expression, variety of moods & themes, dynamic variances
Investment/Motivation	Willingness to build musical experience or conversation, sustaining involvement in the musical-verbal dialogue
Use of Structure	Reaction to space-boundaries, adherence/resistance to formatted theme, and improvisation
Integration	How forms (music, words, feelings, songs, thoughts) are put together
Self-Esteem	Evaluation of the created themes—response to self-recordings
Risk-Taking	Experimenting, trying something new, playing alone & together w/others
Independence	Ability to separate self/others—musically & verbally

APPENDIX D

MUSIC THERAPY ASSESSMENT FORM

Louis & Lucille Armstrong Department of Music Therapy

_____Individual _____Family _____Group

Referred by:_____

Reason for referral:

Instruments / Activity:

Voice:

Description of the music:

Significant Issues:

Follow-up plan:

Music Therapist:_____Ext. Beeper: _____

Date:_____ Time:_____

APPENDIX E

NICU MUSIC THERAPY ASSESSMENT FORM

Beth Israel Medical Center
The Louis & Lucille Armstrong Department of Music Therapy

Patient:_____Date of Birth:_____

Average Heart Rate:

      Sleeping: _____bpm   Awake: _____bpm   Stress: _____bpm

Respiratory:

      Does infant become tachypneic? [ ] YES   [ ] NO

Define stressors:

Crying/Comfort Sounds:

      Pitch: [ ] HIGH   [ ] LOW   [ ] AVERAGE

      Absence of Cry: [ ] YES   [ ] NO

      Colic: [ ] YES [ ] NO

      Irritable? [ ] YES   [ ] NO

Feeding Noise: _____

Psycho-Social Needs:

      ACS Hold: [ ] YES   [ ] NO

      Intrauterine exposure to drugs/alcohol? [ ] YES   [ ] NO

      If yes, what? _____

How can music therapy benefit the infant? _____

Who in this family can help the infant benefit? _____

Family's religious preference: _____

Feeding / Intake / Weight Gain / Voiding:

      [ ] Breast   [ ] Reflux

      [ ] Gavage   [ ] Bottle

Is the patient's suck response in need of assistance? [ ] YES   [ ] NO

Is Physical or Occupational Therapy involved? [ ] YES   [ ] NO

Can the infant self regulate? [ ] YES   [ ] NO

Feed Schedule: _____

Sleep: Irritable   [ ] YES   [ ] NO

Stimulation:

      Does the baby like proprioceptive stimulus? [ ] YES   [ ] NO

Pain: Please describe physiological indicators, location and perceived level (1-10):

_____

_____

Ongoing Procedures: (which may benefit from music therapy assistance)

_____

Development: Is the infant organized in:

      Sound [ ] YES   [ ] NO

      Touch [ ] YES   [ ] NO

      Movement [ ] YES   [ ] NO

Is the infant developing appropriate muscle tone?

      [ ] YES   [ ] NO

Sedation: Is the infant on a sedative?

      [ ] YES   [ ] NO

      Medication(s): _____

      Time(s): _____

Music therapist: _____ Extension or beeper _____

Date: _____Time:_____

APPENDIX F

CHAKRA VOWELS FOR BREATH ENTRAINMENT

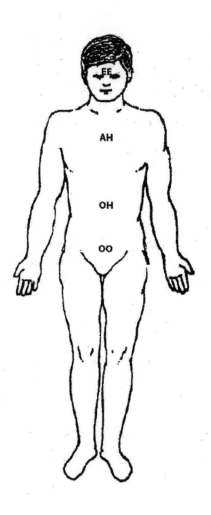

APPENDIX G

WIND CLEANING PROTOCOL

Infection Control

Louis and Lucille Armstrong Department of Music Therapy
5.5 Cleaning of Wind Instruments

The following procedure was developed for the cleaning of wind instruments at the Petrie Campus of Beth Israel Medical Center. This policy was the result of consultation and a meeting Wednesday, April 9, 2003, with Susan Marchione RN and David Crimmins RN, from Infection Control and Joanne Loewy DA, MT-BC and Jisun Kim (NYU) from the music therapy program with oversight from Brian Koll MD. The policy and procedure for cleaning wind instruments is as follows.

     Step 1: wash instruments in soap and water
     Step 2: wipe dry
     Step 3: soak instruments in bleach for approximately 20 minutes
     Step 4: rinse with soap and water, wipe dry
     Step 5: air-dry overnight

CLEANING LOG

The music therapy team will maintain a weekly written log of the use of winds, documenting specifically each use of the instruments, and when it was cleaned, with a checklist, date and signature ensuring that the above procedure for instrument use is maintained.

Wash in soap & water	Rinse with water & wipe dry	20 minute soak in 1:10 solution of bleach	Rinse thoroughly with water	Air dry	Date & initials

Chapter 12

Medically Fragile Children in Low Awareness States

Jennifer Townsend

INTRODUCTION

Children who have suffered an accident, have a chronic illness or congenital disorder, or have been abused or neglected are sometimes left in a condition that requires them to receive life-sustaining medications, treatments, or equipment. These children are considered to be medically fragile and require assistance with activities of daily living. This chapter will focus on medically fragile children in low awareness states.

An overview of diagnostic information and definitions as well as assessment and treatment options will be given. This chapter is aimed at providing the reader with the basic tenets of medical and psychosocial care, as well as guidelines for music therapy interventions for the child and his family as they learn to live with a person in a low awareness state.

DIAGNOSTIC INFORMATION

Determining Consciousness

In order to be conscious, one must first be aware. Consciousness has been defined as the quality or state of being aware, while awareness is having or showing realization, perception, or knowledge (Webster, 2003). At first glance, these definitions seem easy enough to understand. However, when attempting to determine consciousness in a person with a brain disorder, the shift between unconscious and conscious states can be difficult to discern. This is especially prevalent in patients whose neurological course is developing slowly. These persons must be able to access awareness at the time of assessment and exhibit some behavior to communicate that awareness to the assessor, a trying task for someone with severe neurologic deficit.

Because there is no suitable biological probe for consciousness, medical professionals rely on behavior as the primary means to determine consciousness in patients with brain dysfunction. However, Andrews (1996) details many factors that can inhibit behavioral assessment of persons in low awareness states. These factors include the physical ability of the patient to respond, the desire or will to respond, observer-patient rapport, the ability to observe accurately, the time available for observation and assessment, and the lack of available and reliable assessment tools. Even if all of these issues were optimized, there would still be ambiguities in deciding whether certain individuals are truly unconscious.

The American Academy of Neurology practice parameter (1995) points out that some clinical signs such as visual tracking and fixation can demonstrate conscious behavior but can also occur in people in prolonged vegetative states. So how are we to understand consciousness as it relates to patients? For instance, how is the conscious mental state related to the body? Can consciousness be explained in terms of brain activity? Several scientists have attempted to answer this question through *MRI*s and *PET* scans (Crick, 1994; Kock, 2004). Scientists observe brain activity and then try to match it with first-person reports of conscious experiences. The basic tenet is that consciousness becomes a mental state when large numbers of neurons all fire in synchrony with one another. Specifically, two areas of the brain must be intact for a person to obtain consciousness: the *cerebral cortex* and the *brain stem.*

Neuroscience research suggests important differences between children and adults in the area of cognitive control. The American Academy of Neurology (1988) defined persistent vegetative state (PVS) as a condition in which a person has progressed past the state of coma into a state of wakefulness without demonstrable awareness, and classified artificial nutrition and hydration as medical treatment. A survey by the Child Neurology Society (Ashwal et al., 1992) uncovered differences in opinion among neuroscience professionals regarding the treatment of adults versus children in a PVS. These differences stem from the belief that the extent of damage and period of recovery is less predictable in children (The Medical Task Force on Anencephaly, 1990). In addition, even if conscious, a child may have more difficulty than an adult in presenting such awareness due to development. Children show greater brain activation in the *prefrontal cortex* during attention and awareness activities, while adults show more brain activation in the brain stem area (The Multi-Society Task Force on Persistent Vegetative State, 1994). This difference in location of information processing may play a role in the child's ability to respond to commands and environment while in a low awareness state. Moreover, a child's brain may have more *neuroplasticity,* or ability to reorganize neural pathways based on new information, than the brain of an adult (Gopnik, Meltzoff, & Kuhl, 1999). This would allow a child better chances for some functional recovery than an adult. Further research into the differences between the child and adult brain in the area of consciousness is required if we are to successfully understand disorders of consciousness.

The problem of how to determine consciousness is arguably the most central issue to diagnosing and treating persons in low awareness states such as brain death, coma, persistent vegetative, minimally conscious state, and locked-in syndrome. Some studies have shown that synaptic connections occur in people who are unconscious, proving that synaptic connections alone are not enough to determine a state of awareness (Drubach, 2000). The next section of this chapter will give current explanations of low awareness state disorders in the midst of a continuous quest for defining consciousness.

Disorders of Consciousness

Brain Death. Brain death is the irreversible end of all brain activity due to total necrosis or death of the cerebral neurons. People who are brain dead are unable to carry out the necessary involuntary functions required to live such as breathing and maintaining a heartbeat. A brain dead individual has no clinical evidence of brain function upon physical examination. They do not respond to pain, and preservation of reflexes is absent (Sullivan, Seem, & Chabakewski, 1999).

Brain death is used as a legal indicator of death in the U.S. and many other countries (Waters, French, & Burt, 2004). It is important to distinguish between brain death and states that may mimic brain death. Some comatose patients may initially present similarly to patients who are brain dead. In a person who is brain dead, electrical brain activity can stop completely or drop to such low levels that the *electroencephalogram* (EEG) equipment cannot detect it. However, little to no EEG reading is not enough to diagnose brain death alone. There have been cases where patients showed no brain wave readings on an EEG but when disconnected from life support continued living independent of the machines. This is especially common in pediatric patients. The American Electroencephalographic Society (1986) defines this state of brain death without somatic or physical death as electrocerebral inactivity.

Coma. Coma is a state of prolonged unconsciousness in which a person cannot be awakened; fails to respond normally to painful stimuli, light, and sound; lacks a normal sleep-wake cycle; and does not initiate voluntary actions (Weyhenmyeye, James, Eve, & Gallman, 2007). The comatose patient may appear to be awake. However, they are unable to consciously feel, speak, eat, or move (Bordini, Luiz, Fernandes, Arruda, & Teive, 2010). In contrast to brain death, a comatose patient has electrical impulses in response to auditory and tactile stimulus that are recognizable on scans.

There are many events that may cause a person to go into a coma: traumatic brain injury, brain tumor, drug or alcohol intoxication, or even underlying illness such as diabetes or an infection. The most common cause of coma results from drug poisoning followed by *anoxic brain injury* (Leversedge & Hirsch, 2010). Anoxic brain injury occurs when a person is without oxygen for an extended period of time.

Coma is a serious medical condition and requires medical help immediately in order to preserve life and brain function. Comas seldom last longer than several weeks. People who are unconscious for longer than several weeks can transition to a persistent vegetative state.

Persistent Vegetative State. A person in a vegetative state is in a state of partial arousal rather than true awareness. People with this diagnosis differ from those in a coma in that they have easily detectable sleep-wake cycles. A person in a vegetative state has survived a coma and is medically stable but has not gained awareness. This diagnosis differs from that of brain death in that the patient has brain functioning and is able to sustain breathing and heart rate without medical intervention. After four weeks in a vegetative state, the patient is classified as in a persistent vegetative state (PVS) (The Multi-Society Task Force on PVS, 1994). Although the medical field accepts this definition, there are issues of legal clarity with this diagnosis. It is important for music therapists to understand the legal ramifications when a patient is classified as PVS. Unlike brain death, PVS is not recognized by statute as death in any legal system. In the US and UK, courts have required petitions before termination of life support that demonstrate that any recovery of cognitive functions above a vegetative state is assessed as impossible by authoritative medical opinion for patients in a PVS (Jennette, 1999). Because of this legal gray area, two themes of advocacy work for persons experiencing PVS have been established. One is that a person in PVS should be allowed to die. These people believe that the person in a PVS will have no quality of life and, therefore, is essentially dead. Others argue that if there is at all a possibility for recovery, care should be continued. Because history has shown cases of recovery when such was thought impossible, legal entities have been unable to issue consistent rulings in cases involving people in PVS and requests to terminate life (Cranford, 1994).

Minimally Conscious State. It has been widely recognized that many patients display a clinical condition that does not fit the criteria for vegetative state and yet they are not fully conscious (American Congress of Rehabilitative Medicine, 1995; Andrews, 1996). These patients maintain partial preservation of conscious awareness and are diagnosed as being in a minimally conscious state (MCS). Although patients in an MCS have severely altered consciousness, they possess definitive behavioral evidence of self or environmental awareness (Giacino, Ashwall, Childs, Cranford, & Katz, 2002). These patients are able to demonstrate, although unreliably and inconsistently, some level of awareness to environmental stimulation. Like other low awareness states, MCS is caused by severe damage to multiple areas of the brain. Because of the major differences in prognoses, it is crucial that MCS be diagnosed correctly. Incorrectly diagnosing MCS as a vegetative state may lead to serious repercussions related to clinical management.

Studying people in minimally conscious states from a neuroimaging perspective may hold the key to determining consciousness. Preliminary studies have shown that overall cerebral metabolism in people in a minimally conscious state is less than in those with conscious awareness and is slightly higher but comparable to those people in a vegetative states. During conscious waking, activation in the *medial parietal cortex* and *posterior cingulate cortex* seem to differ between patients in MCS and those in a vegetative state (Giacino & Zasler, 1995). Of importance to music therapists is the finding that auditory stimulation induces more widespread activation in the primary and prefrontal associative areas of MCS patients than in vegetative state patients (Laureys, Owen, & Schiff, 2004).

Akinetic Mutism. Akinetic mutism, also known as coma vigil, is a term used to describe patients lacking the ability to move, speak, or respond to stimulation (Cartlidge, 2001). The patient with akinetic mutism is conscious but unable to respond to stimulation in any way. This disorder is a result of severe frontal lobe damage in which the pattern of inhibitory control is increased and speech and motion decreased.

Causes of this disorder include: olfactory groove meningioma or a condition where tumors grow along the nerve between the nose and the brain; encephalitis lethargica or inflammation of the brain along with paralysis of extrinsic eye muscles and extreme muscular weakness; and stroke to both anterior cerebral arteries. Neurotoxicity due to immunosuppressant drugs such as *Tacrolimus* and *Cyclosporine* can also cause akinetic mutism (Cartlidge, 2001).

Locked-in Syndrome. Locked-in syndrome is a condition in which a patient is aware and awake as evidenced by communicating through eye blinks, but cannot move or communicate verbally due to complete paralysis of nearly all voluntary muscles in the body except for the eyes. People who are paralyzed in the eyes as well are known to be in a total locked-in state (Bauer, Gerstenbrand, & Rumpl, 1979). Unlike people in a vegetative state, where portions of the upper brain are damaged, people in a locked-in state have damage to the lower portion of the brain and brain stem with no damage to the upper brain (Bauer et al, 1979).

Most people in a locked-in state are quadriplegic and unable to speak but are otherwise cognitively intact individuals. Communication with a person with locked-in syndrome can sometimes occur through eye blinking or eye movements. Some patients may have the ability to move certain facial muscles, most often some or all of the *extra ocular eye muscles*. Individuals with locked-in syndrome lack coordination between breathing and voice. This inhibits them from producing voluntary sounds, even though the vocal cords themselves are not paralyzed (Fager, Hux, Baukeleman, & Karantounis, 2006).

Figure 1 below graphically represents the different states of awareness.

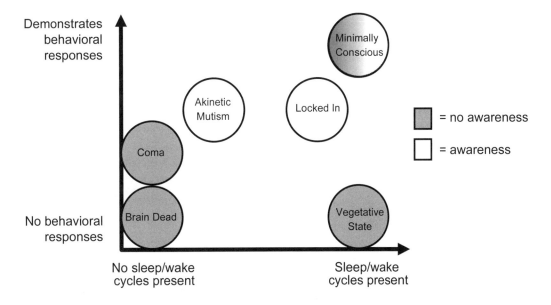

Figure 1. Levels of Awareness

NEEDS AND RESOURCES

Needs

Disorders of consciousness require special care from both a medical and psychosocial perspective. The most important goal for children in low awareness states is to attempt arousal. Because arousal is so important to the diagnosing process and assessment process and is the basis for many of the treatments offered to a child, it should be attempted at every session.

Motivation to participate can be low for children in a low awareness state. Agitation and restlessness can be common in children emerging from a low awareness state. Similarly, patients who maintain low awareness states such as those in a minimally conscious state may display agitation. Factors that contribute to agitation for these patients include having a limited attention span, lack of reasoning skills, and limited memory. These cognitive issues make it difficult for the child to stay focused on a particular task or topic. Additionally, it is challenging for them to figure out what to do if a problem arises. Add to this the inability to communicate wants and needs, and the chances of agitation multiply. Agitation can lead to decreased motivation for these individuals. Therefore, success-oriented interventions should be provided whenever possible.

Since children in low awareness states have limited to no mobility, muscle tone can play an important role in their care. Nursing and rehabilitation staff will often provide stretching treatments to help maintain muscle flexibility and fight off muscle atrophy. During these exercises, it is important that the child remain relaxed so that the stretching and passive movement can be achieved. Relaxation can play an important role in this area of care.

Because of low cognitive skills, it is difficult for the child in a low awareness state to connect with their environment, including people, places and favorite toys. Recognizing people, places, familiar sounds, or toys can help increase arousal, bring about awareness, and build hope for both the child and the family.

When working with patients in low awareness states, the needs extend beyond the patient. Family members of these patients are often faced with challenging decision-making about the care of their loved one. Additionally, family members may find it difficult to interact with the patient since he is no longer able to do things he used to do. Supportive services should be offered to family members during the hospital stay and after. Family members are experiencing great loss, sadness, and pressure in making decisions about the care of their loved one. The sights, sounds, and smells of the hospital can frighten siblings. Hospital equipment and the patients' diagnoses should be explained to siblings in a developmentally appropriate manner. Additionally, family members may require assistance in bonding to their loved one, as they may have a difficult time knowing how to respond to their child's current state. They may require assistance in finding ways to bond since many of the bonding activities that they formerly did (e.g., throwing a ball together, doing a puzzle, playing tag,) are no longer accessible to the child.

Music therapy can play an essential role in teaching families to communicate with their severely brain-damaged child. Furthermore, the physiological effects of music can provide unique insight into the abilities of the patient. Music is a powerful stimulus that can activate the central nervous system, promote memory, and enhance connections both inter- and intrapersonally.

Resources

Families play a very important role in identifying the optimal conditions and best responses for assessment of patients in low awareness states. While there are some relatives who interpret reflex responses as being meaningful, there is no doubt that members of the family are often more sensitive to early changes than experienced clinical staff. The rapport between family members and pediatric patients should remain an essential part of the treatment plan. Parents and siblings have relationships with these patients that may elicit stronger responses than efforts by the medical team. Family bonding, especially during traumatic times, can build strength and support for each family member. This is true for the patient in a low awareness state as well. Ylvisaker (1985) suggests that patients show increased responsiveness to stimulation provided by family members.

Research on auditory processing has indicated that patients, regardless of whether suffering from coma, vegetative state, minimally conscious state, akinetic mutism, or locked-in syndrome, maintain the ability to process auditory information (Boly et al., 2005). The ability to continue processing auditory information as well as knowledge of how auditory information is processed in the brain provides a strong theoretical foundation for the use of music therapy in treatment of these patients. Perhaps the most important fact is that auditory information passes through the *thalamus* as it is processed. The thalamus is responsible for relaying motor and sensory information as well as regulating consciousness, sleep, and alertness (Sherman, 2006).

Physiologic responses to music are also not lost for people in low awareness states. Heart rate, breath patterns, and respiration rates can all be affected by external auditory stimulation. Children in low awareness states may respond to exciting music with an increase in heart rate, just as their heart rate may slow down to a lullaby. This ability to regulate vital organ function by an external auditory source can be a significant resource for this patient population.

REFERRAL AND ASSESSMENT PROCEDURES

Referral Criteria

Any number of reasons can trigger the need for a music therapy referral for a child in a low awareness state. Early on in treatment, music therapy may be sought for assistance with assessment. If the child's cognition, communication, or movement abilities are unknown, music therapy may lead to behavioral responses to help define the child's status in these areas. Patients who were musicians prior to loss of consciousness may be a priority for music therapy services since music will inevitably hold special meaning for that person. However, care should be taken when working with such patients, as they may have difficulty in adjusting to their lack of current ability to play the way that they did prior to their change in consciousness.

The music therapist can be essential in determining the parameters of sound that are most offensive to a child who is agitated by environmental stimuli. Music, in this case, may be used to mask unwanted environmental sounds and provide relaxation for the child. Music therapy can also play an important role in the treatment of a person demonstrating emotionally driven behaviors. Music can provide a nonverbal means of expression and can be validating to the child struggling with the confusion that often occurs when in a low awareness state. Strong rhythmic cues and melodic contour can assist the child who is having difficulty initiating speech or movement. These children may also benefit from music as a means of exciting neurologic pathways that can lead to improvement in brain functioning.

Finally, music therapy can be beneficial in developing family-shared experiences. Music can be a social activity that leads to bonding and positive family leisure time. Family members who are struggling with how to engage in play and activities with their loved one should be referred to music therapy.

Assessment

Disorders of consciousness are among the most difficult medical disorders to diagnose. These diagnoses carry a great deal of weight for the treatment and resources that a person receives. Current assessment relies heavily on behavioral observation. The observations must be clear responses to questions asked or directives given during the assessment and must be repeatable over time. For those patients who lack communication and movement skills, behavioral responses can be quite limited.

The sensitivity of these scales is often lacking in that they are unable to capture the minute changes in functional behavior that is typical of recovery in patients in low awareness states. Andrews (1996) showed that a lack of sensitivity in the area of functional behavior led to 42% of patients being misdiagnosed. Poor diagnoses with this patient population can lead to ineffective or withdrawal from treatment, incorrect prognosis, and an overall lack of motivation for treatment (Magee, 2007). Furthermore, the diagnoses of vegetative state can be difficult for families to accept. While the term refers to the fact that organ function and growth continue during this state, many people associate this term with "vegetable." This derogatory term implies that there is no hope and that treatment is pointless (Andrews, 1996).

Legal implications of misdiagnosis include withdrawal of tube feeding. Legal criteria vary, but in general most countries require neurological examinations by two independent physicians. The exams must show complete and irreversible absence of brain function. This can be shown through two *isoelectric EEGs* 24 hours apart or a *radionuclide cerebral blood flow scan* that shows complete absence of intracranial blood flow. In either case, the patient should have a normal temperature and be free of drugs that can suppress brain activity (Erbengi et al., 1991).

Assessment Procedures

Music Therapy. Music, when applied in a planned clinical manner, has been shown to be effective in stimulating a range of behavioral, physiological, and expressive responses in patients with disorders of consciousness (Magee, 2005; Magee, 2007). Music is naturally emotional, can be highly motivating, uses visually stimulating instruments, and is nonverbal. These characteristics make music a primary resource for interaction with patients in low awareness states. Furthermore, live music can be adjusted in volume, pitch, melodic contour, and rhythm in order to assess a patient's responses to specific auditory information.

The emotional content of music may provide the multidisciplinary team with information about a patient's cognitive functioning. In order to produce emotional behaviors, one must possess cognitive functioning (Magee, 2007). Music may be instrumental in triggering emotional responses in people diagnosed with a disorder of consciousness. However, the practicing music therapist should note that limbic and emotional responses look very similar. It is easy for the therapist and multidisciplinary team to confuse one for the other. *Limbic responses* may consist of crying, laughing, or smiling as a reaction to specific sounds, pitches, or volume levels. While emotional behaviors also include crying, laughing, and smiling, when produced as an emotional response, the behavior must be seen over repeated presentation of emotional stimuli.

Another reason why music may be so effective in assessing and treating disorders of consciousness is its primitive association with language. Early communication is dependent on musical elements such as pitch, melody, articulation, timing, and phrasing. Within these musical parameters are the organizational beginnings of communication. Music may provide a structured experience for nonverbal dialogue with even the most minimal of movements or sounds from the patient. Furthermore, musical characteristics can be used to determine the optimal pitch, dynamic, and direction of stimulation to best allow patients with receptive communication issues. People in low awareness states may have encountered physical changes that affect hearing, such as with inner ear fluid or damage to the inner ear. Through the use of music's characteristics, a trained therapist can assess appropriate dynamics, pitch, and direction of stimulus to optimize hearing.

Neuroimaging. Although neuroimaging techniques are not yet sophisticated enough to determine diagnoses, they may offer assistance in establishing levels of consciousness. Functional imaging describes a variety of techniques used to assess brain function from a physiological, as opposed to anatomical, perspective. One of the most common forms of functional imaging is the *functional magnetic resonance imaging* (fMRI). This technique looks at blood oxygenation fluctuation to determine active regions in the brain. The fMRI image has been used to examine activation differences between normal speech and reversed speech, making it possible to note which regions are involved in higher-level auditory processing (Schiff et al., 2005).

Other tests, such as the *fluorodexyglucose* (FDG), *positron emission tomography* (PET), and *single-photon emission computerized tomography* (SPECT), measure resting state metabolism and its change over time comparative to clinical improvement. These scans observe the absorption of small quantities of *radioactive glucose* in the brain. Since brain cells use glucose as fuel, PET works off of the theory that if brain cells are more active, they will consume more of the radioactive glucose, and if less active, they will consume less. A computer uses the absorption data to show levels of activity in the brain through a color-coded brain map.

As neuroimaging techniques continue to be used, scientists hope to learn more about the brain and cognition. This information may lead to doctors being able to more accurately diagnose disorders of consciousness in people without volitional motor or speech abilities. However, the primary source of assessment at this time remains behavioral.

Behavioral Assessments. Because consciousness cannot formally be measured by any machine, clinicians and medical professionals rely heavily on clinical signs of wakefulness and awareness to determine conscious states. Many measures and scales have been developed to quantify and standardize behavioral assessment of consciousness. For the music therapist working with this population, it is imperative that they understand what the scores of these scales mean. Scale scores are often used in medical charts as well as in care plan meetings. A physician may refer to a scale score when describing a patient's current level of consciousness. The therapist must understand what level of consciousness the score refers to and what type of tasks were involved in achieving that score. The next section describes the most commonly used tools, as well as a newly developed tool specific to music therapy.

Measures of Consciousness

Los Ranchos Amigos Levels of Cognitive Functioning. The Los Ranchos Amigos Cognitive Scale (Hagen, Malkmus, & Durham, 1972) is an evaluation tool used by rehabilitation teams to help determine when the patient is progressing toward cognitive awareness. This scale has eight levels representing the typical progression of recovery from a severe brain injury. However, individuals will progress at different rates and may plateau at any stage of recovery. The lower the number at which they plateau, the more likely the patient is to be in a vegetative state or brain dead.

Patients are scored based on combinations of the following criteria: responsiveness to stimuli, ability to follow commands, presence of nonpurposeful behavior, cooperation, confusion, attention to environment, focus, coherence of verbalizations, appropriateness of verbalizations and actions, memory recall, orientation, and judgment and reasoning. These scores are used by the health care team to standardize communication about a patient's status and can be used as a basis for treatment. The Los

Ranchos scale is for patients 14 years of age and older. It is one of the most commonly used scales and is often paired with the Glasgow Coma Scale.

Glasgow Coma Scale (GCS). The GCS (Teasdale & Jennett, 1974) aims to give a reliable, objective way of recording the conscious state of a person. The test can be used for both initial and subsequent assessment. The scale has points assigned to different criteria. The resulting points give the patient a score between 3 and 15. The lower the score, the more unconscious a person is, while high numbers represent high levels of consciousness.

The GCS has limited applicability to children. The test is highly dependent on verbal performance, which is expected to be poor even in a healthy child. The Pediatric Glasgow Coma Scale (PGCS) is a modified version of the GCS to meet the needs of children. The primary changes in the PGCS are in the area of verbal response. Instead of verbal responses, the test focuses on facial affect, crying, and ability to be consoled. The PGCS is most commonly used in emergency medical situations.

Full Outline of UnResponsiveness Scale (FOUR). The FOUR was developed to replace the Glasgow Coma Scale in assessment of severely brain-injured patients in intensive care (Wijdicks, 2006). The scale involves assessment under four subscales that consider skill levels in the areas of motor responses, ocular or eye responses, brainstem reflexes, and breathing. Unlike the GCS, the FOUR does not assess verbal communication but instead focuses on ocular responses. This allows the test to have better success with intubated patients in the intensive care setting. The focus on ocular movement makes this test exceptionally good at diagnosing locked-in syndrome (Schnakers, Giacino, & Laureys, 2012).

The total score of the FOUR ranges from 0 to 16. A patient who scores a 0 is assumed to have no brain stem activity and can therefore, when paired with EEG results that show no electrical brain activity, be diagnosed as brain dead. *Autonomic functions* are tracked with this test and can help establish emergence of VS.

JFK Coma Scale–Revised (CSR–R). This scale, developed by investigators at the JFK Johnson Research Institute in 1991 (Giacino, Kezmarsky, DeLuca, & Cicerone, 1991), consists of 23 items that include six subscales. The subscales address auditory, visual, motor, aural motor, communication, and arousal skills. The lowest behavioral item on each subscale represents reflexive or unconscious responses, while the highest item represents purposeful or conscious responses. Patients receive scores based on operationally defined behavioral responses to specific sensory stimuli. Scores on this scale range from 0 to 16. The scale has been shown to be effective in discriminating between patients in MCS and VS and is commonly used to further assess and monitor a patient's functioning level.

Wessex Head Injury Matrix (WHIM). The Wessex Head Injury Matrix or WHIM (Sheil et al, 2000), is most commonly used with patients in MCS or VS. The tool was developed to measure changes in patients in low awareness states such as VS and is particularly helpful in determining if a patient is in VS or MCS. The assessment has proven useful in detecting slow recovery. Patients who are static on other scales are often found to have change on the WHIM because of its ability to recognize minute changes in behavior.

There are 62 items on the WHIM, and, much as in the JFK Coma Scale–Revised, they are broken down into five subcategories. The subcategories for the WHIM are arousal level and concentration, visual consciousness, communication, cognition (i.e., memory and spatiotemporal orientation), and social behaviors (Schnakers, Giacino, & Laureys, 2012). Patients receive a score based on the most complex behaviors observed; therefore, a higher score represents a higher level of consciousness.

Sensory Modality Assessment and Rehabilitation Technique (SMART). The SMART focuses on three areas of assessment: the sensory, motor, and communicative responses. Each area receives a score based on the SMART's five-point hierarchical scale. A structured and regulated sensory program is introduced in order to test the patient's skill in these three areas. The scale is consistent across all sensory modalities with the following range of scores: level 1—no response, level 2—reflexive, level 3—

withdrawal, level 4—localizing, and level 5—discriminating. This five-point scale relates directly to the description of the Los Ranchos Amigos levels 1–4 (Gill-Thwaites, 1997). A patient is diagnosed as being in a minimally conscious state or higher if they receive consistent level 5 scores in any one of the sensory modalities.

Perhaps the most unique aspect of the SMART is that it involves collecting data from family and caregivers about observed behaviors outside of the formal assessment time. This includes learning about the patient's interests, likes, and dislikes as they were before brain damage. This component ensures that all responses are recorded and categorized, encourages family and caregiver participation, and optimizes the opportunity for meaningful response to stimuli.

Music Therapy Assessment Tool for Low Awareness States (MATLAS). Unlike the other assessment tools discussed above, the MATLAS (Magee, 2007) does not rely on the patient's ability to process language. Instead, the procedure uses live music in order to focus on the auditory processing capabilities of the patient (the test includes presenting single musical characteristics such as tones, harmony, improvised melodies, musical instruments, and precomposed songs) to elicit behavioral responses. This musical focus, along with offering emotionally significant stimuli, allows the patient exceptional opportunities to demonstrate awareness.

The MATLAS is composed of 14 items that cover five areas of behavior. These behavior areas are similar to behavior responses in other tools. Behavior response categories for the MATLAS are visual, auditory, awareness of musical stimuli, verbal commands, and arousal. The 14 items that are used to stimulate behavioral responses are completed during four assessment sessions provided within an 8- to 10-day span and are given a numerical grade. Grades range from zero (equaling no response) to somewhere between three and seven (indicating highest level of response) in each category. The highest possible score for this assessment is 45, which is achieved by observing a number of intentional responses across several categories. The test also includes pre- and post-observation periods in order to assess resting state behaviors of the patient.

For each behavior response area, Magee (2007) has developed interventions to assess the category. Two example areas will be discussed here. Intervention items within the auditory domain provide information regarding the patient's ability to hear. These interventions include the playing of a single musical sound to complex musical phrases. Each intervention can be manipulated in terms of pitch and volume. Further assessment is done through an item that breaks down the pulse/rhythm, melody/pitch, timbre, dynamics/intensity, and tempo of the musical stimuli. The information gained from this assessment item provides important insight into the best sound environment for the patient.

The second area of assessment measures communicative intent. Research shows that during musical interventions, a high incidence of spontaneous vocal sounds may occur. Because of this, spontaneous vocal sounds are a major focus of the communicative intent assessment area. An item is included in the assessment that specifies the amount of vocal response given by the patient. This hierarchical rating begins with "no vocalization to stimulus" and ends with "sang all the words to the song." Additionally, a level nine indicates "unable to vocalize." Level nine is used when a *fibrotic endoscopic* evaluation has shown impairment on a physiologic level, which is unlikely to be repaired. Nonverbal communication, choice-making, and responses to verbal commands are also measured during the communicative intent portion of the assessment. The nonverbal and motivational characteristics of music provide an alternate medium to assessment, which may lead to different results than those observed in a language-based assessment.

Magee (2007) suggests that the MATLAS be used in conjunction with other standardized assessments such as those listed above in order to provide a full multimodal assessment. It is difficult to know what stimuli are most powerful in eliciting behaviors that show awareness in patients in low awareness states. The most powerful and salient stimulus for one patient may have a different effect on another. The MATLAS provides visual, tactile, and auditory sensory stimuli throughout the assessment, giving it the advantage of multimodal stimulation.

INTRODUCTION TO MUSIC THERAPY METHODS

Music therapy with the child in a minimally conscious state can be challenging. The therapist working with this population should enter sessions with the realization that she may receive little to no feedback from the client. This lack of feedback can cause the therapist to feel insecure about the work that she is doing. Furthermore, the lack of literature supporting music therapy with this population may add to feelings of insecurity and questioning of how the client is benefiting from services. Although these challenges can seem overwhelming at times, there are many guidelines and interventions that can be used to counteract such difficulty. Before discussing specific music therapy interventions, some general goals, instructions, and contraindications for working with this population are presented.

The music therapist, skilled in interacting nonverbally with clients, can support the emotional experiences of a person in a low awareness state by providing both support for and exploration of emotion states. Opportunities for spontaneous interaction allow for rehabilitation to happen in a creative and functional manner. Creating emotion-centered music aims to promote brain activity in the limbic system while simultaneously engaging the *hippocampus,* encouraging cognitive performance (Magee, 2007).

The music therapist uses music to reach deep into the psyche of a person (Wheeler, 1981). Bruscia (1987) explains that communication begins by matching the client's inner condition with music. This matching creates an environment in which the child can begin making connections. Music, as a tonal language, may provide the beginnings for contact with the unconscious child and stimulate communication at emotional, social, and cognitive levels (Jochim, 1994).

Regardless of treatment paradigm, one goal is constantly present for the music therapist working with people in low awareness states: awareness. Awareness is the basis for all other goals and treatment. Without awareness, no other goals can be worked toward. Throughout the music therapy session, the therapist should vigilantly watch the child for any signs of arousal. Eye opening, eye movement, finger tapping, foot movement, and head movement are often the most common indicators of arousal. However, a change in breath pattern or heart rate may also reflect arousal (The Multi-Society Task Force on PVS, 1994). In this author's clinical work, it has been evident that children diagnosed with coma or persistent vegetative state are more likely to produce behavioral responses such as change in breath pattern or heart rate, whereas children in a minimally conscious state may respond through eye opening or small movements.

Contraindications for treatment of people in low awareness states are primarily centered on medical stability. The therapist must keep close watch on the child's oxygen saturation and heart rate. If the child wavers in saturation of oxygen or changes in heart rate to a degree which is deemed unsafe by the medical team, music should quickly be faded out and stopped for the session. Another contraindication is related to music as a trigger of emotion-laden memories. There is debate within the music therapy field about using familiar music since music listening may provoke traumatic memories that cannot be resolved due to the person's cognitive state (Anderson, 1994; Segall, 2007). If possible, the therapist should interview family members to learn about the child's musical preferences, important life events, and songs that may conjure negative or sad memories.

When conducting the music therapy session, there are several communicative and environmental aspects that the therapist should keep in mind.

- Always use a social greeting and introduce yourself. Even if you have worked with the child daily for several weeks, they may not remember you due to memory issues.

- Speak slowly and clearly. A child in a low awareness state may need additional time to process your verbal cues and instructions. Be sure to give commands in a direct and brief manner. For example, "Open your eyes" as opposed to "Can you open your eyes for me today?"
- Create a safe environment. Too much stimulation, such as TV, loud conversations, and large groups of people, can decrease arousal in a person with a low awareness state. Since processing of stimuli is often slow and difficult for the child, it is important that the environment be free of all extraneous sound and stimuli.
- Formally end your contact. Often individuals with impaired cognition are not aware of cues that suggest that the session is ending. It is important to state your intentions in a direct manner, "I have to leave now, [patient's name]."

Music has long been associated with parent-child interactions and bonding. Lullaby singing is one of the earliest shared experiences between a parent and child (Papousek, 1996). Music is a fun activity that most children enjoy and to which parents can relate. Music can also be normalizing. It is a common cultural phenomenon that encourages social interaction within family life (Oldfield & Bunce, 2001). Many music therapy interventions utilize these musical characteristics to help families bond during times of difficulty. The music therapy guidelines provided in this chapter clearly indicate that the music therapist working with children who have disorders of consciousness plays an essential role in assisting their families during the grieving and healing process. Many of the interventions provide opportunities for caregivers to overcome their insecurities of being able to have a relationship with the child in a low awareness state. Music therapy interventions directed at caregivers provide mutual benefit for the caregiver and the child, as relationship-building carries over to visits outside of the music therapy session.

OVERVIEW OF MUSIC THERAPY METHODS AND PROCEDURES

Receptive Music Therapy

- Music Listening for Arousal: playing live or recorded music to promote arousal and wakeful states in a child in a low awareness state.
- Improvised Music Based on Vital Functions: the use of improvised music to match, accentuate, and react to a child's responses, facilitating internal integration of physiological body rhythms, awareness of self, environment, and others, and facilitation of communicative contact through music.
- Music Entrainment of Physiological Functions: altering a child's physiological response by first matching the music to the tempo of his respiratory or heart rate, and then gradually changing the tempo to either decrease or increase the rate of the response.
- Vibrotactile/Vibroacoustic Stimulation: the use of vibrotactile equipment that emphasizes the vibrations produced by music in order to facilitate relaxation and reduction in muscle tone, blood pressure, and heart rate.
- Contingent Music: the use of music as a reinforcement to stimulate communication through small movements.
- Musicokinetic Therapy: the combination of vestibular motion with a synchronized beat to trigger activation of the central nervous system and increase awareness.

Improvisational Music Therapy

- Music Improvisation for Sibling Support: the use of music improvisation with the patient's sibling(s) to help express thoughts and feelings, master situational factors, and process the changes that are likely happening in the family dynamics.
- Sound Bath: A sound bath consists of a patient receiving music played by others, typically the therapist and family members. The fluid nature of the music creates a sense of the sound washing over the person, enhancing relaxation and creating an atmosphere of calm.

Re-creative Music Therapy

- Family Singing/Song Dedication: singing and song dedication by family members to explore the emotional side of living with a child who has a disorder of consciousness and help build new memories and connections with that child.
- CD Creation: recording of the family member(s) speaking or singing to the child to express their thoughts and feelings to their loved one. The recording is played to the child with the caregivers present or during times when they are not able to be present.

Compositional Music Therapy

- Family Songwriting: creation of songs to promote bonding among family members as well as help families process the grief of their child's loss of abilities, hospitalization, and the loss of hopes and wishes that they had for their child.

GUIDELINES FOR RECEPTIVE MUSIC THERAPY

Music for listening can be a powerful tool when working with children in low awareness states. Children are naturally drawn to music. They seem to thrive off of energizing beats and sweet lullabies. There are several ways in which music listening can be an effective treatment for children experiencing disorders of consciousness.

Music Listening for Arousal

Overview. Playing live or recorded music to a person in a low awareness state can facilitate the awakening of the *central nervous system* and promote *synaptic connections.* The more individualized and meaningful the music is to the child, the more likely it is to connect the child with past memories, thereby further encouraging recovery of the central nervous system (Lancioni et al., 2010). Music listening for arousal can be used with children with any diagnoses of a disorder of consciousness. The primary goal is to promote arousal and wakeful states.

Preparation. Musical choices should be prepared prior to the session, and when using live music, it should be memorized in order to eliminate unnecessary distraction and stimulation. The therapist should be able to focus her attention on the child in order to recognize subtle movements during the music stimulation.

Procedures. The therapist should begin with a minimum of five minutes of silence. During this silence, the therapist can observe nonvolitional movements and behaviors. After the silence, the therapist should introduce herself and the music listening intervention. The therapist can then begin playing the music. Music should be played with a simple accompaniment pattern and melody line. Too many sound sources may confuse the child or be too much for him to process (Magee, 2008). At the close of each song, the therapist should allow silence to fill the room. This may be a time when the child shows behavioral signs of arousal due to a delay in auditory processing and/or change in environment from sound to no sound (Wilson, Cranny, & Andrews, 1992). Before beginning the next music listening experience, watch for any changes in the child. If it seems that he is having difficulty with processing the accompaniment instrument and melody as shown through unhealthy changes in vital signs, the therapist should try using only voice. All stimulation, including music listening, should be provided for short durations of time. This author recommends 10 to 15 minutes, as tolerated by the child. Once music listening is complete, the therapist should observe the patient quietly for five minutes in order to note any changes after the music stops.

Improvised Music Based on Vital Functions

Overview. Improvised music is flexible and can be altered in the moment to match, accentuate, and react to patient responses. It is created in the moment, and the therapist is given freedom to respond in the real time to any change or contribution from the patient (Ansdell, 1991). Music improvisation can therefore be used to encourage active participation and communication (Tamplin, 2000). Goals of improvisational music therapy with children in a low awareness state include internal integration of physiological body rhythms, awareness of self, environment and others, and facilitation of communicative contact through music.

Jochim (1994) speaks of "preverbal emotionally focused tonal language" (p.) having the ability to establish contact and stimulate communication at emotional, social, and cognitive levels with the patient in a low awareness state. Bruscia (1987) states that by matching the patient's inner condition, the music therapist can establish communicative contact. The trained music therapist can recognize a person's inner experience through their outward behavior and physiologic responses. The following intervention details how the music therapist may use improvised music as a means to achieve human contact and elicit communication with an unconscious or semiconscious person.

Preparation.   Prior to conducting the session, the therapist should meet with the child's family and friends to learn what the child was like prior to the accident. This knowledge helps the therapist to feel a sense of connection with the child. The therapist should also contact nursing staff to ensure that no invasive procedures are planned and interruptions will be minimal. The therapist should ask nursing staff not to provide any procedures or unnecessary care for 10 minutes after the intervention in order to allow the child rest and processing time.

What to observe. Any response shown by the child should be recognized and a musical reaction should be provided.

Procedures. Before providing improvised music, the therapist should introduce herself to the child and explain that she will sing to the child at the tempo of the child's pulse and /or breath rhythm. If the child is being monitored, the therapist can use the heart rate or respiratory rate from the monitor as a starting tempo. If there is no monitoring of physiological responses, the therapist can take the child's pulse either by placing two fingers on his wrist and counting his pulse for one minute or by counting how many times the child's chest rises and falls in one minute. The therapist can then proceed with singing wordless music for 8 to 12 minutes at the determined tempo. The singing should be clearly phrased so that if a reaction is noted from the child, the phrase can easily be repeated (Aldridge, Gustorff, & Hannich, 1990). The therapist may choose to change the characteristics of the music when repeating the phrase to match the child's response. For example, if the child coughs during a phrase of music, the therapist may repeat the phrase in a more staccato style matching that of the child's cough.

At the end of the 8 to 12 minutes, or when the child displays signs of overstimulation such as closing eyes, turning head away from therapist and sound source, or a grimaced affect, the therapist should fade the music to a close. Before leaving the room, it is important that the therapist explain that the music session is finished for the time being, bringing closure to the session.

Music Entrainment of Physiological Functions

Overview. Although entrainment and improvisation based on vital signs both start by observing and matching music to the tempo of the child's heart rate or respiratory rate, the two techniques are quite different. Once the initial tempo of the song based on the child's current state is established, entrainment aims to change that tempo to either stimulate or relax the patient into a more stable state. Entrainment can also be used to adjust an emotional state.

Agitation is a common characteristic of people in low awareness states. As it usually occurs as a side effect to the confused state when waking up from a coma, it is typically seen as a positive sign of recovery. However, it can be detrimental to therapy progress. When in an agitated state, it may difficult for the child to respond to cues, focus on tasks, and process information. Music entrainment has been used by music therapists to alter heart rates and increase oxygen by changing breath rhythms, thereby helping the child to relax (Bradt, 2009; Chlan, 1998; Hilliard, 2005). Aldridge (1996) and Rider (1985) suggest that humans are musical and that there is an underlying rhythmicity that helps to regulate each bodily system. These systemic rhythms can be upset by stress or trauma, causing disorganization throughout the body. For the patient in a low awareness state, the disorganized rhythms can become a static state. When this happens, music therapy can support stimulation and reorganization. Music entrainment is achieved by matching the physiological rhythm of the patient and then slowly adjusting the rhythm to achieve a desired state (Bradt, 2009).

Children with respiratory difficulty or irregular heart rhythms may benefit from music entrainment. Music entrainment can also be useful during acute episodes of increased agitation to help the child relax. Roederer explained that sound stimuli are able to manipulate physiological functions, such as heart rate and respiration pattern, by resonating with the "natural clocks" of the brain (as cited in Bradt, 2009). Another explanation of how entrainment works relates to auditory processing. Auditory stimuli are processed first in the *medulla* of the brain. This part of the brain manages autonomic function, including heart rate and respiration (Scartelli, 1991, as cited in Bradt, 2009).

What to observe. The therapist will be observing the child's vital rhythms, namely heart rate and respiration rate. She should also take care to notice signs of overstimulation.

Procedures. Bradt (2009) describes the following process for musical entrainment. Prior to beginning the session, the therapist should consult with the medical team to determine the appropriate range for the individual child's heartbeat or respiratory count. Typically, the child's nurse and or respiratory therapist will have this information. The treatment begins by observing the respiration or heart rate of the child and determining the direction in which the rate should change. Should it get faster or slower? What meter would best suit the child's current rhythm? If working on breath rhythms, what is the breath pattern? Is it even or syncopated? It is recommended that the therapist practice recognizing breath pattern prior to the session. This can be done during outings with friends, or while people watching at the park.

The music therapist then plays or sings a melody that matches the rhythm of the physiological response. If focusing on breath pattern, it is important to provide a rhythmical cue for when the next inhale will happen. The recommended pattern is to use a grouping of three eighth notes just before the downbeat that aligns with the next exhale. If working on heart rate, the music's tempo is matched to the rate of the child's heartbeat. This author has found that a nonsyncopated beat works best when using entrainment for heart rate. Once the tempo is set and consistent, the therapist can gradually slow her tempo and the child's vitals will follow. The eighth notes discussed earlier provide a melodic pull to the downbeat and are used to adjust the tempo. When the child is in a calm state, the therapist can slowly fade out the music.

Vibrotactile/Vibroacoustic Stimulation

Overview. Vibrotactile instruments that emphasize the vibrations produced by music in order to be felt in the patient's body have been reported anecdotally to produce relaxation and reductions in muscle tone, blood pressure, and heart rate (Punkanen & Ala-Ruona, 2012; Wigram, 1993). Furthermore, tactile input from these instruments can add an important dimension to the treatment of a person in a low awareness state.

Vibroacoustic or vibrotactile therapy involves the use of a stimulus that combines a sedative music with a pulsed, sinusoidal low-frequency tone played through a bed or chair (Wigram, 1993). *Sinusoidal low frequency tone* refers to a bass tone played between 20Hz and 70Hz that creates a sound wave in a particular curve (Webster, 2003; Wigram, 1993). Some of the more commonly used devices among music therapists are Somatron™ and Soundwave™. Patients lie on the bed or sit in the chair and experience vibration from the music and sinusoidal tones while simultaneously hearing the stimuli. Skille (1989a, 1989b) proposed three principles of sound vibration and music. The first is that low frequencies can relax and high frequencies can raise tension. The second states that rhythmical music can stimulate and nonrhythmical music can pacify. Finally, loud music can create aggression and soft music can act as a sedative.

Some patients experience nausea, headaches, and discomfort when receiving vibroacoustic stimulation. It is theorized that the nausea may stem from the patient experiencing a motion effect during the treatment. The motion effect may be caused by the difference in tone, which occurs when a tone is pulsed by matching two tones closely together (Griffin, 1983; Yamada et al., 1983). Vibroacoustic therapy may also reduce blood pressure and therefore may be contraindicated as a treatment for the following conditions (Wigram, 1993):

- When being treated for an acute condition (e.g., *thrombosis*)
- When being treated for active or acute inflammation
- When suffering from a recently prolapsed *invertebral disc*
- After an accident (e.g., when suffering a physical head or neck injury, broken bone)
- During internal or external bleeding
- In cases of psychotic, prepsychotic, or borderline psychotic conditions
- When suffering from *hypotension*
- After a recent *myocardial infarction*

Regression has also been noted in cognitively delayed populations during use of vibroacoustic therapy (Bergström-Isacsson, 2011). Regression may be difficult to assess in a person in a low awareness state and could cause increased agitation and disorientation after vibroacoustic treatment has stopped. Given these contraindications and the potential for negative side effects, vibroacoustic therapy should be used with caution.

Procedures. The process of vibroacoustic therapy can be defined in six stages (Wigram, 1993):

1) Presession preparation: The vibroacoustic equipment, the bed or chair, should be prepared in order to meet the positioning needs of the child. The therapist should consult with rehabilitation and nursing staff to determine the best positioning for the child and should supply the correct amount of support with pillows, wedges, and bolsters. Volume controls on playback equipment should be turned down to zero. If the recording started with the volume turned up, the child would be subjected to a sudden jolt of sound that could be alarming and perhaps uncomfortable from a vibration standpoint. For this reason, the sound stimulus should be introduced gradually.

2) Introduction: The therapist should inform the child that they will be feeling vibrations from the chair and hearing sounds from the speakers or instrument. Although the child may not be able to understand the information being given, a calm tone of voice can set the scene and create an environment for a successful session.

3) Starting the treatment: As mentioned previously, the sound should be introduced gradually and increased to a volume that seems to be most beneficial for the child. A short amount of response time should be provided before introducing the bass frequencies.

4) Monitoring the treatment: The therapist must watch carefully for overstimulation as indicated by increased heart rate, shallow breathing, or facial grimace. These changes can alert the therapist that the stimulus is too much. The first course of action should be to lower the bass tones. Although the low tones can often be perceived as subtle in the beginning, over time they feel stronger even without any change to the volume level. This author recommends that vibroacoustic sessions be short, a maximum of 15 minutes, so as not to overstimulate or cause discomfort to the child.

5) Ending the treatment session: Sometimes during vibroacoustic therapy, patients go into a quiet, deep state of relaxation. The therapist should fade out the vibroacoustic stimulation, leave one to two minutes of silence, and proceed by singing the child's name and, if appropriate, providing gentle touch to the hands and feet of the child. This change in stimulation is provided to assist the child in becoming aware of their environment once again. If scheduling permits, the end of the vibroacoustic session may be an optimal time for rehabilitation staff to provide passive range of motion since the child is likely to have reduced muscle tone.

When working with a 16-year-old male with anoxic brain injury, this author found that a vibroacoustic session seemed to relax his muscle tone. The therapist consulted physical therapy, and the physical therapist began seeing the patient just after the vibroacoustic session. The physical therapist reported that the patient was able to achieve as much as 15 degrees more in passive range of motion than in sessions not paired with vibroacoustics.

Contingent Music

Overview. Music can be a powerful motivator. This technique harnesses music's motivational power to achieve communication through small movements (Larsen & Ayllon, 1990; Standley, 2000). Children who demonstrate some level of awareness, such as those in a minimally conscious state, benefit most from this exercise. Contingent music can be used to achieve communication as well as return control back to the patient.

What to observe. The therapist should observe the child for signs of communication as discussed below.

Procedures. Targeted communication responses should be established by the team and already be a part of the child's behavioral repertoire. Possible responses include eye squeezing, finger movement, and mouth movement. The therapist should request that the child produce the communication response. Each time the child completes the movement requested, he receives 15 seconds of patient-preferred music. Once the communication response is produced consistently, the therapist can ask the child to do the movement when he hears the song he would like to listen to in order to work on choice-making abilities. Family members can be taught this technique as a way for them to interact with their child. Some children in a minimally conscious state may be able to activate a switch device. If this is the case, the child can be provided with a switch-activated music player that can allow him to listen to music at his leisure.

Musicokinetic Therapy (MKT)

Overview. MKT, developed by Noda, Maeda, and Yoshino (2003), is an intervention designed to trigger activation of the central nervous system and increase awareness through environmental stimuli. The therapist combines vestibular motion with a synchronized beat. The movement stimulates sensorimotor pathways while the music is meaningful and familiar to the child.

This technique is most successful when provided within six months of injury regardless of diagnoses (Noda et al., 2003). It is important that the child be cleared for vestibular motion by the medical team prior to conducting this intervention. The therapist will need assistance from the rehabilitation or nursing team to carry out the intervention.

What to observe. The therapist should observe signs of awareness as well as signs of discomfort in the child. If the child demonstrates discomfort through change in heart rate or grimace of facial expression, the therapist should stop the intervention and provide relaxation for the child until he reaches homeostasis.

Procedures. In order to provide this intervention, the therapist will need a quiet room with a trampoline. Positioning equipment may also be needed such as pillows, wedges, and bolsters. The rehabilitation staff can supply these items.

With the assistance of the rehabilitation team, the therapist should transfer the child to the trampoline and provide necessary supports so that the child is comfortable and safe. A pair of caregivers or rehabilitation therapists supports the child in a sitting position on the trampoline. The caregivers stimulate the child through vertical, soft bounces on the equipment. At the same time, the music therapist begins providing live music that matches the beat of the bounces. After 5 to 10 minutes of vestibular and musical stimulation, the caregivers lay the child down while the therapist plays slow and soft music for three to five minutes. During this relaxation period, the rehabilitation staff can provide massage or passive range of motion. This process is repeated for 30 minutes (Noda et al., 2003). If a trampoline is not readily accessible, a physioball that allows for soft bouncing motion can be used in its place.

During musicokinetic therapy, signs of awareness may become more apparent. One clinical example is that of a five-year-old girl participating in musikokinetic therapy who showed anticipation of start and stop in the song "Bringing Home a Baby Bumble Bee" through a change in facial affect.

GUIDELINES FOR IMPROVISATIONAL MUSIC THERAPY

Improvisational techniques are not commonly used with children in low awareness states as most of these children are not able to participate in improvising due to physical inability and decreased cognitive understanding. However, siblings and family members of children in low awareness states can participate in such sessions. Nonverbal expression through improvisation can help family members become more aware of the emotions that they are feeling around the illness of their loved one. Once these emotions are identified, the family member(s) can then work toward building coping skills and processing the hospital experience, and they oftentimes have a better of understanding of the reality of the situation.

Music Improvisation for Sibling Support

Overview. Music improvisation can be useful as an approach to emotional expression and coping for siblings of children with disorders of consciousness. Children often have difficulty expressing their emotions due to lack of verbal skills and abstract thinking (Schirrmacher, 1988). The nonverbal medium of music can allow a child to express thoughts and emotions without needing to find the words.

The sibling who fears entering a patient's room, becomes withdrawn, or is exhibiting increased behavioral problems is a prime candidate for music therapy. Music therapy can provide opportunities for the sibling to express thoughts and feelings, master situational factors, and process the changes that are likely happening in his family dynamics (Hilliard, 2001).

Preparation. Before working with the sibling of a patient, it is important to get parental approval. The music therapist should explain what music therapy is and discuss the benefits of the service to parents, explain and show them the space where you will conduct the session, and then ask for permission to bring their child in for a session. Since siblings are not always at the hospital, it can also be helpful to schedule a date and time for the session.

What to observe. The music therapist should be tuned in to the sibling, noticing facial affect, changes in musical patterns, scales, and instruments, as well as any vocal- or verbalizations expressed during music-making.

Procedures. A safe and private space should be provided for music therapy sessions. This can be accomplished through a child-friendly, private room that has a door and no windows to internal hallways. It is important that the room be free of people peering in so that the child feels comfortable expressing himself. The room should be equipped with a variety of instruments to cover a full range of expression. It is also beneficial to have other play items in the room, such as dolls, trucks and cars, pretend guns and swords, medical equipment, and costumes.

At the beginning of the session, the music therapist allows the child to explore all materials to facilitate a sense of safety in the child. The music therapist's role is to validate, support, and help the sibling process his family's situation. This can happen in the music or during discussion about the music. Depending on the need of the client and what he chooses to express during each session, supporting the child may take on different forms.

At times it may be that the therapist provides musical grounding and holding for the child's emotions. Grounding helps a patient to stay present (or, for some, become present in the first place). The music therapist may ground the child through keeping a steady beat, helping to maintain the emotion so that it does not grow into a state of uncontrolled emotions or overwhelming catharsis. Like grounding, holding is used to create an environment that has a therapeutic ambiance or setting which permits the patient to experience safety, thereby facilitating psychotherapeutic work. For example, a repeated musical pattern, often in a 3/4 time signature, can create a holding feeling similar to a mother's rocking during lullabies. Through the holding, the child may be able to maintain a sense of presence that allows him to better process the emotions that he is feeling.

A child who had recently experienced the death of a sibling began the music improvisation session on the xylophone that was set up in a C pentatonic scale. As she played, this author quietly strummed her guitar in a 3/4 pattern, alternating between Am and E. As the child continued to play, her slow, jazzy melodies expressed sadness and fear. The child began to cry during the music but did not stop playing. After some time, she brought the song to a close and stated that her song was titled "Angels Dancing." Through verbal processing, the child expressed that she imagined her sister dancing with the other angels and, even though she was sad that she could not dance with them, she was happy that her sister was not alone.

In other sessions, the therapist may repeat or mimic motifs and themes that the child produces in his play. These repetitions can bring light to the emotion behind the phrase and help the child center on that emotion in order to gain a greater awareness of it. Sometimes the child will choose to play with the toys only. Music can be a powerful soundtrack for this play and can be used to emphasize emotion. Oftentimes, the child will correct the therapist in her playing, stating that "the music should be soft now" or "now you play this instrument." This direction can help the therapist to better understand what the child is feeling and can lead to discussion around how and why the music is changing. There are many ways that improvisation and play can manifest in the music therapy session. The therapist is encouraged to be creative and adapt to the needs of the sibling.

Improvised Sound Bath

Overview. An improvised sound bath consists of a patient receiving sound being played by others. The fluid nature of the music often creates a sense of the sound washing over the person and can be very relaxing. The improvised sound bath lends itself easily to family involvement and can provide a forum for family bonding while building awareness of self, environment, and others for the patient. It can also help with agitation because of its relaxing nature. Because creating a sound bath often involves the family members in improvisational music-making, it is categorized under improvisational methods. However, since the child is listening to music in this intervention, it could also be categorized under receptive methods.

Preparation. Before beginning the session, the therapist should collect a variety of instruments to be used during the sound bath. This author has identified the following instruments as useful for sound bathing with patients in low awareness states: singing bowls, ocean drum, shruti box, resonators or xylophones, tone bars, rain stick, and voice.

What to observe. If working with a family to provide a child with a sound bath, the therapist should help the family learn to look for cues that the child is responding. Oftentimes, families are unaware of responses from their loved one because they are so minor and difficult to notice.

Procedures. The procedural steps described here are based on this author's clinical experience of using improvised sound baths with children in low awareness states. The therapist should start by explaining to the family what an improvised sound bath is and how the child may benefit from it. The therapist then helps each family member choose an instrument to play during the bath and shows them how to play it. It may be helpful to meet with the family in a private room where they can practice playing the instruments at relaxing volume levels and rhythms for a sound bath prior to entering the child's room. Once in the child's room, the family members are asked to stand or sit around the child and are invited to begin the improvisation softly. During the improvisation, the therapist should provide rhythmic grounding for the family group. The therapist may want to incorporate some reflection into the improvisation, whereby she musically reflects moods and feelings as family members produce them in their music. This can be done through mimicking phrases or repeating motifs.

There is no set time for how long the improvisation should last, as long as the family is emotionally able to maintain the improvisation and the child in a low awareness state is not getting overstimulated. Many times, the improvisation will naturally come to a close as family members feel that they have experienced or provided enough for the child. However, if the child seems to be getting overstimulated or some family members are beginning to look overwhelmed, the therapist can lead the improvisation to a close by increasing the volume, gaining eye contact with the family members, and then fading our the music by slowing her tempo and decreasing her volume. When the improvisation is complete, the therapist should encourage the family to allow silence to fill the space. The therapist then processes the improvised sound bath experience with the family members, giving them opportunities to share their thoughts and feelings about the sound bath as well as any movements or changes in the child they may have observed. If family is not available to participate, the therapist can create the sound bath by using an electric shruti box or drone sound and layering instruments and voice over the top of the drone.

GUIDELINES FOR RE-CREATIVE MUSIC THERAPY

Singing precomposed songs and performing them on instruments can promote family bonding, give voice to messages, feelings, and thoughts that loved ones want to share with their child in a low awareness state, and provide family with a means of interacting with their child. This section of the chapter will discuss two interventions using re-creative music therapy.

Family Singing/Song Dedication

Overview. As mentioned earlier in this chapter, families of a child with a disorder of consciousness can often feel disconnected from that child. Family members may have a hard time interacting with and providing care for the child. The feelings and emotions that they experience are similar to those of people who have lost a loved one. Music therapy literature points to how music therapy can assist with relationship completion (Dileo & Magill, 2005). According to Byock (2004), relationships are complete when we feel reconciled, whole, and at peace. Byock (1997) states that there are five sentiments that permit relationships to reach completion once they are expressed: "I love you," "Thank you," "Forgive me," "I forgive you," and "Good-bye." These are sentiments that can be expressed to complete various types of relationships including interpersonal, intrapersonal, and those with a spiritual connection. Music therapy can offer support and encouragement to develop family bonds during times of difficulty, thereby promoting relationship completion (Bradt & Dileo, 2010; Dileo & Parker, 1997).

Families that are struggling with staying involved in their ill child's care or are feeling as if they have nothing to offer him benefit most from this intervention. Family singing and song dedication can be used to assist families in exploring the emotional side of living with a child who has a disorder of consciousness and help them to build new memories and connections with that child.

Preparation. Building rapport with the family and having a repertoire of familiar music ready for the session is important presession work.

What to observe. The music therapist should observe family members' reactions and responses throughout the session. This will provide a basis for discussion after singing. Also, it is important to document and share with the multidisciplinary team any signs of awareness or change in the patient during the session.

Procedures. The music therapist can invite family members to sing songs to the child and give opportunities for song dedication throughout the session. Some families will readily accept invitations, while others may feel hesitant about singing in front of others or the therapist. The therapist should be sensitive to these feelings and offer a variety of experiences so that the family member(s) can choose what is best for them. For instance, it may be more comfortable for the family if the therapist steps to the side or back of the room while the family sings to their child, or the family may find it helpful for the therapist to sing along with the family. Cultural differences may also play a role in song dedication. For example, families from the Islam faith may believe that music is reserved only for religious ceremony, while others find it permissible to sing songs during specific occasions. The clapping of hands in public performances and music created for dancing or with dancing are two musical forms that the prophet Mohammed did not approve.

As the therapist leads the family in song or in choosing songs, she helps them to recognize any positive changes in the patient that may indicate awareness. Also, the therapist observes changes in expression or affect of the family members during the session and offers support in talking about the feelings they experienced during the song. Music can help people express emotions for which it is difficult to find words (Dileo & Magill, 2005). This release of emotion often leads to an ability to connect with a loved one and build a relationship.

The mother of a three-year-old in a low awareness state was encouraged to sing lullabies to her child in the music therapy session. After the session, the mother reported feeling like she was contributing to her child's care through the singing. This was significant since the mother had previously expressed feelings of guilt and sadness that the nursing staff seemed to provide more care for her child than she did.

CD Creation

Overview. There are many reasons a family member may choose to create a CD rather than speak directly to their child. Perhaps it is too overwhelming, and the remoteness of the CD recording gives them just enough space to begin expressing their thoughts to their loved one. Some families feel that the CD allows for more privacy since sessions in hospital settings are often interrupted by medical staff needing to provide patient care. Finally, parents of children in a low awareness state may choose to create a CD so that their voices can be heard even when they are not able to be present with their child. Any family that has a child in a low awareness state will benefit from creating a CD message for that child. Although the parent or family member does not need to be present during the CD playback, it is important that when the family is not available a staff member be present in order to observe signs of overstimulation or discomfort.

Preparation. Many recording devices can be used to capture the family members' voices. A computer with GarageBand™ or a digital voice-recorder are two examples. Sometimes a small device, such as a digital voice recorder, is less intimidating for family members than a computer, since it can simply sit on a table in the room and be almost unnoticeable. It is vital to the session that the therapist has a good understanding of how the recording system works in order to both teach the family member(s) and solve simple technology glitches that may occur during the session. If a child has an MP3 device, the recording can be transferred onto the device rather than burning a CD. In this case, oftentimes the family will know how to transfer the recording onto the MP3 device, but the therapist must know how to make the recording MP3-compatible. This can easily be done through iTunes™. The help feature in iTunes™ will explain to the therapist how to change the format of the recording to an MP3 format.

The family should be provided with a quiet, private room in which to create their recording. A sign is placed on the door to notify staff that recording is in progress. Any books or songs that the family members have requested should be readily accessible so that recording is not stalled.

What to observe. The therapist must be an active listener during the family recording. In order to assist the family member in overcoming their barriers to bond with their child, the therapist should be attentive to changes in voice or emotion during the recording. These changes may help the therapist identify areas of discussion after the recording is completed.

Procedures. The steps outlined below were developed by the music therapy team at the Elizabeth Seton Pediatric Center (ESPC) in New York upon realization of the need for family members to have a private expression of emotions to their child since most children shared a room with three other patients.

Prior to introducing the technique to the family, the therapist should assess for each child the most appropriate way to play the recording for the child. The recording must be able to be played in a private manner that is well tolerated by the child. Some children in a low awareness state will have difficulty tolerating headphones due to sensitive touch responses and positioning. The team at ESPC found that speaker pillows are often a useful alternative for children who cannot tolerate the tactile stimulation of headphones.

Once a suitable playback option is identified, the therapist can introduce to the family the idea of making a recording. When describing the intervention, the therapist should be sure to explain to the family that they are welcome to read stories, sing songs, or simply speak to their child. The therapist should remain flexible in order to provide the best support for the family members. Some families may require multiple recording sessions in order to get the recording just right. Families may prefer that the therapist be present during the recording or playback session or may decide that recording in private without the therapist present feels more comfortable. If the family chooses to record in private, the therapist should be accessible to the family in the event that they have questions or need assistance. Finally, the family may request that the therapist provide background music or accompaniment to songs during the recording. By offering choices to the family, the therapist is giving the family control over their creation in a time when they may feel that they have little control of the care of their child.

The therapist should always take the family through a short trial recording to make sure that everything is working properly. When the family is ready to record, the therapist can either press the Record button for them or show them where it is so that they can press it in their own time. Once the recording is complete, the therapist should listen to the recording to make sure that the voices and music were captured and are understandable and that the volume levels are audible. If the therapist completed a trial recording before the actual recording, the settings for capturing the voices and music should have been optimized, and therefore few problems should occur. Some families will choose to listen back to the recording while others will choose not to. At this point, the family can re-record sections of the recording or the entire thing if there is a problem with sound or legibility or if the family is not satisfied with the product. Please note that it will be possible for families to access previous GarageBand™ recordings (unless they have been deleted), including those made by other patients and families. The therapist must take care to ensure that the family only accesses their recordings so that confidentiality of work is maintained.

Once the recording is complete, the therapist offers time for discussion or musical expression around the recording process. Before the end of the session, the family and the patient each receive a CD with the recording or an MP3 file, depending on their playback preferences. The therapist should then discuss with the interdisciplinary team appropriate times for the recording to be played, ensuring that a staff member is present during playback in order to observe for signs of distress in the patient as well as turn the recording off when it has finished playing. Sometimes family members will record over an hour of music. It is recommended that stimulation for a person in a low awareness state be provided for short durations of time (Wilson, Cranny, & Andrews, 1992). Therefore, the recording should be played for only 15 to 30 minutes at a time, depending on the patient's ability to tolerate the stimulation. Staff should be encouraged to take note of the track number or time that the recording was stopped in order to have a starting place for the next listening session.

GUIDELINES FOR COMPOSITIONAL MUSIC THERAPY

Songwriting has been shown to improve grief processing, promote expression of emotion, develop self-awareness, and assist with coping (Baker & Wigram, 2005; Baker, Wigram, Scott, & McFarren, 2008; Dalton & Krout, 2005). Although children in a low awareness state cannot participate in songwriting, it can be a useful method of assisting family members in coping with the emotions and grief around having a loved one in such a state.

Family Songwriting

Overview. Family songwriting can promote bonding among family members as well as help families process the grief of their child's loss of abilities, hospitalization, and the loss of hopes and wishes that they had for their child. Through the course of writing a song, emotions are explored and feelings are released (Baker & Wigram, 2005). This release and exploration of emotions can be a valuable tool for the families of children in a low awareness state, as they are often faced with many questions, difficult decisions, and fear of what their child's future will look like.

Songwriting can be most helpful to families that have recently been given the news that their loved one is unlikely to recover from a lowered state of consciousness. These families are at risk for losing all hope and distancing themselves from the child. Songwriting can assist them in expressing and learning to cope with the many changes that they are facing (Dileo & Parker, 2005).

The music therapist providing songwriting experiences for these families requires special training in grief and loss. This author recommends that the therapist receive professional supervision during the time of working with the family as they may express severe grief and anger. The music therapist needs to be prepared to effectively work with these emotions and be able to provide support during and after cathartic experiences that may arise.

Preparation. The songwriting sessions should take place in a private room. The therapist should have all recording equipment set up and ready for use. Additionally, notebooks, pens, and art materials should be in the room for family members to write down or explore ideas for their song, and a variety of instruments should be available to promote creativity (Baker & Wigram, 2005).

What to observe. It is important that the music therapist be well informed of signs that may indicate depression, suicidal tendencies, and post-traumatic stress disorder. If a family member demonstrates actions or verbalizes these thoughts, there may be a need for referral to a medical professional for further assessment and medication.

Procedures. A variety of techniques can be used to help facilitate songwriting. Fill-in-the-blank, piggybacking, and original compositions are among the most common (Baker & Wigram, 2005). Fill-in-the-blank songs provide a structured experience and allow family members to simply complete sentences in the songwriting process. Templates for fill-in-the-blank songs can be found in books such as *Songwriting for the Music Therapist* (Brunk, n.d.). Therapists can also use familiar songs, deleting a portion of the actual words and leaving that portion blank for the patient to fill in. A third method of fill-in-the-blank songwriting is for the therapist to develop original songs that are composed with blanks in them (Baker & Wigram, 2005). Such therapist-composed song offers the advantage of using lyrics that target specific needs of individual families. Piggyback songs provide families with a musical structure that is familiar to them. The family works together to change the lyrics of an existing song to express their own thoughts and feelings (O'Callaghan, 1996; Salmon, 1993; Slivka & Bailey, 1986). This author has found that this type of songwriting is often a good warm-up for families and is especially successful with young children. Finally, original compositions allow for complete creative freedom (Baker & Wigram, 2005). The family chooses the musical motifs and song structure either through loops in a music software program such as GarageBand™ or by examples played by the therapist. If there is a musician in the family, they can be invited to create an instrumental part of the song.

Once a type of songwriting intervention has been chosen, the therapist's role is to support the family through the process both emotionally and musically. The therapist uses counseling and musical skills to ground, validate, and support the emotions expressed in the song (Baker & Wigram, 2005). If the family members choose to write a song for the child, the therapist should guide the process so that it does not become too emotional. Song with emotionally intense lyrics and/or performances can be traumatizing for the patient. This author has found that encouraging family members to give messages to their child is often helpful in reducing the amount of emotional content in the song. This type of guidance can also be beneficial when family members are at different stages of grieving or acceptance.

Once the song is written for the child, the therapist can approach individual family members about writing a song that describes their unique feelings surrounding the diagnosis of their loved one. Songwriting has been used in the palliative care setting to offer patients opportunities to connect with and express their feelings at their own pace. For the individual family member, songwriting may present an opportunity for portraying feelings about the patient (Bruscia, 1991); exploring images, dreams, and fantasies (Magill-Leverault, 1993); and creating lasting memories (Bruscia, 1991).

RESEARCH EVIDENCE

Very few studies exist that examine the effectiveness of music therapy techniques with patients in low awareness states. However, results of the few available quantitative studies show great benefit. An overview of these studies is discussed below. No qualitative studies were identified in the literature.

Receptive Music Therapy

Perhaps the area with the most amount of research related to music therapy and disorders of consciousness is that of physiologic arousal. Several studies make recommendations for placing people in low awareness states in stimulation-rich environments (Ansdell, 1991; Mitchell, Bradley, Welch, & Britton 1990). It is typical for patients in low awareness states to reside in sensory-deprived environments; they are often isolated in hospital rooms and sometimes have limited visitors. Sounds and events may be absent. Unless an active effort is made to provide appropriate sensory stimulation, these patients may not receive a sufficient amount of stimulation to foster neurologic and cognitive recovery. Researchers have investigated the use of stimulation to promote changes in the awareness level and responsiveness of individuals in low awareness states. Whereas some of this research suggests that sensory stimulation positively affects the responsiveness of comatose, PVS, and MCS patients (Kater, 1989; Mitchell et al, 1990; Sison, 1990; Wilson, Powell, Elliott, & Thwaites, 1991), other studies found that sensory stimulation may not affect arousal (Wilson, Cranny, & Andrews, 1992). In addition to the inconsistent results of these studies, controversy exists over determining the most effective amount of stimulation.

Ansdell (1991) and Mitchell et al. (1990) reason that exposure to frequent and varied sensory stimulation facilitates *dendritic* growth and improves synaptic connections, even in people with severe nervous system damage. Therefore, sensory stimulation may promote cognitive functioning as well as awareness. In a study with 24 coma patients (Mitchell et al., 1990), the experimental group (n = 12) received stimulation to all five senses, with wood blocks, tuning forks, and voice used for auditory stimulation. When compared to a no–sensory stimulation control group, patients in the experimental group came out of the coma earlier [$t(11)$ = 2.38, p = 0.05].

Wilson et al. (1992) studied four individuals receiving multimodal stimulation. The participants received two stimulation sessions a day for a period of 23 days. Results suggested that two patients showed statistically significant improvements in behavioral responses to stimulation from pre- to posttest [$t(14)$ = 2.47, p < 0.025 and $t(14)$ = 3.53, p < 0.005], while two patients did not demonstrate any statistically significant changes.

Some research has demonstrated a connection between arousal and memory facilitation. Kater (1989) suggests that because of the frequent memory impairments of brain injury survivors, stimulation should focus on experiences and behaviors learned prior to injury. The underlying principle is that personalized sensory stimulation, like recordings of favorite music, may help the patient connect the stimulus to a past experience. Kater studied 30 adult participants divided into two groups. The experimental group received two 45-minute sensory stimulation sessions per day for up to three months. Sensory stimulation was provided based on an experience and interest questionnaire filled out by patients' families. When compared with the control group, which received typical interaction by nursing staff, the experimental group showed a statistically significant improvement in cognitive functioning scores [$t(28)$ = 2.20, p < .05].

Many of the studies on sensory stimulation include a musical component in their experimental design. Thaut and colleagues (2009) point to evidence that music connects attention networks through the analysis of perceptual patterns in music. Adult participants in this study (N = 63) were divided into two groups. Both groups received the Digit Span subset of the Wechsler Adult Intelligence Scale–III, Auditory Verbal Learning Test, Part B of the Trail Making Test, the Global Severity Index from the Brief Symptom Inventory 18, the Multiple Affect Adjective Check List, and an adapted Self-Efficacy Questionnaire test measuring cognitive skills and emotional adjustment prior to and after the session. The treatment group took part in 30 minutes of neurologic music therapy (NMT) techniques aimed at promoting attention, memory, executive functioning, emotional adjustment, self-efficacy, and patient satisfaction. The control group was given 30 minutes of rest. The results suggested that neither group showed improvement in attention skills. However, the authors reported a statistically significant pre- to posttest difference in executive functioning skills for the treatment group [$t(18)$ = 3.82, p < 0.01], but not for the control group [$t(15)$ = 1.63, p = 0.06]. Emotional adjustment improved significantly for both the control group [$t(14)$ = 2.64, p = 0.01] and the NMT group [$t(22)$ = 3.60, p < 0.02]. No improvements were found for memory skills.

Rosenfeld and Dun (1999) used a combination of live and familiar music listening experiences to accelerate emergence from coma and help orient children with severe brain injury (N = 10). Anecdotally noted responses included changes in heart rate, orienting to sounds, and vocalizing in songs. They theorized that music therapy might directly influence the injured brain because of its influence on the *cerebral cortex, limbic system, basal ganglia, hypothalamus,* and *reticular activating system.*

Musicokinetic therapy, as discussed in the guidelines for receptive music therapy section above, was designed to promote simultaneous activation of multiple neurologic pathways in order to encourage awareness of the patient. In a study by Noda, Maeda, and Yoshino (2003), outcomes were measured by an assessment tool for PVS developed by the Society for Treatment of Coma in Japan. The authors reported that patients (N = 26) achieved better scores after musicokinetic treatment (18.77 ± 7.68) than before (10.5 ± 4.74), and this difference was statistically significant (p < .0001). They also found that treatment was most effective when initiated within six months of injury.

One article on contingent music shows the potential benefit of such an intervention. Boyle and Greer (1983) provided contingent music therapy interventions to three patients in vegetative and semicomatose states. Although the research had great variability and requires further investigation, clinical significant findings for two out of the three behaviors were determined. Eye squeeze and finger or head movement showed greater behavioral responses in all three subjects with the use of contingent music. One participant showed a mean eye squeeze of .9 at baseline and 4.7 during contingent music. Another participant demonstrated a baseline of .5 and a contingent music mean of 3.5, and the third participant's baseline mean was .44, whereas his contingent music mean was 2. Small movement (finger or head movement) data for the participants showed baselines of 1.9, .75, and .17, with 4.6, 2.5, and 1.1 during contingent music. The third behavior observed was mouth movement. Although all three participants demonstrated increased frequency of mouth movements during the contingent music intervention, the results were less than those of eye squeeze and small body movements. Participants demonstrated a baseline mean of 1.9, .34, and 0. Contingent music means improved to 3.8, .5, and .31. Furthermore, one participant showed great success in learning that producing a behavior resulted in musical reward. This success demonstrates that contingent music is most effective with patients in a less deteriorated state.

Overall, the studies on effectiveness of sensory stimulation, including music, in patients in low awareness states show a trend toward improvement of functioning. However, there are a number of studies that suggest a lack of improvement (Zasler, Kruetzer, & Taylor, 1991). Therefore, further research is needed to determine the true benefit of sensory stimulation, and more specifically musical stimulation, for people in low awareness states.

Improvisational Music Therapy

Aldridge, Gustorff, and Hannich (1990) provided improvised vocal music based on the pulse tempo and breathing patterns of five coma patients with GCS scores ranging between 4 and 7. During the eight- to twelve-minute music therapy interventions, the authors measured brain waves through EEG. Although these authors did not report statistical data, their anecdotes showed an increase in a range of reactions such as change in breath rhythms, fine motor movement, turning of the head, and eye opening. Additionally, the authors discussed the EEG findings. EEG measurements demonstrated that desynchronized theta rhythms (47 cycles per second, representing dream states) became alpha (8 to 12 cycles per second) or beta rhythms (18 to 40 cycles per second) that were synchronized. This type of synchronization represents arousal and perceptual activity in the brain. The changes in brain activity faded out when the music therapy stopped. Additional changes in breathing, fine motor movements, grabbing movements of the hand, head turning, eye opening, and even regaining consciousness were documented.

Re-creative Music Therapy

Re-creative music therapy research literature does not include work done specifically with children or families of children in low awareness states. Research shows that families dealing with the trauma and hospitalization of a child are at risk for experiencing circumstances that impact their ability to bond and interact with their children (Kelly, Buehlman, & Caldwell, 2000; Morton & Brown, 1998). Family relationships as well as the personal, social, and economic resources of the family impact each individual's physical, social, and emotional well-being (Sanders, 1999). Yet, this has not received attention in the music therapy research literature.

One phenomenological qualitative study used family-centered music therapy within a play group setting with children at risk for developmental delay. The program was meant to nurture creative expression and enjoyment in family members and help build mothers' confidence in creating any kind of music. Results of the study demonstrated that music was able to support families in developing skills to enhance their relationships with their children (Shoemark, 1996). In a descriptive article by Oldfield and Bunce (2001), music therapy treatment was successful in engaging mothers and their children in positive interactions like play and intimacy. Their interventions included greeting songs, instrument playing, mother and toddler solos, and action songs.

The success of music therapy in supporting and promoting interpersonal bonding has been shown to be effective through the above studies. Families working to develop new bonds with their child in a low awareness state can benefit from the same approaches and interventions. At this time, research on the impact of music therapy on family-child bonding in children in low awareness states is urgently needed.

SUMMARY AND CONCLUSIONS

Diagnoses and treatment of children in low awareness states is ever changing. As research continues to define disorders of consciousness and establish appropriate treatment methods, music therapists will need to adjust their protocols and treatment plans to reflect this new knowledge. Furthermore, music therapy researchers may play a vital role in developing evaluations and interventions for children in such states with respect to music and its interaction with the brain.

Currently, music therapists working in a pediatric setting that treats low awareness states should be cautious in their treatment. A child emerging from consciousness or with limited consciousness requires special treatment in order to ensure that overstimulation does not occur. Observation skills must be honed and flexibility within the session must be present. These therapists should also pay close attention to family needs. Music therapy interventions as outlined in this chapter can assist the family in bonding, feeling empowered, and expressing emotions centered on their loved one's state and care.

It is recommended that the novice therapist seek support through professional supervision when working with patients in low awareness states, as this type of work can lead to many ethical and existential questions. In addition, therapists will be confronted with difficult situations and must explore their own emotional reactions in order to support those of the child's family.

Unfortunately, children in low awareness states may not be considered prime candidates for music therapy services because of their inability to produce overt responses or participate in music-making. Yet, brain research shows that auditory stimulation, specifically music stimulation, offers unique opportunities for arousal and communication in patients with low awareness states. Therefore, music therapists have the ethical responsibility to bring music therapy services to these children, and the music therapy research community needs to take up the challenge to carefully investigate the efficacy of music therapy for arousal and awareness in these children.

Glossary

The following definitions are based on *The Merriam-Webster Online Dictionary* (n.d.) and *The American Heritage Medical Dictionary* (2007).

Amygdala: One of the four basal ganglia in each cerebral hemisphere that is part of the limbic system and consists of an almond-shaped mass of gray matter in the roof of the lateral ventricle —also called *amygdaloid body* or *amygdaloid nucleus*

Anoxic Brain Injury: Hypoxia or deprivation of oxygen in the brain of such severity as to result in permanent damage

Autonomic Functions: Bodily functions that occur involuntarily or are controlled by the autonomic nervous system

Basal Ganglia: A region of the base of the brain that consists of three clusters of neurons that are responsible for involuntary movements such as tremors, athetosis (uncontrolled rhythmic writhing movement), and chorea (involuntary jerky movements)

Brain Stem: The part of the brain composed of the midbrain, pons, and medulla oblonggata that connects the spinal cord with the forebrain and cerebrum

Central Nervous System: The part of the nervous system which, in vertebrates, consists of the brain and spinal cord. The central nervous system is responsible for sending, receiving, and interpreting information from all parts of the body. It receives information from and sends information to the peripheral nervous system.

Cerebral Cortex: The layer of unmyelinated neurons (the grey matter) forming the cortex of the cerebrum. The cerebral cortex is largely responsible for higher brain functions, including sensation, voluntary muscle activity and learning, language, and memory.

Cingulate Cortex: A component of the limbic system of the brain, responsible for producing emotional responses to physical sensations of pain

Cyclosporine: An immunosuppressive drug used to prevent rejection of transplanted organs

Dentrite: A short branched extension of a nerve cell, along which impulses received from other cells at synapses are transmitted to the cell body

Electroencephalogram: The tracing of brain waves made by an electroencephalograph or a piece of equipment that measures brain waves

Extraocular Eye Muscles: The six voluntary muscles that move the eyeball: superior, inferior, middle, and lateral recti, and superior and inferior oblique muscles

Fibrotic Endoscopy: Diagnosis and treatment of swallowing disorders by means of a flexible fiberoptic endoscope introduced transnasally into the hypopharynx

Fluorodexyglucose (FDG): A radio-fluorine derivative used to trace metabolic activity or detect malignant tissue; commonly used as the agent in positron emission tomography (PET)

Functional Magnetic Resonance Imaging (fMRI): Magnetic resonance imaging used to detect physical changes (as of blood flow) in the brain resulting from increased neuronal activity

Hippocampus: A ridge in the floor of each lateral ventricle of the brain that consists mainly of gray matter and has a central role in memory processes

Hypotension: Abnormally low blood pressure

Hypothalamus: The area of the brain that secretes substances that influence pituitary and other gland function and is involved in the control of body temperature, hunger, thirst, and other processes that regulate body equilibrium

Invertebral Disc: A fibrocartilaginous disc serving as a cushion between all of the vertebrae of the spinal column (except between the first two)

Isoelectric EEG: An EEG in which no brain waves are recorded, indicating a complete lack of brain
    activity, consistent with brain death

Limbic: Of, relating to, or being the limbic system of the brain

Limbic System: A group of subcortical structures (the hypothalamus, the hippocampus, and the
    amygdala) of the brain that are concerned especially with emotion and motivation

Magnetic Resonance Imaging (MRI): A noninvasive diagnostic technique that produces computerized
    images of internal body tissues

Medulla: The part of the brain that contains the centers controlling involuntary vita functions

Myocardial Infarction: An acute episode of heart disease marked by the death or damage of heart muscle
    due to insufficient blood supply to the heart usually as a result of a coronary thrombosis or a
    coronary occlusion and that is characterized especially by chest pain; a heart attack

Neuroplasticity: Capacity of neurons and neural networks in the brain to change their connections and
    behavior in response to new information, sensory stimulation, development, damage, or
    dysfunction

Parietal Cortex: Part of the brain, specifically the section of the cerebral hemisphere that lies beneath the
    parietal bone, the main side bone of the skull

Positron Emission Tomography (PET): A sectional view of the body constructed by positron-emission
    tomography

Prefrontal Cortex: Of, relating to, or situated in the anterior part of the frontal lobe of the brain

Radionuclide Cerebral Blood Flow Scan: A scan that tests for a specific type of atom that exhibits
    radioactivity

Regression: A relapse to a less developed state

Reticular Activating System: The network in the reticular formation that serves an alerting or arousal
    function

Single-Photon Emission Computerized Tomography (SPECT): The recording of internal body images at a
    predetermined plane by means of the tomograph

Sinusoidal Low Frequency Tone: A low-frequency tone that is of, relating to, shaped like, or varying
    according to a sine curve or sine wave

Synaptic Connections: A connection made between two synapses

Tacrolimus: An immunosuppressive drug used in combination with corticosteroids to prevent rejection
    of organ transplants

Thalamus: A large, ovoid mass of gray matter that serves chiefly to relay sensory impulses to and from the
    cerebral cortex

Thrombosis: The formation or presence of a blood clot within a blood vessel

REFERENCES

Aldridge, D. (1996). From out of the silence. Music therapy: Breaking new ground .*AMTA Conference
    Collection, 2,* 41–51.

Aldridge, D., Gustorff, D., & Hannich, H. J. (1990). Where am I? Music therapy applied to coma patients.
    Journal of the Royal Society of Medicine, 83, 345–346.

American Congress of Rehabilitation Medicine. (1995). Recommendations for the use of uniform
    nomenclature pertinent to patients with severe alterations in consciousness. *Archives of Physical
    Medicine and Rehabilitation, 76,* 205–209.

Anderson, R. (1994). *Practitioner's guide to clinical neuropsychology.* New York, NY: Plenum Press.

Andrews, K. (1996). International working party on the management of the vegetative state: Summary
    report. *Brain Injury, 10,* 797–806.

Ansell, B. J. (1991). Slow-to-recover brain injured patients: Rationale for treatment. *Journal of Speech and Hearing Research, 34* (5), 1017–1022.

Ashwal, S., Bale, J. F. Jr., Coulter, D. L., Elbin, R., Garg, B. P., Myer, E. C.,...Sunder, T. R. (1992). The persistent vegetative state in children: Report of the child neurology society ethics committee. *Annals of Neurology, 32,* 570–576.

Baker, F., & Wigram, T. (2005). *Songwriting: Methods, techniques and clinical applications for music therapy.* Philadelphia, PA: Jessica Kingsley.

Baker, F., Wigram, T., Stott, D., & McFerran, K. (2008). Therapeutic songwriting in music therapy. *Nordic Journal of Music Therapy, 17*(2), 105–123.

Bauer, G., Gerstenbrand, F., & Rumpl, E. (1979). Varieties of the locked-in syndrome. *Journal of Neurology, 221* (2), 77–91.

Bergstrom-Isacsson, M. (2011). Music and vibroacoustic stimulation in people with Rett Syndrome: A neurophysiological study. Unpublished doctoral dissertation. Aalborg University, Denmark.

Boly, M., Faymonville, M. E., Peigneux, P., Lambermont, B., Damas, F., Luxen, A.,...Laureys, S. (2005). Cerebral processing of auditory and noxious stimuli in severely brain-injured patients: Differences between VS and MCS. *Neuropsychological Rehabilitation, 15,* 283–289.

Bordini, A. L., Luiz, T. F., Fernandes, M., Arruda, W. O., & Teive, H. A. (2010). Coma scales: A historical review. *Arquivos de Neuro-psiquiatria,* 930–937.

Boyle, M., & Greer, R. (1983). Operant procedures and the comatose patient. *Journal of Applied Behavior Analysis, 16* (1), 3–12.

Bradt, J. (2009). Music for breathing regulation. In J. Loewy (Ed.), *Music, the breath & health: Advances in integrative music therapy.* New York, NY: Louis Armstrong Center for Music & Medicine.

Bradt, J., & Dileo, C. (2010) Music therapy for end-of-life care *Cochrane Database of Systematic Reviews,* 2010, 1. Art. no.: CD006787. DOI: 10.1002/14651858.CD006787.pub2.

Brunk, B. (n.d.). *Songwriting for the music therapist.* University of California: Prelude Music Therapy.

Bruscia, K. (1987). *Improvisational models of music therapy.* Illinois: Charles C. Thomas.

Bruscia, K. E. (1991). The fundamentals of music therapy practice. In K. E. Bruscia (Ed.), *Case studies in music therapy* (pp. 3–13). Gilsum, NH: Barcelona Publishers.

Byock, I. (1997). *Dying well: The prospect for growth at the end of life.* New York, NY: Riverhead Books.

Byock, I. (2004). *The four things that matter most: A book about living.* New York, NY: Free Press.

Cartlidge, N. (2001). States related to or confused with coma. *Journal of Neurology, Neurosurgery, and Psychiatry, 71* (1), 18–19.

Chlan, L. (1998). Effectiveness of a music therapy intervention on relaxation and anxiety for patients receiving ventilatory assistance. *Heart & Lung, 27* (3), 169–176.

Cranford, R. (1994). Medical aspects of the persistent vegetative state. *New England Journal of Medicine, 330,* 1499–1508.

Crick, F. H. (1994). *The astonishing hypothesis: The scientific search for the soul.* New York: Scribners.

Dalton, T., & Krout, R. (2005). Development of the grief process scale through music therapy songwriting with bereaved adolescents. *The Arts in Psychotherapy, 32* (2), 131–143.

Dileo, C., & Magill, L. (2005). Songwriting with oncology and hospice adult patients from a multicultural perspective. In F. Baker & T. Wigram (Eds.), *Songwriting: Methods and clinical applications for music therapy clinicians, educators and students* (pp. 226–245). Philadelphia, PA: Jessica Kingsley.

Dileo, C., & Parker, C. (2005). Final Moments: The use of song in relationship completion. In C. Dileo & J. Loewy (Eds.), *Music therapy at the end of life.* Cherry Hill, NJ: Jeffrey Books.

Drubach, D. (2000). *The brain explained.* Upper Saddle River, NJ: Prentice-Hall.

Erbengi, A., Erbengi, G., Cataltepe, O., Topcu, M., Erbas, B., & Aras, T. (1991). Brain death: Determination with brain stem-evoked potentials and radionuclide isotope studies. *Acta Neurochirurgica, 112* (3–4), 118–125.

Fager, S., Hux, K., Beukelman, D. R., & Karantounis, R. (2006). Use of safe-laser access technology to increase head movements in persons with severe motor impairments: A series of case reports. *Augmentative and Alternative Communication, 22* (3), 222–229.

Giacino, J., Kezmarsky, M., DeLuca, J., & Cicerone, K. (1991). Monitoring rate of recovery to predict outcome in minimally responsive patients. *Archives of Physical Medicine and Rehabilitation, 72* (11), 897–901.

Giacino, J. T., Ashwal, S., Childs, N., Cranford, R., Jennett, B., & Katz, D. I. (2002). The minimally conscious state: Definition and diagnostic criteria. *Neurology, 58* (3), 349–353.

Giacino J. T., & Zasler, N. D. (1995). Outcome after severe traumatic brain injury: coma, the vegetative state and the minimally responsive state. *Journal of Head Trauma and Rehabilitation, 10,* 40–56.

Gill-Thwaites, H. (1997). The Sensory Modality Assessment Rehabilitation Technique: A tool for assessment and treatment of patients with severe brain injury in a vegetative state. *Brain Injury, 11* (10), 723–734.

Gopnik, A., Meltzoff, A. N., & Kuhl, P. K. (1999). *The scientist in the crib*: M*inds, brains, and how children learn.* New York, NY: Morrow.

Griffin, M. J. (1983). Effects of vibration on humans. In R. Lawrence (Ed.), *Proceedings of internoise, 1,* (pp. 1–14). Edinburgh: Institute of Acoustics.

Hagen, C., Malkmus, D., & Durham, P. (1972). Original Rancho Los Amigos Cognitive Scale. Rancho Los Amigos Hospital.

Hilliard, R. (2001). The effects of music therapy-based bereavement groups on mood and behavior of grieving children: A pilot study. *Journal of Music Therapy, 38* (4), 291–306.

Hilliard, R. (2005). Music therapy in hospice and palliative care: A review of empirical data. *Evidence-Based Complementary and Alternative Medicine, 2* (2), 173–178.

Jansen, E. (1993). *Singing bowls: A practical handbook of instruction and use.* Holland: Binkey Kok Publications.

Jennett, B. (1999). Should cases of permanent vegetative state still go to court? Britain should follow other countries and keep the courts for cases of dispute. *British Medical Journal* (Clinical research ed.), *319,* 796–807.

Jochim, S. (1994). Establishing contact in the early stage of craniocerebral trauma: Sound as the bridge to mute patients. *Rehabilitation, 35,* 8–13.

Jones, J. D. (2005). A comparison of songwriting and lyric analysis techniques to evoke emotional change in a single session with people who are chemically dependent. *Journal of Music Therapy, 42* (2), 94–111.

Kater, K. M. (1989). Response of head-injured patients to sensory stimulation. *West Journal of Nursing Research, 1,* 20–33.

Kelly, J. F., Buehlman, K., & Caldwell, K. (2000). Training personnel to promote quality parent-child interaction in families who are homeless. *Topics in Early Childhood Special Education, 30* (3), 174–189.

Koch, C. (2004). *The Quest for consciousness: A neurobiological approach.* Englewood, CO: Roberts and Company.

Lancioni, G. E., Bosco, A., Belardinelli, M. O., Singh, N. N., O'Reilly, M. F., & Sigafoos, J. (2010). An overview of intervention options for promoting adaptive behavior of persons with acquired brain injury and minimally conscious state. *Research in Developmental Disabilities, 31* (6), 1121–1134.

Larsen, K., & Ayllon, T. (1990). The effects of contingent music and differential reinforcement on infantile colic. *Behavior Research and Therapy, 28,* 119–125.

Laureys, S., Owen, A. M., & Schiff, N. D. (2004). Brain function in coma, vegetative state, and related disorders. *The Lancet Neurology, 3* (9), 537–546.

Lehrer, P. M., Vaschillo, E., & Vaschillo, B. (2000). Resonant frequency biofeedback training to increase cardiac variability: Rationale and manual for training. *Applied Psychophysiology and Biofeedback, 25* (3), 177–191.

Liversedge, T., & Hirsch, N. (2010). Coma. *Anesthesia & Intensive Care Medicine, 11* (9), 337–339.

Magee, W. (2005). Music Therapy with patients in low awareness states: Approaches to assessment and treatment in multidisciplinary care. *Neuropsychological Rehabilitation, 15* (3–4), 522–536.

Magee, W. (2007). Music as a diagnostic tool in low awareness states: Considering limbic responses. *Brain Injury, 21* (6), 593–599.

Magee, W. (2008). Using music in leisure to enhance social relationships with patients with complex disabilities. *NeuroRehabilitation 23* (4), 305–311.

Magill-Levreault, L. (1993). Music therapy in pain and symptom. *Management Journal of Palliative Care, 9* (4), 42–48.

Mitchell, S., Bradley, V. A., Welch, J. L., & Britton, P. G. (1990). Coma arousal procedure: A therapeutic intervention in the treatment of head injury. *Brain Injury, 4* (3), 273–279.

Morton, N., & Brown, K. (1998). Theory and observation of attachment and its relation to child maltreatment: A review. *Child Abuse and Neglect, 2* (1), 1093–1104.

Noda, R., Maeda, Y., & Yoshino, A. (2003). Effects of musicokinetic therapy and spinal cord stimulation on patients in a persistent vegetative state. *Acta Neurochirurgica, 87,* 23–26.

O'Callaghan, C. (1996). Lyrical themes in songs written by palliative care patients. *Journal of Music Therapy, 33* (2), 74–92.

Oldfield, A., & Bunce, L. (2001). 'Mummy can play too….' Short-term music therapy with mothers and young children. *British Journal of Music Therapy, 15* (1), 27–36.

Papousek, M. (1996). Intuitive parenting: A hidden source of musical stimulation in infancy. In I. Deliege & J. Sloboda (Eds.), *Musical beginnings.* Oxford: Oxford University Press.

Punkanen, M., & Ala-Ruona, E. (2012). Contemporary vibroacoustic therapy: Perspectives on clinical practice, research, and training. *Music and Medicine, 4* (3), 128–135.

Rider, M. (1985). Entrainment mechanisms are involved in pain reduction, muscle relaxation and music-mediated imagery. *Journal of Music Therapy, 22* (4), 183–192.

Rosenfeld, J., & Dun, B. (1999). Music therapy and children with severe traumatic brain injuries. In R. R. Pratt & D. E. Grocke (Eds.), *Proceedings of the 1998 ISMM conference.* Melbourne: The University of Melbourne Press.

Salmon, D. (1993). Music and emotion in palliative care. *Journal of Palliative Care, 9* (4), 48–52.

Sanders, M. (1999). The triple P-positive parenting program: Towards an empirically validated multilevel parenting and family support strategy for the prevention of behaviour and emotional problems in children. *Clinical Child and Family Psychology Review, 2* (2), 71–90.

Schiff, N., Rodriguez-Moreno, D., Kamal, A., Kim, K. H., Giacino, J., Plum, F., & Hirsch, J. (2005). fMRI reveals large-scale network activation in minimally conscious patients. *Neurology, 64,* 514–523.

Schirrmacher, R. (1988). *Art and creative development for young children.* Albany, NY: Delmar Publishers. Schnackers, C., Giacino, J., & Laureys, S. (2012). Coma: Detecting signs of consciousness in severely brain injured patients recovering from coma. *International Encyclopedia of Rehabilitation.* Retrieved from: http://cirrie.buffalo.edu/encyclopedia/en/article/133/

Segall, L. (2007). The effect of patient preferred live versus recorded music on non-responsive patients in the hospital setting as evidence by physiological and behavioral states. Unpublished master's thesis. Florida State University, Tallahassee, FL.

Sherman, S. (2006). Thalamus. *Scholarpedia, 1* (9), 1583.

Shiel, A., Horn, S., Wilson, B., Watson, M., Campbell, J., & McLellan, D. (2000). The Wessex Head Injury Matrix (WHIM) main scale: A preliminary report on a scale to assess and monitor patient recovery after severe head injury. *Clinical Rehabilitation, 14* (4), 408–416.

Shoemark, H. (1996). Family-centred early intervention: Music therapy in the playgroup program. *Australian Journal of Music Therapy, 7,* 3–15.

Sisson, R. (1990). Effects of auditory stimuli on comatose patients with head injury. *Heart & Lung: The Journal of Acute and Critical Care, 19,* 373–378.

Skille, O. (1989a). Vibroacoustic research. In R. Spintge & R. Droh (Eds.), *Music medicine.* St. Louis, MO: Magna Music Baton.

Skille, O. (1989b). Vibroacoustic therapy. *Music Therapy: Journal of the American Association for Music Therapy, 8,* 61–77.

Slivka, H., & Bailey, L. (1986). The conjoint use of social work and music therapy with children of cancer patients. *Music Therapy, 6* (1), 30–40.

Standley, J. (2000). The effect of contingent music to increase non-nutritive sucking of premature infants. *Pediatric Nursing, 26* (5), 493–499.

Sullivan, J., Seem, D. L., & Chabalewski, F. (1999). The brain explained. *Critical Care Nurse, 19* (2), 37–44.

Tamplin, J. (2000). Improvisational music therapy approaches to coma arousal. *Australian Journal of Music Therapy, 11,* 38–51.

Teasdale, G., & Jennett, B. (1974). Glasgow Coma Scale. The University of Glasgow.

Thaut, M., Gardiner, J., Holmberg, D., Horwitz, J., Kent, L., Andrews, G.,...McIntosh, G. (1990). Neurologic music therapy improves executive function and emotional adjustment in traumatic brain injury rehabilitation. *The Neurosciences and Music III–Disorders and Plasticity: Annals of the New York Academy of Sciences, 1169,* 406–416.

The American Academy of Neurology. (1988). Position of the American Academy of Neurology on certain aspects of the care and management of the persistent vegetative state patient: Adopted by the Executive Board, American Academy of Neurology, *Neurology, 39,* 125–126.

The American Academy of Neurology. (1995). Practice parameters: Assessment and management of patients in the persistent vegetative state. *Neurology, 45,* 1015–1018.

The American Electroencephalographic Society. (1986). Guidelines in EEG and evoked potentials. *Journal of Clinical Neurophysiology, 3* (supplement), 43.

The Medical Task Force on Anencephaly. (1990). The infant with anencephaly. *New England Journal of Medicine, 322,* 669–674.

The Multi-Society Task Force on PVS. (1994). Medical aspects of the persistent vegetative state—second of two parts. *New England Journal of Medicine, 330* (22), 1572–1579.

Waters, C. E., French, G., & Burt, M. (2004). Difficulty in brainstem death testing in the presence of high spinal cord injury. *British Journal of Anesthesia, 92* (5), 762–764.

Webster, Inc. (2003). *Merriam-Webster's collegiate dictionary* (11th ed.). Springfield, MA: Merriam-Webster, Inc.

Weyhenmyeye, J. A., & Gallman, E. A. (2007). *Rapid review neuroscience* (1st ed.), 177–179. Philadelphia: Elsevier, Health Sciences Division.

Wheeler, B. (1981). The relationship between music therapy and theories of psychotherapy. *Music Therapy, 1* (1), 9–16.

Wigram, T. (1993). "The Feeling of Sound"—The effect of music and low-frequency sound in reducing anxiety in challenging behaviour in clients with learning difficulties. In H. Payne (Ed.), *Handbook of enquiry in the arts therapies: "one river, many currents"* (pp. 177–197). Philadelphia, PA: Jessica Kingsley.

Wijdicks, E. F. (2006). Clinical scales for comatose patients: The Glasgow Coma Scale in historical context and the new FOUR Score. *Reviews in Neurological Disease, 3* (3), 109–117.

Wilson, S., Cranny, S., & Andrews, K. (1992). The efficacy of music for stimulation in prolonged coma: Four single case experiments. *Clinical Rehabilitation, 6* (3), 181–187.

Wilson, S., Powell, G., Elliott, K., & Thwaites, H. (1991). Sensory stimulation in prolonged coma: Four single case studies. *Brain Injury, 5,* 393–400.

Yamada, S., Ikugi, M., Fujikata, S., Watanabe, T., & Kosaka, T. (1983). Body sensation of low-frequency noise of ordinary persons and profoundly deaf persons. *Journal of Low Frequency Noise and Vibration, 2* (3), 32–36.

Ylvisaker, M. (1985). Head injury rehabilitation: Children and adolescents. London: Taylor & Francis.

Zasler, N. D., Kruetzer, J. S., & Taylor, D. (1991). Coma recovery and coma stimulation: A critical review. *NeuroRehabilitation, 1* (3), 33–40.

Chapter 13

Children in General Inpatient Care

Christine Neugebauer

INTRODUCTION

Music therapists working in a pediatric medical setting, whether in a stand-alone children's hospital or in a pediatric unit within a hospital, will most likely encounter a general pediatric medicine service. This unit services children, ranging from newborns to adolescents, with a variety of diagnoses who are in stable condition and require a lower level of care (less critical) compared to children in an intensive care unit or intermediate care unit. Depending upon multiple factors, including diagnosis, treatment needs, psychosocial issues, and availability of outpatient services, length of stay in this unit can range from less than 24 hours to several weeks. Although these children are not in critical condition, they still hold many significant physiological and psychosocial needs that music therapists can help to address with the goal of decreasing the deleterious effects of hospitalization and illness.

Regardless of one's philosophical orientation, having a strong foundation in child development as well as a child-centered approach will only enhance the therapeutic process when working with hospitalized children. The therapeutic relationship maintains an important function and serves as a vehicle to learn and communicate and fosters an environment conducive to healthy growth and development (Aldridge, Gustroff, & Neugebauer, 1995). Because children and adolescents seem to have an innate ability to sense when someone is inauthentic or disingenuous, the music therapist needs to be self-aware. Clinical supervision and consultation are highly suggested for novice or inexperienced clinicians working in this setting. Even experienced music therapists will benefit from supervision and guidance from colleagues and seasoned professionals. Personal therapy for the music therapist can also be helpful for enhancing self-awareness and in assisting in coping with personal reactions that may arise when working with this population. As with many clinical populations, routine practice of self-care strategies will enable the music therapist to maintain professional boundaries and decrease the risk of burnout or vicarious stress. Self-care practices such as healthy eating habits, regular exercise, adequate sleep, and balance between work and recreation should be an ongoing commitment. Ultimately, pediatric music therapists have an ethical responsibility to provide the highest level of quality care.

DIAGNOSTIC INFORMATION

According to the Agency for Healthcare Research and Quality, nearly 17 percent of all hospital stays in 2009 were for children age 17 and younger, accounting for one out of every six discharges from US hospitals (Yu, Wier, & Elixhauser, 2011). A wide variety of diagnoses may warrant an inpatient admission to a general pediatric unit. Acute onset illnesses such as viral infections (e.g., influenza, viral bronchitis), as well as flare-ups or exacerbations of chronic conditions such as *sickle cell disease, inflammatory bowel disease,* and *asthma,* are common. This unit may also include children undergoing diagnostic testing and observation. Depending upon the facility, the general pediatric unit may also include children transferred from other units, such as an intensive care unit or surgical unit, who are stabilized and require a lower level of critical care. Although it is not unusual for trauma patients and surgical patients to be in a general pediatric service, this chapter will focus primarily on acute and chronic conditions frequently encountered in a general pediatric inpatient unit. Although music therapy in pediatric surgery and procedural support will be covered in separate chapters, it is important to be aware that children in the general pediatric unit may have previously undergone surgery or may require various invasive and noninvasive procedures as part of their treatment.

For many children hospitalized in the general pediatric unit, this may be their first and only hospitalization experience. Many common acute ailments, such as *bronchitis, influenza, gastroenteritis, osteomyelitis, appendicitis,* and *pneumonia,* could result in an inpatient hospital stay. Acute medical conditions can be defined as diseases having an "abrupt onset and usually a short course" of treatment or an "illness of short duration, rapidly progressive, and in need of urgent care" (Acute illness: MedicineNet.com, n.d.). In some cases, an acute illness could indicate an underlying chronic condition. The general pediatric unit may be the first place where a child becomes diagnosed with a medical condition such as *epilepsy* or *type 1 diabetes.*

Children with chronic ailments may have frequent inpatient hospitalizations throughout their childhood. A chronic condition is an illness that "has persisted for a long period of time," generally lasting "three months or more" (Chronic illness: MedicineNet.com, n.d.). According to the National Health Interview Survey, the prevalence of chronic illnesses that limit activities of daily living continues to increase in the United States, with approximately 7% of children meeting this criterion (Perrin, Bloom, & Gortmaker, 2012).

Chronic illnesses, as well as some genetic disorders including *cystic fibrosis, sickle cell disease, diabetes, asthma*, and many gastrointestinal disorders, necessitate ongoing treatment. In addition, many infants born prematurely or medically fragile infants previously in the NICU may be admitted to the general pediatric service due to line infections, dehydration, or other ailments.

In addition to encountering many different diagnoses, a music therapist working in the general pediatric unit will also service children ranging in age from newborns to older adolescents, who come from varied socioeconomic, ethnic, cultural, and spiritual backgrounds. Depending upon the location of the hospital facility, the primary language for children and families may not necessarily be English. Family systems will include both traditional and alternative family structures, including blended families, extended families, adoptive families, foster families, and families with gay parents. Moreover, the developmental level of the pediatric patient will also vary extensively. Due to frequent hospitalizations, children with chronic medical conditions are at increased risk for delays in various domains of development (Pao, Ballard, & Rosenstein, 2007). It is also not unusual for children with developmental disorders to have associated medical conditions. For example, many children on the autism spectrum suffer from gastrointestinal dysfunctions, such as constipation, that could require an inpatient hospital stay (Gorrindo et al., 2012). Other medical conditions commonly associated with developmental delays include *cerebral palsy, hydrocephalus, spina bifida,* and seizure disorders. In some cases, the child's illness or injury caused a disruption in the developmental process, resulting in developmental regression.

Failure to thrive (FTT) is another condition that can hinder normal growth and development. FTT "refers to children whose current weight or rate of weight gain is significantly lower than that of other children of similar age and gender" (Failure to thrive: MedlinePlus Medical Encyclopedia, n.d.). Causes for FTT can be of medical origin ranging from premature birth to genetic disorders (e.g., *Trisomy 21*) or due to environmental factors, such as poverty or neglect. Unfortunately, children may be admitted to the pediatric unit due to known or suspected abuse, neglect, and/or medical neglect. These additional psychosocial stressors can certainly complicate the child's emotional and physical recovery and overall well-being. One form of abuse deserving special mention is factitious disorder, or Munchausen syndrome by proxy. Munchausen syndrome by proxy (MSbP) is a "form of child abuse in which a parent or caregiver, usually the mother, intentionally creates or feigns an illness in order to keep the child (and therefore the adult) in prolonged contact with health providers" (Criddle, 2010, p.23). MSbP is difficult to confirm, and when the medical team suspects MSbP, a trial separation involving the child's removal from the family for a period of time usually occurs upon approval by a court of law. During this period of trial separation, the child will generally not be allowed contact with the family and will remain in the hospital and be closely monitored as medications and treatments are weaned. The music therapist can serve a vital role in offering the child emotional support and a safe outlet for self-expression during this separation period.

Finally, it is important to mention that some children admitted to the general pediatric unit may have more than one diagnosis or medical condition or have a concurrent psychiatric disorder. A music therapist may work with children or adolescents who have eating disorders, depression, anxiety disorders, or even suicidal ideations. Some of these children may be awaiting transfer to a psychiatric unit, while others may require having their medical condition stabilized prior to discharge. In cases of suicidal patients, there may be a "sitter" in the room accompanying the patient at all times.

The reasons and range of diagnoses necessitating general inpatient care are unending and can be as simple as a routine case of bronchitis or as complex as diagnosing *mitochondrial disorder*. The music therapist working in this setting can be an important member of the child's treatment team. The music therapist will frequently interact with many members of the child's health care team, including physicians, nurses, case managers, social workers, child life specialists, chaplains, dieticians, and rehabilitation therapists, including physical, occupational, and speech therapists. It is an ethical responsibility of the music therapist to continue learning about the various diagnoses and medical conditions encountered and have an ongoing dialogue with the team in order to provide the highest quality of music therapy services.

NEEDS AND RESOURCES

Even though the illness may be less critical than that of a child on the intensive care unit, the medical, psychosocial, and developmental needs of this population can be multifaceted. Children in the general pediatric unit vary widely in their physical abilities and limitations and medical needs. They may need medical equipment, including leads to vital signs monitors, an IV *(intravenous line)*, a PICC line *(peripherally inserted central catheter)*, a G-tube *(gastrostomy tube)*, a *colostomy bag*, and even a *nasal cannula* for supplemental oxygen. Some of the children may be on isolation precautions restricting them to the hospital room. Isolation precautions may be contact (requiring gown and gloves), airborne (requiring mask), or both. Proficiency in playing the guitar while wearing gloves is an important skill to develop in this environment. Being mindful of what equipment to bring into the music therapy session, especially for patients in isolation, will be necessary. All music therapists working in this setting need to be fully informed and adhere to the infection control guidelines established by the facility, and use hospital-approved cleaners when disinfecting music therapy equipment, including the music therapist's guitar.

In addition to the restrictions related to being connected to monitors, IV medications or oxygen, or restrictions due to isolation precautions, the medical condition or disease process itself may have negative effects on the child's energy level, physical independence, endurance, ability to focus and concentrate, quality of sleep, mental status, developmental skills, pain tolerance, and even mood. Music therapy sessions should be paced according to the child's energy level and, when possible, conducted at a time of day when the child can receive the most benefit from the music therapy intervention. Some children may have pain issues, such as those in sickle cell crisis, exhibit hospital-related anxiety, or, in many cases, experience an interrelated combination of both pain and anxiety. Moreover, medications and treatments may have side effects such as headaches, nausea, and sleepiness. The music therapist should keep current on basic knowledge of disease processes and the potential side effects of medications. The illness, treatments, invasive and noninvasive procedures, and a combination can result in the child having a distorted body image or poor self-concept (Walker, 2009). Offering music therapy interventions that are successful and focus on what the child *can do* may help to improve self-identity both internally and externally.

The hospital environment itself, regardless of the illness, can have an impact, negative or positive, on the child. For children who are experiencing hospitalization for the first time, many aspects of the hospital experience may seem scary, strange, chaotic, unpredictable, and painful (Pao & Bosk, 2011). For these same children, hospitalization could also be a time for them to discover inner strengths, develop constructive coping skills, learn about themselves and the world around them, and develop positive relationships. First-time experiences in the hospital can strongly influence responses to future hospitalizations. Therefore, an opportunity exists for the music therapist to play a viable role through offering the child therapeutic music experiences that empower the child to express feelings, enhance locus of control, foster constructive coping skills, and stimulate developmental skills. For children who have had a previous negative hospitalization experience, increased anticipatory and hospital anxiety may be a consequence. The music therapist can serve a significant role in ameliorating the negative effects of previous hospitalizations by helping the child develop constructive coping skills (Edwards, 2005).

From a developmental perspective, the hospital environment is generally not conducive to normal growth and development. Children who are hospitalized only once or for a short duration of time are at low risk for any negative impact on their developmental skills. However, for children who are hospitalized for a prolonged period of time or are frequently in and out of the hospital due to chronic medical conditions, the risk of deleterious effects on development increases. The risk also increases when the child is hospitalized during a critical phase of development, such as during the first two years of life or during puberty, when the brain is experiencing a rapid growth spurt (Blakemore, Burnett, & Dahl, 2010; Pao et al., 2007). Not only does the hospital environment include aversive stimulation such as monitors beeping, interruption of sleep, and non-nurturing touch (e.g., needle sticks, physical examinations), but it also does not offer the normalized stimulation necessary for healthy development. Since children are away from home, school, and peers, they have limited opportunities to master developmental tasks or undergo the sequential developmental process necessary for healthy development (Pao et al., 2007). Providing opportunities throughout the course of a child's hospitalization to practice and master developmental tasks is vital and certainly possible. Music as a modality has the unique ability to stimulate all domains of development, including social, cognitive, communication, motor, and emotional skills.

As previously mentioned, hospitalized children are separated from their normal routine, daily activities at home and school, and network of social support. Some children may have a parent or caregiver present with them throughout the hospitalization, others may have family/caregivers visit occasionally, and others are alone or unaccompanied. Limited social engagement as well as other stressors related to illness can negatively impact the quality of life in hospitalized children (Manificat, Guillaud-Bataille, & Dazord, 1993; Payot & Barrington, 2011; Taylor, Gibson, & Franck, 2008; Wallander & Varni, 1998). Assisting the child in developing a network of social support within the hospital and providing opportunities for participation in developmental activities can enhance the coping process, decrease feelings of isolation, and enhance quality of life. Music therapists can further help children identify and discover their inner strengths and empower them to more effectively cope and adjust.

There are many characteristics common to hospitalized children through the shared challenges associated with illness and medical treatment. However, each child brings a set of personal characteristics and life experiences that makes one individual and unique in responding to illness and hospitalization. Musically, there is not one specific song, instrument, or music therapy method that can be applied to all pediatric patients. Music therapists cannot make assumptions about a child's musical preferences based upon age, gender, or any other characteristic. Musical preferences, exposure to music, and previous musical experiences will vary greatly among hospitalized children. For some children, a music therapy session may be the child's first exposure to having an authentic musical experience.

As previously mentioned, one of the advantages of using music therapy with hospitalized children is the ability of the music therapist to capitalize on the strengths of the child and family. Whereas the traditional medical model often targets symptom management and focuses upon what is ailing the body, the music therapist can center on what the child and family can do within a successful and supportive framework. Having a strength-based perspective can empower children and families by building upon individual strengths and actively engaging them through the recovery process (Smith, 2006). Regardless of the child's physical level of functioning, the music therapist can engage the child in the moment by listening to music, feeling the sensation of music, moving to music, creating music, or even choosing not to have music. The smallest action of movement, such as a wiggling finger, can become the rhythmic cue for a music improvisation or the movement needed to successful play a musical instrument such as the chimes. The music therapy session can also serve as a consistent and predictable period for joy and playfulness in the child's daily routine. With consistency, even the most highly anxious child can begin to associate "music time" as a safe part of his day. The music therapist can also integrate the child's nonmusical interests and talents into the session as a way to maximize his inner capabilities. For example, if the child has a hobby or knowledge base (e.g., cars, dinosaurs, Disney movies) in a particular subject area, then songs can be composed or improvised drawing upon interests or themes.

CAREGIVERS AND FAMILY-CENTERED CARE

When working with hospitalized children, one must consider the child's family system in the context of a family-centered care framework. Family-centered care is a philosophy of care that is adopted by most pediatric institutions and recognizes "that the family is the constant in the child's life while the service systems and personnel within those systems fluctuate" (Shelton, Jeppson, & Johnson, 1987). Practicing family-centered care means focusing on the strengths of the family and respecting individual beliefs, values, and different methods of coping (Abraham & Moretz, 2012). Within the hospital setting, one will encounter diversity in family structure, culture, ethnicity, religious or spiritual affiliation, socioeconomic background, and community environment (e.g., rural or urban). Therefore, music therapists have an obligation to understand the unique needs and perspectives of families, keep families informed about music therapy services, and respect the decisions and choices made by families even when those decisions are incongruent with one's own belief or value system.

The degree of family involvement and level of participation in music therapy sessions will vary according to the needs of the family, the availability of the family, and the goals for the patient. In cases of abuse or neglect, some children may not have family or caregivers present due to the child having been placed into protective services or into custody of the state. Inflexibility with work schedule, financial or transportation limitations, and having other children at home needing care can also inhibit caregivers from staying at the hospital or limit visitation opportunities. In those situations, the music therapist can leave notes at the bedside or make telephone calls to the family informing them and keeping them updated about music therapy services.

During music therapy sessions, the music therapist may have one or more members of the family present. Range of family involvement will vary, with some actively participating while others passively observe. For some caregivers, music therapy sessions may be one of the only times to take a "break" in order to shower, eat lunch, or have respite. For others, music therapy offers an opportunity for caregivers to have a normalized and nonmedical interaction with their child, especially for parents who are involved in performing tasks such as administering medications or performing dressing changes. There may also be times when the role of the music therapist is to facilitate positive parent-child interaction (Jacquet,

2011). Some caregivers may be unsure or uncomfortable in knowing how to interact with their ill child. The music therapist can engage the child and caregiver together through positive musical and playful interactions. Occasionally, siblings, cousins, and even friends of the child may be present and actively involved during a session. Interacting with families, offering emotional support to families, advocating for families, and providing ongoing information to families about music therapy services are all important elements in practicing family-centered music therapy.

REFERRAL AND ASSESSMENT PROCEDURES

Referral

The music therapy assessment begins at the moment of referral. The referral process for music therapy services will vary according to facility policy and how the music therapy program is structured. Some facilities may require that only physicians make referrals, while others allow referrals to come from any member of the treatment team or even the child's family. For many chronic patients who require frequent admissions, music therapy services may be requested upon each admission. The format for a referral, or consult, will also vary per facility, with some programs using an electronic referral process while others use referral sheets, verbal referrals, or a combination of these formats. The referral most often includes the name and room number of the child as well as the reason for the consult. Educating staff about identifying children who would benefit from music therapy services is helpful in increasing appropriate referrals. Common reasons for referrals include alleviating pain and anxiety; facilitating adjustment to a new diagnosis or illness; improving coping skills, such as when a child is withdrawn or lashing out in anger; providing developmental stimulation; increasing compliance or motivation to participate in treatments; and enhancing quality of life.

Assessment

When possible, the music therapist should gather information about the child from various sources prior to implementing the first music therapy session. Although assessment procedures will vary per facility, it will often include one more of the following methods: review of the medical record; discussion with the child's treatment team, including the team member who made the referral; meeting with the parent or caregiver; and, finally, observing and interacting with the child, both musically and nonmusically. It is important to note that in some instances, the music therapist may have little opportunity to conduct a formal assessment or gather significant information about the child prior to the initial session. In this situation, the music therapist should use caution as well as judgment when interacting with the hospitalized child. Talking with the nurse prior to interacting with the child can provide sufficient information and insight as to the child's current medical, emotional, and physical state.

When the child's parent or primary caregiver is available, the music therapist can learn additional information about the child while also building a positive working relationship with the family. Useful questions to caregivers include asking about the child's coping style, previous hospitalization experiences, current hospitalization issues, play interests, hobbies, musical experiences and preferences, and developmental level of functioning. For hospitalized children who have concurrent developmental disabilities, it is important to know what services the child receives at home or at school so that the music therapist can help the child maintain those skills while hospitalized. Finally, the music therapist may wish to observe the child outside the context of the music therapy session, such as when the child is interacting in the hospital playroom or working with other therapists and health care professionals, such as child life specialists. The purpose of the assessment process is to gather relevant information, identify the significant needs of the patient, and implement the most beneficial treatment plan to target those needs (Sabbatella, 2004).

General items to include in a pediatric music therapy assessment include the following: demographical and medical background of the patient, source and reason for referral, estimated length of hospitalization, previous hospitalizations, medical equipment, precautions and physical restrictions of the patient (e.g., isolation), level of physical functioning, demeanor and range of affect, expressions of pain/discomfort (including procedural and chronic pain), expressions of anxiety (e.g., anticipatory, generalized, hospital-related, separation), attitude toward illness, coping style and comfort methods, attention level, receptive and expressive communication (including nonverbal), developmental level (include sensory integration issues when applicable), energy/endurance level, level of participation (e.g., passive, active, etc.), degree of motivation, level of engagement (e.g., withdrawn, uninterested, partially active, spontaneous, etc.), family availability and involvement, support networks (including community and spiritual), other stressors (e.g., grief or loss issues), leisure interests, musical background and preferences, and description of musical interaction and responsiveness.

The last two items listed are, of course, what makes the assessment unique to music therapists and should be a significant component of the music therapy assessment process. Assessing musical responses, responses to music, interactions, and expressivity may include the following types of observations: ability or desire to explore musical elements when playing music; changes in affect with musical interaction; ability to follow, imitate, or respond to musical cues; emotional reactions to music; changes or improvements in attention; motor responses (voluntary and involuntary); changes in nonverbal communication (e.g., body tension); description of interaction (verbal or nonverbal) with music; ability to tolerate musical stimulation; interest in discussing musical interests; and/or associations when listening to music. In addition to asking/learning about musical preferences and musical background, the music therapist should ask children what music energizes and calms them. Also, asking them *when* they listen to music can provide significant information. Additional information related to referral and assessment procedures in the medical setting can be found in the Standards of Clinical Practice document established by the American Music Therapy Association (AMTA Standards of Clinical Practice, n.d.).

After the informational component of the assessment is completed, a treatment plan is established based upon the knowledge acquired from the assessment. The treatment plan includes goals, interventions or methods, type(s) of session, and intended frequency of music therapy sessions. The following list includes treatment goals commonly addressed in the pediatric medical setting: enhance or improve coping skills (including anxiety and pain management), emotional adjustment, self-concept development, quality of life, developmental skills, emotion regulation, and motivation to participate in the recovery process. The music therapist then needs to determine the type of session most applicable for the child's needs. Types of sessions include individual sessions; cotherapy sessions in which one collaborates and works simultaneously with another health care professional such as physical therapist or occupational therapist; group sessions; family sessions; and procedural support. In some cases, more than one session type will be incorporated into the child's treatment plan. The plan then includes the specific methods that will be used to target the goals stated in the treatment plan. Finally, the music therapist determines an established frequency of music therapy treatment, meaning how often the child will be seen for music therapy services. This frequency will be dependent upon many factors, including the child's estimated length of stay, goals, and amount of support systems within the hospital setting, as well as the music therapist's availability. Some children may necessitate receiving music therapy services on a daily basis, while others may need only once or twice per week. The following is an example of a summarized treatment plan based upon an assessment:

Music therapist will visit with patient approximately 2x/week for 1:1 music therapy sessions using music-facilitated dramatic play as an outlet for coping with feelings related to illness/hospitalization. Will encourage participation in weekly group music therapy sessions to provide opportunities for social interaction with peers. Music therapy sessions will continue throughout the duration of the patient's hospital stay.

As previously mentioned, the general pediatric unit may include children hospitalized for one day, a few days, or even several weeks. Therefore, some children may receive one music therapy session during their hospitalization stay, while other patients receive several visits. It is important to remember that even one music therapy session can have significant benefit to the hospitalized child (Lane, 1994). Time spent with patients during sessions will also vary and could range from 15 minutes to over an hour in some circumstances. Children with low physical energy levels may only tolerate 15 to 20 minutes, whereas a verbally engaging adolescent may require at least an hour-long session. Location of music therapy sessions will also vary. Not every music therapy session needs to or should occur at the child's bedside. For children who are not on isolation, leaving the hospital room can provide psychological benefits. Music therapy sessions can occur in the hospital playroom, a music therapy room, or in other locations in the hospital. Even for children who are on isolation, it may be beneficial to have the child seated in a chair or positioned on a floor mat, if the child does not require bed rest. Talking with the child's nurse as well as family will help determine the ideal location and position in which to conduct the music therapy session.

Although the initial assessment is the one that is documented in the medical record, the music therapist working in the pediatric medical setting needs to assess the child on an ongoing basis. The nature of some illnesses and medical treatments can cause sudden changes in the child's physical and emotional status. One day, the child may display a high level of physical energy, while the next day, the child is experiencing pain or fatigue. The music therapist needs to have flexibility in adjusting to the child's current emotional state and physical status to address the immediate needs of the child.

INTRODUCTION TO MUSIC THERAPY METHODS

The following section outlines 11 music therapy methods that can be applied when working with hospitalized children in the general pediatric unit. The methods outlined below are based upon the music therapy clinical and research literature as well as the author's extensive experience working in the pediatric medical setting. It is important to keep in mind that this is not a prescriptive classification system but an interconnected tapestry. Within a single music therapy session, a therapist may integrate two or more methods as part of the overall therapeutic music experience in order to better respond to the child's needs and interactions. When applicable, a brief discussion about group considerations is included.

Prior to going into any child's room, it is strongly recommended that the therapist talk with the nurse in order to have the most up-to-date information on the child's status, significant occurrences related to the child's care, and any necessary physical restrictions and precautions. Although overstimulation may be a concern for some hospitalized children, particular attention should be given to children with seizure disorders. Prior to the session, the therapist should know what sensitivities the child has, what induces seizure activity, and what signs indicate seizure activity for that particular child. Also, the music therapist should be careful not to overly fatigue the child and should adhere to the child's energy and endurance level throughout the session. In addition, the music therapist needs to be aware of the physiological needs of the child and adjust the musical elements accordingly. For example, if the child's respiration rate needs to remain stable and not increase, then maintaining a tempo entrained to the child's baseline respiration rate should be considered. Following up with the nurse after the music therapy session will not only offer the nurse valuable information about the child's involvement in music therapy, but also provide an additional way to educate the team about the benefits of music therapy services.

Finally, some practical considerations are offered when working in this setting. Although most hospitals offer private rooms for patients, some sessions may occur in hospitals where the child has a roommate. The music therapist needs to be respectful to the roommate in considering the timing of the session as well as volume level. Some hospital music therapy programs may have a separate treatment room or area to conduct music therapy sessions. As previously mentioned, each pediatric music therapist needs to be trained in and implement the infection control practices established by the facility. Proper care and maintenance of music therapy equipment, including the therapist's guitar, requires cleaning with hospital-approved disinfectants. Choosing equipment to transport instruments to and from sessions is another consideration. Some therapists use a portable cart with wheels, while others prefer to carry items in a plastic tote bag that can be wiped down with disinfectant. For children who are on isolation, the therapist needs to become proficient in playing guitar and/or keyboard while wearing gloves.

OVERVIEW OF MUSIC THERAPY METHODS AND PROCEDURES

Receptive Music Therapy

- Music Listening for Normalization and Anxiety Reduction: the use of music listening to decrease anxiety through the familiarity and containment of the music.
- Music to Facilitate Movement and Body Awareness: the use of music-guided therapeutic movement experiences, including free and/or structured movement, to promote body awareness and positive self-image.
- Music-Based Sensory Stimulation: integrating the elements of music with other sensory experiences, including tactile, visual, vestibular, proprioceptive, and olfactory stimulation as a means to enhance body awareness, awareness of environment, and/or self-regulation, and/or facilitate states of alertness or relaxation.

Improvisational Music Therapy

- Active Music Engagement: a developmental and reciprocal approach to music-making that uses the components of structure, autonomy, and support to enhance coping skills.
- Music-Based Developmental Stimulation: the use of specific music activities such as exploring sound through instruments, mirroring, imitating, movement, and vocal play to target developmental skills in children who display developmental regression or are at risk for falling behind in meeting developmental milestones.
- Music-Facilitated Dramatic Play: a child-centered approach that uses music improvisation as a means to musically reflect and validate the underlying themes and emotional content of a child's dramatic play or narrative stories.
- Music Improvisation for Emotional Expressivity: the process of creating music in the moment, including instrumental, vocal, or the combination of both to stimulate and reflect nonverbal and/or verbal expression of thoughts and feelings experienced during hospitalization.

Re-creative Music Therapy

- Singing for Normalization and Anxiety Reduction: engaging the child in singing familiar songs to enhance coping, promote relaxation, provide distraction, normalize the environment, and decrease the body's stress response.
- Therapeutic Music Instruction: the process of teaching a child or adolescent to play a musical instrument, such as guitar or keyboard, for the purpose of enhancing self-esteem as well as stimulating executive functioning skills.

Compositional Music Therapy

- Songwriting for Self-Expression and Coping: the use of songwriting approaches including song parody, fill-in-the blank, song collage, and original composition to provide opportunities for self-expression, enhance coping and adjustment, and facilitate identification of individual strengths and support systems.
- Music Video Creation: a process, including planning, decision-making, and designing, that uses technology and media to create an original music video composition that conceptualizes one's thoughts and emotions into a contained product.

GUIDELINES FOR RECEPTIVE MUSIC THERAPY

Music Listening for Normalization and Anxiety Reduction

Overview. Music listening for normalization and anxiety reduction involves music listening at the bedside to decrease the child's anxiety through the familiarity and emotional containment of the music. Science has shed some insight into the benefits of music listening, including music's ability to decrease cortisol levels, a stress hormone that can inhibit the healing process (Khalfa, Bella, Roy, Peretz, & Lupien, 2003; McCraty, Atkinson, Rein, & Watkins, 1996). In the pediatric medical setting, listening to either recorded or live music has been shown to decrease anxiety by normalizing the environment and enhancing a state of relaxation. Playing music at the bedside provides a nonthreatening way to establish rapport with an infant, child, or adolescent who is highly anxious. Because the medical environment and treatments can be unfamiliar, overstimulating, unpredictable, or even painful, the music therapist offers a unique modality that can provide normalcy to an abnormal and emotionally vulnerable situation. The goal of music listening at the bedside is to decrease the child's generalized anxiety through the familiarity and containment of the music and establish a therapeutic relationship between the music therapist and the child (including the child's family). The music therapist needs to be aware that there are some instances when a procedure, treatment, or medical condition requires limited physical activity or bed rest (e.g., after a lumbar puncture). Because music has the ability to stimulate and arouse motor responses, there exists a risk of increasing active movement for those children. Certain types of music or music in general may be contraindicated in this situation.

Preparation. This method requires little preparation and equipment. Generally, a guitar or portable keyboard will be used for accompaniment. The music therapist should have a repertoire of songs to reflect a range of musical preferences for infants through adolescents and demonstrate proficiency in performing these songs with the ability to vary musical elements (e.g., tempo, dynamics, timbre, style, meter) according to the responses of the child. The music therapist may choose to bring a binder filled with song lyrics and chords or may use an electronic device such as an iPad™ to maintain song files.

Before starting the music therapy session, it is important that the music therapist consult with the nurse as to the current status and needs of the child.

During the session, the music therapist should position herself in a manner that facilitates eye contact with the child but is not confrontational. The child may be lying in bed, seated on a caregiver's lap, or sitting up in a chair. Caregivers of infants may choose to hold and rock the infant to the beat of the music. When possible, the music therapist should ask the child or family if they prefer to have the lights on or off and the room door open or closed. Hospital rooms are personal spaces, and demonstrating respect to the child's environmental preferences can enhance the establishment of trust. Generally, it is best to have any other distractions removed, such as televisions turned off, although one should first ask the child's permission.

What to observe. There are several observable behaviors that can indicate decreased anxiety and positive rapport-building. These behaviors include the child's ability to make choices, degree of reciprocal verbal interaction (does the child respond to questions, initiate verbal interaction, or not respond?), level of eye contact, affective changes in facial expression, and degree of tension in the body/posture. In cases where the child is connected to a monitor, the music therapist should be alert to the child's vital signs and routinely check the monitor throughout the session.

It will also be important to observe whether certain songs, phrases within a song, or moments in the music seem to evoke increased responsiveness such as smiling, tearfulness, mouthing words/singing, or increased active movement (e.g., clapping hands). In situations where family members are present, the therapist should observe family interactions and degree of involvement/participation.

Procedures. Upon entering the child's room and preparing the environment, the music therapist can offer some choices of songs for the child to listen to. Songs offered will depend upon the child's age, developmental level, and musical preferences. Adolescents may enjoy looking through a songbook, while younger patients may choose popular melodies from cartoons or traditional children's songs. It is not uncommon for a child or adolescent to respond by saying something like, "I don't care, whatever you want." In this circumstance, the music therapist can ask if he prefers a musical style or mood such as fast, slow, relaxing, upbeat, etc. If he is highly anxious or too overwhelmed to make a choice, then the music therapist can take suggestions from family members or make a selection for him.

Once a song has been selected, the music therapist plays the song for the child while observing his responses. The music therapist should demonstrate flexibility vs. rigidity when "performing" the song. For example, consider repeating certain phrases when that part of the song or music seemed meaningful to the child. Discussing song lyrics and other aspects of the music may be beneficial for some children. The songs may facilitate sharing of memories or discussing aspects of their life both within and outside of the hospital. Others, however, may demonstrate resistance to probing questions related to the lyrics or their experience of the song. When conducting the session, the music therapist needs to be attuned to the needs and responses of the child.

The music therapist then continues the process of song selection, performing, and discussion. The benefit of this method is that it offers flexibility with time, is appropriate for all developmental levels, and can be adjusted according to the child's energy level. Some children may become calm and relaxed to the degree that they fall asleep. In this case, the music therapist can use a fade-out approach with the music when transitioning out of the room.

Adaptations. This intervention allows much opportunity for adaptation. The music therapist should consider moving from "structured" performance of a song to an "improvisational" experience when certain events occur during the session. For example, when a monitor starts to beep during the music listening experience, the therapist can immediately begin to integrate the "beeps" into the song either by improvising lyrics about the machine beeping or by matching the tempo/pitch of the beeping into the musical experience. "Normalizing" the hospital environment through the musical interaction can be an effective tool to decrease hospital-related anxiety. An improvisational response by the music therapist may then lead into an improvisational method such as active music engagement for coping or a compositional method such as songwriting.

Another adaptation is to specifically provide music listening for relaxation (Edwards, 1999a, 1999b). In this case, it is recommended that the music therapist entrain the music to the child's breath rate. Entraining to breath rate, as opposed to heart rate, is recommended because heart rate is an involuntary function whereas breathing can be self-paced (Haas, Distenfeld, & Axen, 1986). Gradually slowing the tempo and using the music to cue deeper breaths (e.g., inhale on the dominant chord and exhale on the tonic chord), can facilitate a relaxation response. Using imagery within the listening experience, appropriate to the child's cognitive and developmental level, may also be indicated (Abad, 2003; Wolfe & Waldon, 2009). When working with infants, live music, including the therapist's improvised music, can be combined with rocking to facilitate sleep for hospitalized infants and toddlers (Marley, 1984, 1996).

Live music is generally preferred over recorded music due to the ability of the therapist to have immediacy in manipulating the musical elements based upon the responses of the child. However, recorded music may be better suited when the music therapist is unable to replicate the child's preferred songs in a way that is satisfying to the child. Playing the recording, listening attentively with the child, and understanding the meaning of the music from the child's perspective will convey respect and genuine caring as a means to develop trust. Some hospitals provide music listening libraries offering a variety of CDs, including relaxation music, for families to borrow during their hospital stay (Wolfe & Woolsey, 2003).

This method can also be a useful warm-up in music therapy groups. In a general pediatric setting, most children attending groups will arrive without knowing any of the other participants. Playing familiar songs can be an inviting way for children to gather and socially connect with others. With adolescents, music listening to familiar songs can stimulate discussion about lyrics while facilitating a connection with one another through the shared experience.

Music to Facilitate Movement and Body Awareness

Overview. Music listening to facilitate movement and body awareness involves music-guided therapeutic movement experiences, including free and/or structured movement, to promote body awareness and positive self-image. Because illness and disease often result in physical dysfunction, therapeutic movement can improve the child's body image and awareness, thus facilitating coping and adjustment. Medical equipment, such as an IV line, seems to become a temporary extension of the child's body. Learning how to move safely and function successfully while connected to monitors, IV pumps, and other medical equipment can be a challenge for children. In addition, children may be overwhelmed by all the medical equipment and the physical restrictions imposed upon them. Furthermore, they may be fearful that movement will result in (increased) pain or discomfort. Some children and adolescents may hold tension within the body (e.g., clenching fists), and releasing that tension through therapeutic music experiences can promote relaxation and enhance the healing process. The goal of this method is to develop a healthier self-image, increase awareness of body sensations, and identify how the body can move, function, and feel without disturbing any medical equipment or causing discomfort.

It is important that the music therapist check with the nurse about the child's limits and capabilities in regard to active movement. When applicable, the music therapist should also consult with the child's physical therapist. There are some children who may be required to wear restrictive devices around arms, wrists, and hands to keep from pulling out tubes and lines. When able to remove those devices during the session, the music therapist needs to maintain vigilant attention so that the child does not reach or pull at lines. Also, there may be circumstances where active movement can be unsafe or contraindicated, such as after a lumbar puncture procedure. Finally, during the session, the music therapist needs to be careful that IV lines do not become twisted or caught, which can result in an occlusion.

Preparation. Before entering the child's room, the music therapist needs to be fully aware as to what medical equipment the child is connected to, what parts of the body the child can and cannot move, and how the child is positioned. All of this information will determine additional session preparation. For example, for children who can leave their hospital room, the music therapy session can be conducted in an open space. The music therapist may wish to bring props such as scarves, balls, and ribbon sticks to enhance the movement experience by integrating tactile and visual stimuli for expressive purposes (Barrickman, 1989; McDonnell, 1984). Music may be played live or recorded. If the music therapist needs to attend to the physical safety of the child, then recorded music may be more practical. Choice of music will be dependent upon the child's developmental level, his music preferences, and the pace and manner of the desired movement (e.g., slower-paced music may ease fluidity of movement).

What to observe. Foremost, the music therapist needs to be observant and attentive to the safety of the child and the medical equipment. It is necessary for the therapist to observe the child's level of participation, resistance to moving any specific areas of the body, and degree of comfort to freely and actively move. Therapists should notice the child's awareness and attentiveness to medical lines and tubes as well as receptivity to learn ways to move safely. As in every clinical situation, it is important that the therapist observe affective responses and verbal and nonverbal interaction. When working with an older child or adolescent, the therapist should be attuned to the words used in describing body sensations as well as any other comments made about his body, either positive or negative.

Procedures. When working with younger children, there are many ways to begin the session, including asking the child to point out lines and tubes connected to his body, having him choose a scarf or ribbon stick, or even singing a song about how parts of the body can move (e.g., waving with hands, wiggling toes, scrunching the nose). With singing a song about the body, the music therapist can assess the child's body awareness by having him point to the body part mentioned in the song. You can then distinguish which parts of the child's body can move freely and which parts should move carefully or not at all. You can use props such as a scarf, ribbon stick, or even a stuffed toy belonging to the child to be used for movement. This method allows for much creativity and spontaneity on the part of the music therapist, as well as immediacy in responding to the child's interactions. The session can be as structured as singing or adapting a movement song such as "Head, Shoulders, Knees, and Toes" or as free as moving or tossing ribbons to melodically flowing music.

In working with older children and adolescents, one way to begin the session is for the therapist to ask the child to describe how his body is feeling at that moment. The therapist can ask the child to identify where he feels tense as well as relaxed. Discussion can include how emotions are sometimes experienced as sensations within the body (Koshland & Curry, 1996) and that keeping tense emotions within the body can make it more difficult for the body to heal. The therapist can then use relaxation exercises, such as tension and relaxation of muscles, to release tension and stress. Active movement such as dancing to preferred pop music can also provide an emotional release. For children and adolescents with the physical capability to participate, dancing video games may be more motivating.

Adaptations. For infants, having a parent or caregiver hold and rock an infant while the music therapist plays live music provides vestibular stimulation necessary for infants to develop balance and body awareness. Also, for children who cannot actively move, combining nurturing, playful, or intentional touch within the context of a song can decrease some of the negative effects of invasive and aversive touch often experienced during medical procedures. Scarves can be used to playfully touch parts of the body (e.g., toes, arms, and tummy) as music is sung or played to support the interaction.

Music-guided movement experiences in a group setting can provide a sense of normalcy and cohesiveness among children. A parachute can be a wonderful tool for movement because children can have varied abilities and still actively participate. Children who cannot tolerate the continuous movement in holding the parachute can assist with tossing soft balls inside the parachute or enjoy the sensation of the breeze of the parachute's movements. When implementing any movement experience, attention to safety precautions is essential (e.g., children with an IV should use the hand without the IV to hold on to the parachute).

Music-Based Sensory Stimulation

Overview. Music-based sensory stimulation is a technique that integrates the elements of music with other sensory experiences, including tactile, visual, vestibular, proprioceptive, and olfactory stimulation as a means to enhance body awareness, awareness of environment, and/or self-regulation, and/or facilitate states of alertness or relaxation. This method is indicated for children who have minimal to no verbal skills, have moderate to profound developmental and cognitive impairment, or have *sensory integration disorder*. Oftentimes these children are unable to participate in other routine play opportunities provided for hospitalized children. However, these children still need an outlet to cope with the stressors of hospitalization. The overstimulating and aversive environment of the hospital, as well as the sudden change from their normalized routine, can be challenging for these children to process, resulting in increased agitation or developmental regression. The goal of this method is to provide normalized sensory stimulation as a means to decrease agitation and discomfort while enhancing quality of life. This method may not be suitable for all children with severe cognitive impairments, as music may overstimulate or overly excite some children.

Preparation. This method can be implemented at the bedside or while the child is positioned in a wheelchair or wagon. In some cases, the therapist can work with the child on a floor mat. Some children may have specialized wheelchairs brought from home that offer increased range of positioning. The therapist should bring a guitar as well as a variety of musical instruments, such as chimes, rain stick, ocean drum, tambourine, and/or cabasa. Bringing items that provide visual as well as tactile sensory input, including scarves, ribbons, O-balls, and other sensory integration tools (e.g., fiber-optic light-up toys, textured balls, soft toys that crinkle or have bells inside, vibrating toys) are also recommended. Minimizing other stimulation in the room, such as turning off the television, dimming lights, and closing the room door, may allow the child to better process the music-based stimulation.

What to observe. Throughout the session, the music therapist will need to look keenly for responses from the child, including subtle ones. Caregivers can provide the music therapist with valuable information as to the child's baseline responses and what certain behavioral responses may indicate. Be sure to monitor what type of musical and nonmusical sensory stimuli seem to arouse, excite, calm, indicate pleasure, and increase purposeful/reciprocal interaction. Responses may include but are not limited to visual tracking, eye contact, sound localization, increased activation of movement, purposeful reaching, and social interaction such as smiling (Hannan, 2008). Other observations include monitoring the child's vital signs, including heart rate and respiration rate. Because an increase in heart rate may indicate excitement or overstimulation, the therapist needs to know the child's baseline range of vital signs.

Procedures. The music therapist can start with a transitional or welcome song to indicate the therapist's presence in the room. One approach may be to begin by singing the child's name entrained to the child's breath rate and then gradually adding the guitar accompaniment. Providing the same transitional songs at the beginning and end of the session may help the child to associate time for music therapy, indicating a safe and pleasurable part of the day. Throughout the session, the music therapist can assist the child in exploring auditory, visual, and tactile sensory stimuli. Initially, the therapist may introduce one stimulus at a time and then, as the child tolerates the stimulus, add a secondary stimulus. For example, the therapist can first allow the child time to explore the tambourine visually and tactilely and then start singing with the child as the tambourine is played. Some children may require hand-over-hand playing of instruments, while others have the ability to reach and play independently. Placing the child's hand on the guitar as the therapist strums can provide tactile and proprioceptive input while associating cause and effect. Musical instruments can also be placed against the child's skin to stimulate interest and purposeful responsiveness to nonaversive sensory stimuli (McCauley, 1996). Moving chimes over the child's fingers may provide a physical and auditory cue, thus activating movement in fingers or eliciting the child to reach. Parents and caregivers can also be involved by providing some of the hand-over-hand assistance while the music therapist plays guitar to reinforce the reciprocal interaction between child and caregiver.

Adaptations. There may be times when the music therapist can implement this method while the child is receiving another treatment or therapy. For example, offering pleasant musical stimulation while the child is receiving a passive range of motion exercises by a physical therapist may help him better tolerate the exercises. When medically safe and approved by the treatment team, some children may enjoy having scented lotion rubbed on upper and lower extremities, including hands and feet. In this case, the therapist can ask the family to bring favorite lotions from home and the therapist can provide music as the caregiver provides nurturing touch and comfort through the lotion massage.

GUIDELINES FOR IMPROVISATIONAL MUSIC THERAPY

Music Improvisation for Emotional Expressivity

Overview. Music improvisation for emotional expressivity is the process of creating music in the moment, including instrumental, vocal, or the combination of both to stimulate and reflect nonverbal and/or verbal expression of thoughts and feelings experienced during hospitalization. Music improvisation offers a creative and nonverbal outlet where emotions can be safely expressed, contained, and validated through the musical interaction as well as in the music itself. This method can be beneficial for children having difficulty verbally expressing thoughts and feelings related to illness/hospitalization, thus inhibiting adjustment and coping. It also provides an alternative means to constructively and safely explore emotions for those children who are expressing confusion, anger, depression, or frustration in a way that impedes their recovery or treatment regimen. Since the structure of music can start from a basic layer and grow to a complex portrait of sound, music improvisation is applicable for both children and adolescents. A young child may express frustration through intense beating on a drum, whereas an older teen may create an intricate melodic motif on the keyboard to represent one's illness. The primary goal is to facilitate emotional adjustment through the immediate release of feelings, thoughts, and emotions manifested through musical expression, while building upon the child's inner strengths (Turry, 1999; Turry & Turry, 1999).

Music improvisation is not something that all children feel comfortable or open to experiencing. Some children may find the freedom to create music "in the moment" overwhelming, which may increase the child's stress response, a reaction that could inhibit healing and recovery. If the music therapist notices significant resistance when trying to engage a child to improvise, then this method may not be appropriate.

Preparation. Music improvisation offers much flexibility in application and can therefore occur at the bedside with the child positioned sitting up or lying down. It is recommended to select instruments that are age appropriate and encompass a broad spectrum of musical timbre, with consideration to both melodic and percussive resonance. The music therapist should also take into account the child's level of physical independence when selecting instruments to use during the session (e.g., if the child has use of only one hand).

What to observe. Throughout the session, the music therapist needs to be highly attuned to the musical expressivity of the child, including choice of instrument(s). The therapist can attend to musical motifs and the integration/use of musical elements such as tempo, dynamics, rhythmic structure, harmony, and melody, while observing nonverbal cues, such as eye contact. The therapist can also listen to the degree of intensity in the child's music, which may provide insight into the child's emotional state. For example, if the child chooses to improvise "feeling happy" yet plays loudly and in a chaotic manner while displaying an aggressive facial expression (e.g., furrowed eyebrows and clenched teeth), the music therapist may use this incongruence as a therapeutic opportunity to explore this disconnect with the child. When improvisations include verbal and vocal expressions, listen to key words and phrases, especially those that are repeated.

Procedures. There are multiple ways to engage a child in music improvisation, including instrumental improvisation, vocal improvisation (using one's voice without words), song improvisation, or a combination of these. Improvisations can be loosely or highly structured, begin through a spontaneous musical interaction, or purposefully be initiated by the child or music therapist. In highly structured improvisational experiences, the music therapist may provide an underlying rhythm, word, phrase, theme, or song to structure the musical experience. Referential improvisation involves an improvisation based upon a specific experience, event, object, person, sensation, or emotion (Bruscia, 1987; Hannan, 2008). Sometimes the improvisational experience can be based upon a specific theme or subject matter, such as feelings about treatment, a word such as "hospital," or sources of strength for the child. The child chooses an instrument for himself and the therapist and creates music to represent that one specific concept. This process may facilitate discussion about significant events in the child's life or hospitalization experience and the meaning surrounding those events as applied to his current situation. Another example of a structured improvisation is to create music or songs from the perspective of the child's medical equipment, such as the child's IV (Froehlich, 1996a). For example, a child may choose to create an improvisation that explores the concept of having an injection. As part of the improvisational music-making, the therapist may ask the child, "What do you think the needle would say to you if it could talk?" (either as a rhythmic chant or melodic phrase). The child has the opportunity to respond to the question through the music. For younger children, having visual aids, such as pictures of faces reflecting different emotions such as happy, sad, angry, and scared, may elicit the child's exploration to play out those emotions through music. The therapist can explore verbally or through the music moments when the child feels and experiences these emotions in the hospital.

An unstructured improvisation is done without or with little verbal instruction, guidance, or theme. The improvisation is undefined, purely reflecting the child's emotions in the here-and-now. The music therapist may encourage the child to just begin playing, or the child may begin an improvisation spontaneously as he explores an instrument such as the keyboard. Free and unstructured improvisation may invoke anxiety in some children and adolescents who may feel emotionally exposed, are unsure of what they are supposed to do, or think they need to have musical talent to participate. In this writer's experience, children and adolescents with prior musical experience or exposure, either through school or family, have seemed more readily open to this type of improvisational experience.

Once engaged in music improvisation, the music therapist needs to maintain focus on the child's ongoing musical creation and continuously support, validate, reflect, and respond musically. Responding musically may be through supporting the child's melody with a harmonic structure, imitating/reflecting musical motifs with or without variation, or matching dynamics. During the improvisational experience, the person guiding the "groove" may fluctuate between child and therapist or be simultaneous. A call-and-response interaction may also occur. An improvisation can be brief or carry on uninterrupted for as long as the child needs to maintain. Informing the child at the beginning of the session as to how long the music therapist can stay may help to ease the transition in closing improvisational music-making when the music therapist needs to leave. Verbal processing may or may not occur as part of the improvisational experience and will depend upon treatment goals, the child's interest or ability to engage in verbal processing, and the trust level between child and therapist.

Adaptations. Music improvisation may serve as a catalyst for compositional methods such as songwriting. Certain children may benefit from having improvisations audio recorded and made into a CD to take home with them upon discharge. Music improvisation can also be combined with other expressive modalities such as art, poetry, storytelling, and movement.

Music improvisation can be a powerful therapeutic tool when working within a group. Depending upon group dynamics and cohesiveness, the type of the improvisational experience could be a group jam session or reflect a specific feeling, topic, or theme that is introduced to or chosen by the group. A structured group improvisation facilitated by the music therapist could be in the form of a 12-bar blues with each child or teen in the group shouting out in the moment what "gives them the blues" in the hospital as the group continues to jam. Finding commonalities among the group participants (e.g., having to be awoken in the middle of the night by the nurse to have vital signs taken) may also provide a theme for an improvisation experience. In general, the less cohesive the group is, the more structure the music therapist may need to provide in order to create a successful musical experience.

Active Music Engagement

Overview. Active music engagement (AME), initially described by Robb (2000), is a developmental and reciprocal approach to music-making that uses the components of structure, autonomy, and involvement to elicit constructive coping behaviors in hospitalized children (Robb, 2000, 2003a). Music provides the organization (structure) to normalize a chaotic environment, allows opportunities for the child to make choices (autonomy), and facilitates reciprocal interaction (support) between the therapist and child (Robb, 2003a). This method often combines re-creative approaches by allowing the child to choose familiar songs and structured music activities, especially when building rapport with a child. AME is included as an improvisational method because it requires the therapist to musically respond to the child's actions as well as the "in the moment" occurrences that can arise during a session. Although the initial part of the session may include active music-making to familiar and structured songs, the session often evolves into an improvisational music experience using the songs and music activities as the initial or thematic foundation. Although some overlap exists between AME and music improvisation for emotional expressivity, the primary focus of AME is to allow the child increased opportunity for choice and control.

AME is indicated for children who are experiencing anxiety, stress, or lack of control, or are having difficulty adjusting to and coping with the hospitalization experience. The primary goal is to help the child develop constructive coping skills through music experiences that allow the child to have increased control over the environment, engage in positive reciprocal social interaction, and express feelings verbally and/or nonverbally. The importance of offering choices (Hannan, 2008; McDonnell, 1984) and promoting engagement through music (Marley, 1984) is often mentioned in the literature about music therapy with hospitalized children. Researchers and clinicians have successfully applied this method to hospitalized infants and children, as well as adolescents (Barrera, Rykov, & Doyle, 2002; Ghetti, 2011; Marley, 1996; Robb, 2000, 2003b).

There are few circumstances when this method would be contraindicated in the general pediatric unit, such as for children who are not in an alert state or are medically unstable. In rare instances, some children may display such a high degree of anxiety that anxiety worsens even in the presence of the music therapist. In this case, the music therapist can provide the family and caregivers with resources, such as age-appropriate musical instruments and toys, as a means to allow the child opportunities for play and interaction.

Preparation. This intervention can be done with the child in any position or location. Preparation of the session will depend upon the child's chronological age, developmental level, medical condition, and isolation status. Generally, it is helpful to bring a variety of musical instruments and activities from which the child can make choices. For younger children, including toddlers and preschoolers, song storybooks or other types of visual aids may be helpful in engaging the child. The music therapist should also be prepared to sing the child's preferred songs (if known) for rapport-building.

What to observe. There are many behaviors and responses that indicate a child's level of responsiveness to this method. The music therapist should observe the child's ability to make choices, level of interaction, duration of engagement, range of affect, degree of initiative, and communication style. For example, when offered a choice of which instrument to play, the child may respond in a number of ways: not answering or acknowledging the therapist, pointing to an instrument, nodding to communicate yes or no, verbalizing, or immediately grabbing an instrument. Observing the changes in the child's demeanor and body posture over the course of the session can also be significant. Some children may initially be withdrawn or hiding under the covers and by the end of the session are initiating musical interaction with the therapist.

Procedures. Although the music therapist's role is one that is "safe" and "nonthreatening," the hospitalized child may still display uncertainty and anxiety when meeting the music therapist for the first time. Being attuned to the child's initial response to the music therapist's presence will determine the music therapist's approach with the child. Sometimes the music therapist may need to stand at the child's door while singing and then gradually move closer, while at other times, the music therapist can greet the child at the bedside. The initial musical interaction may have a structured beginning, such as singing a greeting song (or the child's favorite song) while the child plays a shaker or other instrument of choice. The music therapist can then become more improvisational by singing about what the child is doing in the moment or by following the musical cues (e.g., dynamics and tempo) expressed through the child's playing. One of the most effective ways to empower a child through control of the music is to immediately follow and respond to the child's music-making. For example, if the child stops or pauses in the middle of the song, the music therapist should immediately stop as well, preferably, simultaneously with the child. Often, the child will notice that the therapist is closely listening to him and test the theory, meaning that the child will alternate playing and pausing again to see if the therapist does the same. This musical attunement to the child can evolve into a follow-the-leader improvisational experience with the therapist following all of the child's musical cues such as fast, slow, loud, soft, stop, and go. If the child chooses not to actively participate or has limited mobility, the therapist can encourage the child to select instruments for others in the room to play (e.g., parent or nurse). The child can then direct everyone in the room when to play and when to stop, which brings independence and control back to the child. Another version of this is to have the child play music to make the therapist (or a puppet) dance (Sheridan & McFerran, 2004) or have the child select specific musical instruments to designate how the music therapist moves (e.g., moves arms when the child plays the tambourine; turns around when the child plays the glockenspiel).

Some children may require more structure within the musical engagement experience than others. For example, the song "Down by the Bay" can be changed to "Down at the Hospital," where the child identifies things and/or people in the hospital and the therapist creates the rhymes for the song. Another structured approach is to sing a familiar song that the child chose and improvise creative ways to perform the song such as singing it fast, slow, using a low voice, high voice, etc. Having a playful and creative approach in manipulating the musical elements will help maintain the child's interest and attention throughout the session (Robb, 2003b). Throughout the session, the music therapist should continue to offer choices to the child and follow the child's lead during the musical interaction.

Adaptations. It is not unusual for other staff members to routinely enter the child's room throughout the duration of a music therapy session. This interruption is a highly common occurrence in the medical setting. Displaying immediacy to the situation by acknowledging the staff person as part of the musical interaction can not only normalize the situation, but also facilitate positive rapport between the child and staff member. This can be done by improvising songs with the staff in the room or by encouraging the staff person to play along with the child, even if only for a brief period of time.

There are many therapeutic music experiences and activities that are applicable in group music therapy with hospitalized children. Group music therapy naturally facilitates peer interaction and offers creative expression within a supportive network. In ensemble playing, children can take turns being a "musical leader," can have opportunities for making choices of instruments to play, and can find joy in exploring musical elements such as fast, slow, loud, and soft. When leading a group in improvisational music-making, the therapist may initially need to take an active and direct role in facilitating the musical experience. For example, the therapist can provide verbal and musical cues indicating when to play fast, slow, loud, and soft, as well as when to stop/pause. As musical cohesion develops, the therapist can pass on the leader/facilitator role to other children in the group and encourage each leader to cue when to play and when to stop. With the luxury of two music therapists as coleaders, one of the therapists can provide a steady rhythmic beat on a drum while the other music therapist facilitates other rhythmic patterns for the group to play or use a call-and-response approach. Overall, the therapist needs to be attuned to the developmental level of the group participants and adjust the degree of musical complexity within the improvisational experience accordingly.

Music-Based Developmental Stimulation

Overview. Music-based developmental stimulation is the use of music activities such as exploring sound through instruments, mirroring, imitating, movement, and vocal play to target developmental skills in children who display developmental regression or are at risk for falling behind in meeting developmental milestones (Kennelly, 2000; Marley, 1984, 1996). Although this approach may integrate previously written songs as part of the intervention, it is was included as improvisational because the music therapist is continuously adapting and improvising therapeutic interactions based upon the child's responses throughout the session. This method is applicable for those children who are regressing in their developmental skills or at risk for falling behind in meeting milestones due to prolonged hospitalization, frequent hospitalizations, or complications from the illness and/or treatments. Infants and toddlers are the primary age group for this intervention due to their being in a critical phase of growth and development. The primary goal is to maintain or facilitate the attainment of developmental milestones, with particular attention to the domain area(s) at greatest risk for delay. Since music-based developmental stimulation can be carefully adjusted to the child's physical limitations, endurance level, and medical status, there are few instances when this intervention would be contraindicated. However, the therapist should be aware that certain degenerative diseases, such as *spinal muscular atrophy*, will cause gradual loss of neurological functioning over time. In these cases, the goal may be to assist the child in maintaining function or assist the child in meeting his developmental potential to enhance quality of life.

Preparation. The music therapist should have knowledge of child development and the specific developmental milestones achieved at various stages of development in all domains including motor, communication, social-emotional, and cognitive. Using a developmental assessment tool, such as the Hawaii Early Learning Profile (Teaford, Wheat, & Baker, 2010), can assist in assessing the child's current level of functioning. Consulting with other members of the team such as rehabilitation therapists may also offer insight into what specific developmental tasks to address during music therapy sessions. Of course, the child's primary caregiver can serve as the most valuable source of information. The music therapist should bring to the session musical instruments and toys that can be used to target those specific developmental skills. In addition to bringing a guitar, useful items to bring include egg shakers and a small drum for dump-and-fill play, various instruments (e.g., rain stick, ocean drum, tambourine, chimes, O-ball rattle) for cause-and-effect learning, small plastic maracas for fine motor grasping, a mirror, and a scarf for peek-a-boo play. All instruments should be developmentally appropriate and child-safe. Ideally, positioning the child on a floor mat will provide increased freedom of movement and options for working with the child in different positions (e.g., sitting, side-lying, prone). However, depending upon the child's medical status, the child may be required to remain in a bed or crib. When possible, to provide increased mobility, conduct the session when the child is not connected to lines such as IV medication treatments or tube feedings.

What to observe. The therapist should observe which songs, instruments, toys, reciprocal play activities, and other developmental interactions seem to capture and sustain the child's attention and elicit the most desired developmental responses. Knowing what engages the child can increase motivation for attention, reaching, positive affect, and vocalizing, and elicit other developmental responses. When caregivers are present, observe the interaction between caregiver and child. When a child is emerging in a specific skill area, such as reaching to grasp a musical toy, the therapist should take note of the frequency and duration of the child's emerging developmental skill.

Procedures. When possible, it is important to involve the caregivers or parents in developmental music therapy sessions. Modeling interactive developmental musical play experiences can assist parents in taking an active and productive role in their children's developmental growth (Abad & Edwards, 2004). Structuring the session with opening and closing songs can help the young child with transitioning as well as associate that music therapy is a safe part of the child's daily hospital routine. Session contour should be structured in the following sequential manner: warm-up time to establish trust and enhance positive mood, followed by targeting the desired developmental skill(s), and closing with relaxing, quiet-time play.

Repetition and breaking down the desired task into smaller and more attainable steps are excellent ways to master and reinforce emerging and new skills. Examples of developmental play experiences that can be integrated with music include imitative play, vocal play, mirror play, peek-a-boo play, cause-and-effect play, reaching/exploring play, vestibular movement, and reciprocal social interaction (Barrickman, 1989). Movement games and action songs are also ways to increase activation of muscle movement and improve body awareness (Marley, 1996). The therapist can sing standard children's songs or improvise simple songs in the moment to coincide with the child's musical play and interactions. For example, using colored egg shakers and a small drum, the therapist can begin a cause-and-effect learning activity known as dump-and-fill. The therapist first demonstrates how to empty the shakers from the drum and then demonstrates putting the egg shakers back inside the drum. Modeling the skill first through demonstration is a key part of the learning process. The therapist can then dump the shakers again and observe whether the child initiates or needs assistance in putting the shakers back into the drum. While engaging in dump-and-fill play, the therapist can improvise a simple "in and out" song to musically reinforce the developmental concept.

An example to develop auditory perception skills is a sound localization activity. Using a musical instrument such as bells or a shaker, the therapist first plays the sound away from the child's visual field. The therapist observes if the child demonstrates facial recognitioan to the sound (such as opening eyes wider), tries to localize the sound with his eyes, or turns his head toward the direction of the sound. A variation is to show the child the instrument, play it, and then hide it. The therapist observes if the child continues to search for the instrument after it is hidden. Instruments can also be used to practice visual tracking skills, including horizontal and vertical directions, as well auditory perception skills by hearing the difference in how the instrument sounds when it is played close to or far from the child. Since it impossible in this brief overview to include the numerous ways music can be used to facilitate attainment of developmental milestones, the music therapist is encouraged to read additional articles and resources such as *Music, Therapy, and Early Childhood: A Developmental Approach* by Schwartz (2008).

Adaptations. This method can be conducted in collaboration with other disciplines such as physical, occupational, or speech therapy. Also, offering group music therapy sessions specifically designed for hospitalized infants and toddlers may provide normalized developmental play experiences within a social context. Each child who attends the group should have an accompanying adult, whether a parent, staff person, or trained hospital volunteer, so that group activities can be specifically tailored to the individual needs of the infant.

Music-Facilitated Dramatic Play

Overview. Music-facilitated dramatic play integrates concepts from child-centered play therapy (VanFleet, Sywulak, & Sniscak, 2010) by using music improvisation as a means to musically reflect and validate the underlying themes and emotional content of a child's dramatic play or stories. This method is well suited for children who are verbally expressive, creative, and drawn to dramatic play. Props such as puppets are used to help the child express thoughts and emotions and provide insight into the child's perception of the world around them, such as the hospitalization experience (Brounley, 1996; Ghetti, 2011; Hanson-Abromeit & Colwell, 2008; Loveszy, 1991). Preschool-age children and school-age children tend to be the ideal candidates for this intervention due to their cognitive phase of development. It can be of particular benefit for children who are having a difficult time adjusting to a new illness or diagnosis, have undergone many medical procedures and treatments, or are frequently in and out of the hospital due to a chronic illness. The purpose is to offer the child respect and unconditional positive regard through attending and using music to reflect thoughts, feelings, and needs as expressed through nondirected play. The primary goal is to allow children the freedom to express themselves through music and play as a means to understand, cope with, and resolve problems.

The music therapist needs to be cautious when using this method for children who have a history of abuse or other trauma, especially if the therapist does not have the training, experience, or qualifications for trauma work. Like any projective technique, the music therapist needs to be well-trained and cognizant about opening emotional wounds that the child may not be ready to explore. It would also be potentially harmful for the child if the music therapist begins exploring trauma issues that cannot be followed through due to the child being discharged from the hospital. Moreover, this method is not recommended for children who have limited cognitive ability or are unable to engage in imaginative play. Finally, this method should be facilitated in the child's primary language, with the therapist fluent in that same language.

Preparation. The music therapist should have available an assortment of "figurines" such as plastic finger puppets and/or action figures to serve as "characters" in the child's story. Figurines may include animals, dinosaurs, superheroes, fairies, monsters, and people (including doctor figures). Play medical kits can also be used to draw out dramatic play experiences specific to hospitalization themes. The therapist may also choose to bring a variety of musical instruments, such as an ocean drum, thunder tube, drum, xylophone, and rain stick, that could serve as sound effects or musical moments within the story. For younger children, animal-shaped instruments, such as animal castanets, could be used. The music therapist should use either a guitar or keyboard to musically reflect and facilitate the emotional tone of the child's story. The session may take place in the child's room, at the bedside, or in another area of the hospital such as a playroom, if the child is able to leave the room. As long as the child has space to manipulate the characters chosen for the story, little preparation of the therapeutic environment is required.

What to observe. First, it will be important to take note of which figurines and props the child chooses to use for the story, as well as which items are purposefully "avoided" or cast aside. Throughout the session, the therapist must take mental note of the themes of the story, especially themes that are repeated over the course of several sessions. Also, therapists should listen carefully to what the child says with specific attention to words and phrases the child uses. It is also recommended to observe the level of emotional intensity and tone of the stories while observing nonverbal cues such as facial expressions, tone of voice, and bodily actions and movements.

Procedures. This method may occur spontaneously with the child initiating storytelling during a music therapy session or by the music therapist introducing the concept of creating a musical story. When not initiated by the child, the therapist can encourage the child to choose "characters" for a story and explain how music can be added for the story, as in a movie. As the child begins to create a story, the music therapist, playing guitar or keyboard, improvises music with and without lyrics to reflect and validate the underlying emotional tone and words, phrases, and themes of the story (Hannan, 2008). The improvisational music may be primarily instrumental or can include meaningful key words and phrases mentioned in the child's narration of events. In cases where the child begins to improvise a song for the story, the music therapist should musically support the child. Also, the therapist should respect the child's choices on how musical instruments are incorporated into the story. Instruments may be played for sound effects but may also be used creatively as props for the story (e.g., a boomwhacker is used as a "tunnel," or egg shakers become "medicine").

In general, it is recommended that the music therapist be a part of the child's story only when the child initiates it by assigning the music therapist a role or character. When role-playing a character within the child's story, the therapist can improvise responses or use a "stage whisper" voice and ask the child, "What does he/she say?" or "What does he/she do now?" Throughout the session, the therapist should avoid interrupting the child's story with too many questions, and, if needing clarification or additional information, should try to integrate it within the musical improvisation, as in a call-and-response format. The therapist should also refrain from placing judgment, criticism, praise, or other value statements upon the child, such as "What a good story!" or "That animal shouldn't kill" (VanFleet, Sywulak, & Sniscak, 2010). The therapist is encouraged to trust the creative process of the child and the child's need to release various emotions as a means to work through difficult feelings (Curry, 1988; Haiat, Bar-Mor, & Shochat, 2003; Hendon & Bohon, 2008).

Adaptations. Some children may choose to videotape or audio record the musical story. Another adaptation is to integrate other expressive modalities such as drawing pictures of story scenes and then improvising music (with or without words) for each scene. Some children may also be interested in using clay or Play-Doh™ to make characters directly from their imagination. Creative possibilities for adaptation are limitless. One approach is for the therapist to create a story based upon the music improvised by the child (Sheridan & McFerran, 2004). Another adaptation is for the therapist to select storybooks that reflect situations or emotions the hospitalized child is experiencing and encourage the child to create music to accompany the story (Froehlich, 1996b).

GUIDELINES FOR RE-CREATIVE MUSIC THERAPY

Singing for Normalization and Anxiety Reduction

Overview. Singing for normalization and anxiety reduction involves actively engaging the child in singing preferred songs to enhance coping, promote relaxation, provide distraction, normalize the environment, and decrease the body's response to stress. Although singing has been integrated into improvisational methods such as active music engagement and song improvisation, singing as an independent re-creative method has been less explored in the general pediatric setting. Engaging the child in singing familiar songs can serve several purposes. First, singing during hospitalization can be an effective technique to enhance coping, promote relaxation, and provide distraction, especially during invasive procedures (Edwards, 1995, 1999b; Malone, 1996; Prensner, Yowler, Smith, Steele, & Fratianne, 2001). Second, singing familiar songs normalizes the environment by offering an organic and nonmedical experience that focuses on the child's preferences (i.e., music tastes). Third, singing can facilitate controlled as well as diaphragmatic breathing, which can decrease the body's stress response by improving oxygen intake and lowering heart rate, blood pressure, and respiratory rate (Bonilha, Onofre, Vieira, Prado, & Martinez, 2009; Irons, Kenny, McElrea, & Chang, 2012; Leanderson & Sundberg, 1988). This method is applicable for children as young as two years of age and older, as long as the child has the expressive ability to sing.

Caution needs to be taken with certain children who have respiratory illnesses or other issues such as those with a *tracheostomy.* In those cases, the music therapist should consult with the medical team, including respiratory therapists, to ensure that singing will not exacerbate the medical condition. The reader may also refer to the chapter on music therapy in respiratory care for more in-depth information related to this topic. Accordingly, children on mechanical ventilation will not be able to participate in this intervention. As in the cases of other music therapy methods, some children may feel uncomfortable, self-conscious, or inhibited to sing, especially in front of other people. In this instance, engaging the child in singing could potentially increase anxiety and may not be the best initial music therapy intervention.

Preparation. The therapist should be prepared to play the child's preferred songs on the guitar, portable keyboard, or other accompaniment instrument. The therapist may bring a capo or have solid transposition skills so that songs can be sung in a key ideal for the child's vocal range. Having song lyrics readily available is also recommended. Many therapists have binders containing a variety of songs (with lyrics and chords) in different genres which children and teens can use to select songs for singing.

What to observe. When accompanying, the therapist needs to listen to the child's singing pace, observe when the child needs to take breaths, and adjust the tempo and volume accordingly. While the child is singing, observe facial expressions, variance in intensity, and musical expressivity to gain insight as to what parts of the song seem most meaningful to the child.

Procedures. Procedures for implementing this method will be similar to music listening, under receptive methods. In many cases, music listening may naturally lead into singing. As in music listening, the child should make choices when selecting songs. Initially, the music therapist may sing along with the child and then occasionally fade out and let the child sing independently. If the child does not have the endurance or respiratory strength to sing the entire song, ask the child to sing along only to the chorus or pause before the end of a phrase and cue the child to complete it. As the therapist plays the song, be sure that the accompaniment is not overly complicated or difficult to follow. The therapist provides rhythmic support, balanced volume, and cues when necessary, musically or verbally, for taking breaths, such as before a chorus or phrase. When singing with adolescents, the therapist should use a therapeutic voice vs. a performance voice to prevent overshadowing or intimidating the teen, who may already feel self-conscious or inhibited to sing. Adolescents may also readily engage in discussion about the lyrics and the personal meaningfulness of the song. Throughout the process, the therapist should be mindful to provide musical reinforcement and verbal encouragement in a way that empowers the child or teen. For example, instead of responding, "Nice singing," the therapist can give a more meaningful response by saying something specific about the musical experience: "I noticed your voice became stronger with each verse" or "I can tell this part of the song brought you some joy because your entire face lit up with a smile. Let's sing that section again."

Adaptations. Children may benefit from recording the sessions and creating their own music CD to take home upon discharge. Singing can also serve as a catalyst for improvisation or songwriting. Some music therapists use therapeutic singing to improve lung capacity and respiratory strength as a primary goal (Hurt-Thaut & Johnson, 2003; Rudenberg & Royka, 1989).

Therapeutic Music Instruction

Overview. Therapeutic music instruction is the process of teaching a child or adolescent to play a musical instrument, such as guitar or keyboard, for the purpose of enhancing self-esteem while also stimulating executive functioning skills. Learning to successfully play favorite songs on a musical instrument can promote a sense of empowerment and control and can be an ideal intervention for preteens and adolescents who have recurrent or prolonged hospitalizations (Abad, 2003). Adolescence is a critical stage of development marked by an exploration of self-identity and rapid cognitive development. Teaching an adolescent to play an instrument such as the guitar, ukulele, dulcimer, harmonica, or keyboard can not only provide necessary cognitive stimulation, but also enhance positive self-concept through having a successful experience. The primary goal is to facilitate emotional and cognitive adjustment by mastering the new skill of learning to play a musical instrument. The process of learning and mastering a new skill that is personally meaningful can facilitate positive self-perception (Shields, 2001). Particularly during adolescence when identity development remains a significant milestone, positive identity development and personal growth can serve as aids in coping and adjusting to illness (Berntsson, Berg, Brydolf, & Hellstrom, 2007; Luyckx et al., 2008).

Before implementing this method, the adolescent needs to have the cognitive and motor skills to learn a musical instrument; otherwise, he may become frustrated due to lack of success. When physical limitations restrict his ability to learn an instrument using traditional methods, the music therapist can use adaptive devices and alternative methods of instruction (Clark & Chadwick, 1980). Other resources, such as *Therapeutic Guitar* (Krout, 2011), can provide the music therapist with additional suggestions for adaptive instruction. However, the music therapist should be sensitive in approaching the topic of adaptive methods, as some teenagers may feel "different" and discouraged that their illness prevents them from learning a desired skill in a traditional way.

Preparation. Therapeutic music instruction can occur at the bedside or in another location such as a hospital "teen room." Positioning of the instrument will depend upon the adolescent's positioning (sitting in a chair or bed) and location of IVs and other lines that may impede mobility. Portable keyboards can be placed on an adjustable tray-table found in the hospital room. After the session, be sure to return items back onto the tray-table, such as water, tissues, or other items that were removed. If the adolescent is in isolation, it is beneficial to leave the instrument in the room throughout hospitalization to decrease the need to repeatedly disinfect the instrument. Loaning the instrument offers the adolescent the opportunity to practice skills learned. The therapist can bring a note pad, pen, and a folder to keep notes, as well as any necessary teaching tools, including staff/tablature paper and any adaptive devices. It is recommended to structure and pace the session according to the adolescent's physical abilities and limitations, learning style, attention level, and musical interests. For general pediatric units that do not have private rooms but rather shared patient rooms, the music therapist needs to be respectful of the roommate. The degree of tolerance in listening to one's roommate "practice" an instrument will vary. Possible solutions to resolving this concern are to provide the teen with headphones (if using an electronic instrument), schedule an agreeable time during the day for "practicing," or offer the roommate an opportunity to participate in learning an instrument if clinically appropriate.

What to observe. During the session, the music therapist should be attentive to the teen's level of participation and motivation. Some may initiate asking questions and be actively involved in the learning process, while others appear hesitant, unsure, or frustrated or demonstrate little assertiveness and independence. Observing how the teen responds to the challenge of learning an instrument, either with perseverance or apprehension, can be a reflection on how he copes with his own illness. Listening to self-statements made by the teen, both positive and negative, will also provide insight into his view of self.

Procedures. In many ways, the session will have similarities to teaching music lessons although the purpose is more process-oriented vs. product-oriented. To foster self-concept, adolescents should be encouraged to establish their own goals (e.g., learn three guitar chords to play one song, learn to play the melody of a chorus on the keyboard, or learn to play a blues riff on the harmonica), keeping in mind a realistic time frame. In teaching, the music therapist should cater to the teen's skill level (from simple to complex musical concepts) and focus on learning one concept at a time while reinforcing previously learned concepts. For a pleasing musical experience, the therapist should also consider musically reinforcing and supporting the adolescent, such as by playing guitar chords as the patient plays a melody on the keyboard. Throughout the session, focusing on the successes, big and small, and providing positive feedback that is immediate and specific will help to build the adolescent's self-confidence. For example, to say "You learned to play that chord in only two minutes" brings the accomplishment back to the adolescent. In ending the session, guide the teen to verbally acknowledge his own successes as a means for him to internalize self-validation.

Adaptations. When an adolescent has successfully mastered learning a song or riff, an opportunity arises for the teen to demonstrate this accomplishment to others. For teens who are hospitalized for prolonged periods of time, a music performance may be a possibility. Music performances can enhance positive self-concept development, whether performing composed songs or showcasing new skills learned on the guitar (Abad, 2003; Neugebauer, 2008). Encouraging teens to perform or play what they learned can be an additional way to enhance self-esteem. A "performance" can be done informally for just a few people or done on a larger scale with the teen planning the program, creating invitations, and choosing the time and location.

GUIDELINES FOR COMPOSITIONAL MUSIC THERAPY

Songwriting for Self-Expression and Coping

Overview. Songwriting is most likely the most applied compositional method in music therapy when working with hospitalized children, particularly, children with cancer (Kennelly, 2001; Robb, 1996; Turry, 1999; Turry & Turry, 1999). Songwriting involves several approaches, including song parody, fill-in-the blank, song collage, and original composition, to provide opportunities for self-expression, enhance coping and adjustment, and facilitate identification of individual strengths and support systems. Songwriting is a technique that can be tailored for many hospitalized children, including preschoolers, school-age patients, and adolescents. It is indicated for those who need an outlet or venue to communicate thoughts, express feelings, find meaning, and process what they are experiencing. The goal is to provide the opportunity for self-expression in order to enhance coping and adjustment. Songwriting can also be used to help the child to identify specific internal and external strengths, support systems, and approaches to aid in coping.

Songwriting may prove challenging or frustrating for children who are nonverbal or have profound limits in cognitive ability. In these cases, the therapist may use adaptive communicative devices or other technology to communicate words or ideas for songwriting. The music therapist may also use a closed-ended question approach (yes/no questions) if the child can respond by using body language, such as blinking his eyes or raising a finger. Another alternative is to involve the child's family in the songwriting experience and have families share what they know about the child so that the music therapist can use this in the songwriting process.

Preparation. One of the benefits of songwriting is that it can be done easily at the bedside, regardless of the child's positioning or degree of physical limitations. Session preparation will depend in part on the songwriting method. When using structured formats for songwriting, such as song parody, fill-in-the-blank, or mad-lib, the music therapist will need to bring prepared materials to the session. For most sessions, the music therapist will need to bring a guitar or keyboard as well as a pen and pad of paper. In situations where the song will have original music as well as lyrics, bringing a recording device to remember the melodic and harmonic arrangement may be useful.

What to observe. Throughout the session, the therapist should observe the child's level of involvement/participation, motivation, assertiveness, creativity, mood, emotional responses (e.g., does the child get frustrated with the process?), depth of personal disclosure, and song topics/subjects.

Procedures. Songwriting is flexible and can be easily modified according to the child's musical tastes, preferences, endurance level, developmental level, and cognitive ability. Structured songwriting experiences such as song parody or fill-in-the blank formats can serve as a warm-up to writing an original song. Lyric substitution or song parody approaches provide a flexible structure while promoting opportunities to express strong emotions such as feelings of isolation or frustration with illness-related challenges (Abad, 2003; Sheridan & McFerran, 2004). Another structured option is a technique referred to as song collage (Tamplin, 2006). In this method, the child selects specific words, phrases, or verses from different songs which are then combined into an entirely new song. Sometimes the songwriting process can occur spontaneously, such as when the child makes a statement during a session and the therapist uses that opportunity to take that comment and create a song lyric. This action may result in a continued collaboration between child and therapist to write a song. When introducing songwriting for the first time, a safe way to begin is to ask the child what topic he would like to write a song about. The subject of the song may be about the hospitalization experience or illness or may be a completely unrelated topic. Persuading children to write songs about difficult emotional topics may cause the child to withdraw, especially if trust has not been established. In assisting children to brainstorm ideas to use in a song, Hannan (2008) uses a tool called a mind map which involves writing down words and ideas clustered around the word or phrase representing the song's central theme. Once the topic has been selected, the songwriting process generally begins with the lyrics. Asking open-ended questions and writing down responses can create a flow of ideas pertinent for lyrics and phrases. The role of the music therapist is to help take the children's words and ideas and put them into the format of a song. Some therapists find it easier to begin with the chorus, as it can provide therapeutic resonance of what the child wants to express. Regardless of the procedure, the majority of the lyrics should come from the child's own words, without judgment or unsolicited influence from the therapist. When composing original music, the child should participate in choosing the stylistic characteristics of the music, including musical genre. The therapist can play sample melodies or chord progressions and ask the child for feedback as to likes and dislikes. When the song is completed, the child can sing along, play along with an instrument (e.g., tambourine), or solely listen to the final product.

Adaptations. Oftentimes, a song written by a child can subsequently be used in creating a music video. Children may also choose to share songs with family members or staff as a means for an additional outlet for communication. When children compose several songs over the course of one or many hospitalizations, one can create a CD and even design a CD cover using the child's original artwork. When making recordings or videotaping, the music therapist may need to have formal permission/written consent from the legal guardian, even when the recording will only be given to the child. The therapist should check with the hospital or institution's legal department prior to making any recordings. Another adaptation is to include the child's family in the songwriting process. As with any group approach to songwriting, the therapist needs to be sure that all family members contribute to the song without any one family member taking over or dominating the process. One approach to preventing this from happening is for the therapist to facilitate a turn-taking approach or assign each family member a line or verse to write. The music therapist can also create an original song for a child based upon information gathered from the child, family, and staff. Whitehead-Pleaux, Clark, and Spall (2011) describe a case example using GarageBand to create a CD for a child soon to be discharged after a long hospitalization. The music therapist created an original composition looping positive messages from staff into the music to create a song the child could listen to upon returning home.

Group songwriting is applicable for school-age and adolescent young people. Generally, the music therapist will need to provide more structure to the process when working with groups vs. individuals to ensure that each child in the group has an opportunity to contribute to the song.

Music Video Creation

Overview. Music video creation is a process, including planning, decision-making, and designing, that uses technology and media to create an original music video composition that conceptualizes one's thoughts and emotions into a contained product. Music video creation is a method that can be particularly beneficial when working with children hospitalized for an extended period of time (Robb & Ebberts, 2003a, 2003b). This projective technique can be an effective tool to provide the child or teen a safe outlet to expressive feelings while providing the therapist insight into the child's or teen's perspective. Although most often used with an adolescent population, this method can be relevant for school-age children as well. The aspect of utilizing technology can be appealing for many children who seem less motivated by or interested in other therapeutic music experiences. The process of creating the video, as well as the completed product, allows the child intellectual stimulation, a motivating leisure interest, and, most importantly, a forum for self-expression. The goals of this method are to enhance coping, facilitate adjustment, and promote positive self-concept development.

Because the process of making a music video can take several sessions to complete, this method is not indicated for short-term hospitalizations. Also, the music therapist needs to consider whether the child has the cognitive ability and patience to participate in such a project.

Preparation. Prior to implementing this method, the music therapist needs to be proficient in using the technology chosen for the project. Depending upon the type of music video that will be created, Internet access may be useful to search for images or pictures to use in the video. Access to purchasing and downloading music from a source such as iTunes™ may be necessary. It is important that the music therapist be up to date regarding copyright laws and legal use of recorded music and how these laws apply to music therapy practice. The music therapist will need to use a laptop or tablet computer with a software program or app that can be used for making videos. Common video-making programs include Windows Movie Maker™, iMovie™, and iDVD™; however, technological advances will certainly elicit additional viable options in the future. Other items that may be needed include a video camera (separate or built into the computer), digital camera, and photo scanner. As songs are chosen for the video, the music therapist needs to be aware of digital music file formatting requirements so that the media file will be compatible with the video software program or application. The therapist may wish to bring a paper and pen for writing down ideas and drawing a conceptual map for the music video. It is also useful to bring a copy of the song lyrics. This author also recommends having a computer file readily available with a variety of photos and images from which the children can select. This is helpful for those children who may have trouble coming up with ideas for the video content. The child may want to film or photograph other areas of the hospital for use within the video. Needless to say, the music therapist needs to take care that no other individuals are captured in this video fragments or pictures unless explicit video or picture releases have been obtained.

What to observe. The music therapist should be attentive to the child's ability to make his own decisions throughout the process of the project. The content of the composition, including the theme/topic and choices for songs, video clips, images, and photos, may be a significant indicator of what the child is experiencing and wants to communicate. Throughout the process, the therapist should attend to the child's level of motivation, thought process, degree of participation, ability to assert independence, ego strength, and view of self.

Procedures. When introducing the idea of making a music video, it can be motivating to share one or two completed examples with the child or teen to aid in conceptualizing the project. The music therapist may wish to create an example on her own or ask former patients for consent to use their videos to share with others. Once interest has been expressed in creating a music video, the first step is to determine what song to use for the audio component. One approach is to ask the child to choose a song that is meaningful, significant, comforting, or empowering or to use an original song that he has composed during a previous music therapy session. Once the song has been chosen, it is helpful to listen to the song and have the child freely express what thoughts come to mind when hearing the song. The music therapist can write down what the child verbalizes so that this can facilitate further brainstorming about the project. The next step is to choose the visual media for the project. Some children may prefer to participate in filming excerpts or taking photos, while others prefer to select images from the Internet or from the therapist's photo file. The child can choose to have photos or clips correspond with specific lyrics in the song or can create a randomized "collage" of images. Throughout the process, if the child appears overwhelmed, the therapist can break the project down into smaller components such as by focusing on one verse per session. The music therapist should offer guidance in facilitating the compositional process but should not influence the child's choices regarding content of the project itself. The final step is to compile the audio, video, photos, and images into the program, begin the editing process, and burn the final version onto a DVD for the child to have. The entire process, from beginning to end, can take several days or even weeks to complete, depending upon the complexity of the video. When the video is complete, the child or teen may wish to show the video to family, friends, or staff.

Adaptations. This method allows for many creative opportunities for additional applications. Children can have an official "viewing" of the music video, similar to a performance experience. Music videos can also provide a means to showcase artwork, using a slide show format, for those children who find drawing, painting, sketching, or other media to be a meaningful outlet for expression. Electronic or digital music, such as music composed using programs like GarageBand™, could be used for the audio component of the video.

This method can be implemented within a group format, especially if the group can work on the project over the course of consecutive sessions. To streamline the process, the music therapist can use a directive approach of assigning a song for the project or have the group choose from a selection of songs. Depending upon time constraints, using a slide show format for the video may serve more practical.

RESEARCH EVIDENCE

Few research studies exist at this time specific to music therapy in general pediatric medicine. However, some are worth highlighting. To learn more about research evidence specific to music therapy in pain management and in pediatric surgical care, the reader should consult Chapters 2 and 6, respectively. In addition, readers should turn to Chapter 8, *Music Therapy in Pediatric Cancer*, as many research findings and clinical approaches are applicable to the general pediatric population.

Two systematic reviews of randomized controlled trials have investigated the evidence base for music with pediatrics. Mrázová and Celec (2010) conducted a systematic review of randomized controlled trials (RCT) specific to music therapy with children. The review included music therapy and music medicine studies as well as studies investigating music with children with depression and autism. The authors identified 28 studies that met the criteria which covered a broad range of diagnoses and types of music interventions. Due to the variability among the studies as well as most studies having a low number of participants or poor control group design, the authors concluded that better-designed studies with stronger statistical power need to be conducted in order to support the evidence base for music in pediatrics. Treurnicht et al. (2011) conducted a review of 17 randomized controlled trials in pediatric health care consisting of both music therapy and music medicine. The authors were unable to pool the data from these studies due to the studies having a wide range of variability as well as poor methodological quality. Instead, the authors provided a narrative synthesis summarizing the studies according to diagnoses and outcomes. In discussing their findings, the authors commented that music therapy may enhance cognition, facilitate communication, and reduce the effects of trauma through enhanced coping strategies for hospitalized children.

Approaches that focus on engagement, choice and control, and reciprocal music interaction as a way to enhance coping have been explored in the music therapy pediatric literature. In an early study by Froehlich (1984), the researcher compared two groups of children's verbalized responses to four questions about hospitalization: interactive music therapy (singing, movement, and instrument-playing) compared to medical play therapy (hospital story, medical play, and free play). Children in the music therapy group were asked questions within the content of a song, whereas children in the medical play group were asked the questions verbally. Children (ages 5–12) were randomized to either the music therapy group (N = 20) or the medical play therapy group (N = 19). Results showed that 90% of children's responses in the music therapy group were coded as "answer," compared to 62% of children's responses in the medical play group. Due to the exploratory nature of the study, the researcher chose a significance level of .10. Using a posttest-only design, a content analysis of the videotaped sessions indicated that children in the music therapy group verbalized "more involved" feelings about hospitalization, compared to children in the medical play group [$\chi^2(13)$ = 31.39, p < .10]. Similarly, Hendon and Bohon (2008) compared music therapy with play sessions in a general hospital setting. Sixty children, ages 13 months to 12 years, were observed either during a music therapy intervention (singing with instrument-playing) or a play therapy intervention (free play). An observer monitored each child for three minutes and documented the number of positive affective responses (smiling) within that interval. Children in the music therapy group demonstrated significantly more positive affect responses (M = 12.43, SD = 4.83) compared to children in the play therapy group (M = 5.83, SD = 3.10)(p < 0.001). Through involving children with singing, instrument-playing, imitative and improvisational music-making, and listening activities, Lane (1994) investigated the effects of a single 30-minute music therapy session compared to a control group (30-minute nonmusic activity) on salivary IgA, an indicator of immune function. Although the study sample was small (N = 38), results suggested that children who received the 30-minute music therapy session showed a significant increase (p < .01) in their salivary IgA after the music treatment condition.

Music technology, especially as a tool for compositional methods, has become a growing specialization within the music therapy field. Colwell, Davis, and Schroeder (2005) conducted a study to measure the effect that creating an art or music composition had on self-concept in 24 hospitalized children, ages 7 to 18. Children were randomly assigned to receive one 45- to 60-minute art session (using standard art media to create a picture) or music session (compositional software program). The results indicated no differences between groups on total self-concept scores. The music composition group showed a significant increase in self-concept subscores in the areas of Intellectual and School Status ($p = .02$) and Physical Appearance and Attributes ($p = .026$). When comparing subscore categories between the two conditions, the music composition group showed more improvement in the Intellectual and School Status category [$F(1,21) = 6.74$, $p = .017$].

SUMMARY AND CONCLUSIONS

The general pediatric unit is one of the most diverse and fascinating areas to work in within the pediatric medical setting. The music therapist working in this setting should possess the full range of skills to deal with the multifaceted psychosocial and medical factors that can either inhibit or facilitate coping, adjustment, development, and quality of life. Because research in pediatric music therapy continuously evolves, the music therapist should keep current on publications in both scientific and clinical journals as well as books and online resources. In addition to the music therapy literature, this author recommends reading the work in related disciplines such as developmental psychology, play therapy, and nursing in order to gain additional insight, increased knowledge, and deeper understanding of theoretical models and approaches in order to better address the needs of hospitalized children. Continuing education courses and professional conferences are additional venues to learn more about pediatric music therapy and hospitalized children. Given the limited amount of research at this time supporting evidence-based practice, music therapists working in this area would benefit from collaboration with seasoned researchers. The music therapist clinician can shed insight into observed outcomes in the clinical setting as the experienced researcher develops well-designed studies, including quantitative, qualitative, and mixed methods, to examine such clinical phenomena. When the evidence base strongly supports the benefits of music therapy in pediatric health care, music therapy will more likely become a standard of care in every children's hospital.

GLOSSARY

Definitions obtained or adapted from: MedicineNet.com, medical-dictionary.thefreedictionary.com, and Medline Plus.

Cerebral palsy: a disability resulting from damage to the brain before, during, or shortly after birth and outwardly manifested by muscular incoordination and speech disturbances.

Colostomy: a surgical procedure where a portion of the large intestine is brought through the abdominal wall to carry stool out of the body.

Colostomy bag: a removable, disposable bag that attaches to the exterior opening of a *colostomy* to permit sanitary collection and disposal of bodily wastes.

Cystic fibrosis: a genetic disease that affects the lungs, digestive system, sweat glands, and male fertility. It is characterized by the production of abnormal secretions, leading to mucus buildup that impairs breathing, the pancreas, and, secondarily, the intestine.

Epilepsy: a brain disorder that causes people to have recurring seizures.

Gastroenteritis: inflammation of the lining membrane of the stomach and the intestines that can cause abdominal discomfort, vomiting, and diarrhea.

Gastrostomy: a surgical opening into the stomach. A gastrostomy may be used for feeding, usually via a feeding tube called a gastrostomy tube.

Hydrocephalus: an abnormal buildup of cerebrospinal fluid (CSF) in the ventricles of the brain that is accompanied by expansion of the cerebral ventricles, enlargement of the skull and especially the forehead, and atrophy of the brain. The fluid is often under increased pressure and can compress and damage the brain.

Inflammatory Bowel Disease: a group of chronic intestinal diseases characterized by inflammation of the bowel—the large or small intestine. The most common types are ulcerative colitis and Crohn's Disease.

Intravenous line: an apparatus used to administer a fluid (as of medication, blood, or nutrients) into a vein.

Mitochondrial disease: a genetic neuromuscular disease caused by damage to the mitochondria—small, energy-producing structures that serve as cells' "power plants." Nerve cells in the brain and muscles require a great deal of energy, and thus appear to be particularly damaged when mitochondrial dysfunction occurs.

Nasal cannula: a device for delivering oxygen by way of two small tubes that are inserted into the nostrils.

Osteomyelitis: an infectious and usually painful inflammatory disease of bone that is often of bacterial origin and may result in death of bone tissue.

Peripherally inserted central catheter (PICC): a long catheter introduced through a vein in the arm and then through the subclavian vein into the superior vena cava or right atrium to administer parenteral fluids or medications or to measure central venous pressure.

Sensory integration disorder: a neurological disorder that results from the brain's inability to integrate certain information received from the body's five basic sensory systems.

Sickle cell disease: an inherited blood disorder characterized by chronic anemia, painful events, and various complications due to associated tissue and organ damage. Because sickle cell diseases are characterized by the rapid loss of red blood cells as they enter the circulation, they are classified as hemolytic disorders, "hemolytic" referring to the destruction of the cell membrane of red blood cells, resulting in the release of hemoglobin.

Spina bifida: a serious birth abnormality in which the spinal cord is malformed and lacks its usual protective skeletal and soft tissue coverings.

Spinal Muscular Atrophy: any of several inherited disorders that are characterized by the degeneration of motor neurons in the spinal cord, resulting in muscular weakness and atrophy, and that in some forms are fatal.

Tracheostomy: an opening through the neck into the trachea through which a tube may be inserted to maintain an effective airway and help a patient breathe.

Trisomy 21 syndrome: a common chromosome disorder, often called Down's Syndrome, due to an extra chromosome number 21 (trisomy 21). The chromosome abnormality affects both the physical and intellectual development of the individual.

Type 1 diabetes: a form of diabetes that usually develops during childhood or adolescence and is characterized by a severe deficiency of insulin secretion resulting from atrophy of the islets of Langerhans and causing hyperglycemia and a marked tendency toward ketoacidosis (a condition due to starvation or uncontrolled Type I diabetes that causes abdominal pain, vomiting, rapid breathing, extreme tiredness, and drowsiness).

References

AMTA Standards of Clinical Practice. (n.d.). *American Music Therapy Association.* Retrieved November 1, 2012, from http://www.musictherapy.org/about/standards/

Abad, V. (2003). A time of turmoil: Music therapy interventions for adolescents in a paediatric oncology ward. *Australian Journal of Music Therapy, 14,* 20–33.

Abad, V., & Edwards, J. (2004). Strengthening families: A role for music therapy in contributing to family centered care. *Australian Journal of Music Therapy, 15,* 3–17.

Abraham, M., & Moretz, J. G. (2012). Implementing patient and family-centered care: Part I—understanding the challenges. *Pediatric Nursing, 38*(1), 44–47.

Acute illness: *MedicineNet.com.* (n.d.). Retrieved from http://www.medterms.com/script/main/art.asp?articlekey=2134

Aldridge, D., Gustroff, G., & Neugebauer, L. (1995). A pilot study of music therapy in the treatment of children with developmental delay. *Complementary Therapies in Medicine, 3*(4), 197–205.

Barrera, M. E., Rykov, M. H., & Doyle, S. L. (2002). The effects of interactive music therapy on hospitalized children with cancer: A pilot study. *Psycho-oncology, 11*(5), 379–388.

Barrickman, J. (1989). A developmental music therapy approach for preschool hospitalized children. *Music Therapy Perspectives, 7,* 10–16.

Berntsson, L., Berg, M., Brydolf, M., & Hellstrom, A. (2007). Adolescents' experiences of well-being when living with a long-term illness or disability. *Scandinavian Journal of Caring Sciences, 21,* 419–425.

Blakemore, S., Burnett, S., & Dahl, R. (2010). The role of puberty in the developing adolescent brain. *Human Brain Mapping, 31*(6), 926–933.

Bonilha, A. G., Onofre, F., Vieira, M. L., Prado, M. Y. A., & Martinez, J. A. (2009). Effects of singing classes on pulmonary function and quality of life of COPD patients. *International Journal of Chronic Obstructive Pulmonary Disease, 4,* 1–8.

Brounley, N. (1996). Puppet and drama therapy with hospitalized and abused children. In M. A. Froehlich (Ed.), *Music therapy with hospitalized children: A creative arts child life approach* (pp. 177–193). Cherry Hill, NJ: Jeffrey Books.

Bruscia, K. E. (1987). *Improvisational models of music therapy.* Springfield, IL: Charles C. Thomas.

Chronic illness: *MedicineNet.com.* (n.d.). Retrieved May 5, 2012, from http://www.medterms.com/script/main/art.asp?articlekey=2731

Clark, C., & Chadwick, D. (1980). *Clinically adapted instruments for the multiply handicapped: A sourcebook.* St. Louis, MO: Magnamusic-Baton.

Colwell, C. M., Davis, K., & Schroeder, L. K. (2005). The effect of composition (art or music) on the self-concept of hospitalized children. *Journal of Music Therapy, 42*(1), 49–63.

Criddle, L. (2010). Monsters in the closet: Munchausen syndrome by proxy. *Critical Care Nurse, 30*(6), 46–55.

Curry, N. E. (1988). Enhancing dramatic play potential in hospitalized children. *Children's Health Care, 16*(3), 142–149.

Edwards, J. (1999a). Anxiety management in pediatric music therapy. In C. Dileo (Ed.), *Music therapy and medicine: Theoretical and clinical applications* (pp. 69–76). Silver Spring, MD: American Music Therapy Association.

Edwards, J. (1999b). Music therapy for children hospitalised for severe injury or illness. *British Journal of Music Therapy, 13*(1), 21–27.

Edwards, J. (2005). Special feature: A reflection on the music therapist's role in developing a program in a children's hospital. *Music Therapy Perspectives, 23*(1), 36–44.

Failure to thrive: *MedlinePlus Medical Encyclopedia*. (n.d.). Retrieved May 28, 2012, from http://www.nlm.nih.gov/medlineplus/ency/article/000991.htm

Froehlich, M. A. (1984). A comparison of the effect of music therapy and medical play on the verbalization behavior of pediatric patients. *Journal of Music Therapy, 21*, 2–15.

Froehlich, M. A. (1996a). Orff-Schulwerk music therapy in crisis intervention with hospitalized children. In M. A. Froehlich (Ed.), *Music therapy with hospitalized children: A creative arts child life approach* (pp. 25–36). Cherry Hill, NJ: Jeffrey Books.

Froehlich, M. A. (1996b). Bibliotherapy and creative writing as expressive arts with hospitalized children. In M. A. Froehlich (Ed.), *Music therapy with hospitalized children: A creative arts child life approach* (pp. 195–206). Cherry Hill, NJ: Jeffrey Books.

Ghetti, C. M. (2011). Active music engagement with emotional-approach coping to improve well-being in liver and kidney transplant recipients. *Journal of Music Therapy, 48*(4), 463–485.

Gorrindo, P., Williams, K. C., Lee, E. B., Walker, L. S., McGrew, S. G., & Levitt, P. (2012). Gastrointestinal dysfunction in autism: Parental report, clinical evaluation, and associated factors. *Autism Research: Official Journal of the International Society for Autism Research, 5*(2), 101–108.

Haas, F., Distenfeld, S., & Axen, K. (1986). Effects of perceived music rhythm on respiratory patterns. *Journal of Applied Physiology, 61*(3), 1185–1191.

Haiat, H., Bar-Mor, G., & Shochat, M. (2003). The world of the child: A world of play even in the hospital. *Journal of Pediatric Nursing, 18*(3), 209–214.

Hannan, A. (2008). General pediatrics medical/surgical. In D. Hanson-Abromeit & C. Colwell (Eds.), *Medical music therapy for pediatrics in hospital settings* (pp. 107–146). Silver Spring, MD: American Music Therapy Association.

Hanson-Abromeit, D., & Colwell, C. (Eds.). (2008). *Medical music therapy for pediatrics in hospital settings*. Silver Spring, MD: American Music Therapy Association.

Hendon, C., & Bohon, L. M. (2008). Hospitalized children's mood differences during play and music therapy. *Child: Care, Health and Development, 34*(2), 141–144.

Hurt-Thaut, C., & Johnson, S. (2003). Neurologic music therapy with children: Scientific foundations and clinical application. In S. L. Robb (Ed.), *Music therapy in pediatric healthcare: Research and evidence based practice* (pp. 81–100). Silver Spring, MD: American Music Therapy Association.

Irons, J. Y., Kenny, D. T., McElrea, M., & Chang, A. B. (2012). Singing therapy for young people with cystic fibrosis: A randomized controlled pilot study. *Music and Medicine, 4*(3), 136–145.

Jacquet, C. (2011). Music therapy and pediatrics: Impact on the parent-child relationship. *Canadian Journal of Music Therapy, 17*(1), 95–103.

Kennelly, J. (2000). The specialist role of the music therapist in developmental programs for hospitalized children. *Journal of Pediatric Health Care, 14*(2), 56–59.

Kennelly, J. (2001). Music therapy in the bone marrow transplant unit: Providing emotional support during adolescence. *Music Therapy Perspectives, 19*(2), 104–108.

Khalfa, S., Bella, S. D., Roy, M., Peretz, I., & Lupien, S. J. (2003). Effects of relaxing music on salivary cortisol level after psychological stress. *Annals of the New York Academy of Sciences, 999*, 374–376.

Koshland, L., & Curry, L. (1996). Dance/movement therapy with hospitalized children. In M. A. Froehlich (Ed.), *Music therapy with hospitalized children: A creative arts child life approach* (pp. 161–176). Cherry Hill, NJ: Jeffrey Books.

Krout, R. E. (2011). *Therapeutic guitar*. Van Nuys, CA: Alfred Music Publishing Co., Inc.

Lane, D. (1994). Effects of music therapy on immune function of hospitalized patients. *Quality of Life—A Nursing Challenge, 3*(4), 74–80.

Leanderson, R., & Sundberg, J. (1988). Breathing for singing. *Journal of Voice, 2*(1), 2–12.

Loveszy, R. (1991). The use of latin music, puppetry, and visualization in reducing the physical and emotional pain of a child with severe burns. In K. E. Bruscia (Ed.), *Case studies in music therapy* (pp. 153–161). Gilsum, NH: Barcelona Publishers.

Luyckx, K., Seiffge-Krenke, I., Schwartz, S. J., Goossens, L., Weets, I., Hendrieckz, C., & Groven, C. (2008). Identity development, coping, and adjustment in emerging adults with a chronic illness: The sample case of type 1 diabetes. *Journal of Adolescent Health, 43,* 451–458.

Malone, A. B. (1996). The effects of live music on the distress of pediatric patients receiving intravenous starts, venipunctures, injections, and heel sticks. *Journal of Music Therapy, 33*(1), 19–33.

Manificat, S., Guillaud-Bataille, J. M., & Dazord, A. (1993). Quality of life in children with chronic disease. Review of the literature and conceptual aspects. *Pediatrie, 48*(7–8), 519–527.

Marley, L. (1984). The use of music with hospitalized infants and toddlers: A descriptive study. *Journal of Music Therapy, 21*(3), 126–132.

Marley, L. (1996). Music therapy with hospitalized infants and toddlers in a child life program. In M. A. Froehlich (Ed.), *Music therapy with hospitalized children: A creative arts child life approach* (pp. 77–86). Cherry Hill, NJ: Jeffrey Books.

McCauley, K. (1996). Music therapy with pediatric aids patients. In M. A. Froehlich (Ed.), *Music therapy with hospitalized children: A creative arts child life approach* (pp. 233–240). Cherry Hill, NJ: Jeffrey Books.

McCraty, R., Atkinson, M., Rein, G., & Watkins, A. (1996). Music enhances the effect of positive emotional states on salivary IgA. *Stress Medicine, 12,* 167–175.

McDonnell, L. (1984). Music therapy with trauma patients and their families on a pediatric service. *Music Therapy, 4*(1), 55–63.

Mrázová, M., & Celec, P. (2010). A systematic review of randomized controlled trials using music therapy for children. *Journal of Alternative and Complementary Medicine, 16*(10), 1089–1095.

Neugebauer, C. T. (2008). Pediatric burn recovery: Acute care, rehabilitation, and reconstruction. In D. Hanson-Abromeit & C. M. Colwell (Eds.), *Medical music therapy for pediatrics in hospital settings* (pp. 195–230). Silver Spring, MD: American Music Therapy Association.

Pao, M., Ballard, E. D., & Rosenstein, D. L. (2007). Growing up in the hospital. *JAMA®: The Journal of the American Medical Association, 297*(24), 2752–2755.

Pao, M., & Bosk, A. (2011). Anxiety in medically ill children/adolescents. *Depression and Anxiety, 28*(1), 40–49.

Payot, A., & Barrington, K. J. (2011). The quality of life of young children and infants with chronic medical problems: Review of the literature. *Current Problems in Pediatric and Adolescent Health Care, 41*(4), 91–101.

Perrin, J. M., Bloom, S. R., & Gortmaker, S. L. (2012). The increase of childhood chronic conditions in the United States. *Public Health, 297*(24), 2755–2759.

Prensner, J. D., Yowler, C. J., Smith, L. F., Steele, A. L., & Fratianne, R. B. (2001). Music therapy for assistance with pain and anxiety management in burn treatment. *Journal of Burn Care & Rehabilitation, 22*(1), 83–88.

Robb, S. L. (1996). Special feature: Techniques in song writing: Restoring emotional and physical well-being in adolescents who have been traumatically injured. *Music Therapy Perspectives, 14*( ), 30–37.

Robb, S. L. (2000). The effect of therapeutic music interventions on the behavior of hospitalized children in isolation: Developing a contextual support model of music therapy. *Journal of Music Therapy, 27*( ), 118–146.

Robb, S. L. (2003a). Designing music therapy interventions for hospitalized children and adolescents using a contextual support model of music therapy. *Music Therapy Perspectives, 1*( ), 27–40.

Robb, S. L. (2003b). Coping and chronic illness: Music therapy for children and adults with cancer. In S. L. Robb (Ed.), *Music therapy in pediatric healthcare: Research and evidence-based practice* (pp. 101–136). Silver Spring, MD: American Music Therapy Association.

Robb, S. L, & Ebberts, A. G. (2003a). Songwriting and digital video production interventions for pediatric patients undergoing bone marrow transplantation, part I: An analysis of depression and anxiety levels according to phase of treatment. *Journal of Pediatric Oncology Nursing, 20*(1), 2–15.

Robb, S. L, & Ebberts, A. G. (2003b). Songwriting and digital video production interventions for pediatric patients undergoing bone marrow transplantation, part II: An analysis of patient-generated songs and patient perceptions regarding intervention efficacy. *Journal of Pediatric Oncology Nursing, 20*(1), 16–25.

Rudenberg, M. T., & Royka, A. M. (1989). Promoting psychosocial adjustment in pediatric burn patients through music therapy and child life therapy. *Music Therapy Perspectives, 7,* 40–43.

Sabbatella, P. E. (2004). Assessment and clinical evaluation in music therapy: An overview from literature and clinical practice. *Music Therapy Today* (online), *5*(1), available at http://musictherapyworld.net

Schwartz, E. (2008). *Music, therapy, and early childhood: A developmental approach.* Gilsum, NH: Barcelona Publishers.

Shelton, T. L., Jeppson, E. S., & Johnson, B. H. (1987). *Family-centered care for children with special health care needs.* Washington, DC: Association for the Care of Children's Health.

Sheridan, J., & McFerran, K. (2004). Exploring the value of opportunities for choice and control in music therapy within a paediatric hospice setting. *Australian Journal of Music Therapy, 15,* 18–31.

Shields, C. (2001). Music education and mentoring as intervention for at-risk urban adolescents: Their self-perceptions, opinions, and attitudes. *Journal of Research in Music Education, 49*(3), 273–286.

Smith, E. J. (2006). The strength-based counseling model: A paradigm shift in psychology. *The Counseling Psychologist, 34*(1), 134–144.

Tamplin, J. (2006). Song collage technique : A new approach to songwriting. *Nordic Journal of Music Therapy, 15*(2), 177–190.

Taylor, R. M., Gibson, F., & Franck, L. S. (2008). The experience of living with a chronic illness during adolescence: A critical review of the literature. *Journal of Clinical Nursing, 17*(23), 3083–3091.

Teaford, P., Wheat, J., & Baker, T. (Eds.). (2010). *HELP 3-6 Assessment Strands* (2nd ed.). Palo Alto, CA: CORT Corporation.

Treurnicht, N. K., Kingsnorth, S., Lamont, A., McKeever, P., & Macarthur, C. (2011). The effectiveness of music in pediatric healthcare: A systematic review of randomized controlled trials. *Evidence-Based Complementary and Alternative Medicine, 2011,* 1–18.

Turry, A., & Turry, A. E. (1999). Creative song improvisations with children and adults with cancer. In C. Dileo (Ed.), *Music therapy and medicine: Theoretical and clinical applications and clinical applications* (pp. 167–177). Silver Spring, MD: American Music Therapy Association.

Turry, A. E. (1999). A song of life: Improvised songs with children with cancer and serious blood disorders. In T. Wigram & J. De Backer (Eds.), *Clinical applications of music therapy in developmental disability, paediatics and neurology* (pp. 13–31). Philadelphia, PA: Jessica Kingsley.

VanFleet, R., Sywulak, A. E., & Sniscak, C. C. (2010). *Child-centered play therapy.* New York, NY: The Guilford Press.

Walker, A. (2009). The role of body image in pediatric illness: Therapeutic challenges and opportunities. *American Journal of Psychotherapy, 63*(4), 363–376.

Wallander, J. L., & Varni, J. W. (1998). Effects of pediatric chronic physical disorders on child and family adjustment. *Journal of Child Psychology and Psychiatry, and Allied Disciplines, 39*(1), 29–46.

Whitehead-Pleaux, A. M., Clark, S. L., & Spall, L. E. (2011). Indications and counterindications for electronic music technologies in a pediatric medical setting. *Music and Medicine, 3*(3), 154–162.

Wolfe, D. E., & Waldon, E. G. (2009). *Music therapy and pediatric medicine.* Silver Spring, MD: American Music Therapy Association.

Wolfe, D. E., & Woolsey, W. (2003). Information sharing: Developing a music listening/relaxation program for parents of children in pediatric care. *Music Therapy Perspectives, 21*(1), 41–43.

Yu, H., Wier, L. M., & Elixhauser, A. (2011). Statistical brief #118: Hospital stays for children, 2009. *Agency for Healthcare Research and Quality, 374,* 1–13. Rockville, MD.

INDEX

A

Aasgaard, T.   189, 191, 195, 313, 320, 337, 347, 349, 351

Abad, V.   121, 144, 295, 320, 488, 500-2, 508

ABI (acquired brain injury)   170, 356-8, 362-9, 371, 373-4, 376, 378, 380, 382-3, 385-8, 392, 394-7, 473

Active Sleep   148-9

Adaptations   16, 130, 223, 228-30, 233, 235-7, 240, 242, 261, 268, 271-3, 276-7, 279-81, 283-4, 302, 304, 307, 309, 378-9, 392, 413, 487, 497-8, 500-1, 503-4

Aldridge, D.   87, 96, 321, 351, 429, 455-6, 468, 471, 477, 508

AME (active music engagement)   13, 197, 316, 323, 485, 488, 493, 499, 509

Anderson, V.   68, 96, 104, 206-9, 246, 356, 358-60, 362, 369, 373, 376, 386, 388, 395, 397, 452, 471

ASD (Acute Stress Disorder)   154, 255-6, 269, 287

Asthma Initiative Program   409, 411, 422-3, 429

Azoulay, R.   101, 144, 146, 196-8, 227, 247, 249-50, 405, 428-31, 441

B

Baker, F.   27, 59, 97, 103, 145, 169-70, 188-9, 191, 193, 195-6, 199, 249, 326, 352, 367, 369-70, 382-3, 388, 390, 393-7, 400, 402, 429, 465, 471-2

Baker & Tamplin   358, 361, 364, 366, 369-71, 374-5, 379, 380, 381-90

Baker & Wigram   190, 465-6

Barry, P.   13, 240, 245, 247, 292, 313-14, 317, 320, 322

Baryza, M.   52, 59, 245, 251, 285-6, 289

Behavioral Assessments   442, 449

Bishop , B.   24, 33-5, 39, 49, 54, 58, 237, 245, 247, 263, 285, 288-9

Blosser, J.   357, 360, 362, 364, 382-3, 389, 395-6

BMGIM (Bonny Method of Guided Imagery)   343

Bower, J.   369, 371, 392-3, 396

Brain injuries in children   356-402

Bradt, J.   3-14, 15-65, 165-6, 196, 242-3, 247-8, 456, 472

Bruscia, K.   10, 12, 180, 196, 198, 232, 247, 309, 321, 379, 396, 430, 452, 455, 466, 472, 492, 508-9

Burn Care for Children   252-289

C

Cancer, children with   290-323

Cassidy, J.   56, 59, 92-3, 97, 103, 146

Cevasco, A.   89, 94-5, 97, 103, 123, 142, 146, 199

Children in General Inpatient Care   477, 479, 481, 483, 485, 487, 489, 491, 493, 495, 497, 499, 501, 503, 505, 507, 509, 511

Christenberry, A.   34, 54, 237, 245, 247, 252, 263, 287-8

Chronic Lung Disease (CLD)   117, 141, 350

CI (cognitive impairment)   28-9, 57-8, 71, 490

Clark, S.   50, 59, 152, 199, 266, 278, 289, 366, 398, 503, 508, 512

Cochrane Database of Systematic Reviews   12, 52, 55, 196, 250, 396

Coleman, K.   92-4, 98, 360, 395

Color Analysis Scale (CAS)   26-7

Colwell , C. 13, 57, 99, 115, 143, 180, 197, 288, 321, 428, 506, 508-10

Compositional Music Therapy, Guidelines for

      Brain Injuries and Rehabilitation   388-92

      Burn Care   278-81

      Cancer   312-4

      Full-term Hospitalized Newborns   137-8

      Medically Fragile Children (Low Awareness)   465-6

      Inpatient Care, General   501-5

      Intensive Care, Pediatric   188-91

      Pain Management   49-51

      Palliative/End of Life Care   347-8

      Surgical and Procedural Support   238-42

Congenital Diaphragmatic Hernia (CDH)   117, 122, 141

Continuous Pressure Air Pathway *see* CPAP

COPD (chronic obstructive pulmonary disease)   350, 404-5, 508

CPAP (Continuous Pressure Air Pathway)   108-9, 113, 124, 132, 141, 155, 194

Creative music therapy (CMT)   10, 31, 48, 80-1, 87-9, 100-1, 128, 131, 136, 160, 182, 221, 236-7, 240, 245, 265, 274, 278, 281, 300, 309, 368, 393-4, 462, 468

D

Daveson, B.   199, 245, 248, 288, 315, 321, 329, 351, 362, 367, 396-7

Dileo, C.   12, 45-6, 55-6, 143, 165, 196, 198, 200, 242, 248-50, 288, 323, 349, 351, 392, 396, 429, 472, 508, 511

Dileo & Bradt   7, 132, 226

Dileo & Magill   462-3

Disorders of consciousness   446, 448

Down's Syndrome   117, 141, 507

Dun, B.   13, 153, 175-6, 191, 196, 200, 290-323, 361, 398, 467, 474

E

Ebberts , A.   13, 191, 200, 316, 323, 511

ECMO (Extra Corporeal Membrane Oxygenation)   117, 132, 141, 150

Edwards, J. 100-1, 145, 153, 155, 167, 169-70, 182-3, 191, 196, 198, 263, 266, 274, 288, 313, 320, 360, 365, 367, 396-7, 480, 488, 499, 508

Edwards & Kennelly 157, 159, 183, 185, 363, 365

EEG 198, 244-5, 443, 468, 470, 475

EMTs (electronic music technologies) 50, 59, 86, 230-1, 266, 275, 277-8, 280-1, 283, 398, 512

EMU (Epilepsy Monitoring Unit) 237, 243, 245

End of Life *see Palliative*

Epilepsy Monitoring Unit (EMU) 237, 243, 245

Evidence-Based 14, 164, 201, 251, 322, 473, 511

Extra Corporeal Membrane Oxygenation (ECMO) 117, 132, 141, 150

F

Fagen, T. 177, 179, 196, 332, 349, 352

Fragile Children in Low Awareness States 12, 442-476

Froehlich, M. 24, 32, 54-5, 177-8, 181, 196-7, 199, 288, 322, 349, 352, 492, 498, 505, 508-10

Full-Term Hospitalized Newborns 4, 116-151

G

GA (gestational age) 66, 70-1, 74, 76, 79, 82, 85, 87, 102, 107-8, 112, 124, 145, 398, 415

GarageBand 44, 50-1, 177, 185, 189, 241, 278, 281, 366, 388, 399, 463-4, 466, 504

Gate Control Theory 8, 17-18, 32

Gato box 80, 84-5, 105

GCS (Glasgow Coma Scale) 364, 450, 475

General Inpatient Care, Children in 4, 477,-512

Ghetti , C. 7-8, 11, 13, 18, 55, 152-204, 242-3

Ghetti & Walker 174, 177, 179, 292, 295, 298-9, 306, 309-10

Gilbertson, S. 356, 367, 393, 395-7

Graft vs. Host Disease (GVHD) 293, 304, 319

Grocke, D. 12, 36, 39, 56, 101-2, 146, 156, 165, 196, 198, 200, 247, 292, 320-1, 324, 335-6, 339, 341, 349, 352-3, 398, 474

Grocke & Wigram 32, 34, 36, 38-9, 301, 303, 305

GVHD (Graft vs. Host Disease) 293, 304, 319

H

Hannan, A. 13, 157-8, 180, 187, 197, 490, 492-3, 498, 502, 509

Hanson-Abromeit , D. 6, 13, 57, 69, 75-9, 81, 83, 92, 95, 99, 108, 115, 123, 140, 143, 180, 184, 197, 288, 509-10

Haslbeck, F. 87, 93, 95, 99-100

Heart rate (HR) 5, 33-4, 42, 44, 58, 72, 74-5, 82, 84-5, 89-90, 92-5, 154-5, 162, 170-1, 193, 225-6, 228-9, 285-6, 304, 411-12, 447, 452-3, 455-9, 488, 490

Heidelberg Music Therapy Manual for Pediatric Migraine 31, 46

Herndon, D. 253-4, 288-9

HIE (hypoxic ischemic encephalopathy) 117-18, 122, 142

Hilliard, R. 314, 321, 332, 336, 347, 349, 352, 456, 460, 473

HSCT (Hematopoietic Stem Cell Transplant) 293, 296, 303-4, 312-13

I

ICUs (Intensive Care Units) 66, 120, 145, 152, 155, 193, 195, 200, 230-1, 233, 250, 257, 297, 391

Improvisational models of music therapy 321, 396, 472, 508

Improvisational music therapy, Guidelines for

        Brain Injuries and Rehabilitation 378-82

        Burn Care 274-8

        Cancer 305-9

        Full-term Hospitalized Newborns 128-32

        Medically Fragile Children (Low Awareness) 460-2

        Inpatient Care, General 491-9

        Intensive Care, Pediatric 175-82

        Pain Management 39-48

        Palliative/End of Life Care 343-6

        Premature Infants 87-9

        Surgical and Procedural Support 232-6

IMTAP (Individual Music Therapy Assessment Profile) 365, 396

Infant Behavior and Development 98, 101-2, 143-4

Injuries, Brain 4, 12, 117, 356-7, 359, 361, 363, 365, 367, 369, 371, 373, 375, 377, 379, 381, 383, 385, 387, 389, 391, 393-5, 397, 399, 401\

Inpatient Care, General 477-512

Instrumental Improvisation to Decrease Perseveration 380

Instrumental Improvisation to Reduce Perseverations 368

Integrative Models 55, 205, 248-50, 430-1

Iso principle 8, 34, 268, 273

K

Keith, D. 93-4, 100, 123, 139, 144

Kennelly, J. 356-402

Klassen, J. 9, 13, 243, 249

Knapp, C. 324, 326-7, 348-9, 352

L

Late preterm infant 67, 87, 102

Lindenfelser, K. 156, 173-5, 191, 198, 324-355

Loewy, J. 13, 37, 39-43, 55-9, 75-7, 81, 84-6, 93-5, 97-103, 115, 131-2, 143-4, 166, 174-7, 184-5, 196-8, 200-1, 226-8, 243-7, 249-51, 403-441

Loewy & Stewart 166, 173-9, 218, 418
Loveszy, R. 157, 175-6, 179, 184-5, 187-8, 198, 497, 509

M

MAE (Music Alternate Engagement) 49, 221, 237
Magee, W. 165-9, 199, 278, 288-9, 367, 370, 376, 392, 396-7, 448, 451-2, 455, 474
Marley, L. 182-3, 199, 488, 493, 495-6, 510
MATLAS 451
McFerran, K. 122, 145, 156, 198, 305, 313, 322, 324, 329, 335, 338, 349, 351, 353, 471, 511
McGrath, P. 21-5, 28, 39, 54, 57, 65, 102
MCS (minimally conscious state) 198, 443-4, 446-7, 450-2, 459, 472-3
Medically Fragile Children *see* Fragile
MedicineNet.com 478, 506, 510
Melzack, R. 17-18, 55, 57
MMIT (Modified Melodic Intonation Therapy) 368, 382-3
MMS (Music and Multimodal Stimulation) 80, 82-3, 93
Mondanaro, J. 5, 19, 30, 55-6, 121, 137, 144, 205-251, 430-1
Motor activity 93, 148-9
MP3 devices 51, 366, 463
MRI (Magnetic Resonance Imaging) 53, 208, 225, 293, 320, 470
MSbP (Munchausen syndrome by proxy) 478-9, 508
Multiple (Combined) Methods of Music Therapy, Guidelines for
        Respiratory Care 417-23
Music and Medicine 12, 54-5, 59, 97, 101-3, 143, 146, 196, 199, 200, 247, 249, 251, 288-9, 321,
        396-8, 407, 408-411, 422-23, 428-9, 431, 472, 474, 509, 512
Music-Assisted Reality Orientation and Awareness 160, 168
Music-Assisted Relaxation and Sedation 410, 413
Music-Based Sensory Stimulation 485, 490
Music Entrainment for Pain Management 31, 44
Music Entrainment of Physiological Functions 453, 456
Music-Facilitated Dramatic Play 160, 177, 485, 497
Music-Facilitated Psychoeducation 220, 223
Music for Stimulation and Comfort 300, 304
Music-Guided Imagery for Relaxation 335, 340
Music Improvisation for Active Engagement and Exploration 31, 43
Music Improvisation for Emotional Expressivity 485, 491
Music Improvisation for Sibling Support 454, 460
Music Improvisational-Play Opportunities 221, 233
Music Listening for Arousal 453-4
Music Listening for Emotional Support 367, 376
Music Listening for Normalization and Anxiety Reduction 485-6
Music Listening for Orientation and Arousal 367, 369
Music Listening for Refocusing 220, 224

Music Listening for Relaxation 300-1
Music Listening for Sustained Focus 30, 32
Music psychotherapy assessment 56, 408, 429, 441
Music Therapy Assessment 115, 321, 364,365, 396, 436
Music to Facilitate Movement and Body Awareness 485, 488
Musical Characteristics of Term Infants 118
Musical sedation 101, 144, 198, 413, 429
Musicokinetic Therapy (MKT) 453, 459-60, 467, 474
MVT (music vibration table) 55

N

NAPI (Nursing Assessment of Pain Intensity) 285-6
Neonatal Network 55, 97-8, 104, 146
Neugebauer , C. 18, 34, 57, 250, 264, 288-9, 477-512
Neurologic Music Therapy (NMT) 197, 366, 368, 386, 397-9, 467, 475, 509
Neurology 104, 198, 323, 396, 473-5, 511
Neuropsychological Rehabilitation 199, 472, 474
NeuroRehabilitation 474, 476
NICU (Neonatal Intensive Care Unit) 66-9, 72-7, 79-81, 85, 88, 91-3, 95-101, 103-4, 115-17,
        120-1, 123, 126, 132, 134-5, 138, 140, 144, 146, 150, 158, 182, 197, 251, 410, 415
NICU environment 66-7, 69, 78, 86, 88-9, 94
NICU music therapy 88, 92, 103, 431
Nöcker-Ribaupierre , M. 4, 13, 66-115
Nolan, P. 6, 13, 39, 52, 57, 93, 98, 410
Nonreferential improvisations 160, 180-1, 274-5

O

O'Callaghan, C. 9, 13, 247, 292, 305, 314, 317, 320, 322, 466, 474

P

Pain management with children 15-65
PAL (Pacifier-Activated Lullaby) 80, 84, 94, 97, 103, 113, 409
Palliative and End-of-Life Care for Children 12, 324-355
PATTERNS 81, 88-9, 103, 415, 431
Pediatric Intensive Care 152-3, 155, 157, 159, 161, 163, 165, 167, 169, 171, 173, 175, 177, 179, 181,
        183, 185, 187, 189, 191, 193, 195, 197, 199, 201
Pediatric Pain Profile (PPP) 29
Pediatric Pain Questionnaire (PPQ) 27, 59
Pediatric traumatic brain injury 395-7
PEF (peak expiratory flow) 425-6, 431
Perinatology 96, 99, 102, 143-4, 248

PET (positron emission tomography) 449, 470-1

Pharmacological interventions 230, 258

Phenomenological observations 212-13

Philbin, M. 73, 81, 97, 99, 102, 123, 126, 143, 145, 430

PICU (Pediatric Intensive Care Unit) 52, 116-17, 126, 143, 152-204, 216, 344, 362-3, 420

PICU environment 116, 138, 176, 180, 183-4, 187-8

PICU setting 153, 155, 157, 159, 184-5, 193-4

PMR (progressive muscle relaxation) 34-5, 271, 303, 414, 425

PPQ (Pediatric Pain Questionnaire) 27, 59

Premature Infant Pain Profile (PIPPS) 28, 58

Premature Infants 66-115

Procedural Support for Children 205-251

PT/OT 113-14, 264-5, 272-4

PTSD (Post-Traumatic Stress Disorder) 255-6, 261, 269, 287, 465

PVS (persistent vegetative state) 198, 361, 443-4, 452, 466-7, 471-2, 474-5

R

RAS (Rhythmic Auditory Stimulation) 368, 371, 380, 386-7, 397

RDS (Respiratory Distress Syndrome) 85, 109, 141, 154, 185, 404, 415-16

Receptive Music Therapy, Guidelines for
    Brain Injuries and Rehabilitation 369-78
    Burn Care 265-74
    Cancer 301-5
    Full-term Hospitalized Newborns 132-6
    Medically Fragile Children (Low Awareness) 454-60
    Inpatient Care, General 486-91
    Intensive Care, Pediatric 161-75
    Pain Management 31-9
    Palliative/End of Life Care 336-43
    Premature Infants 81-7
    Respiratory Care 411-7
    Surgical and Procedural Support 221-32

Re-creative music therapy 31, 48, 81, 89, 128, 131, 136, 160, 182, 221, 236-7, 240, 245, 265, 281, 300, 309, 318, 335, 346, 368, 375, 380, 382, 394

Re-creative Music Therapy, Guidelines for
    Brain Injuries and Rehabilitation 382-8
    Burn Care 281-5
    Cancer 309-12
    Full-term Hospitalized Newborns 136-7
    Medically Fragile Children (Low Awareness) 462-5
    Inpatient Care, General 499-501
    Intensive Care, Pediatric 182-8
    Pain Management 48-9

Palliative/End of Life Care 346-7
Surgical and Procedural Support 236-8
Referential improvisation 180-1, 265, 274, 492
Referral Procedures 25, 105, 122, 157, 212, 261, 298, 363, 407
Rehabilitation in Children 12, 356-402
Research Evidence, Music therapy for
Brain Injuries and Rehabilitation 392-4
Burn Care 285-6
Cancer 314-8
Full-term Hospitalized Newborns 138-40
Medically Fragile Children (Low Awareness) 466-9
Inpatient Care, General 505-6
Intensive Care, Pediatric 191-4
Pain Management 51-3
Palliative/End of Life Care 348-50
Premature Infants 92-5
Respiratory Care 424-6
Surgical and Procedural Support 242-6
Respiratory Care for Children 403-441
Robb, S. 5, 7-8, 13-14, 23-4, 32-5, 54, 57-8, 140, 145, 191, 193, 197, 200, 237, 245, 288-9, 295-6, 307, 310, 316-17, 323, 365, 397-8, 493, 509-11
Robb & Ebberts 190-1, 503
Rubin-Bosco, J. 177, 179-80, 200, 306, 323, 430

S

SCD (Sickle Cell Disease) 19, 36, 47, 50, 55, 239, 248, 294
Schneider, S. 103, 156, 163-4, 200, 230, 250-1
Schwartz, E. 67, 94, 102, 183, 200, 416, 431, 497, 510-11
SCT (stem-cell transplantation) 317, 321
Sedation/Sleep/Pain 107, 434
Sheridan , R. 52, 59, 245, 251-7, 285-6, 289, 353, 511
Shoemark, H. 11, 75-9, 81, 83, 86, 89, 94, 97, 99, 102-3, 115, 116-151, 184, 197, 200, 396, 415-16
Shoemark & Dearn 121, 123, 137, 156, 183
Shoemark & Grocke 119, 123, 127, 129, 139
Songs of kin 81, 84, 86, 128, 136-7, 185
Spall, L. 50, 59, 266, 278, 289, 366, 398, 503, 512
SPECT (single-photon emission computerized tomography) 449, 471
Standley, J. 7, 14, 55, 72, 75-7, 79, 81-3, 92-4, 97, 101, 103, 115, 123, 127, 146, 183, 199-200, 248, 285, 288, 323, 459, 475
Standley & Walworth 4, 76, 82, 94, 139, 167, 183
Stewart , J. 8, 13, 78, 85-6, 88-9, 101, 103, 124, 136, 146, 175, 180, 198, 200, 249, 251, 290, 296-7, 323, 415-16, 430-1, 441
Stewart & Schneider 86, 95, 163-4, 230

Stimulative Listening During Joint PT/OT Services   265, 272
Stouffer, J.   13, 165-6, 192, 200-1, 323
Stouffer & Shirk   152-3, 155, 165-6, 191-2
Super Dooper Music Looper   366, 388, 399
Surgical and Procedural Support for Children   205-251
Sweeney, C.   306, 323, 346, 349, 353

T

Tamplin, J.   155, 168-9, 188, 196, 201, 367, 388, 390, 393-7, 402, 455, 475, 502, 511
TBI (traumatic brain injury)   168, 196, 356-60, 362, 367, 376, 392-8, 444
Thaut , M.   187, 201, 302, 321, 366, 371, 380, 384-8, 397-8, 467, 475
Therapeutic Music Instruction   160, 187, 486, 500
Townsend, J.   278, 288, 361, 442-476
Trisomy   117, 141, 332, 347, 351, 478, 507
Turry, A.   5, 37, 39, 49, 59, 175-6, 180-1, 201, 218, 232, 251, 309, 323, 491, 501, 511

V

VAS (Visual Analogue Scale)   26, 28, 60

W

Walworth, D. 14, 103, 115, 123, 146, 171, 183, 199-201, 224, 244-6, 251
Whipple , J.   7, 14, 59, 77, 79, 82-4, 94-5, 104, 123, 147, 199-200
Whitehead-Pleaux, A.   29, 50, 52, 59, 245, 251, 252-289, 366, 398
Wigram, T.   36, 39, 56, 58, 189, 191, 195-6, 321-3, 352, 395-6, 457, 465, 471-2, 475, 511
Wolfe, D.   14, 81, 97, 325-6, 352, 512

X

X-rays   208-9, 292-3, 320

Guidelines for Music Therapy Practice
A Four Volume Series

GUIDELINES FOR MUSIC THERAPY PRACTICE IN DEVELOPMENTAL HEALTH
Edited by Michelle R. Hintz
1) Introduction: *Michelle R. Hintz*
2) Early Intervention: *Elizabeth K. Schwartz*
3) Autism: *Michelle R. Hintz*
4) Rett Syndrome: *Jennifer M. Sokira*
5) Developmental Speech and Language Disorders: *Kathleen M. Howland*
6) Attentional Deficits in School Children: *Michelle R. Hintz*
7) Learning Disabilities in School Children: *Michelle R. Hintz*
8) Behavioral and Interpersonal Problems in School Children: *Patricia McCarrick*
9) Children with Hearing Loss: *Christine Barton*
10) Visually Impaired School Children: *Paige A. Robbins Elwafi*
11) Mild to Moderate Intellectual Disability: *Douglas R. Keith*
12) Severe to Profound Intellectual and Developmental Disabilities: *Donna W. Polen*
13) Physical Disabilities in School Children: *Jennifer M. Sokira*
14) Individuals with Severe and Multiple Disabilities: *Barbara Wheeler*

GUIDELINES FOR MUSIC THERAPY PRACTICE IN MENTAL HEALTH
Edited by Lillian Eyre
1) Introduction: *Lillian Eyre*
2) Adults with Schizophrenia and Psychotic Disorders: *Andrea McGraw Hunt*
3) Adult Groups in the Inpatient Setting: *Lillian Eyre*
4) Adults in a Recovery Model Setting: *Lillian Eyre*
5) Children and Adolescents in an Inpatient Psychiatric Setting: *Bridget Doak*
6) Foster Care Youth: *Michael L. Zanders*
7) Survivors of Catastrophic Event Trauma: *Ronald M. Borczon*
8) Women Survivors of Abuse and Developmental Trauma: *Sandra Lynn Curtis*
9) Adult Male Survivors of Abuse and Developmental Trauma: *Jeffrey H. Hatcher*
10) Children and Adolescents with PTSD and Survivors of Abuse and Neglect: *Penny Rogers*
11) Adults with Depression and/or Anxiety: *Nancy A. Jackson*
12) Adults and Adolescents with Borderline Personality Disorder: *J. M. Dvorkin*
13) Adults and Adolescents with Eating Disorders: *Peggy Tileston*
14) Adults with Substance Use Disorders: *Kathleen M. Murphy*
15) Adolescents with Substance Use Disorders: *Katrina Skewes McFerran*
16) Adult Males in Forensic Settings: *Vaughn Kaser*
17) Adult Females in Correctional Facilities: *Karen Anne Litecky Melendez*
18) Adjudicated Adolescents: *Susan Gardstrom*
19) Juvenile Male Sexl Offenders: *Lori L. De Rea-Kolb*
20) Elderly Residents in Nursing Facilities: *Elaine A. Abbott*

21) Persons with Alzheimer's and Other Dementias: *Laurel Young*
22) Professional Burnout: *Darlene M. Brooks*
23) Stress Reduction and Wellness: *Seung-A Kim*
24) Musicians: *Gro Trondalen*
25) Spiritual Practices: *Annie Heiderscheit*

GUIDELINES FOR MUSIC THERAPY PRACTICE IN PEDIATRIC CARE
Edited by Joke Bradt

1) Introduction: *Joke Bradt*
2) Pain Management with Children: *Joke Bradt*
3) Premature Infants: *Monika Nöcker-Ribaupierre*
4) Full-Term Hospitalized Newborns: *Helen Shoemark*
5) Pediatric Intensive Care: *Claire Ghetti*
6) Surgical and Procedural Support for Children: *John Mondanaro*
7) Burn Care for Children: *Annette Whitehead-Pleaux*
8) Children with Cancer: *Beth Dun*
9) Palliative and End-of-Life Care for Children: *Kathryn Lindenfelser*
10) Brain Injuries and Rehabilitation in Children: *Jeanette Kennelly*
11) Respiratory Care for Children: *Joanne Loewy*
12) Medically Fragile Children in Low Awareness States: *Jennifer Townsend*
13) Children in General Inpatient Care: *Christine Neugebauer*

GUIDELINES FOR MUSIC THERAPY PRACTICE IN ADULT MEDICAL CARE
Edited by Joy Allen

1) Introduction: *Joy Allen*
2) Surgical and Procedural support: *Annie Heiderscheit*
3) Pain Management with Adults: *Joy Allen*
4) Adults in Critical Care: *Jeanette Tamplin*
5) Adults in Cardiac Care: *Christine Pollard Leist*
6) Adults with Stroke: *Simon Gilbertson*
7) Adults with Traumatic Brain Injury: *Victoria Policastro Vega*
8) Adults with Neurogenic Communication Disorders: *Nicki Cohen*
9) Adults with Neurogenerative Diseases: *Wendy Magee*
10) Adults with HIV/AIDS: *Douglas Keith*
11) Adults with Cancer: *Joy Allen*
12) Adults in Palliative/Hospice Care: *Amy Clement-Cortes*
13) Caring for Caregivers: *Barbara Daveson*

THE BARCELONA COLLECTION
OF PRINT AND E-BOOKS
2013

ANALYTIC MUSIC THERAPY
- Essays on Analytical Music Therapy (Priestley)
- Music Therapy in Action (2nd Edition) (Priestley)
- The Dynamics of Music Psychotherapy (Bruscia)
- Group Analytic Music Therapy (Ahonen-Eerikäinen)

CASE STUDIES
- Case Examples of Guided Imagery and Music (Bruscia)
- Case Examples of Improvisational Music Therapy (Bruscia)
- Case Examples of Music Therapy for____ (Bruscia):
  - Alzheimer's Disease
  - Autism and Rett Syndrome
  - Children and Adolescents with Emotional or Behavioral Problems
  - Developmental Problems in Learning and Communication
  - End of Life
  - Event Trauma
  - Medical Conditions
  - Mood Disorders
  - Multiple Disabilities
  - Musicians
  - Personality Disorders
  - Schizophrenia and other Psychoses
  - Self-Development
  - Substance Use Disorders
  - Survivors of Abuse
- Case Examples of the Use of Songs in Psychotherapy (Bruscia)
- Studies in Music Therapy (Bruscia)
- Inside Music Therapy: Client Experiences (Hibben)
- Psychodynamic Music Therapy: Case Studies (Hadley)

CHILDREN WITH SPECIAL NEEDS
- Alike and Different: The Clinical and Educational Uses of Orff-Schulwerk – Second Edition (Bitcon)
- The Miracle of Music Therapy (Boxill)
- Music for Fun, Music for Learning (Birkenshaw-Fleming)
- Music: Motion and Emotion: The Developmental-Integrative Model in Music Therapy (Sekeles)
- Music, Therapy, and Early Childhood (Schwartz)
- Music Therapy in Special Education (Nordoff & Robbins)

- Therapy in Music for Handicapped Children (Nordoff & Robbins)

COMMUNITY MUSIC THERAPY
- Elaborations Toward a Notion of Community Music Therapy (Stige)
- Culture-Centered Music Therapy (Stige)

INFANCY AND EARLY CHILDHOOD
- Music, Therapy, and Early Childhood (Schwartz)
- Music Therapy for Premature and Newborn Infants (Nöcker-Ribaupierre)

END OF LIFE
- Music Therapy: Death and Grief (Sekeles)

FEMINISM
- Feminist Perspectives in Music Therapy (Hadley)

FIELDWORK AND INTERNSHIP TRAINING
- Clinical Training Guide for the Student Music Therapist (Wheeler, Shultis & Polen)
- Music Therapy: A Fieldwork Primer (Borczon)
- Music Therapy Supervision (Forinash)

GROUP WORK
- Music Therapy: Group Vignettes (Borczon)
- Music Therapy Improvisation for Groups: Essential Leadership Competencies (Gardstrom)

GUIDED IMAGERY AND MUSIC (BONNY METHOD)
- Guided Imagery and Music: The Bonny Method and Beyond (Bruscia & Grocke)
- Music and Consciousness: The Evolution of Guided Imagery and Music (Bonny)
- Music and Your Mind: Listening with a New Consciousness (Bonny & Savary)
- Music for the Imagination (Bruscia)

GUITAR
- Guitar Skills for Music Therapists and Music Educators (Meyer, De Villers, Ebnet)
- Use of the Guitar in Music Therapy (Oden)

IMPROVISATIONAL MUSIC THERAPY
- The Architecture of Aesthetic Music Therapy (Lee)
- Essays on Analytical Music Therapy (Priestley)
- Creative Music Therapy: A Guide to Fostering Clinical Musicianship – Second Edition with Four CDs (Nordoff & Robbins)
- Group Analytic Music Therapy (Ahonen-Eerikäinen)
- Healing Heritage: Paul Nordoff Exploring the Tonal Language of Music (Robbins & Robbins)
- Improvising in Styles: A Workbook for Music Therapists, Educators, and Musicians (Lee & Houde)
- Music as Therapy: A Dialogal Perspective (Garred)
- Music-Centered Music Therapy (Aigen)
- Music Therapy: Improvisation, Communication, and Culture (Ruud)
- Music Therapy Improvisation for Groups: Essential Leadership Competencies (Gardstrom)
- Paths of Development in Nordoff-Robbins Music Therapy (Aigen)

- Playin' in the Band: A Qualitative study of Popular Music Styles as Clinical Improvisation (Aigen)
- Sounding the Self: Analogy in Improvisational Music Therapy (Smeijsters)

MUSIC FOR CHILDREN TO SING AND PLAY

- Distant Bells (Levin & Levin)
- Learning Songs (Levin & Levin)
- Learning Through Music (Levin & Levin)
- Learning Through Songs (Levin & Levin)
- Let's Make Music (Levin & Levin)
- Music for Fun, Music for Learning (Birkenshaw-Fleming)
- Snow White: A Guide to Child-Centered Musical Theatre (Lauri, Groeschel, Robbins, Ritholz & Turry)
- Symphonics R Us (Levin & Levin)

NORDOFF-ROBBINS MUSIC THERAPY (CREATIVE MUSIC THERAPY)

- The Architecture of Aesthetic Music Therapy (Lee)
- Being in Music: Foundations of Nordoff-Robbins Music Therapy (Aigen)
- Conversations on Nordoff-Robbins Music Therapy (Verney & Ansdell)
- Creative Music Therapy: A Guide to Fostering Clinical Musicianship – Second Edition with Four CDs (Nordoff & Robbins)
- Healing Heritage: Paul Nordoff Exploring the Tonal Language of Music (Robbins & Robbins)
- Here We Are in Music: One Year with an Adolescent Creative Music Therapy Group (Aigen)
- A Journey into Creative Music Therapy (Robbins)
- Music Therapy in Special Education (Nordoff & Robbins)
- Paths of Development in Nordoff-Robbins Music Therapy (Aigen)
- Playin' in the Band: A Qualitative study of Popular Music Styles as Clinical Improvisation (Aigen)
- Therapy in Music for Handicapped Children (Nordoff & Robbins)

MUSIC THERAPY PRACTICE

- Guidelines for Music Therapy Practice in Mental Health (Eyre)
- Guidelines for Music Therapy Practice in Developmental Health (Hintz)
- Guidelines for Music Therapy Practice in Pediatric Care (Bradt)
- Guidelines for Music Therapy Practice in Adult Medical Care (Allen)

MUSIC PSYCHOTHERAPY

- The Dynamics of Music Psychotherapy (Bruscia)
- Essays on Analytical Music Therapy (Priestley)
- Emotional Processes in Music Therapy (Pellitteri)
- Group Analytic Music Therapy (Ahonen-Eerikäinen)
- Guided Imagery and Music: The Bonny Method and Beyond (Bruscia & Grocke)
- Music and Consciousness: The Evolution of Guided Imagery and Music (Bonny)
- Music and Your Mind: Listening with a New Consciousness (Bonny & Savary)

- Music Therapy: Group Vignettes (Borczon)
- Psychodynamic Music Therapy: Case Studies (Hadley)

ORFF-SCHULWERK
- Alike and Different: The Clinical and Educational Uses of Orff-Schulwerk – Second Edition (Bitcon)

PIANO
- Functional Piano for Music Therapists and Music Educators (Massicot)
- Improvising in Styles: A Workbook for Music Therapists, Educators, and Musicians (Lee & Houde)

PROFOUND MENTAL RETARDATION
- Age-Appropriate Activities for Adults with Profound Mental Retardation – Second Edition (Galerstein, Martin & Powe)

PSYCHODRAMA
- Acting Your Inner Music (Moreno)

PSYCHIATRY – MENTAL HEALTH
- Music Therapy in the Treatment of Adults with Mental Disorders: Theoretical Bases and Clinical Interventions (Unkefer & Thaut)
- Psychiatric Music Therapy in the Community: The Legacy of Florence Tyson (McGuire)
- Psychodynamic Music Therapy: Case Studies (Hadley)
- Resource-Oriented Music Therapy in Mental Health Care (Rolvsjord)

RACE
- Experience Race as a Music Therapist: Personal Narratives (Hadley)

RESEARCH
- A Guide to Writing and Presenting in Music Therapy (Aigen)
- Multiple Perspectives: A Guide to Qualitative Research in Music Therapy (Smeijsters)
- Music Therapy Research: Quantitative and Qualitative Perspectives – First Edition (1995) (Wheeler)
- Music Therapy Research – Second Edition (2005) (Wheeler)
- Playin' in the Band: A Qualitative study of Popular Music Styles as Clinical Improvisation (Aigen)
- Qualitative Inquiries in Music Therapy: A Monograph Series (Free Downloads Available Here)
- Qualitative Music Therapy Research: Beginning Dialogues (Langenberg, Frömmer & Aigen)

SUPERVISION
- Music Therapy Supervision (Forinash)

THEORY
- Culture-Centered Music Therapy (Stige)
- Defining Music Therapy – Second Edition (Bruscia)
- Emotional Processes in Music Therapy (Pellitteri)
- Music and Life in the Field of Play: An Anthology (Kenny)

- Music as Therapy: A Dialogal Perspective (Garred)
- Music-Centered Music Therapy (Aigen)
- Music Therapy and its Relationship to Current Treatment Theories (Ruud)
- Music Therapy: A Perspective from the Humanities (Ruud)
- Music Therapy: Improvisation, Communication, and Culture (Ruud)
- Music—The Therapeutic Edge: Readings from William W. Sears (Sears)
- The Music Within You (Katsh & Fishman)
- Readings on Music Therapy Theory (Bruscia)
- Resource-Oriented Music Therapy in Mental Health Care (Rolvsjord)
- The Rhythmic Language of Health and Disease (Rider)
- Sounding the Self: Analogy in Improvisational Music Therapy (Smeijsters)

VOICE

- Authentic Voices, Authentic Singing (Uhlig)
- Psychiatric Music Therapy in the Community: The Legacy of Florence Tyson (McGuire)